Urticaria and Angioedema

Urticaria and Angioedema

Second Edition

Edited by

Allen P. Kaplan
Medical University of South Carolina
Charleston, South Carolina, USA

Malcolm W. Greaves
St. Johns Institute of Dermatology
St. Thomas' Hospital
London, UK

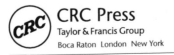

CRC Press
Taylor & Francis Group
Boca Raton London New York

CRC Press is an imprint of the
Taylor & Francis Group, an **informa** business

CRC Press
Taylor & Francis Group
6000 Broken Sound Parkway NW, Suite 300
Boca Raton, FL 33487-2742

First issued in paperback 2019

© 2009 by Taylor & Francis Group, LLC
CRC Press is an imprint of Taylor & Francis Group, an Informa business

No claim to original U.S. Government works

ISBN-13: 978-1-4200-7784-1 (hbk)
ISBN-13: 978-0-367-38594-1 (pbk)

This book contains information obtained from authentic and highly regarded sources. While all reasonable efforts have been made to publish reliable data and information, neither the author[s] nor the publisher can accept any legal responsibility or liability for any errors or omissions that may be made. The publishers wish to make clear that any views or opinions expressed in this book by individual editors, authors or contributors are personal to them and do not necessarily reflect the views/opinions of the publishers. The information or guidance contained in this book is intended for use by medical, scientific or health-care professionals and is provided strictly as a supplement to the medical or other professional's own judgement, their knowledge of the patient's medical history, relevant manufacturer's instructions and the appropriate best practice guidelines. Because of the rapid advances in medical science, any information or advice on dosages, procedures or diagnoses should be independently verified. The reader is strongly urged to consult the relevant national drug formulary and the drug companies' and device or material manufacturers' printed instructions, and their websites, before administering or utilizing any of the drugs, devices or materials mentioned in this book. This book does not indicate whether a particular treatment is appropriate or suitable for a particular individual. Ultimately it is the sole responsibility of the medical professional to make his or her own professional judgements, so as to advise and treat patients appropriately. The authors and publishers have also attempted to trace the copyright holders of all material reproduced in this publication and apologize to copyright holders if permission to publish in this form has not been obtained. If any copyright material has not been acknowledged please write and let us know so we may rectify in any future reprint.

Library of Congress Cataloging-in-Publication Data

Urticaria and angioedema / edited by Allen P. Kaplan, Malcolm W. Greaves.
– 2nd ed.
    p. ; cm.
Includes bibliographical references and index.
ISBN-13: 978-1-4200-7784-1 (hardcover : alk. paper)
ISBN-10: 1-4200-7784-8 (hardcover : alk. paper) 1. Urticaria.
2. Angioneurotic edema. I. Greaves, M. W. II. Kaplan, Allen P.
[DNLM: 1. Angioedema. 2. Urticaria. WR 170 U812 2009]

RL249.U77 2009
616.5'17–dc22

                                                                      2008039024

Visit the Taylor & Francis Web site at
http://www.taylorandfrancis.com

and the CRC Press Web site at
http://www.crcpress.com

Preface

Urticaria and angioedema affect at least 20% of the population and frequently become chronic and persistent, causing significant personal, domestic, social, and occupational disability. That "urticaria" encompasses a group of very different disorders is incompletely understood by many clinicians who nevertheless confidently make this diagnosis. For this reason and because, until recently, little progress has been made in understanding the pathomechanisms of the chronic forms, progress in diagnosis and treatment has been disappointingly slow. Nevertheless the past 10 to 15 years have been a time of considerable development with many new approaches, and interest has accelerated since publication of the first edition.

The first edition of *Urticaria and Angioedema* owes its outstanding success to its ability to satisfy a previously unmet need for a scholarly yet essentially practical handbook combining insights into recent exciting developments in the pathogenesis of urticaria and angioedema with practical advice on investigation and management based on our authors' wide personal clinical experience. But now a pressing need has emerged for a second edition, prompted by important recent advances, including, at a cellular level, the realization of the importance of HLA class II—expressing dermal dendritic cells in immune responses in skin, the role of cross-talk between dermal mast cells and PAR-2 receptors expressed by unmyelinated C neurons in pruritus, and the development of screening tests for autoimmune urticaria based upon expression of activation markers such as CD203c upon exposure of donor basophils to serum from patients with autoimmune urticaria. Furthermore, treatment of recalcitrant chronic urticaria by anti-IgE receptor antibody (omalizumab) and anti-CD 20 monoclonals (e.g., rituximab) or physical urticarias by anti-TNFα and angioedema by novel anti-kallikrein or anti-bradykinin drugs are now being actively explored.

We believe this second edition reflects all these new developments in the field and much more besides, with major revision and augmentation of all chapters plus new ones added where advances have warranted it. We begin with a discussion of the relevant biology of the skin and then describe the mediator cascades and effector cells of the inflammatory response relevant to the pathogenesis of the various forms that urticaria and angioedema can take. Then all of the clinical entities that one is likely to encounter are explored in depth including new chapters on epidemiology, anaphylaxis, mastocytosis, and the hypereosinophilic syndrome. Emphasis is given to new data regarding autoimmune mechanisms that appear to initiate chronic urticaria and angioedema in about 45% of patients, as well as to abnormalities of signal transduction that may be found in both the autoimmune and "idiopathic" subgroups.

We believe the book will be an important addition to the armamentarium of allergists and dermatologists and that it will also intrigue immunologists, cell biologists, and pharmacologists with an interest in clinical immunology and allergy. The unraveling of the ways in which dermal mast cells and basophil leucocytes become promiscuously activated, the interactions of the multiple inflammatory mediators thus released, and the ensuing cavalcade of cellular pruritic and vascular responses represent a paradigm for immunologically driven diseases. Moreover, urticaria and angioedema are models potentially accessible for study in human skin.

However, in many patients with chronic urticaria and especially in the physical urticarias, causation of dermal mast cell activation at the molecular level still remains elusive, and we have endeavored, in the relevant chapters, to point the way forward to future developments in these fields.

Overall we hope we have achieved a reasonable balance—satisfying both the clinician, who requires reassurance that recommended clinical practice is scientifically soundly based, and the investigator, who sees a secure clinical context for research in his or her important and challenging area.

Allen P. Kaplan
Malcolm W. Greaves

Contents

Contributors

Anne Kobza Black   St. John's Institute of Dermatology, St. Thomas' Hospital, London, U.K.

Heidi P. Chan   Department of Dermatology, UCSF School of Medicine, San Francisco, California, U.S.A.

Liliana Cifuentes   Division Environmental Dermatology and Allergy GSF/TUM, Department of Dermatology and Allergy Biederstein, Technical University of Munich, Munich, Germany

Elie Cogan   Department of Internal Medicine, Erasme Hospital, Université Libre de Bruxelles, Brussels, Belgium

Berhane Ghebrehiwet   Division of Allergy, Rheumatology, and Clinical Immunology, Department of Medicine, Health Sciences Center, Stony Brook University, Stony Brook, New York, U.S.A.

Gerald J. Gleich   Departments of Dermatology and Medicine, The University of Utah Health Sciences Center, University of Utah, Salt Lake City, Utah, U.S.A.

Michel Goldman   Institute for Medical Immunology, Université Libre de Bruxelles, Gosselies, Belgium

Clive Grattan   Dermatology Centre, Norfolk and Norwich University Hospital, and St. John's Institute of Dermatology, St. Thomas' Hospital, London, U.K.

Malcolm W. Greaves   St. John's Institute of Dermatology, St. Thomas' Hospital, London, U.K.

Hal M. Hoffman   Division of Rheumatology, Allergy, and Immunology, University of California, San Diego, La Jolla, California, U.S.A.

Allen P. Kaplan   Department of Medicine, Medical University of South Carolina, Charleston, South Carolina, U.S.A.

Esther Kim   Department of Dermatology, UCSF School of Medicine, San Francisco, California, U.S.A.

Kristin M. Leiferman   Departments of Dermatology and Medicine, The University of Utah Health Sciences Center, University of Utah, Salt Lake City, Utah, U.S.A.

Donald MacGlashan, Jr.   Johns Hopkins Asthma and Allergy Center, Baltimore, Maryland, U.S.A.

Howard I. Maibach   Department of Dermatology, UCSF School of Medicine, San Francisco, California, U.S.A.

Barbara A. Martinez   Laboratory of Allergic Diseases, National Institute of Allergy and Infectious Diseases, National Institutes of Health, Bethesda, Maryland, U.S.A.

Dean D. Metcalfe   Laboratory of Allergic Diseases, National Institute of Allergy and Infectious Diseases, National Institutes of Health, Bethesda, Maryland, U.S.A.

Matthias Möhrenschlager   Division Environmental Dermatology and Allergy GSF/TUM, Department of Dermatology and Allergy Biederstein, Technical University of Munich, Munich, Germany

Timo Reunala   Tampere University and University Hospital, Tampere, Finland

Johannes Ring   Division Environmental Dermatology and Allergy GSF/TUM, Department of Dermatology and Allergy Biederstein, Technical University of Munich, Munich, Germany

Florence Roufosse   Department of Internal Medicine, Erasme Hospital, Université Libre de Bruxelles, Brussels and Institute for Medical Immunology, Université Libre de Bruxelles, Gosselies, Belgium

Ruth A. Sabroe   Department of Dermatology, Barnsley Hospital NHS Foundation Trust, Sheffield, U.K.

Sarbjit Saini   Johns Hopkins Asthma and Allergy Center, Baltimore, Maryland, U.S.A.

Lawrence B. Schwartz   Division of Rheumatology, Allergy & Immunology, Department of Internal Medicine, Virginia Commonwealth University, Richmond, Virginia, U.S.A.

F. Estelle R. Simons   Department of Pediatrics & Child Health, Department of Immunology, CIHR National Training Program in Allergy and Asthma, Faculty of Medicine, University of Manitoba, Winnipeg, Canada

Keith J. Simons   Faculty of Pharmacy and Faculty of Medicine, University of Manitoba, Winnipeg, Canada

Nicholas A. Soter   The Ronald O. Perelman Department of Dermatology, New York University School of Medicine; Charles C. Harris Skin and Cancer Pavilion; and Tisch Hospital, The University Hospital of NYU, New York, New York, U.S.A.

Lori Wagner   Departments of Dermatology and Medicine, The University of Utah Health Sciences Center, University of Utah, Salt Lake City, Utah, U.S.A.

Alan A. Wanderer   Department of Pediatrics–Allergy, University of Colorado Health Sciences Center, Allergy and Asthma Consultants of Montana, Bozeman, Montana, U.S.A.

Todd M. Wilson   Laboratory of Allergic Diseases, National Institute of Allergy and Infectious Diseases, National Institutes of Health, Bethesda, Maryland, U.S.A.

Michael C. Zacharisen   Department of Pediatrics, Medical College of Wisconsin, Milwaukee, Wisconsin, U.S.A.

Wei Zhao   Division of Allergy, Immunology & Rheumatology, Department of Pediatrics, Virginia Commonwealth University, Richmond, Virginia, U.S.A.

1

What Is Urticaria? Anatomical, Physiological, and Histological Considerations and Classification

Ruth A. Sabroe
Department of Dermatology, Barnsley Hospital NHS Foundation Trust, Sheffield, U.K.

Malcolm W. Greaves
St. John's Institute of Dermatology, St. Thomas' Hospital, London, U.K.

INTRODUCTION

This chapter explains the structural, physiological, and molecular correlates of the symptoms and visible changes in the skin of the patient with urticaria and angioedema.

The lesions of urticaria are, at first sight, straightforward. Localized vasodilatation causes redness, increased blood flow causes warmth, enhanced vascular permeability leads to swelling (edema)—the features of Lewis's "Triple Response"(1)—and itch is the dominant symptom. Similar processes underlie angioedema, but in this case, increased vascular permeability predominates, leading to massive dermal and subcutaneous edema. Itching and visible redness are more variable. However, it is evident to anyone who deals with these patients regularly that there is more to urticaria and angioedema than this. What determines the distribution of the lesions of urticaria and angioedema? Why do wheals of chronic "idiopathic" urticaria (other than delayed pressure urticaria and dermographism) often develop at sites of pressure such as around the waistband? Why does angioedema show a predilection for the eyelids and lips? Why do individual lesions in "idiopathic" chronic urticaria last for 12 hours or more, in contrast with wheals of most physical urticarias, which last no more than an hour? Why is itching worse at night? Why do patients usually rub the itch of urticaria rather than scratch it? Why does chronic urticaria characteristically flare-up at times of stress? We do not pretend we can answer these and other puzzling questions to the readers' (or our own) entire satisfaction, but we will address them.

ANATOMICAL AND PATHOPHYSIOLOGICAL CONSIDERATIONS

Urticaria and angioedema are inflammatory and predominantly dermal processes. Patients rub the intense itch of urticaria, and this may result in bruising, but the epidermis is unscathed, and even scratch marks are rare despite the severe pruritus. Thus inflammatory skin lesions which peel on resolution (desquamation) are not due to urticaria or angioedema, and, in such cases, other causes such as urticarial dermatitis (2) or cellulitis should be sought. Besides the epidermis, the dermoepidermal junction is spared, the pathology being mainly mid- or deep dermal. Therefore blistering, or bulla formation, is exceptionally rare, and if present, should prompt consideration of alternative diagnoses, including autoimmune bullous dermatoses, some of which (e.g., bullous pemphigoid) may manifest prodromal urticaria–like skin changes.

Although itch is usually the dominant symptom of urticaria, pain and tenderness are occasional features of straightforward urticaria and occur not infrequently in patients with the less common urticarial vasculitis and also in angioedema.

THE DERMAL MAST CELL

Inappropriate activation of the dermal mast cell is thought to be the prime pathophysiological event in most forms of urticaria. The detailed pathophysiology of the mast cell in urticaria will be dealt with in a later chapter.

Dermal mast cells are derived from CD34+ pluripotent bone marrow stem cells and express receptors for the growth factor c-kit (3). In some forms of cutaneous mastocytosis (urticaria pigmentosa) in adults, mutations in the tyrosine kinase c-kit gene (e.g., codon D816V mutation) lead to over-activation of c-kit causing proliferation of dermal mast cells. Upregulation of the BCL2 apoptosis-preventing protein may also be important (4). Such mutations have not been described in urticaria or angioedema. Indeed there is controversy about whether mast cell numbers alter in urticarial wheals (see section "Inflammatory Infiltrate").

In the skin, mast cells are located throughout the dermis, but with a predilection for the vicinity of appendages, including pilosebaceous follicles, nerve fibers, and blood vessels. The turnover of dermal mast cells is slow. They can be almost entirely ablated by repeated prolonged potent topical corticosteroid application (5), and it takes about 24 weeks for re-establishment of the dermal mast cell population (6). This finding has been used as a treatment option in urticaria pigmentosa (7).

Skin mast cells differ from pulmonary mast cells, being responsive to opioid peptides, and neurone-derived substance P. Of interest, the optimum temperature for skin mast cell activation is as low as 30°C, whereas the same figure for lung mast cells is closer to 37°C (8). Unlike pulmonary mast cells, dermal mast cells possess complement C5a receptors. They can also be activated by other basic non-immunological stimuli such as compound 48/80 (8). Immunological activation occurs via cross-linking of receptor-bound IgE by specific antigen. Cross-linking due to IgG anti–high affinity IgE receptor (FcεR1) autoantibodies leading to activation also occurs in autoimmune urticaria (described in a later chapter). Although the pathways for activation differ, the end result—mast cell degranulation and release or secretion of mediators—is the same. However, the types of mediators released may differ, depending on the stimulus (9,10). Besides histamine, mediators released from human dermal mast cells include eicosanoids (prostaglandin D_2, leukotriene C_4), cytokines, including tumor necrosis factor-α (TNF-α), interleukins (IL) 4, 6, and 8/CXCL8, fibroblast growth factors, and proteases including chymase, tryptase, and granzyme B (11–17). More recently, it has been shown that if endogenous proteases are inhibited, then additionally, IL 5 and 13, and granulocyte macrophage-colony stimulating factor (GM-CSF) can be detected 24 to 48 hours after human skin–derived mast cell activation by cross-linkage of FcεR1 (18). Of note, human lung mast cells have been reported to be a source of IL 4, 5, 6, and 13, TNF-α GM-CSF and monocyte chemoattractant protein-1 (MCP-1/CCL2) (19–22). Human mast cell leukemia cell lines and murine mast cells secrete a number of additional factors, including IL 3 and 16, regulated upon activation normal T-cell expressed and secreted (RANTES/CCL5), macrophage inflammatory protein-1α (MIP-1α/ CCL3), vascular permeability factor/ vascular endothelial cell growth factor (VPF/VEGF), and oncostatin M (23–27).

It has recently been shown that human and rodent mast cells express toll-like receptors (TLRs) [recently reviewed (28)], which provides a new mechanism by which mast cells may respond to both microbial molecules and endogenous mediators of tissue damage. Urticaria may be triggered or exacerbated by various infective agents, and mast cell expression of TLRs may provide a link between the two.

Of considerable interest is the close anatomical and functional relationship between dermal mast cells and protein gene product (PGP) 9.5 positive neurones (29). This relationship is recognized as a plausible pathway for the familiar association of stress with exacerbations of urticaria.

It is reasonable to suppose that the different appearance and duration of wheals occurring in different types of urticaria are due to stimulus–specific combinations of the above mediators, or those released from incoming inflammatory cells. The susceptibility of an individual to get urticarial wheals, or to produce autoantibodies in autoimmune urticaria, may also be influenced by the mediators released.

THE CUTANEOUS VASCULATURE AND THE ROLE OF HISTAMINE

The visible signs of urticaria and angioedema are due to local vasodilatation, increased blood flow, and increased vascular permeability. Lymphatic drainage contributes a modulating influence on the degree of local edema (whealing). The extent to which angioedema and urticaria develop depends on the severity of capillary leakage and efficiency of its clearance by lymphatics. The pale halo of blanching, which can frequently be observed surrounding the red wheal, testifies to the role played by increased blood flow. It is the result of a "steal" effect and is best seen in cholinergic urticaria (Fig. 1). The

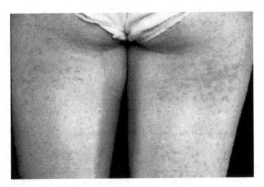

Figure 1 (*See color insert*). Cholinergic urticaria in a 12-year-old female. The prominent blanching surrounding the wheals is due to a vascular "steal" effect (see text).

redness of the wheal itself is caused by engorgement of the sub-papillary venous plexus, although by analogy with the axon reflex flare of the histamine wheal (1) it is probable that neurovascular reflex mechanisms also play a part, at least in acute urticarial lesions. The main site of increased vascular permeability is the post capillary venule. Increased blood flow raises the intraluminal pressure within post-capillary venules, altering the homeostatic balance between intraluminal hydrostatic pressure forcing fluid out and osmotic forces keeping it in (Starling's Law). This process is augmented by increased leakiness of the venular endothelial cells.

That histamine, via H1 and H2 receptors (30), is the principal mediator of these vascular changes is probably true for most physical urticarias, in which the wheal is short-lived and manifests the features of a histamine wheal. Although increased tissue levels of histamine have been demonstrated in involved skin in chronic idiopathic urticaria (CIU) (31), the role of this mediator in the pathogenesis of the wheal in CIU is less clear for the following reasons: (*i*) The visible vascular changes of CIU last for at least 12 hours, whereas histamine manifests rapid tachyphylaxis with respect to its vascular effects (32). (*ii*) Unlike the itch, the wheal of CIU is poorly responsive to H1 antihistamines. (*iii*) The cellular infiltrate seen histologically in the affected skin of CIU implies the involvement of other mediators. (*iv*) Lack of systemic manifestations of histamine release in patients with widespread CIU. Indeed, the wheal may be initiated by histamine, but it is likely that its perpetuation is attributable to additional mediators (see below). Kinetic data support this view (33).

If one cannot fully explain the itch of CIU by histamine acting through H1 and H2 receptors, then perhaps other histamine receptors might be involved, although their role in urticaria has yet to be defined. All histamine receptors are G-protein-coupled to intracellular signal transduction systems. All possess constitutive activity in the absence of ligand binding. H1 antihistamines act as inverse agonists, resulting in stabilization of the inactive state of the receptor (34). Recently described H3 and H4 receptors (35,36) are also believed to mediate pruritus, and both are potential targets for novel anti-itch drugs. H3 receptors are predominantly expressed in the central nervous system and act pre-synaptically on histaminergic neurones to regulate, by feedback inhibition, histamine release and biosynthesis. The location and function of H4 receptors is unclear but they are distributed in the CNS and expressed by some cell types. Indeed, H4 but not H3 receptors are expressed on human mast cells (37), and H4 receptors also appear to be expressed on human eosinophils (38). In mice, H4 receptor antagonists have been shown to be effective in relieving experimental pruritus (36). Also of note, in mice, histamine, depending on whether it acts through H1 or H2 receptors, also has the potential to alter the balance between Th1 and Th2 responses, which may be of relevance in urticaria (39).

THE POTENTIAL ROLE OF OTHER MAST CELL MEDIATORS IN WHEAL FORMATION

The role of non-histamine mast cell mediators in CIU has yet to be defined, but they may be important in the regulation of cell recruitment and the development of the urticarial wheal. PGD_2 and LTC_4 are vasodilators and increase vascular permeability, and similarly, VEGF increases the permeability of human endothelial cells in vitro (40). TNF-α, IL 4, and LTC4 (probably after conversion to LTD4) upregulate adhesion molecule expression on endothelial cells, and promote leukocyte rolling and adhesion (12,41–43). Indeed, of interest, there is some evidence to suggest that cultured foreskin mast cells, when stimulated by serum containing anti-FcϵR1 autoantibodies from patients with chronic urticaria, secrete mediators including TNF-α, which in turn increase the expression of intercellular cell adhesion molecule-1, vascular cell adhesion molecule-1, and E-selectin on human dermal endothelial cells (44). Immunohistochemical studies of urticarial wheals have provided some support for the increased expression of adhesion molecules in vivo (45,46).

MIP-1α /CCL3 and RANTES/CCL5 are variably effective chemoattractants for eosinophils in vitro (47) and can cause eosinophil and T lymphocyte accumulation in human skin in vivo (48). PGD2, acting via the recently identified CRTH2 receptor, may also be important in regulating the recruitment and/or activation of eosinophils, basophils and Th2–type T cells (49). Mast cell interactions with other cell types such as fibroblasts may regulate the generation of other chemokines such as eotaxin/CCL11, a potent stimulus of eosinophil, basophil, and perhaps Th2-type T cells (50). Additionally, IL 8/CXCL8 can cause neutrophil accumulation in human skin in vivo (51), and IL 16 is chemoattractant for human T lymphocytes in vitro (24). IL 3, 5 and GM-CSF are important in the proliferation, differentiation, maturation, viability, and priming of eosinophils, and GM-CSF is also important in neutrophil priming (52). In human B lymphocytes, IL 4 is an essential cofactor for IgE synthesis (53), and similarly IL 13 can induce IgE synthesis independent of IL 4 (54). IL 4 also directs the development of naïve CD4+ T lymphocytes into Th2 cells in mice and humans (55,56). The relative contribution of these mediators to both the susceptibility of patients to have urticaria and the development of individual wheals requires further investigation.

ITCHING

The 19th century Scottish physician, William Heberden, wrote of urticaria that "by far the greatest number (of patients) experience no other evil besides the intolerable anguish arising from the itching" (57). Itch in urticaria is classified as pruritoceptive (58). This means it is generated within the skin, and the contribution of central (neurogenic) components is minimal. Histamine appears to be the main, if not the only, cause of itching in most forms of urticaria, including CIU, since application of histamine to human skin reproduces the symptom convincingly, and H1– antihistamines are usually effective in suppressing this symptom (59). The pruritic response to histamine is due to activation of neuronal H1 and possibly H3 and H4 (shown in mice to date), but not H2, receptors (36,59,60) associated with free nerve endings in skin. Pruritus is transmitted via unmyelinated histamine-sensitive and histamine-independent C or A δ neurons to the gray matter of the dorsal horn of the spinal cord. There, secondary neurones transmit the sensation via the contralateral spinothalamic tracts to higher centers. Recent application of microneurographic technology (61,62) has clearly demonstrated the existence of a subset of dedicated itch-transmitting C neurones and lateral spinothalamic neurones, distinct from those transmitting pain.

Neuroimaging techniques have enabled localization of cerebral itch processing. In these studies, the anterior cingulate cortex, pre/supplementary motor area, pre-frontal and inferior parietal cortex have been found to have important roles in the perception of itch (63).

Studies of the diurnal distribution of pruritus in chronic urticaria revealed that itching is most prominent in the evening and at night—an important consideration when outlining a treatment strategy. The cause of the nocturnal preponderance is unclear but may be due to warmth of the skin and to psychophysiological factors. Perception of itch is downregulated by sensory input from higher centers via inhibitory descending pathways from the periacqueductal gray matter. Such distracting stimuli may be reduced in the evening and at night. Patients rub rather than scratch the itch of urticaria. Rubbing activates myelinated fast-conducting A neurones. This leads to activation of inhibitory neuronal circuits within the substantia gelatinosa of the spinal cord, modulating the traffic of itch. These proposed mechanisms have recently been reviewed (64,65).

INFLAMMATORY INFILTRATE

The significance of the cellular infiltrate in different types of urticaria has been under-investigated. There are qualitative data, but the functional and dynamic aspects are largely unknown. Histologically, the classical features of the urticarial wheal are dermal edema, vasodilatation, including dilatation of lymphatics, and an inflammatory infiltrate consisting of mononuclear cells, mainly lymphocytes, with a variable number of neutrophils and eosinophils (Fig 2A). Unlike in urticarial vasculitis (Fig. 2B), there is no evidence of endothelial cell damage although these cells may be swollen. Erythrocyte extravasation and nuclear dust (karyorrhexis)—other major features of urticarial vasculitis—are absent.

Surprisingly, despite their central role in the pathogenesis of urticaria, light microscope examination of dermal mast cells usually shows no remarkable changes with

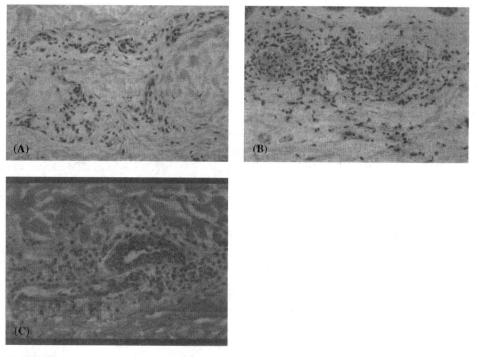

Figure 2   (**A**) Histological appearances of a skin biopsy of a wheal of chronic idiopathic urticaria. There is no evidence of endothelial damage or leukocytoclasia (H&E). (**B**) Histological appearances of a skin biopsy of a wheal of urticarial vasculitis. The endothelial cells are clearly damaged, there is prominent leukocytoclasia and red blood cell diapedesis (H&E). (**C**) Histological appearances of a skin biopsy of a wheal of neutrophilic urticaria. There is no endothelial cell damage or leukocytoclasia, but the walls of the post-capillary venules show marked invasion by neutrophils ("polys in the wall"). *Source*: Photomicrograph courtesy of Dr. RK Winkelmann.

no visible degranulation. Additionally, there is controversy about whether or not mast cell numbers alter in urticarial wheals, with some authors describing a reduced number and others describing a 10-fold increase (66–69).

Use of monoclonal antibodies and enzyme immunohistochemistry has enabled characterization of the mononuclear infiltrate. In chronic urticaria, Kaplan's group (66) reported that about 40% of the infiltrating cells were T lymphocytes, with a ratio of CD4 helper-inducer: CD8 cytotoxic-suppressor cells similar to that in normal healthy blood. In a recent joint publication, Kaplan's and Kay's groups, have demonstrated increases in intradermal CD3+, CD4+, CD8+ and CD25+ T lymphocytes. The cells had a Th0 cytokine profile with significant increases in IL 4, IL 5 and interferon γ mRNA (70).

Our group (71) carried out timed biopsies from involved and uninvolved skin in 22 patients with CIU and from normal skin of 12 healthy control subjects. Biopsies from wheals aged <4 hours or >12 hours showed increased numbers of EG2+ activated eosinophils, neutral elastase+ neutrophils, and to a lesser extent CD3+ T cells compared with uninvolved skin. There was no difference between the healthy skin of normal control subjects and uninvolved skin of CIU patients. However when biopsies of patients whose chronic urticaria was shown to have an autoimmune basis due to anti-FcεR1 or anti-IgE autoantibodies were compared with those without autoanti-bodies, there was little difference, except that the latter were found to have more activated eosinophils in wheals of >12 hours' duration. The explanation for this finding is unclear, although it would suggest that eosinophil activation may occur later or persist for longer in these patients.

That peripheral blood basophil leukocytes are depleted in chronic urticaria has long been recognized (72). More recently, we (73) have shown that this abnormality is associated with the presence in the peripheral blood of autoantibodies against the high-affinity IgE receptor or against IgE—the hallmarks of autoimmune urticaria. As suggested by Grattan (74), active recruitment of basophils into lesional skin of patients with autoimmune urticaria may not only explain this phenomenon but may also be a key factor in the pathogenesis of the disease. There is now evidence to support basophil accumulation in lesional skin (70,75). However, circulating basophils could also be reduced by trapping in the reticuloendothelial system.

Winkelmann (76) has delineated on histological grounds 15.8% of cases of chronic urticaria that have either a diffuse dermal neutrophil infiltrate or neutrophils investing the post-capillary venules, or in some cases invading the wall of the venules or any combination of these changes (76). There was no vasculitis (Fig. 2C). He was unable to attach any particular clinical significance to these findings, which were observed not only in CIU but also in physical urticarias, and believed them to be representative of an "intense stimulus response pattern" in urticaria (77). This conclusion was also reached by Henz's group (78), which believed neutrophilic urticaria to be an acute phase urticarial reaction not restricted to any specific type of urticaria. The present authors have observed the histological pattern of neutrophilic urticaria in several cases of Schnitzler's syndrome (79). In timed biopsies from wheals in patients with CIU, we found that in wheals of <4 hours duration neutrophils were predominantly in or close to vessels, whereas in wheals of >12 hours' duration, they were predominantly in the interstitium (71). Neutrophil accumulation may represent a phase of wheal evolution and as recently proposed (80), may be associated with treatment-resistant disease.

It is the authors' view that much potentially fruitful research could be done on clinicopathological correlates by use of currently available monoclonal antibodies as cell markers and by focusing on the evolution of the cellular infiltrate in sequential biopsies from different subtypes of acute and chronic urticaria and in urticarial vasculitis.

THE LESIONAL DISTRIBUTION OF URTICARIA AND ANGIOEDEMA

In physical urticarias the distribution is determined by the physical provoking factors. Solar and cold urticaria occur predominantly in exposed areas and pressure urticaria or symptomatic dermographism mainly at sites of pressure or friction (waist band, soles, palms). Urticarial vasculitis also often occurs at pressure sites, probably due to the predilection of immune complex deposition for conditions of vascular stasis. Although sites of local pressure on the skin are often involved in the wheals of chronic idiopathic urticaria, this may be due to the high incidence of concurrent delayed pressure urticaria (81). Angioedema frequently affects the skin of the eyelids, lips and genitalia, probably due to the relatively scanty connective tissue in these areas, which offers low resistance to exudation and accumulation of tissue fluid. Lymphatic clearance of rapidly accumulating tissue fluid may also be less effective in these areas. Whether differences in the cutaneous blood vascularization at different sites also play a role is unclear. There is no consensus on whether dermal mast cell population density is altered in chronic urticaria, and so this is probably not a determining factor in the distribution of lesions (66,67,69). Sites at which wheals of CIU were present less than about 72 hours previously are usually spared further whealing. This may be due to refractoriness of dermal mast cells to renewed activation, or to tachyphylaxis manifested by the cutaneous vasculature to vasoactive mediators (32), or both.

PSYCHOSOMATICS AND URTICARIA

Emotional factors can cause flare-ups of urticaria; serious emotional disturbance can also be a consequence of the disease. Of course, in many patients, both may occur concurrently. Awareness of these factors is an essential component of a holistic approach to the patient with chronic urticaria and angioedema.

Although stress itself does not cause urticaria, anyone who deals regularly with patients with chronic urticaria will be aware of the powerful influence of "stress" on the frequency and severity of relapses. The most straightforward example of this is found in patients with the very common physical urticaria, cholinergic urticaria. These patients regularly report that a stressful event, such as speaking in public, a confrontation at work, or troublesome circumstances at home, brings an immediate outbreak of intense itching and typical monomorphic pinhead-like wheals. However, patients with CIU typically report flare-ups when traveling on business trips, during examinations, and during major personal life events. The possible neurophysiological basis for stress-induced exacerbation of urticaria has already been alluded to (29).

On the other hand the impact of chronic urticaria and its associated pruritus on family harmony and on occupational performance, through irritability and depression from impaired sleep and loss of self-esteem as a result of continuous rubbing, should not be underestimated. Recent studies of the effect of chronic urticaria on quality of life (QOL) using recognized QOL instruments (82,83) have underscored the impact of chronic urticaria on personal, social, occupational, and domestic activities. Several patients under the care of one of the authors (MWG) have admitted recourse to alcohol abuse on the (no doubt genuine) grounds that it is the only measure that affords them significant relief from the itch. In practice, it is often difficult to tease out cause from effect in an individual patient.

In the chronic urticaria patient, anxiety may express itself as disordered autonomic function. In a recent study (84), evaluation of autonomic function by measurement of

R–R intervals on the ECG during controlled breathing showed that patients with chronic urticaria had altered autonomic function compared with healthy controls. This clinical observation is of special interest since animal studies have demonstrated the increased secretion of salivary mast cell protease in rats in response to visual stimuli (85), suggesting functional links between the nervous system and mast cells. There is convincing evidence to show that psychological factors can participate in immunological responses in man. For example, shifts in the dose–response curve for the Prausnitz–Kustner reaction (transfer of skin-sensitizing antibodies from the serum of an allergic subject eliciting an immediate type hypersensitivity reaction to the appropriate allergen can be carried out by intradermal injection of the allergic donor's serum into a nonallergic recipient) could be brought about by direct suggestion under hypnosis (86).

Stress management and behavioral therapy may be of benefit in the long-term management of patients with chronic urticaria in whom stress is clearly an exacerbating factor (87).

For those patients in whom emotional disturbance is deemed to be the consequence rather than cause of flare-ups of the disease, it is first important to determine if the reaction is one of anxiety or depression or both (88). After attempting to re-channel or reduce stress, adjunctive treatment by anxiolytic and/or antidepressant drugs should be considered. However, drug therapy though often useful, is no substitute for the establishment of a close rapport with the patient, leading to patient education on the nature and causation of the symptoms signs and prognosis.

CLASSIFICATION OF URTICARIA AND ANGIOEDEMA

The definitions of the different subtypes of urticaria will be dealt with in the appropriate chapters. Here we seek to provide for clinicians a user-friendly classification of the main types of urticaria/angioedema, incorporating advances in understanding of pathogenesis, and loosely based upon recently published European guidelines (89). It is not comprehensive.

"Ordinary" urticaria/angioedema consists of wheals/angioedema that occur randomly without local physical provocation.

- Acute urticaria/angioedema: This includes isolated attacks of urticaria lasting <6 weeks, although mainly idiopathic systemic causes include virusus, drugs, and type I hypersensitivity reactions.
- Chronic urticaria/angioedema: Attacks last >6 weeks and the periodicity may be intermittent or persistent daily or almost daily wheals. Idiopathic chronic urticaria and autoimmune urticaria fall into this category.

Physical urticarias/angioedema consist of wheals/angioedema that develop in response to external physical stimuli.

- Symptomatic dermographism (localized response to stroking the skin): no angioedema.
- Delayed pressure urticaria (localized response to pressure applied against the skin): no angioedema.
- Cold contact urticaria (localized response of skin to lowered temperature): may be associated with angioedema and anaphylaxis.
- Heat contact urticaria (localized response of skin to raised temperature): rarely associated with angioedema.

- Solar urticaria (localized response of skin to UV and/or visible light): rarely associated with angioedema.
- Vibratory urticaria (localized response of skin to vibratory stimuli): frequently associated with angioedema.
- Cholinergic urticaria (widespread monomorphic urticarial eruption in response to exercise, rise in body temperature, or emotional provocation): may be accompanied by angioedema; exercise-induced anaphylaxis may occur rarely.
- Aquagenic urticaria (localized response of skin to wetting by water, morphologically resembling cholinergic urticaria): no angioedema.

SPECIAL TYPES OF URTICARIA/ANGIOEDEMA

- Contact urticaria [localized response of skin to contact with an allergen, but response can also be nonallergic (pseudoallergic)]: may be associated with angioedema.
- Urticarial vasculitis (a chronic urticaria with histological evidence of vasculitis in involved skin, and which may be idiopathic or secondary to systemic disease): may be associated with angioedema.
- Urticaria pigmentosa (cutaneous mastocytosis) (urticaria associated with hyperproliferation of dermal mast cells): rarely associated with angioedema.
- C1 esterase inhibitor deficiency is a rare disorder leading to angioedema only. It is usually hereditary, but can be acquired, for example, in association with lymphoproliferative disorders or other malignancy, or with anti-C′1 esterase inhibitor autoantibodies and systemic lupus erythematosus.

REFERENCES

1. Lewis T. The Blood Vessels of the Human Skin and Their Responses. London: Shaw and Sons, 1927:47.
2. Kossard S, Hamann I, Wilkinson B. Defining urticarial dermatitis: A subset of dermal hypersensitivity reaction patterns. Arch Dermatol 2006; 142:29–34.
3. Buttner C, Henz BM, Welker P, et al. Identification of activating c-kit mutations in adult-, but not in childhood- onset indolent mastocytosis: A possible explanation for divergent clinical behavior. J Invest Dermatol 1998; 111:1227–1231.
4. Akin C, Metcalfe DD. Systemic mastocytosis. Annu Rev Med 2004; 55:419–32.
5. Barlow RJ, MacDonald DM, Black AK, et al. The effects of topical corticosteroids on delayed pressure urticaria. Arch Dermatol Res 1995; 287:285–288.
6. Lawlor F, Black AK, Murdoch RD, et al. Symptomatic dermographism: Wealing, mast cells and histamine are decreased in the skin following long-term application of a potent topical corticosteroid. Br J Dermatol 1989; 121:629–634.
7. Guzzo C, Lavker R, Roberts LJ 2nd, et al. Urticaria pigmentosa. Systemic evaluation and successful treatment with topical steroids. Arch Dermatol 1991; 127:191–196.
8. Lawrence ID, Warner JA, Cohan VL, et al. Purification and characterization of human skin mast cells: evidence for human mast cell heterogeneity. J Immunol 1987; 139:3062–3069.
9. Church MK, el-Lati S, Okayama Y. Biological properties of human skin mast cells. Clin Exp Allergy 1991; 21(suppl 3):1–9.
10. Okayama Y, Ono Y, Nakazawa T, et al. Human skin mast cells produce TNF-alpha by substance P. Int Arch Allergy Immunol 1998; 117(suppl 1):48–51.
11. Schwartz LB. Mast cells and their role in urticaria. J Am Acad Dermatol 1991; 25:190–204.

12. Walsh LJ, Trinchieri G, Waldorf HA, et al. Human dermal mast cells contain and release tumor necrosis factor α, which induces endothelial leukocyte adhesion molecule 1. Proc Natl Acad Sci U S A 1991; 88:4220–4224.

13. Bradding P, Feather IH, Howarth PH, et al. Interleukin 4 is localized to and released by human mast cells. J Exp Med 1992; 176:1381–1386.

14. Möller A, Lippert U, Lessmann D, et al. Human mast cells produce Il-8. J Immunol 1993; 151: 3261–3266.

15. Krüger-Krasagakes S, Möller A, Kolde G, et al. Production of interleukin-6 by human mast cells and basophilic cells. J Invest Dermatol 1996; 106:75–79.

16. Artuc M, Steckelings UM, Hentz BM. Mast cell-fibroblast interactions: human mast cells as a source and inducers of fibroblast and epithelial growth factors. J Invest Dermatol 2002; 118:391–395.

17. Strik MCM, de Koning PJA, Kleijmeer MJ, et al. Human mast cells produce and release the cytotoxic lymphocyte associated protease granzyme B upon activation. Mol Immunol 2007; 44:3462–3472.

18. Zhao W, Oskeritzian CA, Pozez AL, et al. Cytokine production by skin-derived mast cells: endogenous proteases are responsible for degradation of cytokines. J Immunol 2005; 175:2635–2642.

19. Bradding P, Roberts JA, Britten KM, et al. Interleukin-4, -5, and -6 and tumor necrosis factor-α in normal and asthmatic airways: evidence for the human mast cell as a source of these cytokines. Am J Respir Cell Mol Biol 1994; 10:471–480.

20. Jaffe JS, Raible DG, Post TJ, et al. Human lung mast cell activation leads to IL-13 mRNA expression and protein release. Am J Respir Cell Mol Biol 1996; 15:473–481.

21. Okayama Y, Kobayashi H, Ashman LK, et al. Human lung mast cells are enriched in the capacity to produce granulocyte-macrophage colony-stimulating factor in response to IgE-dependent stimulation. Eur J Immunol 1998; 28:708–715.

22. Baghestanian M, Hofbauer R, Kiener HP, et al. The c-kit ligand stem cell factor and anti-IgE promote expression of monocyte chemoattractant protein-1 in human lung mast cells. Blood 1997; 90:4438–4449.

23. Wodnar-Filipowicz A, Heusser CH, Moroni C. Production of the haemopoietic growth factors GM-CSF and interleukin-3 by mast cells in response to IgE receptor-mediated activation. Nature 1989; 339:150–152.

24. Rumsaeng V, Cruikshank WW, Foster B, et al. Human mast cells produce the CD4+ T lymphocyte chemoattractant factor, IL-16. J Immunol 1997; 159:2904–2910.

25. Selvan RS, Butterfield JH, Krangel MS. Expression of multiple chemokine genes by a human mast cell leukemia. J Biol Chem 1994; 269:13893–13898.

26. Boesiger J, Tsai M, Maurer M, et al. Mast cells can secrete vascular permeability factor/ vascular endothelial cell growth factor and exhibit enhanced release after immunoglobulin E-dependent upregulation of Fcε receptor I expression. J Exp Med 1998; 188:1135–1145.

27. Salamon P, Shoham NG, Puxeddu I, et al. Human mast cells release oncostatin M on contact with activated T cells: possible biological relevance. J Allergy Clin Immunol 2008; 121:448–455.

28. Stelekati E, Orinska Z, Bulfone-Paus S. Mast cells in allergy: innate instructors of adaptive responses. Immunobiology 2007; 212:505–519.

29. Hagforsen E, Nordlind K, Michelsson G. Skin nerve fibres and their contact with mast cells in patients with palmoplantar pustulosis. Arch Dermatol Res 2000; 292:269–274.

30. Marks R, Greaves MW. Vascular reactions to histamine and compound 48/80 in human skin: suppression by a histamine H2 receptor blocking agent. Br J Clin Pharmacol 1977; 4:367–369.

31. Kaplan AP, Horakova Z, Katz SI. Assessment of tissue fluid histamine levels in patients with urticaria. J Allergy Clin Immunol 1978; 61:350–354.

32. Greaves MW, Shuster S. Responses of skin blood vessels to bradykinin histamine and 5–hydroxytryptamine. J Physiol 1967; 193:255–267.

33. Cook J, Shuster S. Histamine weal formation and absorption in man. Br J Pharmacol 1980; 69: 579–585.

34. Leurs, R, Church MK, Taglialatela M. H1 antihistamines: inverse agonism, anti-inflammatory activities and cardiac effects. Clin Exp Allergy 2002; 32:489–498.

35. Lovenberg TW, Roland BL, Wilson SJ, et al. Cloning and functional expression of the human histamine H3 receptor. Mol Pharmacol 1999; 55:1101–1107.

36. Dunford PJ, Williams KN, Desai PJ, et al. Histamine H4 receptor antagonists are superior to traditional antihistamines in the attenuation of experimental pruritus. J Allergy Clin Immunol 2007; 119:176–183.

37. Lippert U, Artuc M, Grutzkau A, et al. Human skin mast cells express H2 and H4, but not H3 receptors. J Invest Dermatol 2004; 123:116–123.

38. Buckland KF, Williams TJ, Conroy DM. Histamine induces cytoskeletal changes in human eosinophils via the H(4) receptor. Br J Pharmacol 2003; 140:1117–1127.

39. Jutel M, Watanabe T, Klunker S, et al. Histamine regulates T cell and antibody responses by differential expression of H1 and H2 receptors. Nature 2001; 413:420–425.

40. Hippenstiel S, Krull M, Ikemann A, et al. VEGF induces hyperpermeability by a direct action on endothelial cells. Am J Physiol 1998; 274:L678–L684.

41. Iademarco MF, Barks JL, Dean DC. Regulation of vascular cell adhesion molecule-1 expression by IL-4 and TNF-α in cultured endothelial cells. J Clin Invest 1995; 95:264–271.

42. Kanwar S, Johnston B, Kubes P. Leukotriene C_4/D_4 induces P-selectin and sialyl Lewis^x-dependent alterations in leukocyte kinetics in vivo. Circ Res 1995; 77:879–887.

43. Yao L, Pan J, Setiadi H, et al. Interleukin 4 or oncostatin M induces a prolonged increase in P-selectin mRNA and protein in human endothelial cells 1996; 184:81–92.

44. Lee KH, Kim JY, Kang D-S, et al. Increased expression of endothelial cell adhesion molecules due to mediator release from human foreskin mast cells stimulated by autoantibodies in chronic urticaria sera. J Invest Dermatol 2002; 118:658–663.

45. Barlow RJ, Ross EL, MacDonald D, et al. Adhesion molecule expression and the inflammatory cell infiltrate in delayed pressure urticaria. Br J Dermatol 1994; 131:341–347.

46. Zuberbier T, Schadendorf D, Haas N, et al. Enhanced P-selectin expression in chronic and dermographic urticaria. Int Arch Allergy Immunol 1997; 114:86–89.

47. Sabroe I, Hartnell A, Jopling LA, et al. Differential regulation of eosinophil chemokine signaling via CCR3 and non-CCR3 pathways. J Immunol 1999; 162:2946–2955.

48. Beck LA, Dalke S, Leiferman KM, et al. Cutaneous injection of RANTES causes eosinophil recruitment. Comparison of nonallergic and allergic human subjects. J Immunol 1997; 159: 2962–2972.

49. Hirai H, Tanaka K, Yoshie O, et al. Prostaglandin D2 selectively induces chemotaxis in T helper type 2 cells, eosinophils and basophils via seven-transmembrane receptor CRTH2. J Exp Med 2001; 193:255–261.

50. Hogaboam C, Kunkel SL, Strieter RM, et al. Novel role of transmembrane SCF for mast cell activation and eotaxin production in mast cell-fibroblast interactions. J Immunol 1998; 160:6166–6171.

51. Leonard EJ, Yoshimura T, Tanaka S, et al. Neutrophil recruitment by intradermally injected neutrophil attractant/activation protein-1. J Invest Dermatol 1991; 96:690–694.

52. Nicod LP. Cytokines: 1- overview. Thorax 1993; 48:660–667.

53. Gascan H, Gauchat J-F, Roncarolo M-G, et al. Human B cell clones can be induced to proliferate and to switch to IgE and IgG4 synthesis by interleukin 4 and a signal provided by activated CD4$^+$ T cell clones. J Exp Med 1991; 173:747–750.

54. Punnonen J, Aversa G, Cocks BG, et al. Interleukin 13 induces interleukin 4-independent IgG4 and IgE synthesis and CD23 expression by human B cells. Proc Natl Acad Sci U S A 1993; 90:3730–3734.

55. Bonecchi R, Bianchi G, Bordignon PP, et al. Differential expression of chemokine receptors and chemotactic responsiveness of type 1 T helper cells (Th1s) and Th2s. J Exp Med 1998; 187: 129–134.

56. Swain SL, Weinberg AD, English M, et al. IL-4 directs the development of Th2-like helper effectors. J Immunol 1990; 145:3796–3806.

57. Heberden W. Commentaries on the History and Cure of Diseases. London: Payne, 1802.

58. Twycross R, Greaves MW, Handwerker H, et al. Itch: more than scratching the surface. Q J Med 2003; 96(1):7–26.

59. Robertson I, Greaves MW. Responses of human skin blood vessels to synthetic histamine analogues and to histamine. Br J Clin Pharmacol 1978; 5:319–322.

60. Sugimoto Y, Ida Y, Nakamura T, et al. Pruritus-associated response mediated by cutaneous histamine H3 receptors. Clin Exp Allergy 2004; 34:456–459.

61. Schmelz M, Schmidt R, Bickel A, et al. Specific C-receptors for itch in human skin. J Neurosci 1997; 17:8003–8008.

62. Andrew D, Craig AD. Spinothalamic lamina 1 neurons selectively sensitive to histamine: a central neural pathway for itch. Nat Neurosci 2001; 4:72–77.

63. Leknes SG, Bantick S, Willis CM, et al. Itch and motivation to scratch: an investigation of the central and peripheral correlates of allergen and histamine induced itch in humans. J Neurophysiol 2007; 97:415–422.

64. Yosipovitch G, Greaves MW, Schmelz M. Itch: new concepts. Lancet 2003; 361:690–694.

65. Greaves MW. Recent advances in pathophysiology and current management of itch. Ann Acad Med Singapore 2007; 36:788–792.

66. Elias J, Boss E, Kaplan AP. Studies of the cellular infiltrate of chronic idiopathic urticaria: prominence of T-lymphocytes, monocytes and mast cells. J Allergy Clin Immunol 1986; 78: 914–918.

67. Natbony SF, Phillips ME, Elias JM, et al. Histologic studies of chronic idiopathic urticaria. J Allergy Clin Immunol 1983; 71:177–183.

68. Barlow RJ, Ross EL, Macdonald DM, et al. Mast cells and T lymphocytes in chronic urticaria. Clin Exp Allergy 1995; 25:317–322.

69. Smith CH, Kepley C, Schwartz LB, et al. Mast cell number and phenotype in chronic idiopathic urticaria. J Allergy Clin Immunol 1995; 96:360–364.

70. Ying S, Kikuchi Y, Meng Q, et al. TH1/TH2 cytokines and inflammatory cells in skin biopsy specimens from patients with chronic idiopathic urticaria: comparison with the allergen-induced late-phase cutaneous reaction. J Allergy Clin Immunol 2002; 109:694–700.

71. Sabroe RA, Poon E, Orchard GE, et al. Cutaneous inflammatory cell infiltrate in chronic idiopathic urticaria: comparison of patients with and without anti-FcεR1 or anti-IgE autoantibodies. J Allergy Clin Immunol 1999; 103:484–493.

72. Greaves MW, Plummer VM, McLaughlan P, et al. Serum and cell-bound IgE in chronic urticaria. Clin Allergy 1974; 4:265–271.

73. Sabroe RA, Francis DM, Barr RM, et al. Anti-FcεR1 autoantibodies and basophil histamine releasability in chronic idiopathic urticaria. J Allergy Clin Immunol 1998; 102:651–658.

74. Grattan CEH. Basophils in chronic urticaria. J Invest Dermatol Symp Proc 2001; 6:139–140.

75. Hoskin SL, Wilson SJ, Sabroe RA, et al. Basophil infiltration of weals in chronic idiopathic urticaria. J Allergy Clin Immunol 2002; 109:A229.

76. Winkelmann RK, Reizner GT. Diffuse dermal neutrophilia in urticaria. Hum Pathol 1988; 19:330–335.

77. Peters, MS, Winkelmann RK. Neutrophilic urticaria. Br J Dermatol 1985; 113:25–30.

78. Toppe E, Haas N, Henz BM. Neutrophilic urticaria: clinical features, histological changes and possible mechanisms. Br J Dermatol 1998; 138:248–253.

79. Gallo R, Sabroe RA, Black AK, et al. Schnitzler's syndrome: no evidence for autoimmune basis in two patients. Clin Exp Dermatol 2000; 25:281–284.

80. Kim B, Fiorillo A, Fonancier L. Neutrophilic predominant urticaria associated with more resistance to treatment with antihistamines. J Allergy Clin Immunol 2008; 121(suppl 1): S102.

81. Barlow RJ, Warburton F, Watson K, et al. Diagnosis and incidence of delayed pressure urticaria in patients with chronic urticaria. J Am Acad Dermatol 1993; 29:954–958.

82. O'Donnell BF, Lawlor F, Simpson J, et al. The impact of chronic urticaria on quality of life. Br J Dermatol 1997; 136:197–201.

83. Poon E, Seed PT, Greaves MW, et al. The extent and nature of disability in different urticarial conditions. Br J Dermatol 1999; 140:667–671.

84. Hashiro M, Okumura M. Anxiety, depression, psychosomatic symptoms and autonomic nervous function in patients with chronic urticaria. J Dermatol Sci 1994; 8:129–135.

85. MacQueen G, Marshall J, Perdue M, et al. Pavlovian conditioning of rat mucosal mast cells to secrete mast cell protease. Science 1989; 243:83–85.

86. Black S. Shift in dose response curve of Prausnitz–Kustner reaction by direct suggestion under hypnosis. Br Med J 1963; 1:990–992.

87. Koblenzer CS. The urticarias. In: Psychocutaneous Disease. Orlando, FL: Grune & Stratton, 1987:203.

88. Medansky RS, Handler RM. Dermatopsychosomatics: classification, physiology, and therapeutic approaches. J Amer Acad Dermatol 1981; 5:125–136.

89. Zuberbier T, Bindslev-Jensen C, Canonica W. EAACI/GA^2 LEN/EDF guideline: definition, classification and diagnosis of urticaria. Allergy 2006; 61:316–320.

2
Epidemiology

Johannes Ring, Liliana Cifuentes, and Matthias Möhrenschlager
Division Environmental Dermatology and Allergy GSF/TUM, Department of Dermatology and Allergy Biederstein, Technical University of Munich, Munich, Germany

DEFINITIONS

Usual synonyms for urticaria are the terms "hives" or "nettle rash," the latter focussing on the typical reactions following skin contact with the stinging nettle (*Urtica dioica*).

The primary lesions of this monomorphic exanthematous disease are hives or wheals, which are defined as circumscribed white- to pink-colored compressible skin elevations produced by dermal edema. Eruptions of urticarial lesions are usually associated with intense pruritus. If the process involves deeper layers of the dermis or the subcutaneous tissue, it is known as angioedema ("Quincke's edema") (1).

Pathophysiologically the wheal can be characterized by local vasodilatation and increase of permeability of capillaries and small venules followed by transsudation of plasma constituents into the papillary and upper reticular dermis. Among a large number of substances, including kinins, prostaglandins, leukotriens, and proteolytic enzymes, histamine is the best-known elicitor of typical wheal-and-flare reactions.

COURSE

Depending on the duration of symptoms, urticaria can be divided mainly in two groups. It is considered to be acute if it lasts less than six weeks and chronic if the lesions persist beyond six weeks. Patients suffer from chronic intermittent (i.e., recurrent) urticaria when persisting symptoms are interrupted only by short symptom-free intervals of some days (1).

The most frequent episodes of urticaria are acute, with symptoms lasting for a short period, generally a few days to a few weeks (2).

In detail, Wüthrich et al. (3) documented a ratio of 53.2% acute versus 46.8% chronic cases of urticaria in Switzerland, whereas Gaig et al. (4) described an affliction of 969 adults out of 5.003 individuals by acute urticaria (18.9%) in a population-based study from Spain. Signs of chronic urticaria were detected in 30 out of 5003 individuals (0.59%) (4).

Table 1 Classification of Urticaria and Angioedema According to Etiopathophysiological Factors

Allergy	Food, drugs, eroallergens, insect venoms, contact urticaria allergens, serum thickness reaction
Toxicity	Insects, plants, sea animals
Pseudo-allergy	Nonsteroidal anti-inflammatory drugs (e.g., acetylsalicylic acid), antibiotics, opiates, radiocontrast media, food additives (e.g., azo dyes, preservatives)
Focus reactions	Parasites, bacterial, fungal, and viral infections, hormonal disorders, neoplasms
Physical stimuli	Mechanical (dermatographism, pressure, vibration, and others), thermic (cold, heat), cholinergic (sweat), aquagenic, solar, X ray, and others
Enzyme deficiency/ Enzyme inhibition	C1 inactivator (hereditary, acquired), ACE inhibitors
Autoimmune disorders	Urticaria vasculitis, systemic lupus erythematosus, cryoglobulinemia
Mastocytosis	Cutaneous, systemic
Autoimmune Idiopathic	Antibody to IgE receptor or IgE

Source: From Ref. 8.

Nevertheless, a few authors reported a higher prevalence for chronic urticaria compared with acute types (5–7).

CLASSIFICATIONS

Urticaria can be classified according to the time course (acute vs. chronic; see above) or to etiopathophysiological aspects. Table 1 provides an overview on the most important aspects of the latter.

PREVALENCE RATES

Urticarial diseases belong to the 20 most common skin diseases. Up to 20% or more of the general population have at least one episode of urticaria, angioedema, or both during their lives (1,8–11). Nevertheless, published data on prevalence rates differ widely (Table 2).
    Urticaria and angioedema may occur independently or in association. More than 90% of the cases of angioedema are acquired in nature and are caused by the same etiological factors as urticaria. At least 50% of patients with urticaria also suffer from angioedema, 40% do not, while angioedema as the sole clinical finding occurs in between 3.9% and 10% of the cases (26).

AGE

There are different age-related prevalence rates of urticarial diseases according to the two general courses (acute vs. chronic) of the disease. Acute urticaria is one of the most common childhood dermatoses, affecting up to 15% to 20% of children prior to adolescence (27). Nevertheless, urticaria and angioedema are relatively uncommon disorders under the age of six months with only a few case reports covering newborns (28,29). In contrast, Singh et al. (24) report on a prevalence rate of 23.6% among 424 newborns from India. Further studies are needed to clarify this point of interest.

Table 2 Prevalence Rates of Urticaria: General and Childhood(*) Population

Author(s)	Year	Prevalence (%)	n	Country
Lomboldt	1963	0.05	10.984	Faeroe Islands
Hellgren	1983	0.1	35.343	Sweden
Figueroa et al.	1994	0.15	768	Ethopia
Varonier et al.	1968	0.4	4.781	Switzerland
Gaig et al.	2004	0.6	5.003	Spain[a]
Varonier et al.	1981	0.9	3.270	Switzerland
Ronchetti et al.	1998	1.2	1.210	Italy*
Ronchetti et al.	1992	1.3	1.262	Italy*
Popescu et al.	1995	1.9	1.114	Romania*
Freeman et al.	1964	2.1	2.235	USA
Schäfer et al.	1993	2.8	1.503	Germany*[b]
Baghestani et al.	2001	2.8	6.841	Iran
Mahé et al.	1993	3.0	10.575	Mali
Ogunbiyi et al.	2005	3.3	1.066	Nigeria*
Naldi et al.	2003	4.3	3.660	Italy
Bakke et al.	1990	9.0	4.992	Norway
Wang	1990	23.2	10.144	China
Singh et al.	1980	23.6	424	India*

[a]actual prevalence of chronic urticaria.
[b]preschool children (5–6 yr old).
Source: From Refs. 1, 11–25.

Chronic urticaria tends to be more common in middle-aged individuals between the third and the sixth decade, reaching a maximum prevalence during the fourth decade, particularly among women (4,8,30). Within the pediatric age group, chronic urticaria seems to be uncommon with 5% of all patients younger than 24 months (31).

GENDER

Urticaria and angioedema obviously affect women more often than men. Especially middle-aged woman suffer more frequently from chronic urticaria than men (32). Hellgren mentions a concurrent prevalence rate of urticaria of 0.11% in the male population in contrast to 0.14% in the female population (10), whereas Dorner et al. (33) report a female:male ratio of 1.3:1 for urticaria and 1.8:1 for angioedema, respectively.

Similar results can be observed in the analysis of 316 health examinations carried out in Switzerland where women constituted 56.6% of patients (2). These data were supported by observations of a female predominance in reports from Germany and other countries (2,7). Table 3 summarizes the findings.

URTICARIA AND ATOPIC DISEASE

There are conflicting results as to whether urticaria occurs with a greater frequency in those with a personal or family history of atopic disease.

Some authors found an increase of acute urticaria in patients with atopy (13,39,40). In this context, Zuberbier described a 50.2% fraction of atopics suffering from acute urticaria (25). A positive history of atopy and preexisting dermatitis or pollinosis in

Table 3 Prevalence Rates of Urticaria: Gender Distribution

Author(s)	Year	Females (%)	n	Country
Hamilton et al.	1954	47.2	72	UK
Kauppinen et al.	1984	56.0	163	Finland
Dorner et al.	2007	56.5	11949	Austria
Wüthrich et al.	1980	56.6	316	Switzerland
Gaig et al.	2004	61.0	5.003	Spain[a]
Schäfer et al.	1993	61.9	1.503	Germany[b]
Paul et al.	1987	62.2	119	Germany
Juhlin	1981	63.3	320	Sweden
Wallenstein et al.	1984	68.0	200	Germany
Margolis et al.	1985	76.0	79	USA
Gaig et al.	2004	80.0	5.003	Spain[c]
Schäfer et al.	1993	84.4	1.497	Germany[d]

[a]acute urticaria.
[b]children aged 5 to 6 years.
[c]chronic urticaria.
[d]adults.
Source: From Refs. 1–4, 32–38.

children suffering from acute urticaria was found in more than 50% by Wüthrich (41). Nevertheless, a few authors question this association (11).

CAUSES

Although many cases of acute urticaria have probably never been seen by a physician, the etiological factors resulting in physician-handled acute urticaria can often be discovered (13). In contrast, if more stringent criteria are applied, a cause for chronic urticaria is not found in up to 90% of cases (11,13). Table 1 summarizes the etiology of urticaria. In this chapter, a focusation on important causes had to be performed, as outlined below.

Infections

Chronic infections (e.g., tonsils, teeth, sinuses, gallbladder) are found in some cases of urticaria. Removal or treatment of these foci has been helpful in many cases, but not all (42), and whether the infection is causative or a spurious association is not clear (see chapters 12, 17, and 18).

The most frequent reason for acute urticaria is a viral infection in the upper respiratory tract, usually a few days before onset of wheals (25). Furthermore, urticaria is reported as a frequent prodromal symptom of infection with hepatitis B virus in about 20% to 30% of cases (43). In respect to bacterial infections, 15% of urticaria patients have increased anti-staphylolysin titer (13). Worm infestation is also known to be associated with chronic urticaria (1).

In a cohort of 125 patients with chronic urticaria, 17% and 16% of them reported abnormal sinus and dental roentgenograms, respectively (44). Tanphaichtir (42) reports that 50% to 65% of all patients with chronic urticaria suffered from chronic tooth or gingival infections. In 4% to 35% of the affected patients, appropriate treatment of infections resulted in an improvement of urticaria (42), hereby indicating further hidden causes of the disorder. Others disagree that chronic infection has any role in the etiology of chronic urticaria (see chapters 17 and 18).

Food

In acute urticaria, nutritiva may often act as a responsible factor in elicitation of symptoms. In a study by Zuberbier (25), food was suspected as cause for the complaints in 63% of patients. In this context, cow's milk protein seems to be relevant in 10 out of 12 babies suffering from acute urticaria (25). In 5 to 16 year-old acute urticaria individuals, 15% show signs of food intolerance (25).

584 allergologists in the United States found urticaria as a more common manifestation related to food products (45). With regard to chronic urticaria and angioedema, foods seem not so often involved (13).

Nutritiva commonly seen in this kind of skin reaction include nuts, fish, shellfish, eggs, milk, chocolate, tomatoes, and fresh berries (46). Other factors that may trigger urticaria are food additives and preservatives (47,48).

Oral provocation testing in patients demonstrated an intolerance of a food dye or additive in 11% of patients (49).

Drug

Acetylsalicylic Acid and Other Nonsteroidal Anti-inflammatory Drugs
Acetylsalicylic acid (ASA) may play a role both in precipitating and in exacerbating urticaria. The conditions of 21% to 41% of patients with chronic urticaria will worsen with aspirin (50,51). Patients sensitive to aspirin have an increased urticarial reaction rate to other nonsteroidal anti-inflammatory analgesics, such as indomethacin, as well as food additives (like tartrazine and possibly benzoates) (50,52).

Some European studies have shown that 20% to 35% of patients with chronic urticaria have at least one positive reaction to a standard challenge test consisting of aspirin, azo dyes, benzoates, and yeasts (13). Paul and Greilich (2) mention 237 probands with urticaria, which were provoked by aspirin and indomethacin and showed reactions in 45% and 25% of cases, respectively. Nonsteroidal anti-inflammatory drugs (NSAID) were responsible for eliciting urticaria and/or angioedema in 10% to 20% of these patients in the United Kingdom (53).

The prevalence rates for acute angioedema from NSAIDs is estimated between 0.1% and 0.3%. This prevalence rates increase substantially when the patients are asthmatics or atopics (53). Urticaria was the second most commonly adverse cutaneous drug reaction (12.2%) in a prospective analysis of 4785 Mexican hospitalized subjects ().

Angiotensin-Converting Enzyme Inhibitor and Angiotensin II Antagonists
The frequency of angioedema under *angiotensin-converting enzyme* (ACE) inhibitors is estimated at 1 to 7 per thousand (8,13). The majority of cases occur within two months of start of ACE inhibition therapy, but angioedema may be seen at any time during the course of treatment. Angioedema under angiotensin II antagonists seems less frequent than this observed under ACE inhibitors, but data are inconsistent and vary from 7.7% to 50% (55).

Hormonal Disorder

Thyroid Gland Hormones
Abnormal thyroid function tests are relatively common in serum analyses. In a cohort treated for urticaria, 12 of 279 patients (4%) experienced a decrease in the thyroid-stimulating hormone (TSH) (54). Thyroid autoantibodies are also associated with chronic urticaria, although the exact pathomechanisms remain to be elucidated (56).

Hashimoto's Disease

In one study, 1% of chronic urticaria cases had positive thyroid antibodies, but only a small proportion manifested Hashimoto's thyroiditis (54).

Other Findings

With regard to autoimmune disorders, an autoimmune origin of chronic urticaria is postulated in 35% to 40% of cases (55). Systemic lupus erythematosus may show urticarial lesions in up to 9% of patients (57).

. In constrast, a positive rheumatoid factor is found in 5% of patients with urticaria, equivalent to the rate in the general population (13).

In recent years it has been shown that 35% to 40% of the patients with chronic urticaria have a circulating antibody directed against the alpha subunit of the high affinity IgE receptor (58–60), while an additional 5% to 10% possess antibodies against IgE (61). Comparable results were identified in the serum of at least a third of the patients with chronic idiopathic urticaria having functional IgG autoantibodies against the high-affinity IgE receptor (53).

Erythropoietic protoporphyria (EP) manifests sometimes with angioedema (57). Estimates of 1 case in 75.000 to 200.000 EP patients have been reported for some western European populations. EP has been documented most often in people with European ancestry, but also in Japanese and East Indian people (57).

Malignant neoplasms, diseases of the lymphatic system, para- and dysproteinemias can be associated with acute and chronic urticaria to a varying degree ("focus reaction") (1).

EPIDEMIOLOGICAL TRENDS OF URTICARIA AND ANGIOEDEMA

One has to distinguish between hospital data and population-based studies. In a study by Schäfer and Ring (1), conducted between 1988 and 1991 in a sample of unselected Bavarian preschool children (age: 5–6 yr), 1.503 children were examined.

As shown by the authors, a decrease of urticaria prevalence rates in preschool children (1988: 4.8%; 1991: 1.8%) was detected. In contrast, an increase of urticaria prevalence rates in the mothers of these preschool children was found (1988: 2.2%; 1991: 3.3%) (1). Further studies are needed to confirm these observations.

Although the use of hospitalization data will represent only a small proportion of all cases of urticaria and angioedema, changes in admission rates may reflect changes in general incidence rates.

Studies performed in Australia (55), New York State (62), and United Kingdom (63) were consistent with the increase in hospital admissions for urticaria and angioedema during the last decade (Fig. 1).

Between 1994 and 2005, there were significant increases in the rate of hospital admissions for urticaria in all age groups. An average annual increase of 3% was reported for hospitalizations for angioedema. In the same period, hospitalizations for urticaria represented an average annual increase of 5.7% (55).

The rate of hospitalization for angioedema was highest in persons aged 65 years and older and lowest in children aged 5 to 14 years (55). Although the rate of hospital admissions for angioedema remained relatively constant for most age groups, the rate in persons aged 65 years and older doubled. There was no significant change in the rate of hospital admissions for angioedema in those aged less than 15 years or 35 to 64 years (55). Among the factors that may influence the rising incidence in the older group are the

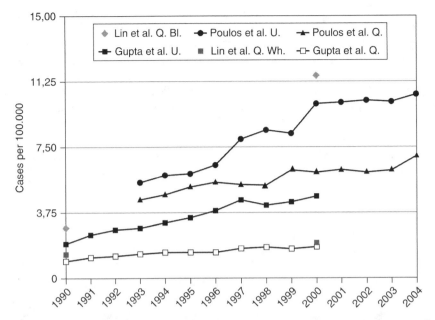

Figure 1 Hospital admissions due to urticaria (U) and angioedema (Q) in Australia (55) and United Kingdom (63) and angioedema in New York State (62). (Bl.: Afro-Americans; Wh.: whites). Diagram by Mr. Andreas Mauermayer, Department of Dermatology and Allergy, Technical University of Munich, Munich, Germany).

increasing exposition to nonspecific and specific aggravating factors such as stress, alcohol, and medicaments with the potential to worsen urticaria and angioedema such as aspirine, codeine, NSAIDs, and ACE inhibitors (55).

The differences between male and female subjects were similar to those seen for urticaria. Among children, rates of admission for these conditions were substantially higher in boys than in girls, which correspond with the sex difference in the prevalence of atopic conditions in this age group. However, among adults, the sex difference was reversed, with higher rates of admission among women than men for most conditions (55).

The prevalence is significantly higher in women than in men with regard to chronic urticaria. One possible explanation could be the 35% to 40% autoimmune origin of chronic urticaria, since women have higher prevalence of autoimmune diseases (55).

SPECIALIZED TYPES OF URTICARIA AND ANGIOEDEMA

Beside acute and chronic urticaria, other types of these entities can be found.

Physical Urticaria

Urticaria can also be triggered by a physical stimulus. These factors are mechanical, thermal, exercise related, solar related, and water related.

Physical urticarias account for 12% to 57% of patients with urticaria and probably represent from 10% to 17% of all cases of chronic urticaria (1,8,13). Predominantly young adults with a more frequent occurrence in the female population are affected by physical urticarias, the peak being between 10 and 40 years (8,13).

Mechanical Stimulus

Pressure. The direct effects of physical agents or trauma might also release histamine by nonimmunological processes, occurring in some persons with urticaria pigmentosa or dermographism, as well as the wheals produced, for example, by a whiplash.

Dermatographism is the most common form of physical urticaria. Its incidence in the general population ranges from 1.5% to 9% of all cases of urticaria (64). Some authors report the same prevalence rate of dermatographism in patients with chronic urticaria as in the general population (25).

Delayed pressure angioedema is characterized by deep, painful swellings developing four to eight hours after exposure to vertical pressure and persisting for the same period of time. It is estimated, that delayed pressure urticaria is present in up to 37% of chronic urticaria cases (65).

Vibration. Vibratory angioedema is a rare form of physical urticaria, encountered for example in motorcyclists. Immediate and delayed forms have been reported. This condition has been described with an autosomal-dominant pattern of inheritance as well as in an acquired type (66,67).

Cholinergic Stimulus

Following often an exercise with sweating or emotional stress, cholinergic urticaria presents with small-sized, disseminated lesions affecting predominately the apical trunk. Cholinergic urticaria is frequent in young adults with a prevalence of more than 10% in the age group of 16 to 35 years (25).

Thermal Stimulus

Cold urticaria. This type constitutes the second most common form of physical urticaria. It manifests especially in countries with a cold climate (68). Both familial and acquired disorders have been recognized. Although cold urticaria may occur at any age, it develops most often in young adults, predominantly young women (25). As many as 90% of these patients have a positive response to an ice cube test (68).

Localized heat urticaria. This very rare disorder is characterized by wheal formation following a circumscribed stimulus within the temperature range of 45°C to 50°C (69).

Electromagnetic Radiation

Visible as well as ultraviolet light and X rays can provoke urticarial skin lesions on exposed areas in rare cases (1).

Solar urticaria occurs throughout the world in all races. Most often light in the range from 280 to 760 nm is responsible for the cutaneous reaction. The total number of patients is quite small, with an involvement of 5 out of 1.000 chronic urticaria cases. In most studies women predominate (8,25).

The age of first consultation varies between 17 and 71 years, with constituting a mean age of onset of 35 years (70).

The symptoms usually commence when patients are young adults, but it has been reported to occur also in infancy. In a patient series from Belgium, 48% of the patients were atopic and 29% had atopy in the immediate family (70).

In contrast, solar angioedema is seldom reported in the French and British literature (71).

Stimulation by Water

Aquagenic urticaria is among the rarest types of physical urticarias. It is assumed that probably a water-soluble autoantigen of the stratum corneum is released to initiate further reactions (72).

Urticarial Vasculitis

When the urticaria is mediated by immune complex deposition in the post-capillary venules, present in 1% of the cases, it is called urticarial vasculitis. About one-third of these patients show hypocomplementemia. The male:female ratio is 1:2. The median age of involvement is around 40 years, with a range of 15 to 90 years. Although, this is primarily a disease of middle-aged adults, it can be seen in persons of any age (8,13).

Adrenergic Urticaria

In 1985 Shelley and Shelley reported two cases in which pruritic hives, as in cholinergic urticaria, were evoked by stress. Blood analysis demonstrated increased plasma noradrenalin and adrenalin levels (73). Adrenergic urticaria may also concomitantly present with cholinergic urticaria (74).

Contact Urticaria

Most of the epidemiological data that are available of contact urticaria originate from occupational field (chromates, latex, other rubber products, and cosmetics).

A frequent combination between irritant contact dermatitis, allergic contact dermatitis, and contact urticaria to latex has been demonstrated in some reports (75,76). Occupational and nonoccupational studies have demonstrated a slightly increased incidence of contact urticaria in female patients. No differences regarding to economic status, geographical location, size of the city, or racial predisposition were demonstrated in the studies conducted by Elpern (77,78), which included persons with white, Asian Filipino, Asian Japanese, and Hawaiian/part Hawaiian origin.

Kanerva gathered statistical data on occupational contact urticaria in Finland (79,80) The incidence more than doubled from 89 reported cases in 1989 to 194 cases in 1994. Between 1990 and 1994, 815 cases were reported. The most common causes (in decreasing order of frequency) were cow dander, natural rubber latex, and flour/grains/feed. These three groups comprised 79% of all cases. Reflecting on this data, the most affected occupations (per 100,000 workers) (in decreasing order of frequency) were bakers, preparers of processed food, and dental assistants.

An older Polish study found that contact urticaria constituted an estimated 1.1% of all urticaria cases seen at the hospital (13). In contrast to the Hawaiian study, in this study, only one out of five patients had a personal or family history of atopy (13).

The duration and time of apparition of a contact urticaria may also vary. Czarnecki et al. (81) reported the case of a contact urticaria resulting from elm, which was delayed and prolonged, disappearing after six days. Other specific publications have described cases of prolonged urticaria caused by vaseline or castor oil (82).

Natural Rubber Latex

Among occupational contact urticarias, natural rubber latex (NRL) is an often found pathogen, although it is much less frequently detected than in occupational eczemas, which account for more than 90% of occupational dermatitis cases. NRL contains several hundred proteins of which 13, Hev b1 to Hev b13 have been recognized by the International Union of Immunological Societies as latex allergens (8).

A high rate of sensitization and clinical allergy to latex has been reported in health care personnel, with an estimated prevalence varying from 4.5% to 10.7% in Europe (83) and up to 17% in some studies in Canada and the United States (84,85), whereas in the general population, the prevalence is estimated to be between 1% and 3% (8,13).

Ownby et al. found an IgE-mediated hypersensitivity of 6.4% to latex (86). The incidence doesn't change in the age groups between the second and eighth decade.

During the years 1997 to 1999, 1.040 health care workers in Italy were evaluated. 3.6% showed evidence of contact urticaria (87). Among subjects with serological and/or skin test evidence for latex sensitization, numerous subjects were asymptomatic for type I hypersensitivity. Some risk factors for the development of clinical manifestations of a latex-related allergy have been identified, including personal history of atopy and exposure to irritants (for example bleach, disinfectants), which can cause hand dermatitis contributing to the skin barrier disruption.

In this context, Elpern demonstrated that 46% of Hawaiian patients with contact urticaria had a personal history of atopy, whereas 44% had a family history of atopy. In contrast, only 21% of patients without contact urticaria had a personal history of atopy (77).

In Germany, powdered NRL products have been banned from the workplace since 1998, with an 80% decrease in occupation contact urticaria in health care workers by 2002 (88). Considering other occupations, most of construction workers with NRL allergy had a concurrent type IV hypersensitivity to chromate or rubber chemicals that facilitated sensitization to latex (89).

In symptomatic latex allergy patients, localized urticaria, sometimes angioedema, and/or generalized reactions are the most frequent reported manifestations. Other encountered disorders include rhinoconjunctivitis, asthma, and systemic anaphylaxis (1,8,13).

Cornstarch powder, which has traditionally been added during glove production to facilitate donning, seems to increase exposure to latex allergens both through direct skin contact and via the respiratory tract (90,91).

Other Causative Substances

The causative substance varies between occupation and country. In Finland, the protein of cattle (*Bos domesticus*) constitute the primary cause of occupational contact urticaria. Among hairdressers hydroxypropyl trimonium hydrolyzed collagen (crotein Q), a modified protein, which is added to shampoos, is often responsible for contact urticaria (92). There have been reports that eugenol—which is a commonly used in various cosmetics, foods, and dental materials—causes acute contact as well as chronic urticaria (92–96).

A special type of photoinduced contact urticaria was described to be elicited by benzophenones, chlorpromazine, methamine hippurate, or formaldehyde. Antibiotics such as cephalosporin may cause contact-type urticaria resulting from an acquired sensitization to cephalosporin compounds (96).

Idiopathic Urticaria

In recent years it has been discovered that in 30% to 50% of patients with idiopathic urticaria, the disease is due to an autoimmune process, and therefore is not strictly "idiopathic" (97).

FAMILIAL DISORDERS WITH AN AUTOSOMAL-DOMINANT INHERITANCE

This is a group of infrequent disorders, which present along with urticaria and angioedema. Among the various disorders, a selection of clinical important disorders was made.

Familial Cold Urticaria

Familial cold urticaria is an uncommon cutaneous and systemic reaction to cold with autosomal dominant inheritance (8).

Muckle-Wells Syndrome

Muckle-Wells syndrome is a rare familial disease characterized by episodes of urticaria, cochlear hearing loss and renal amyloidosis (98).

Hereditary Angioedema

Hereditary angioedema (HAE) is a rare disease affecting probably 1/10.000 to 1/150.000 individuals, reflecting 1% to 2% of all angioedema cases (99). It has been described in all races, and no sex predominance has been found. In two-thirds of patients, HAE will usually manifest during childhood and become more severe after puberty. Nevertheless, HAE may start at any time, even as late as age 70 to 80 years (99).

The autosomal-dominant inheritance pattern would predict equal incidence and severity in men and woman, but most physicians note a preponderance of woman requiring care. Estrogen concentration in serum may increase frequency and severity of HAE. Patients with HAE don't seem to suffer more often from allergies than noted in the general population (13).

It is important to mention that although HAE is an inherited disease, as many as 25% of patients have no family history and presumably suffer from new mutations (100,101).

Schnitzler Syndrome

It is charcterized by chronic urticarial lesions and monoclonal macroglobulinemia, starting around the age of 50 years. Most patients suffering from Schnitzler syndrome are of western European origin. Interestingly, only a few patients of Japanese ancestry have been reported (102,103).

CONCLUSIONS

Urticarial diseases belong to the 20 most common skin diseases. The pathogenesis of urticaria is manifold, and so is the classification of urticarial diseases. Reliable data about the epidemiology of urticaria and angioedema is limited. It is assumed that more than 20% of the general population experience at least one episode of acute urticaria (cumulative prevalence).

Studies performed in Australia, New York State, and United Kingdom found an increase in hospital admissions for urticaria and angioedema, which might reflect an increase in symptomatolgy and number of cases of common urticaria. For the future, more studies on epidemiological aspect of urticaria and angioedema are needed.

REFERENCES

1. Schäfer T, Ring J. Epidemiology of urticaria. In: Burr ML, ed. Epidemiology of Clinical Allergy. Monogr Allergy. Vol. 31. Basel: Karger, 1993:49–60.
2. Paul E, Greilich K-D. Zur Epidemiologie der Urtikariaerkrankungen. Hautarzt 1991; 42(6): 366–375.
3. Wüthrich B, Häcki-Herrmann D. Zur Ätiologie der Urticaria. Z Hautkr 1980; 55:102–111.
4. Gaig P, Olona M, Munoz Lejarazu D, et al. Epidemiology of urticaria in Spain. J Investig Allergol Clin Immunol 2004; 14(3):214–220.
5. Kleine-Natrop HE, Sebastian G. Analyse und Kritik der Urtikaria-Diagnostik. Dermatol Monatsschr 1973; 159:769–778.
6. Hellgren L. Urtikaria, die Prävalenz in Geschlechts-, Alters- und Berufsgruppen in Schweden. Aktuel Dermatol 1983; 9:189–190.
7. Buss YA, Garrelfs UC, Sticherling M. Chronic urticaria – which clinical parameters are relevant? A retrospective investigation of 339 patients. J Dtsch Dermatol Ges 2007; 5:22–29.
8. Ring J. Allergy in Practice. Heidelberg: Springer, 2005.
9. Sheldon JM, Mathews KP, Lovell RG. The vexing urticaria problem: present concepts of etiology and management. J Allergy 1954; 25(6):525–560.
10. Hellgren L. The prevalence of urticaria in the total population. Acta Allergol 1972; 27(3): 236–240.
11. Champion RH, Roberts SO, Carpenter RG, et al. Urticaria and angio-oedema. A review of 554 patients. Br J Dermatol 1969; 81(8):588–597.
12. Lomboldt G. Psoriasis: Prevalence, Spontaneous Course and Genetics. Copenhagen: GEC GAD, 1963.
13. Monroe EW. Urticaria. Curr Probl Dermatol 1993; 5:118–140.
14. Figueroa JI, Fuller LC, Abraha A, et al. Dermatology in southwestern Ethiopia: rationale for a community approach. Int J Dermatol 1998; 37(10):752–758.
15. Varonier HS, de Haller J, Schopfer C. Prevalences of allergies in children and adolescents. Pediatr Acta 1984; 39:129–136.
16. Ronchetti R, Villa MP, Matricardi PM, et al. Association of asthma with extra-respiratory symptoms in schoolchildren: two cross-sectional studies 6 years apart. Pediatr Allergy Immunol 2002; 13(2):113–118.
17. Freeman GL, Johnson S. Allergic diseases in adolescents. Am J Dis Child 1964; 107:549–559.
18. Baghestani S, Zare S, Mahboobi AA. Skin disease patterns in Hormozgan, Iran. Int J Dermatol 2005; 44(8):641–645.
19. Mahé A, Cissé IA, Fave O, et al. Skin diseases in Bamako (Mali). Int J Dermatol 1998; 37(9): 673–676.
20. Ogunbiyi AO, Owoaje E, Ndahi A. Prevalence of skin disorders in school children in Ibadan, Nigeria. Pediatr Dermatol 2005; 22(1):6–10.
21. Naldi L, Colombo P, Placchesi EB, et al. Study design and preliminary results from the pilot phase of the PraKtis study: self-reported diagnoses and selected skin diseases in a representative sample of the Italian population. Dermatology 2004; 208(1):38–42.
22. Bakke P, Gulsvik A, Eide GE. Hay fever, eczema and urticaria in southwest Norway. Allergy 1990; 47:515–522.
23. Wang Z. An allergy prevalence survey in population of 10.144 people. Zhonghua Liu Xing Bing Xue Za Zhi 1990; 11:100–102.
24. Singh M, Arora NK, Sroa HS. Urticaria neonatorum. Indian J Med Res 1980; 71:273–277.
25. Zuberbier T. Urticaria. Allergy 2003; 58(12):1224–1234.
26. Ollert M, Ring J. Urticaria und Angioödem. In: Przybilla B, Bergmann K, Ring J, eds. Praktische allergologische Diagnostik. Darmstadt: Steinkopff, 2000:328–334.
27. Tamayo-Sanchez L, Ruiz-Maldonado R, Laterza A. Acute annular urticaria in infants and children. Pediatr Dermatol 1997; 14:231–234.
28. Carder KR. Hypersensitivity reactions in neonates and infants. Dermatol Ther 2005; 18: 160–175.

29. Miyagawa S, Takahashi Y, Nagai A, et al. Angio-oedema in a neonate with IgG antibodies to parvovirus B19 following intrauterine parvovirus B19 infection. Br J Dermatol 2000; 143: 428–430.

30. Cooper KD. Urticaria and angioedema: diagnosis and evaluation. J Am Acad Dermatol 1991; 25:166–176.

31. Legrain V, Taieb A, Sage T, et al. Urticaria in infants: a study of forty patients. Pediatr Dermatol 1990; 7:101–107.

32. Margolis CF, Nisi R. Urticaria in family practice. J Fam Pract 1985; 20:57–64.

33. Dorner T, Lawrence K, Rieder A, et al. Epidemiology of allergies in Austria. Results of the first Austrian allergy report. Wien Med Wochenschr 2007; 157:235–242.

34. Hamilton NJT, Bendkowski B. Incidence of allergic diseases in general practice. Br J Dermatol 1954; i:1069–1070.

35. Kauppinen K, Juntunen K, Lanki H. Urticaria in children. Allergy 1984; 39:469–472.

36. Paul E, Greilich KD, Dominante G. Epidemiology of urticaria. In: Schlumberger HD, ed. Epidemiology of Allergic Diseases. Monogr Allergy. Basel: Karger, 1987:87–115.

37. Juhlin L. Modern approaches to treatment of chronic urticaria. In: Ring J, Burg G, eds. New Trends in Allergy. Berlin: Springer, 1981:279–282.

38. Wallenstein B, Kersten W. Untersuchungsergebnisse eines Urtikariakollektivs. Allergologie 1984; 7:115–119.

39. Swinny B. The atopic factor in urticaria. South Med J 1941; 34:855.

40. Jones HE, Lewis CW, McMartin S. Allergic contact sensitivity in atopic dermatitis. Arch Dermatol 1973; 107:217.

41. Wüthrich B. Urticaria and Quincke's edema. Ther Umsch 1989; 46(9):641–644.

42. Thanpaichitr K. Chronic urticaria associated with bacterial infections. Cutis 1981; 27(6): 653–656.

43. Hartmann H. Extrahepatic manifestations of HBV and HCV infection. Praxis (Bern 1994) 1997; 86(29–30):1163–1166.

44. Jacobson KW, Branch LB, Nelson JS. Laboratory tests in chronic urticaria. JAMA 1980; 243: 1644–1666.

45. Cruz NV, Wilson BG, Fiocchi A, et al. Survey of physicians' approach to food allergy. Ann Allergy Asthma Immunol 2007; 99(4):325–333.

46. Warin RP. Food factors in urticaria. J Hum Nutr 1976; 30(3):179–186.

47. Juhlin L. Additives and chronic urticaria. Ann Allergy 1987; 59:119.

48. Lockey SD. Reactions to hidden agents in foods, beverages and drugs. Ann Allergy 1971; 29:461.

49. Schäfer T, Ring J. Epidemiology of adverse food reactions due to allergy or other forms of hypersensitivity. In: Eisenbrand G, Aulepp H, Dayan A, eds. Food Allergies and Intolerances. Weinheim: DFG, VCH, 1996:40–54.

50. Doeglas HMG. Reactions to aspirin and food additives in patients with chronic urticaria. Br J Dermatol 1975; 93:135.

51. James J, Warin RP. Chronic urticaria: the effect of aspirin. Br J Dermatol 1970; 93:135.

52. Settipane GA, Chafee FH, Postman MI, et al. Significance of tartrazine sensitivity in chronic urticaria of unknown etiology. J Allergy Clin Immunol 1976; 57:541.

53. Soter NA, Kaplan AP. Urticaria and angioedema. In: Freedberg IM, Eisen AZ, Wolff K, et al. eds. Fitzpatrick's Dermatology in General Medicine. 6th ed. New York: McGraw Hill, 2003:1129–1143.

54. Jimenez Saab NG, Gomez Vera J, Lopez Tiro JJ, et al. Prevalence of chronic urticaria of autoimmune origin at the regional hospital Adolfo Lopez Mateos. Rev Alerg Mex 2006; 53(2): 58–63.

55. Poulos LM, Waters A-M, Hith GDP, et al. Trends in hospitalizations for anaphylaxis, angioedema, and urticaria in Australia, 1993–1994 to 2004–2005. J Allergy Clin Immunol 2007; 120(4):878–884.

56. Leznoff A, Sussman GL. Syndrome of idiopathic chronic urticaria and angioedema with thyroid autoimmunity: a study of 90 patients. J Allergy Clin Immunol 1989; 84:66–71.

57. Braverman IM. Urticaria as a sign of internal disease. Postgrad Med 1967; 41:450.
58. Hide M, Francis DM, Grattan CE, et al. Autoantibodies against the high-affinity IgE receptor as a cause of histamine release in chronic urticaria. N Engl J Med 1993; 328(22):1599–1604.
59. Fiebiger E, Maurer D, Holub H, et al. Serum IgG autoantibodies directed against the alpha chain of Fc epsilon RI: a selective marker and pathogenetic factor for a distinct subset of chronic urticaria patients? J Clin Invest 1995; 96(6):2606–2612.
60. Ferrer M, Kinet JP, Kaplan AP. Comparative studies of functional and binding assays for IgG anti-Fc(epsilon)RIalpha (alpha-subunit) in chronic urticaria. J Allergy Clin Immunol 1998; 101(5):672–676.
61. Gruber BL, Baeza ML, Marchese MJ, et al. Prevalence and functional role of anti-IgE autoantibodies in urticarial syndromes. J Invest Dermatol 1988; 90(2):213–217.
62. Lin RY, Cannon AG, Teitel AD. Pattern of hospitalizations for angioedema in New York between 1990 and 2003. Ann Allergy Asthma Immunol 2005; 95:159–166.
63. Gupta R, Sheikh A, Strachan D, et al. Increasing hospital admissions for systemic allergic disorders in England: analysis of national admissions data. BMJ 2003; 327:1142–1143.
64. Wong RC, Fairley JA, Ellis CN. Dermographism: a review. J Am Acad Dermatol 1984; 11:643.
65. Barlow RJ, Warburton F, Watson K, et al. Diagnosis and incidence of delayed pressure urticaria in patients with chronic urticaria. J Am Acad Dermatol 1993; 29(6):954–958.
66. Kaplan AP, Beaven MA. In vivo studies of the pathogenesis of cold urticaria, cholinergic urticaria, and vibration-induced swelling. J Invest Dermatol 1976; 67:327.
67. Ting S, Reinmann EF, Rauls DO, et al. Nonfamilial, vibration-induced angioedema. J Allergy Clin Immunol 1976; 57:605.
68. Neittaanmaki H. Cold urticaria. Clinical findings in 220 patients. J Am Acad Dermatol 1985; 13(4):636–644.
69. Skrebova N, Takiwaki H, Miyaoka Y, et al. Localized heat urticaria: a clinical study using laser doppler flowmetry. J Dermatol Sci 2001; 26:112–118.
70. Ryckaert S, Roelandts R. Solar urticaria. A report of 25 cases and difficulties in phototesting. Arch Dermatol 1998; 134(1):71–74.
71. Rose RF, Bhushan M, King CM, et al. Solar angioedema: an uncommonly recognized condition? Photodermatol Photoimmunol Photomed 2005; 21(5):226–228.
72. Henz BM. Das Spektrum der Urticaria. In: Henz BM, Zuberbier T, Grabbe J, eds. Urticaria – Klinik, Diagnostik, Therapie. Berlin: Springer, 1996:1–17.
73. Shelley WB, Shelley ED. Adrenergic urticaria: a new form of stress-induced hives. Lancet 1985; 2(8463):1031–1033.
74. Mihara S, Hide M. Adrenergic urticaria in a patient with cholinergic urticaria. Br J Dermatol 2008; 158(3):629–631.
75. de Groot H, de Jong NW, Duijster E, et al. Prevalence of natural rubber latex allergy (type I and type IV) in laboratory workers in The Netherlands. Contact Dermatitis 1998; 38(3):159–163.
76. Holness DL, Mace SR. Results of evaluating health care workers with prick and patch testing. Am J Contact Dermat 2001; 12(2):88–92.
77. Elpern DJ. The syndrome of immediate reactivities (contact urticaria syndrome). An historical study from a dermatology practice. I. Age, sex, race, and putative substances. Hawaii Med J 1985; 44(11):426–428.
78. Elpern DJ. The syndrome of immediate reactivities (contact urticaria syndrome). An historical study from a dermatology practice. III. General discussion and conclusions. Hawaii Med J 1986; 45(1):10–12.
79. Kanerva L, Toikkanen J, Jolanki R, et al. Statistical data on occupational contact urticaria. Contact Dermatitis 1996; 35(4):229–233.
80. Kanerva L, Jolanki R, Toikkanen J, et al. Statistics on occupational dermatoses in Finland. Curr Probl Dermatol 1995; 23:28–40.
81. Czarnecki D, Nixon R, Bekhor P, et al. Delayed prolonged contact urticaria from the elm tree. Contact Dermatitis 1993; 28(3):196–197.
82. Grin R, Maibach HI. Long-lasting contact urticaria from petrolatum mimicking dermatitis. Contact Dermatitis 1999; 40(2):110.

83. Rustemeyer T, Pilz B, Frosch PJ. Contact allergies in medical occupations. Hautarzt 1994; 45(12): 834–844.
84. Smedley J. Occupational latex allergy: the magnitude of the problem and its prevention. Clin Exp Allergy 2000; 30(4):458–460.
85. Yassin MS, Lierl MB, Fischer TJ, et al. Latex allergy in hospital employees. Ann Allergy 1994; 72(3):245–249.
86. Ownby DR, Ownby HE, McCullough J, et al. The prevalence of anti-latex IgE antibodies in 1000 volunteer blood donors. J Allergy Clin Immunol 1996; 97(6):1188–1192.
87. Filon FL, Radman G. Latex allergy: a follow up study of 1040 healthcare workers. Occup Environ Med 2006; 63(2):121–125.
88. Allmers H, Schmengler J, John SM. Decreasing incidence of occupational contact urticaria caused by natural rubber latex allergy in German health care workers. J Allergy Clin Immunol 2004; 114(2):347–351.
89. Conde-Salazar L, Gatica ME, Barco L, et al. Latex allergy among construction workers. Contact Dermatitis 2002; 47(3):154–156.
90. Tomazic VJ, Shampaine EL, Lamanna A, et al. Cornstarch powder on latex products is an allergen carrier. J Allergy Clin Immunol 1994; 93(4):751–758.
91. Brehler R, Kolling R, Webb M, et al. Glove powder–a risk factor for the development of latex allergy? Eur J Surg Suppl 1997; (579):23–25.
92. Niinimaki A, Niinimaki M, Makinen-Kiljunen S, et al. Contact urticaria from protein hydrolysates in hair conditioners. Allergy 1998; 53(11):1078–1082.
93. Grade AC, Martens BP. Chronic urticaria due to dental eugenol. Dermatologica 1989; 178(4): 217–220.
94. Bhalla M, Thami GP. Acute urticaria due to dental eugenol. Allergy 2003; 58(2):158.
95. von Krogh G, Maibach HI. The contact urticaria syndrome–an updated review. J Am Acad Dermatol 1981; 5(3):328–342.
96. Tuft L. Contact urticaria from cephalosporins. Arch Dermatol 1975; 111(12):1609.
97. Greaves M. Chronic urticaria. J Allergy Clin Immunol 2000; 105:664–671.
98. Muckle TJ, Wells MV. Urticaria, deafness and amyloidosis: a new heredo-familial syndrome. Q J Med 1962; 31:235–248.
99. Frank MM, Gelfand J, Atkinson JP. Hereditary angioedema: the clinical syndrome and its management. Ann Intern Med 1976; 84:850.
100. Gelfard JA, Boss GR, Conley CL, et al. Acquired C1 esterase inhibitor deficiency and angioedema: a review. Medicine 1979; 1:39.
101. Möhrenschlager M, Ring J. Male genital oedema—allergy and angio-oedema in the differential diagnosis. J Eur Acad Dermatol Venereol 2008; 22(3):269–270.
102. Eiling E, Schröder JO, Gross WL, et al. The Schnitzler syndrome: chronic urticaria and monoclonal gammopathy – an autoinflammatory syndrome? J Dtsch Dermatol Ges 2008; 6(8):626–631.
103. Sibbald RG, Cheema AS, Lozinski A, et al. Chronic urticaria. Evaluation of the role of physical, immunologic, and other contributory factors. Int J Dermatol 1991; 30(6):381–366.

3

Mast Cells

Wei Zhao
Division of Allergy, Immunology & Rheumatology, Department of Pediatrics,
Virginia Commonwealth University, Richmond, Virginia, U.S.A.

Lawrence B. Schwartz
Division of Rheumatology, Allergy & Immunology, Department of Internal Medicine,
Virginia Commonwealth University, Richmond, Virginia, U.S.A.

INTRODUCTION

Mast cells are generally recognized as the principal cell type to initiate immediate hypersensitivity reactions (Type I), and more recently as a cell that also contributes to innate and acquired immunity and to tissue remodeling (Fig. 1). Mast cells can be activated to release mediators such as histamine by both IgE-dependent and IgE-independent stimuli and are integral to urticaria and associated angioedema. The experimental challenge of an IgE-sensitized host with allergen reveals two phases to the subsequent immediate hypersensitivity reaction. The early phase of the IgE-dependent reactions (5 to 30 minutes post challenge), depending on the target tissue and distribution of allergen, involves local edema from increased permeability of postcapillary venules, smooth muscle contraction, arteriolar vasodilation, mucus secretion, and pruritus. The late phase of an immediate hypersensitivity reaction peaks four to six hours post challenge and involves the recruitment and activation of basophils, eosinophils, and other cell types. These late reactions can persist for at least one day in the lower airway and skin, but eventually appear to completely resolve. In contrast, chronic allergic inflammation results from prolonged allergen exposure, and may provoke changes in the target tissue that resolve much more slowly, if at all.

Mast cells occupy sentinel positions in tissues where noxious substances might attempt entry, and immediate hypersensitivity reactions typically begin. These cells are most concentrated at mucosal sites in the upper and lower airways, conjunctiva and gastrointestinal mucosa, and also in dermal, cardiac, and perivascular sites. Mast cells in human tissues have been divided into two major types based initially on the protease content of their secretory granules (1). Those with tryptase and chymase along with carboxypeptidase and cathepsin G are called MC_{TC} cells; those with only tryptase (lacking chymase protein and mRNA) are called MC_T cells. MC_{TC} cells are the predominant mast cell type in normal and urticaria pigmentosa skin, small bowel

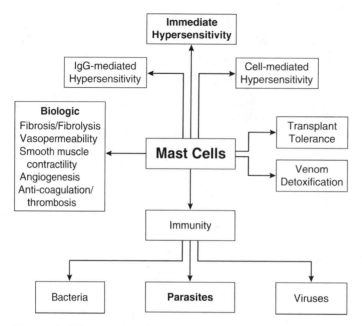

Figure 1 Effector roles of mast cells. Mast cells are the primary effector cells in immediate hypersensitivity reactions in both mice and humans but also participate in innate and acquired immunity, as demonstrated in mice, and exhibit a number of capabilities in vitro, which could be of biologic importance in vivo.

submucosa, conjunctiva, perivascular sites, and cardiac tissue, whereas MC_T cells are the predominant type found in the lung and in the small bowel mucosa.

Elegant studies in mice have indicated important roles for mast cells in the innate immune response against bacteria and in immune complex-mediated hypersensitivity disorders, including classical Arthus reactions. Whether mast cells in humans also extend their capabilities beyond immediate hypersensitivity reactions is uncertain. This chapter will focus on human mast cells and their relevance to urticaria and angioedema.

GROWTH AND DIFFERENTIATION OF MAST CELLS

Mast cells originate from hematopoietic progenitors, as outlined in Figure 2. A cell destined to reside in peripheral tissues as a mast cell will leave the bone marrow as a progenitor, probably with multipotential capabilities, enter a peripheral tissue still without secretory granules and cell surface FcεRI, and then complete its differentiation to a mast cell. Mast cell development and survival is regulated primarily by dimeric stem cell factor (SCF) (2–4), the ligand for Kit, the product of the c-*kit* proto-oncogene (5). SCF binding causes Kit to dimerize and express tyrosine kinase activity.

Various cytokines also influence mast cell development and survival. IL-3 in humans, unlike in rodents, has minimal influence on the differentiation of mast cells other than to expand the pool of hematopoietic progenitor cells (6). This is likely a consequence of mast cells from skin and lung being devoid of IL-3R (7), although it has been found on cord blood–derived (8,9) and intestinal (10) mast cells, where IL-3 partially protects against apoptosis due to SCF withdrawal and enhances degranulation and LTC_4 production (11). IL-9 can enhance the SCF-dependent growth of mast cell progenitors

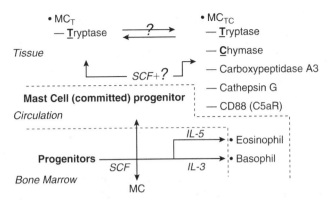

Figure 2 Differentiation of human mast cells. Hematopoietic progenitor cells give rise to both MC$_{TC}$ and MC$_T$ mast cells. Although SCF is critical for the development and survival of mast cells in the bone marrow and peripheral tissues, the factors involved in development of the MC$_{TC}$ and MC$_T$ cells remain to be determined. The most important factors for the development of eosinophils (IL-5) and basophils (IL-3) are different than for mast cells.

from human cord blood (12) but does not protect them from apoptosis due to SCF withdrawal (9). Cell–cell contact may play an important role in mast cell development, because mast developed from cord blood–derived progenitors co-cultured with bone marrow stromal cells in the presence of SCF and IL-6 yielded more mast cells, expressed higher levels of FcεRI, and released more histamine than did those developed in the absence of stromal cells (13).

Certain cytokines divert multipotential progenitors exposed to SCF to non–mast cell lineages. For example, both GM-CSF and IL-4 diminish SCF-dependent development of mast cells from progenitors in vitro but have little effect on more mature mast cells (14,15). The ability of IL-4 to downregulate expression of Kit may help explain the ability of this cytokine to attenuate mast cell development under some circumstances. However, IL-4 exhibits several effects on mast cells, including induction of surface FcεRI on in vitro derived mast cells (16,17), proliferation of intestinal mast cells (18), enhancement of cytokine and arachidonic acid product production of IL-6-stimulated cord blood–derived mast cells (11,19) and apoptosis of cord blood–derived mast cells in the absence of IL-6 (20). IL-33 accelerates the maturation of progenitors into tryptase[+] cells (21). Glucocorticosteroids inhibit mast cell development in vitro, but have minimal effects on mature mast cells. IL-6 also has pleiotropic effects on developing human mast cells that include blocking of IL-4-mediated apoptosis (20). Both IL-4 and IL-6 can enhance the maturation of mast cells expressing chymase (22,23).

Conditions that influence the selective development or recruitment of MC$_{TC}$ and MC$_T$ cells at specific tissue sites are not yet delineated. Of interest is the experimental observation that when intestinal mast cells attach to endothelial cells, the survival and proliferation of MC$_{TC}$ cells are selectively enhanced (24). The expression of CCR3, CCR5, CXCR1, CXCR2 and CXCR4 on cord blood–derived mast cells (25–27) and the CXCR4-dependent migration of these mast cells in response to stromal cell–derived factor-1α (SDF-1α) (28,29) suggest chemokine-dependent pathways for recruitment of mast cells or their progenitors. LTB$_4$, a chemotactic factor for neutrophils, recruits cord blood progenitors, but not cord blood–derived mast cells (30). The neurotransmitter serotonin also has been implicated in the chemotaxis of mast cells derived in vitro from peripheral blood progenitors (31).

Unlike other maturing myelocytes that stop expressing Kit, maturing mast cells express increasing amounts of Kit. Thus, SCF exerts various effects on mast cells throughout their development, including their differentiation, survival, recruitment, activation, and priming. Mice that genetically lack either Kit or SCF have profound mast cell deficiencies. Removal of SCF from cultured murine and human mast cells (32) results in apoptosis. Gain of function mutations in the kinase region of Kit (33) is associated with systemic mastocytosis, while gain of function mutations near the transmembrane region (that cause spontaneous dimerization) is associated with intestinal stromal cell tumors (34,35).

MC$_{TC}$ and MC$_T$ cells appear to be developmentally distinct types of human mast cells. In humans with inherited combined immunodeficiency disease and in those with acquired immunodeficiency syndrome, selective decreases in MC$_T$ cell concentrations occur in the bowel, whereas MC$_{TC}$ cell numbers there are unaffected (36). Lung MC$_T$ cells in culture with SCF and IL-6 fail to develop an MC$_{TC}$ phenotype (37). This suggests that MC$_{TC}$ cell development proceeds independently from that of MC$_T$ cells. Also, even though progenitors can become either an MC$_T$ or MC$_{TC}$ type of mast cell, commitment to a particular mast cell type in vivo appears to occur by the time granules begin to form because granules in immature MC$_T$ cells in tissues have scrolls and tryptase alone, while those in immature MC$_{TC}$ cells have electron dense cores and both tryptase and chymase (38). Once commitment occurs, interconversions between these types of mast cells have not yet been observed. Another distinguishing feature is the surface expression of CD88 (C5aR) on MC$_{TC}$ cells of skin and lung, but not MC$_T$ cells of lung (37).

ACTIVATION AND REGULATED SECRETION

Immunological activation of mast cells typically begins when IgE bound to the high-affinity Fcε receptor (FcεRI, Ka $= 10^9$ M^{-1}) is cross-linked by multivalent allergen (Fig. 3). The complete FcεRI receptor is composed of four subunits, $\alpha\beta\gamma_2$, which appear to float on the cell surface in lipid-based domains called rafts (39,40). The extracellular portion of the α chain binds IgE. The β chain with one immunoreceptor tyrosine activation motif (ITAM) and the two disulfide-linked γ chains, each with two ITAMs, are located primarily in the membrane and cytoplasmic regions. The γ chains also are present in CD16 (FcγRIII).

Regulated secretion by mast cells also may be induced by nonimmunologic agonists. Multivalent lectins, like bivalent concanavalin A, cross-link membrane FcεRI, or IgE. Calcium ionophores activate by translocating calcium. Various neuropeptides such as substance P, vasoactive intestinal peptide, somatostatin, calcitonin gene–related protein, p23 (41), and α-melanocyte-stimulating hormone (42) activate mast cells. Several basic biomolecules such as Compound 48/80, C5a, C3a (43), morphine, codeine, mellitin, and eosinophil-derived major basic protein activate human MC$_{TC}$ cells derived from skin but appear to be inactive against lung mast cells, unless (at least for C5a) the small portion of lung MC$_{TC}$ cells is purified (37). Mast cells from heart respond to atrial natriuretic peptide (44) and C5a, but not to substance P (45). Differences in the secretory response between mast cells isolated from different tissues may relate to micro-environmental influences or to the type of mast cell. Immunologic activation of lung mast cells can be enhanced by adenosine (46), possibly through the adenosine A2b receptor in humans (47). ATP also can enhance mediator release from human lung mast cells (48) by binding to P2Y surface purinoreceptors. IL-4-primed cord blood–derived mast cells express CysLT1, a receptor for sulfidopeptide leukotrienes, and can be

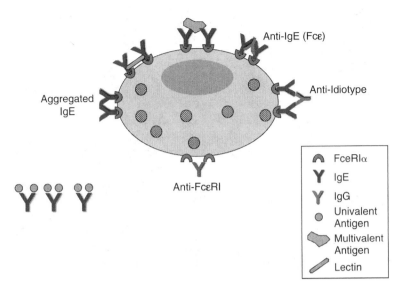

Figure 3 FcεRI-mediated activation of mast cells. Classic IgE-mediated immediate hypersensitivity is represented by multivalent antigen aggregating surface FcεRI by binding to antigen-specific IgE on the surface of mast cells. IgG anti-IgE and anti-FcεRI antibodies can also activate mast cells by aggregating surface FcεRI, as seen in autoimmune chronic urticaria. Aggregated IgE and certain lectins can also activate mast cells by cross-linking FcεRI. On the other hand, univalent allergens fail to activate mast cells, because they do not aggregate FcεRI.

activated by LTC_4 to secrete cytokines without releasing histamine or PGD_2 (49,50). CysLT2, also expressed on cord blood–derived mast cells, seems to downregulate CysLT1 mediated mast cell activation (51).

Pharmacologic responsiveness of mast cells also varies depending on the tissue source. Disodium cromoglycate and nedocromil, each used for the treatment of allergic asthma, rhinitis, and conjunctivitis at high concentrations are weak inhibitors of lung-derived mast cells and do not inhibit those from skin and intestine. β-Adrenoceptor agonists, at concentrations theoretically though transiently achievable on the airway surface with inhaled medication, produce modest inhibition of IgE-dependent histamine release in vitro from dispersed human lung mast cells, and somewhat greater inhibition of LTC_4 and PGD_2 generation. Cyclosporin A, FK-506, and pimecrolimus (52) produce rapid and long-lasting inhibition of IgE-dependent histamine release from human skin- and lung-derived mast cells. Dexamethasone in vitro inhibits cytokine production by lung and cord blood–derived mast cells (37,53,54), but does not inhibit degranulation or production of LTC_4 and PGD_2 from mast cells obtained from human skin, lung, and intestine (55). In vivo, glucocorticosteroids applied topically to the nasal mucosa for several days diminishes mediator release during the early response to a nasal allergen challenge, perhaps because of the capacity for local steroids to reduce mast cell concentrations by suppressing production of SCF (56).

Mast cells undergo regulated exocytosis when FcεRI ($\alpha\beta\gamma_2$) is aggregated on the cell surface by multivalent antigen or anti-receptor antibody. Subsequently, ITAMs on β and γ chains are phosphorylated by associated Src-family protein tyrosine kinases (PTKs) such as Lyn. Fyn also may play an important role in human mast cell activation (57). After FcεRIγ ITAMs have been phosphorylated, they bind and activate Syk tyrosine kinase. This results in downstream signaling events that involved PLCγ, MAP kinase, protein kinase C, and PI-3 kinase. The early events of mast cell activation also are regulated by signal regulatory proteins that contain immunotyrosine inhibition motifs (ITIMs), which act in part by recruiting SH2-bearing protein tyrosine phosphatases (SHP-1 and -2) that dephosphorylate ITAMs on FcεRI-β and -γ, thereby downregulating signal transduction and mediator release (58,59). In contrast, CD45, another protein tyrosine phosphatase, promotes mediator release (60).

Mast cells can also be activated through their pattern recognition receptors, which detect microbial-derived molecules. Among them are mammalian toll-like receptors (TLRs). A total of 11 TLRs have been reported. Bone marrow–derived murine mast cells degranulate and produce cytokines in response to bacterial peptidoglycan via TLR2 (61), while only cytokine production was noticed when they were activated by lipopolysaccharide via TLR4 (62). In addition, murine fetal skin-derived mast cells express functional TLR3, TLR7, and TLR9, which when engaged by ligands, lead to cytokine and chemokine production (63). Human in vitro–derived mast cells express TLRs 1–7, which when occupied by ligands, leads to production of cytokines without degranulation (64).

Human mast cells at rest do not express FcγRI and RIII receptors (65). However, MC_{TC} cells from skin express functional FcγRIIa, aggregation of which leads to degranulation and production of cytokines, PGD_2 and LTC_4 (66). These cells do not express inhibitory FcγRIIb. Treatment with IFN-γ induces the transient expression of FcεRI, which when aggregated also causes mast cells to release histamine, cytokines, PGD_2 and LTC_4 (67,68). These findings suggest human mast cells can be involved in IgG-dependent immune responses and hypersensitivity.

MEDIATORS

Mediators secreted by activated mast cells can be divided into those stored in secretory granules prior to cell activation and those that are newly generated after an activation signal. The former include histamine, proteoglycans, and proteases; the latter include lipid metabolites, cytokines, and chemokines, as summarized in Figure 4.

Biogenic Amine(S)

Histamine is the principal if not sole biogenic amine in human mast cells and basophils and is likely the most important mediator involved in urticaria. Histamine (β-imidazolylethylamine) is formed from histidine by histidine decarboxylase. In mast cells and basophils, histamine is then stored in secretory granules. It is the only preformed mediator of human mast cells with direct potent vasoactive and smooth muscle spasmogenic effects. With degranulation, histamine is released and diffuses rapidly. Extracellular histamine is metabolized within minutes of release, suggesting that it is destined to act quickly and locally. Human mast cells contain 1 to 3 pg of histamine per cell. Histamine concentrations in human plasma are about 1 to 10 nM.

Histamine exerts its biologic and pathobiologic effects through its interaction with cell specific G protein–coupled receptors designated H1, H2, H3, and H4 (69). H1 receptors (H1R) are blocked by chlorpheniramine; H2R by cimetidine; and H3R and H4R by thioperamide. Receptor specific agonists include 2-methylhistamine (H1R), dimaprit (H2R), α-methylhistamine (H3R), and clobenpropit (H4R).

H1R mediate enhanced permeability of postcapillary venules, arteriolar vasodilation, contraction of bronchial, and gastrointestinal smooth muscle, pruritus, and increased mucus secretion at mucosal sites. Increased vasopermeability will facilitate the

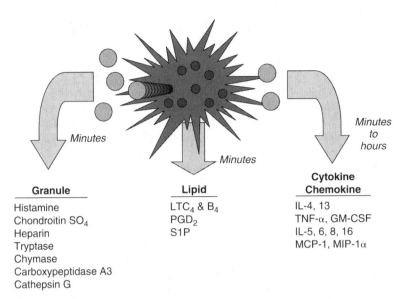

Granule	**Lipid**	**Cytokine Chemokine**
Histamine	LTC$_4$ & B$_4$	IL-4, 13
Chondroitin SO$_4$	PGD$_2$	TNF-α, GM-CSF
Heparin	S1P	IL-5, 6, 8, 16
Tryptase		MCP-1, MIP-1α
Chymase		
Carboxypeptidase A3		
Cathepsin G		

Figure 4 Mediators of activated mast cells. Mast cells release preformed granule and newly-generated lipid mediators within 15 minutes after they are activated, while most cytokines are synthesized and released 4 to 24 hours later. Chymase, cathepsin G, and carboxypeptidase A3 are components of the MC$_{TC}$ type of mast cell. Lung MC$_{TC}$ and MC$_T$ cells produce LTC$_4$ when activated by FcϵRI cross-linking, whereas skin MC$_{TC}$ cells produce little if any of this mediator. Mast cells also produce large amounts of IL-13, but little if any IL-4. TNF-α can be stored in secretory granules and released upon degranulation, but is also newly generated and released with other cytokines.

tissue deposition of factors from plasma that may be important for tissue growth and repair and of foreign material or immune complexes that result in tissue inflammation. H1R-mediated enhancement of P-selectin surface expression by endothelial cells facilitates the recruitment of leukocytes. H1R$^{-/-}$ mice exhibit modest neurologic alterations, but show no developmental abnormalities (70). H2R agonists stimulate gastric acid secretion by parietal cells and inhibit mediator secretion by various leukocytes, enhance epithelial permeability across human airways, stimulate chemokinesis of neutrophils and eosinophils and expression of eosinophil C3b receptors, and activate endothelial cells to release a potent inhibitor of platelet aggregation, PGI$_2$ (prostacyclin). H1R are preferentially expressed on helper T (Th1) cells and stimulate this type of helper T cell, while H2R are preferentially expressed on Th2 cells and inhibit this cell type. H1R$^{-/-}$ mice show a reduced Th1 response and enhanced Th2 response, while H2R$^{-/-}$ mice show increased Th1 and Th2 responses (71). Whether antihistamines used by humans affect their immune response in vivo in a similar manner remains to be determined. Stimulation of H3R affects neurotransmitter release and histamine formation in the central and peripheral nervous system. They are postulated to be involved in cross talk between mast cells and peripheral nerves. Bronchial hyperreactivity in atopics with asthma to irritant stimuli may in part be mediated by histamine-mediated neurogenic hyperexcitability. H4R has been identified on hematopoietic cells and peripheral nerves (72,73). Mast cells express H1R, H2R, and H4R, but not H3R. H4R can directly mediate chemotaxis of mast cells (74) or enhance their migration to CXCL12 (75), indicating the possibility of paracrine recruitment. In animal studies, pharmacological antagonists specific for the H4R have demonstrated their ability to modulate acute inflammation, hapten-mediated colitis, pruritus, and allergic airway inflammation (76,77).

The combined H1R and H2R responses are required for the full expression of histamine vasoactivity. Intradermal injection of histamine causes the "triple response", namely central erythema within seconds (arteriolar vasodilation) is followed by a circumferential erythematous flare (axon reflex vasodilation mediated by neuropeptides) and a central wheal (histamine vasopermeability, edema) that peaks at about 15 minutes. Although the reaction is mostly blocked by H1R antagonists, it is completely blocked only with a combination of H1R and H2R antagonists (78). Analogous results have been observed for the tachycardia, widened pulse pressure, diastolic hypotension, flushing, and headaches resulting from intravenous infusion of histamine (79). Addition of a putative H4R antagonist may be useful for controlling the pruritus of urticaria.

Proteoglycans

The presence of highly sulfated proteoglycans in secretory granules of mast cells and basophils results in metachromasia when these cells are stained with basic dyes. Proteoglycans are composed of glycosaminoglycan side chains (repeating unbranched disaccharide units of uronic acid and hexosamine moieties that are variably sulfated) covalently linked to a single-chain protein core via a specific trisaccharide-protein linkage region consisting of -Gal-Gal-Xyl-Ser. The intracellular proteoglycans of concern to mast cells are *heparin* and *chondroitin sulfate E*, which on average contain 2.5 and 1.5 sulfate residues per disaccharide, respectively. Heparin glycosaminoglycan is selectively expressed by mast cells and is attached to a serglycin peptide core (80). Heparin resides in the secretory granules of all mature mast cells (81) and is exocytosed along with other granule constituents in a complex with positively charged proteases.

The biologic functions of endogenous mast cell proteoglycans include maturation and morphology of secretory granules (57,82–86), and maturation and stabilization of the active form of tryptase (87–89). Heparin and chondroitin sulfate E (to a lesser extent) also have anticoagulant, anticomplement, antikallikrein, and Factor XII activation abilities, at least in vitro. Heparin neutralizes the ability of eosinophil-derived major basic protein to kill schistosomula and enhances the binding of fibronectin to collagen. Heparin protects and facilitates basic fibroblast growth factor activity, which appears to reside in cutaneous mast cells (90) and modulates the cell adhesion properties of matrix proteins. Binding of heparin to L- and P-selectins inhibits inflammation (91), perhaps by blocking leukocyte rolling.

Proteases

Proteases are enzymes that cleave peptide bonds, and certain ones are the dominant protein components of secretory granules in human and rodent mast cells. Some of these enzymes serve as selective markers that distinguish mast cells from other cell types, including basophils, and different mast cell subpopulations from one another. Basophils, compared with mast cells, are deficient in secretory granule protease activity.

Tryptase

Trypsin-like activity was first associated with human mast cells in 1960 (92) and was biochemically characterized and named tryptase in 1981 (93,94). The granule-associated tetrameric enzyme was stabilized by heparin (95). The crystal structure of human β-tryptase precisely defined this tetrameric structure, including the heparin-binding grooves (96,97). All active sites faced into the small, central pore of the planar tetramer, thereby restricting inhibitor (and substrate) access. The crystal structure of human recombinant α-tryptase was solved in 2002, showing a blocked substrate-binding region, which may explain why α-tryptase is proteolytically inactive (98).

Two genes encoding α and β tryptases are clustered on the short arm of human chromosome 16; one gene, named TPSB, is monomorphic for β-tryptase, while the other gene, named TPSAB, is dimorphic and encodes either α or β tryptase (99–101). Each encodes 30 amino acid leader and 245 amino acid catalytic sequences. These α and β tryptases are ∼90% identical by amino acid to one another. Tryptase genotypes exhibit 2:2 (βα/βα), 3:1 (ββ/βα) or 4:0 (ββ/ββ) molar ratios in approximately 25%, 50%, or 25% of individuals, respectively (102,103). A third closely related gene, δ-tryptase, encodes a mRNA for which translation terminates 40 amino acids earlier than α- and β-tryptases, also may be expressed by human mast cells (104), though precise quantitation has not yet been performed. Other trypsin-like enzymes called tryptase are not closely related to the α- and β-mast cell tryptases.

β-Protryptase is processed in two proteolytic steps, pro to pro' by heparin-dependent autocatalysis at acidic pH, and pro' to mature by a dipeptidyl peptidase at acidic pH. The mature peptide then spontaneously forms enzymatically-active tetramers at acidic pH in the presence of heparin (89,105). In contrast, α-protryptase does not undergo autocatalytic processing, and may remain as an inactive proenzyme. α- and β- Protryptases that are not processed to a mature form are spontaneously secreted by human mast cells in vitro and presumably in vivo (106).

The quantity of catalytically active tryptase per mast cell (10–35 pg) (107) is extraordinarily high. What regulates tryptase activity after its release into the extracellular milieu is uncertain, because the enzyme is resistant to classical biologic inhibitors of serine proteases (108). At neutral pH, basic proteins such as antithrombin III can destabilize β-tryptase by displacing it from heparin (108), resulting in the formation of inactive monomers. Inactive monomers at acidic pH, in the presence of heparin, regain activity (87,88). Another related observation is that β-tryptase degrades fibrinogen ∼50-fold faster at pH 6 than at 7.4 (109). Release of β-tryptase at sites of acidic pH (airway mucosal surface, foci of inflammation, and areas of poor vascularity, e.g., solid tumor margins and wound healing sites), might be optimal for the enzyme, while diffusion away from such sites would result in reduced proteolytic activity. Such a mechanism would tend to limit the activity of β-tryptase to its local tissue site of release.

The biologic activities of enzymatically-active tryptase are not obvious from the involvement of mast cells in atopic diseases. On the basis of its activities in vitro, biologic outcomes might include anticoagulation, fibrosis or fibrolysis, kinin generation or kininogen destruction, cell surface PAR-2 activation, and enhancement of vasopermeability, angiogenesis, inflammation, and airway smooth muscle hyperreactivity. Showing the importance of these potential activities in vivo remains a challenge. Studies on mice showed that the numbers of neutrophils increased >100-fold when enzymatically active β-tryptase was instilled into the lungs (110).

Tryptase also has been used as a clinical biomarker, particularly for systemic anaphylaxis and systemic mastocytosis (111). Mature β-tryptase is stored in secretory granules from where it is released by degranulation from activated mast cells. Mature tryptase can be measured by a specific ELISA. Accordingly, mature tryptase levels in serum or plasma are undetectable for healthy subjects (<1 ng/mL), but rise in those with insect sting–induced systemic anaphylaxis according to the clinical severity (hypotension)

Table 1 Characteristics of Immunoassays for Different Forms of Human Tryptase Measured in Serum

Clinical condition	Mature tryptase (ng/mL)	Total tryptase (ng/mL)	Total/mature tryptase ratio
Normal	<1	1–15	Not applicable
Systemic anaphylaxis (within 4 h of onset)	≥1	increased above baseline	≤10
Systemic mastocytosis (nonacute interval)	<1 to low	≥20	≥20 (when mature tryptase is measurable)

(Table 1). Levels of mature tryptase begin to rise within minutes of clinical symptoms, peak approximately one hour after onset and then decline with a half-time of about two hours. In the absence of hypotension, elevated mature tryptase levels are not usually observed. For comparison, histamine levels peak 5 to 10 minutes after onset and then decline with a half-time of 1 to 2 minutes. Also of interest is the observation that anaphylaxis induced by ingestion of foods does not usually result in an elevated level of mature tryptase, suggesting that the pathogenesis of food-induced anaphylaxis may be different than anaphylaxis induced by other stimuli.

Protryptases (α and β) are constitutively released by mast cells at rest. These tryptase precursors can be detected in serum or plasma by an ELISA, which measures all forms of tryptase (mature and pro), referred to as total tryptase. Total tryptase levels in serum from healthy subjects average $\sim$5 ng/mL (1–15 ng/mL range) (Table 1). Individuals with systemic mastocytosis typically have a total tryptase level >20 ng/mL without an elevated level of mature tryptase when their disease is otherwise quiescent, which reflects the increased burden of mast cells. Other conditions associated with an elevated total tryptase level in the absence of an elevated mature tryptase include acute myelogenous leukemia, hypereosinophilic syndrome associated with the FIP1L1-PDGFRA mutation, end-stage renal failure, certain myelodysplastic conditions and refractory anemia, and iatrogenic administration of SCF. Cytoreductive therapy in conditions associated with elevated total tryptase levels can be monitored by following these levels. Interestingly, neither total nor mature tryptase levels are elevated in urticaria (112), unless urticaria is associated with systemic mastocytosis or systemic anaphylaxis. This is consistent with their being modest to no increases in mast cell numbers in cutaneous urticarial lesions (113,114).

Chymase

Chymase, located on human chromosome 14, is one of two principal enzymes accounting for the chymotrypsin-like activity present in human cutaneous mast cells (115,116). Chymase was selectively localized to a subpopulation of mast cells named MC_{TC} cells (1,117). Neither chymotrypsin-like enzymatic activity nor chymase mRNA was detected in lung-derived MC_T cells (118). Dispersed skin-derived MC_{TC} cells contain $\sim$4.5 pg of chymase/mast cell.

Human chymase is a monomer of 30,000 Da whose crystal structure has been solved (119). Similar to tryptase, chymase is a serine esterase that is stored fully active in mast cell secretory granules, presumably bound to proteoglycan. Heparin facilitates processing of prochymase to active chymase by dipeptidyl peptidase I (120), and also modulates substrate accessibility (121). Unlike tryptase, chymase stability is not substantially affected by heparin and its proteolytic activity is inhibited by biologic inhibitors of serine proteinases, such as α_1-antichymotrypsin, α_1-proteinase inhibitor, and α_2-macroglobulin (122). Potential biologic activities of chymase, like those of tryptase, are based on *in vitro* observations. Chymase is a potent activator of angiotensin I, inactivates PAR-1 receptors, stimulates mucus production and leukocyte recruitment, processes procollagen to collagen fibrils, attacks the lamina lucida of the basement membrane at the dermal-epidermal junction of human skin, and degrades growth factors and cytokines such as Kit, pro-IL-18, IL-6, and IL-13 (123–125).

Cathepsin G

Human mast cell cathepsin G, like chymase, is a serine-class neutral protease with chymotryptic substrate specificity that is found in mast cells as well as in neutrophils and monocytes. Its crystal structure shows a similar polypeptide fold to that of rat mast cell proteinase II (126). The enzyme resides with chymase in MC_{TC} cells (127) and exhibits a molecular weight of 30,000. Its proteolytic activity is controlled by serine proteinase inhibitors, α1-antichymotrypsin in particular (128). Cathepsin G cleaves connective tissue and plasma proteins and exhibits modest microbicidal activities and may act in concert with other proteases, such as neutrophil elastase and proteinase 3 (129). Like chymase, it stimulates glandular secretions (130) of possible importance in allergic asthma and rhinitis.

Mast Cell Carboxypeptidase

Human mast cell carboxypeptidase A3, a zinc-dependent exopeptidase, resides with chymase and cathepsin G in secretory granules of MC_{TC} cells (131). Stored fully active, when released, it cleaves the carboxy terminal His^9–Leu^{10} bond of angiotensin I. Human mast cells dispersed from skin contain 5 to 16 pg of carboxypeptidase A3 per cell. Human mast cell carboxypeptidase A3 is a monomer with a molecular weight of 34,500 (132) and substrate specificity for carboxy terminal Phe and Leu residues. Murine bone marrow–derived mast cells showed abnormality in maturation and morphology in the absence of carboxypeptidase A (133). Carboxypeptidase A3, in cooperation with chymase, is also involved in the formation and degradation of angiotensin II (134). Carboxypeptidase A3 also inactivates endogenous endothelin as well as exogenous snake and honeybee venoms (135,136).

Other Proteases and Enzymes

Tissue-type plasminogen activator has been identified in tissue-derived mast cells (137), potentially complementing mast cell antithrombotic and anticoagulant activities with the fibrinolytic properties of this protease. Matrix metalloproteinase-9, a gelatinase, has been identified in cord blood–derived mast cells (138). Mast cells also concentrate various acid hydrolases in their secretory granules, perhaps reflecting the lysosomal origin of this organelle, including β-galactosidase, aryl sulfatase, and β-hexosaminidase, the latter enzyme serving as a marker for degranulation of purified mast cells in vitro (94). Mast cells from human lung tissue and HMC-1 cells reportedly express rennin, which generates angiotensin I from angiotensinogen (139,140). Mast cells also express small amounts of granzyme B in response to FcϵRI-mediated cell activation (141,142).

Lipids

Metabolites of Arachidonic Acid

Human mast cells dispersed and purified from lung incorporate exogenous arachidonic acid into neutral lipids and phospholipids and store these lipids in membranes and cytoplasmic lipid bodies. Liberation of the arachidonic acid destined for oxidative metabolism is dependent upon cytosolic phospholipase A_2 (143). In general, oxidation of arachidonic acid occurs through the cyclooxygenase (Cox) pathways to prostaglandins (PGs) and thromboxanes (TXs), or the 5-, 12-, or 15-lipoxygenase (LO) pathways to monohydroxyl fatty acids, leukotrienes (LTs) that include both LTB_4 and the sulfidopeptides LTC_4, LTD_4, and LTE_4 (*slow reacting substances of anaphylaxis, SRS-A*), and lipoxins. Platelet activating factor is made by acetylating the lysophospholipid remaining after arachidonic acid departs and appears to be a major secretory product of basophils in mice (144) and rabbits (145), but probably not of basophils and mast cells in humans (146,147).

Dispersed and purified preparations of human mast cells obtained from lung, skin, and intestine, upon activation, produce PGD_2 (PGD synthase-dependent). LTC_4 (LTC synthase-dependent) is preferentially produced by lung-derived rather than skin-derived mast cells. LTB_4, a less-abundant product of mast cells, chemoattracts neutrophils as well as progenitors capable of becoming mast cells (30). Also, both leukotriene and prostaglandin production by activated mast cells can be blocked or augmented independently of the release of granule mediators and cytokines.

The biologic importance of mast cell–derived products of arachidonic acid gained support with the advent of inhibitors of 5-lipoxygenase and the CysLT1 receptor (148) for LTD_4, both of which are helpful in atopic and in aspirin-induced asthma (149), each condition also involving activation of mast cells and eosinophils. The importance of PGD_2 production in anaphylaxis was suggested when administration of aspirin inhibited generation of a urinary PGD_2 metabolite in mastocytosis patients with recurrent hypotensive episodes and led to their clinical improvement (150). However, prostaglandin and leukotriene inhibitors exhibit minimal consistent benefit in urticaria.

Metabolite of Sphingosine

Sphingosine-1-phosphate (S1P) is a newly appreciated lipid mediator that is both produced by mast cells and affects mast cell activation and recruitment. S1P is formed from sphingosine and ATP by the action of sphingosine kinases. S1P is produced and secreted by activated mast cells and also acts on mast cells to enhance degranulation through binding to its S1P2 receptor and to enhance recruitment by binding to its S1P1 receptor, both of which are expressed on mast cells (151,152). In mice, S1P levels in the circulation affect the severity of IgE-mediated anaphylaxis (153).

Cytokines and Chemokines

Human mast cells, when activated, produce a diverse array of cytokines and chemokines. These include TNF-α, ILs 3, 4, 5, 6, 8, 10, 13, and 16, lymphotactin, GM-CSF, MCP-1, TGF-β1, MIP-1α (124), and nerve growth factor (154). IL-25 is expressed by murine bone marrow–derived mast cells (155). Cytokines are typically newly generated, being released hours after mast cells are activated. However, in some cases, e.g. TNF-α and IL-8 (156), cytokines also may be stored in secretory granules and released with other preformed mediators. When mast cells reside in secondary lymphoid tissue, these cytokines might influence immunity, and while in tissues, they may serve to recruit and activate other cell types, thereby amplifying and extending the host response during immediate hypersensitivity events.

MAST CELLS IN URTICARIA

Mast cells are a key effector cell in both chronic and acute urticaria. Although classically activated by multivalent allergens, the recognition that cell activation may be caused by or augmented by neuropeptides, autoimmune IgG antibodies against IgE or FcεRIα (157,158), local generation of complement anaphylatoxins (159,160), by IgG immune complexes (66), and by the surface level of FcεRI (161) have enhanced our understanding of the complexity of different presentations of urticaria. For example, the presence of receptors for complement anaphylatoxins on the surface of MC_{TC} (dominant in skin) but not MC_T (dominant in lung) cells (157,158) provides a rationale explanation to why chronic urticaria caused by autoimmune IgG anti-FcεRIα antibodies results in hives without wheezing. Autoimmune IgG levels by themselves may not be sufficient to activate mast cells in vivo but do so together with C5a/C3a that is generated on the surface of mast cells that are decorated with this IgG (159,160). The emerging efficacy of omalizumab (neutralizing IgG anti-IgE monoclonal antibody) in the treatment of chronic urticaria (162) may relate to the decline in FcεRI levels on the surface of mast cells that occurs when free IgE levels are reduced (161). Low levels of surface FcεRI are associated with a shift in the concentration of anti-FcεRI antibody needed to activate mast cells to a higher level. The expression of activating FcγRIIA receptors on the surface of skin MC_{TC} cells (66) may explain why urticaria sometimes occurs in association with autoimmune disorders such as systemic lupus erythematosus and thyroiditis or with an immune response to various infections, conditions in which IgG immune complexes are observed. Finally, the ability of mast cells dispersed from the lung (both MC_T and MC_{TC} types) but not the skin MC_{TC} cells to secrete LTC_4 after aggregation of cell surface FcεRI (37) may explain why leukotriene antagonists are generally ineffective as a therapeutic in chronic urticaria (163). However, modest efficacy of a leukotriene antagonist in a subgroup of chronic urticaria patients with positive skin tests to autologous serum (163) might relate to the ability of skin MC_{TC} cells to secrete LTC_4 when the cells are activated through FcγRIIA receptors (37). Thus, a better understanding of human mast cells will likely improve our understanding of the pathogenesis of urticaria and offer new therapeutic options.

REFERENCES

1. Irani AA, Schechter NM, Craig SS, et al. Two types of human mast cells that have distinct neutral protease compositions. Proc Natl Acad Sci U S A 1986; 83(12):4464–4468.
2. Irani AM, Nilsson G, Miettinen U, et al. Recombinant human stem cell factor stimulates differentiation of mast cells from dispersed human fetal liver cells. Blood 1992; 80(12): 3009–3021.
3. Mitsui H, Furitsu T, Dvorak AM, et al. Development of human mast cells from umbilical cord blood cells by recombinant human and murine c-kit ligand. Proc Natl Acad Sci U S A 1993; 90(2):735–739.
4. Kirshenbaum AS, Goff JP, Kessler SW, et al. Effect of IL-3 and stem cell factor on the appearance of human basophils and mast cells from $CD34^+$ pluripotent progenitor cells. J Immunol 1992; 148:772–777.
5. Zhang Z, Zhang R, Joachimiak A, et al. Crystal structure of human stem cell factor: implication for stem cell factor receptor dimerization and activation. Proc Natl Acad Sci U S A 2000; 97(14):7732–7737.
6. Shimizu Y, Matsumoto K, Okayama Y, et al. Interleukin-3 does not affect the differentiation of mast cells derived from human bone marrow progenitors. Immunol Invest 2008; 37(1):1–17.

7. Valent P, Besemer J, Sillaber C, et al. Failure to detect IL-3-binding sites on human mast cells. J Immunol 1990; 145:3432–3437.

8. Dahl C, Hoffmann HJ, Saito H, et al. Human mast cells express receptors for IL-3, IL-5 and GM-CSF; a partial map of receptors on human mast cells cultured in vitro. Allergy 2004; 59(10): 1087–1096.

9. Yanagida M, Fukamachi H, Ohgami K, et al. Effects of T-helper 2-type cytokines, interleukin-3 (IL- 3), IL-4, IL-5, and IL-6 on the survival of cultured human mast cells. Blood 1995; 86: 3705–3714.

10. Gebhardt T, Sellge G, Lorentz A, et al. Cultured human intestinal mast cells express functional IL-3 receptors and respond to IL-3 by enhancing growth and IgE receptor-dependent mediator release. Eur J Immunol 2002; 32(8):2308–2316.

11. Hsieh FH, Lam BK, Penrose JF, et al. T helper cell type 2 cytokines coordinately regulate immunoglobulin E- dependent cysteinyl leukotriene production by human cord blood-derived mast cells: profound induction of leukotriene C(4) synthase expression by interleukin 4. J Exp Med 2001; 193(1):123–133.

12. Matsuzawa S, Sakashita K, Kinoshita T, et al. IL-9 enhances the growth of human mast cell progenitors under stimulation with stem cell factor. J Immunol 2003; 170(7):3461–3467.

13. Yamaguchi M, Azuma H, Fujihara M, et al. Generation of a considerable number of functional mast cells with a high basal level of FcepsilonRI expression from cord blood CD34+ cells by co-culturing them with bone marrow stromal cell line under serum-free conditions. Scand J Immunol 2007; 65(6):581–588.

14. Du Z, Li Y, Xia H, et al. Recombinant human granulocyte-macrophage colony-stimulating factor (CSF), but not recombinant human granulocyte CSF, downregulates the recombinant human stem cell factor-dependent differentiation of human fetal liver-derived mast cells. J Immunol 1997; 159(2):838–845.

15. Welker P, Grabbe J, Zuberbier T, et al. GM-CSF downmodulates c-kit, Fc(epsilon)RI(alpha) and GM-CSF receptor expression as well as histamine and tryptase levels in cultured human mast cells. Arch Dermatol Res 2001; 293(5):249–258.

16. Xia HZ, Du Z, Craig S, et al. Effect of recombinant human IL-4 on tryptase, chymase, and Fc epsilon receptor type I expression in recombinant human stem cell factor- dependent fetal liver-derived human mast cells. J Immunol 1997; 159(6):2911–2921.

17. Yamaguchi M, Sayama K, Yano K, et al. IgE enhances Fc epsilon receptor I expression and IgE-dependent release of histamine and lipid mediators from human umbilical cord blood-derived mast cells: synergistic effect of IL-4 and IgE on human mast cell Fc epsilon receptor I expression and mediator release. J Immunol 1999; 162(9):5455–5465.

18. Bischoff SC, Sellge G, Lorentz A, et al. IL-4 enhances proliferation and mediator release in mature human mast cells. Proc Natl Acad Sci U S A 1999; 96(14):8080–8085.

19. Ochi H, De Jesus NH, Hsieh FH, et al. IL-4 and -5 prime human mast cells for different profiles of IgE- dependent cytokine production. Proc Natl Acad Sci U S A 2000; 97(19): 10509–10513.

20. Oskeritzian CA, Wang Z, Kochan JP, et al. Recombinant human (rh)IL-4-mediated apoptosis and recombinant human IL- 6-mediated protection of recombinant human stem cell factor-dependent human mast cells derived from cord blood mononuclear cell progenitors. J Immunol 1999; 163(9):5105–5115.

21. Allakhverdi Z, Smith DE, Comeau MR, et al. Cutting edge: The ST2 ligand IL-33 potently activates and drives maturation of human mast cells. J Immunol 2007; 179(4):2051–2054.

22. Kinoshita T, Sawai N, Hidaka E, et al. Interleukin-6 directly modulates stem cell factor-dependent development of human mast cells derived from CD34(+) cord blood cells. Blood 1999; 94(2):496–508.

23. Toru H, Eguchi M, Matsumoto R, et al. Interleukin-4 promotes the development of tryptase and chymase double-positive human mast cells accompanied by cell maturation. Blood 1998; 91(1):187–195.

24. Mierke CT, Ballmaier M, Werner U, et al. Human endothelial cells regulate survival and proliferation of human mast cells. J Exp Med 2000; 192(6):801–811.

25. Ochi H, Hirani WM, Yuan Q, et al. T helper cell type 2 cytokine-mediated comitogenic responses and CCR3 expression during differentiation of human mast cells in vitro. J Exp Med 1999; 190(2):267–280.

26. Nilsson G, Mikovits JA, Metcalfe DD, et al. Mast cell migratory response to interleukin-8 is mediated through interaction with chemokine receptor CXCR2/Interleukin-8RB. Blood 1999; 93(9):2791–2797.

27. Inamura H, Kurosawa M, Okano A, et al. Expression of the interleukin-8 receptors CXCR1 and CXCR2 on cord-blood-derived cultured human mast cells. Int Arch Allergy Immunol 2002; 128(2):142–150.

28. Juremalm M, Hjertson M, Olsson N, et al. The chemokine receptor CXCR4 is expressed within the mast cell lineage and its ligand stromal cell-derived factor-1alpha acts as a mast cell chemotaxin. Eur J Immunol 2000; 30(12):3614–3622.

29. Lin TJ, Issekutz TB, Marshall JS. SDF-1 induces IL-8 production and transendothelial migration of human cord blood-derived mast cells. Int Arch Allergy Immunol 2001; 124(1–3): 142–145.

30. Weller CL, Collington SJ, Brown JK, et al. Leukotriene B4, an activation product of mast cells, is a chemoattractant for their progenitors. J Exp Med 2005; 201(12):1961–1971.

31. Kushnir-Sukhov NM, Gilfillan AM, Coleman JW, et al. 5-hydroxytryptamine induces mast cell adhesion and migration. J Immunol 2006; 177(9):6422–6432.

32. Nilsson G, Miettinen U, Ishizaka T, et al. Interleukin-4 inhibits the expression of Kit and tryptase during stem cell factor-dependent development of human mast cells from fetal liver cells. Blood 1994; 84(5):1519–1527.

33. Nagata H, Worobec AS, Oh CK, et al. Identification of a point mutation in the catalytic domain of the protooncogene c-kit in peripheral blood mononuclear cells of patients who have mastocytosis with an associated hematologic disorder. Proc Natl Acad Sci U S A 1995; 92(23): 10560–10564.

34. Hirota S, Isozaki K, Moriyama Y, et al. Gain-of-function mutations of c-kit in human gastrointestinal stromal tumors. Science 1998; 279(5350):577–580.

35. Kitamura Y, Hirota S, Nishida T. A loss-of-function mutation of c-kit results in depletion of mast cells and interstitial cells of Cajal, while its gain-of-function mutation results in their oncogenesis. Mutat Res 2001; 477(1–2):165–171.

36. Irani AM, Craig SS, DeBlois G, et al. Deficiency of the tryptase-positive, chymase-negative mast cell type in gastrointestinal mucosa of patients with defective T lymphocyte function. J Immunol 1987; 138(12):4381–4386.

37. Oskeritzian CA, Zhao W, Min HK, et al. Surface CD88 functionally distinguishes the MCTC from the MCT type of human lung mast cell. J Allergy Clin Immunol 2005; 115(6): 1162–1168.

38. Craig SS, Schechter NM, Schwartz LB. Ultrastructural analysis of maturing human T and TC mast cells in situ. Lab Invest 1989; 60(1):147–157.

39. Baird B, Sheets ED, Holowka D. How does the plasma membrane participate in cellular signaling by receptors for immunoglobulin E? Biophys Chem 1999; 82(2–3):109–119.

40. Draber P, Draberova L. Lipid rafts in mast cell signaling. Mol Immunol 2002; 38(16–18): 1247–1252.

41. MacDonald SM, Rafnar T, Langdon J, et al. Molecular identification of an IgE-dependent histamine-releasing factor. Science 1995; 269(5224):688–690.

42. Grutzkau A, Henz BM, Kirchhof L, et al. alpha-Melanocyte stimulating hormone acts as a selective inducer of secretory functions in human mast cells. Biochem Biophys Res Commun 2000; 278(1):14–19.

43. Woolhiser MR, Brockow K, Metcalfe DD. Activation of human mast cells by aggregated IgG through FcgammaRI: additive effects of C3a. Clin Immunol 2004; 110(2):172–180.

44. Murray DB, Gardner JD, Levick SP, et al. Response of cardiac mast cells to atrial natriuretic peptide. Am J Physiol Heart Circ Physiol 2007; 293(2):H1216–H1222.

45. Sperr WR, Bankl HC, Mundigler G, et al. The human cardiac mast cell: localization, isolation, phenotype, and functional characterization. Blood 1994; 84(11):3876–3884.

46. Peachell PT, Lichtenstein LM, Schleimer RP. Differential regulation of human basophil and lung mast cell function by adenosine. J Pharmacol Exp Ther 1991; 256(2):717–726.

47. Feoktistov I, Biaggioni I. Pharmacological characterization of adenosine A2B receptors: studies in human mast cells co-expressing A2A and A2B adenosine receptor subtypes. Biochem Pharmacol 1998; 55(5):627–633.

48. Schulman ES, Glaum MC, Post T, et al. ATP modulates anti-IgE-induced release of histamine from human lung mast cells. Am J Respir Cell Mol Biol 1999; 20(3):530–537.

49. Mellor EA, Maekawa A, Austen KF, et al. Cysteinyl leukotriene receptor 1 is also a pyrimidinergic receptor and is expressed by human mast cells. Proc Natl Acad Sci U S A 2001; 98(14):7964–7969.

50. Mellor EA, Austen KF, Boyce JA. Cysteinyl leukotrienes and uridine diphosphate induce cytokine generation by human mast cells through an interleukin 4-regulated pathway that is inhibited by leukotriene receptor antagonists. J Exp Med 2002; 195(5):583–592.

51. Jiang Y, Borrelli LA, Kanaoka Y, et al. CysLT2 receptors interact with CysLT1 receptors and downmodulate cysteinyl leukotriene dependent mitogenic responses of mast cells. Blood 2008; 110:3263–3270.

52. Zuberbier T, Chong SU, Grunow K, et al. The ascomycin macrolactam pimecrolimus (Elidel, SDZ ASM 981) is a potent inhibitor of mediator release from human dermal mast cells and peripheral blood basophils. J Allergy Clin Immunol 2001; 108(2):275–280.

53. Fushimi T, Okayama H, Shimura S, et al. Dexamethasone suppresses gene expression and production of IL-13 by human mast cell line and lung mast cells. J Allergy Clin Immunol 1998; 102(1):134–142.

54. Smith SJ, Piliponsky AM, Rosenhead F, et al. Dexamethasone inhibits maturation, cytokine production and Fc epsilon RI expression of human cord blood-derived mast cells. Clin Exp Allergy 2002; 32(6):906–913.

55. Cohan VL, Undem BJ, Fox CC, et al. Dexamethasone does not inhibit the release of mediators from human mast cells residing in airway, intestine, or skin. Am Rev Respir Dis 1989; 140:951–954.

56. Finotto S, Mekori YA, Metcalfe DD. Glucocorticoids decrease tissue mast cell number by reducing the production of the c-kit ligand, stem cell factor, by resident cells - In vitro and in vivo evidence in murine systems. J Clin Invest 1997; 99(7):1721–1728.

57. Yamashita Y, Charles N, Furumoto Y, et al. Cutting edge: genetic variation influences Fc epsilonRI-induced mast cell activation and allergic responses. J Immunol 2007; 179(2):740–743.

58. Leung WH, Bolland S. The inositol 5'-phosphatase SHIP-2 negatively regulates IgE-induced mast cell degranulation and cytokine production. J Immunol 2007; 179(1):95–102.

59. Lienard H, Bruhns P, Malbec O, et al. Signal regulatory proteins negatively regulate immunoreceptor-dependent cell activation. J Biol Chem 1999; 274(45):32493–32499.

60. Berger SA, Mak TW, Paige CJ. Leukocyte common antigen (CD45) is required for immunoglobulin E-mediated degranulation of mast cells. J Exp Med 1994; 180(2):471–476.

61. Supajatura V, Ushio H, Nakao A, et al. Differential responses of mast cell Toll-like receptors 2 and 4 in allergy and innate immunity. J Clin Invest 2002; 109(10):1351–1359.

62. McCurdy JD, Lin TJ, Marshall JS. Toll-like receptor 4-mediated activation of murine mast cells. J Leukoc Biol 2001; 70(6):977–984.

63. Matsushima H, Yamada N, Matsue H, et al. TLR3-, TLR7-, and TLR9-mediated production of proinflammatory cytokines and chemokines from murine connective tissue type skin-derived mast cells but not from bone marrow-derived mast cells. J Immunol 2004; 173(1):531–541.

64. Kulka M, Alexopoulou L, Flavell RA, et al. Activation of mast cells by double-stranded RNA: evidence for activation through Toll-like receptor 3. J Allergy Clin Immunol 2004; 114 (1):174–182.

65. Okayama Y, Hagaman DD, Woolhiser M, et al. Further characterization of FcgammaRII and FcgammaRIII expression by cultured human mast cells. Int Arch Allergy Immunol 2001; 124 (1–3):155–157.

66. Zhao W, Kepley CL, Morel PA, et al. FcγRIIa, not FcγRIIb, is constitutively and functionally expressed on skin-derived human mast cells. J Immunol 2006; 177(1):694–701.

67. Okayama Y, Kirshenbaum AS, Metcalfe DD. Expression of a functional high-affinity IgG receptor, Fc gamma RI, on human mast cells: Up-regulation by IFN-gamma. J Immunol 2000; 164(8):4332–4339.

68. Okayama Y, Hagaman DD, Metcalfe DD. A comparison of mediators released or generated by IFN-gamma-treated human mast cells following aggregation of Fc gamma RI or Fc epsilon RI. J Immunol 2001; 166(7):4705–4712.

69. Schneider E, Rolli-Derkinderen M, Arock M, et al. Trends in histamine research: new functions during immune responses and hematopoiesis. Trends Immunol 2002; 23(5):255–263.

70. Inoue I, Yanai K, Kitamura D, et al. Impaired locomotor activity and exploratory behavior in mice lacking histamine H1 receptors. Proc Natl Acad Sci U S A 1996; 93(23):13316–13320.

71. Jutel M, Watanabe T, Klunker S, et al. Histamine regulates T-cell and antibody responses by differential expression of H1 and H2 receptors. Nature 2001; 413(6854):420–425.

72. Zhu Y, Michalovich D, Wu H, et al. Cloning, expression, and pharmacological characterization of a novel human histamine receptor. Mol Pharmacol 2001; 59(3):434–441.

73. Nakaya M, Takeuchi N, Kondo K. Immunohistochemical localization of histamine receptor subtypes in human inferior turbinates. Ann Otol Rhinol Laryngol 2004; 113(7):552–557.

74. Hofstra CL, Desai PJ, Thurmond RL, et al. Histamine H4 receptor mediates chemotaxis and calcium mobilization of mast cells. J Pharmacol Exp Ther 2003; 305(3):1212–1221.

75. Godot V, Arock M, Garcia G, et al. H4 histamine receptor mediates optimal migration of mast cell precursors to CXCL12. J Allergy Clin Immunol 2007; 120(4):827–834.

76. Zhang M, Thurmond RL, Dunford PJ. The histamine H(4) receptor: a novel modulator of inflammatory and immune disorders. Pharmacol Ther 2007; 113(3):594–606.

77. Huang JF, Thurmond RL. The new biology of histamine receptors. Curr Allergy Asthma Rep 2008; 8(1):21–27.

78. Davies MG, Greaves MW. Sensory responses of human skin to synthetic histamine analogues and histamine. Br J Clin Pharmacol 1980; 9(5):461–465.

79. Kaliner M, Shelhamer JH, Ottesen EA. Effects of infused histamine: correlation of plasma histamine levels and symptoms. J Allergy Clin Immunol 1982; 69(3):283–289.

80. Kolset SO, Prydz K, Pejler G. Intracellular proteoglycans. Biochem J 2004; 379(Pt 2): 217–227.

81. Craig SS, Irani AM, Metcalfe DD, et al. Ultrastructural localization of heparin to human mast cells of the MCTC and MCT types by labeling with antithrombin III-gold. Lab Invest 1993; 69(5): 552–561.

82. Braga T, Grujic M, Lukinius A, et al. Serglycin proteoglycan is required for secretory granule integrity in mucosal mast cells. Biochem J 2007; 403(1):49–57.

83. Abrink M, Grujic M, Pejler G. Serglycin is essential for maturation of mast cell secretory granule. J Biol Chem 2004; 279(39):40897–40905.

84. Ringvall M, Ronnberg E, Wernersson S, et al. Serotonin and histamine storage in mast cell secretory granules is dependent on serglycin proteoglycan. J Allergy Clin Immunol 2008.

85. Forsberg E, Pejler G, Ringvall M, et al. Abnormal mast cells in mice deficient in a heparin-synthesizing enzyme. Nature 1999; 400(6746):773–776.

86. Humphries DE, Wong GW, Friend DS, et al. Heparin is essential for the storage of specific granule proteases in mast cells. Nature 1999; 400(6746):769–772.

87. Fukuoka Y, Schwartz LB. Human beta-tryptase: detection and characterization of the active monomer and prevention of tetramer reconstitution by protease inhibitors. Biochemistry 2004; 43(33):10757–10764.

88. Ren S, Sakai K, Schwartz LB. Regulation of human mast cell beta-tryptase: conversion of inactive monomer to active tetramer at acid pH. J Immunol 1998; 160(9):4561–4569.

89. Sakai K, Ren S, Schwartz LB. A novel heparin-dependent processing pathway for human tryptase. Autocatalysis followed by activation with dipeptidyl peptidase I. J Clin Invest 1996; 97(4):988–995.

90. Reed JA, Albino AP, McNutt NS. Human cutaneous mast cells express basic fibroblast growth factor. Lab Invest 1995; 72(2):215–222.

91. Nelson RM, Cecconi O, Roberts WG, et al. Heparin oligosaccharides bind L- and P-selectin and inhibit acute inflammation. Blood 1993; 82(11):3253–3258.

92. Glenner GC, Cohen LA. Histochemical demonstration of species-specific trypsin-like enzyme in mast cell. Nature 1960; 185:846–847.

93. Schwartz LB, Lewis RA, Austen KF. Tryptase from human pulmonary mast cells. Purification and characterization. J Biol Chem 1981; 256(22):11939–11943.

94. Schwartz LB, Lewis RA, Seldin D, et al. Acid hydrolases and tryptase from secretory granules of dispersed human lung mast cells. J Immunol 1981; 126(4):1290–1294.

95. Schwartz LB, Bradford TR. Regulation of tryptase from human lung mast cells by heparin. Stabilization of the active tetramer. J Biol Chem 1986; 261(16):7372–7379.

96. Pereira PJ, Bergner A, Macedo-Ribeiro S, et al. Human beta-tryptase is a ring-like tetramer with active sites facing a central pore. Nature 1998; 392(6673):306–311.

97. Alter SC, Metcalfe DD, Bradford TR, et al. Regulation of human mast cell tryptase. Effects of enzyme concentration, ionic strength and the structure and negative charge density of polysaccharides. Biochem J 1987; 248(3):821–827.

98. Marquardt U, Zettl F, Huber R, et al. The crystal structure of human alpha1-tryptase reveals a blocked substrate-binding region. J Mol Biol 2002; 321(3):491–502.

99. Miller JS, Westin EH, Schwartz LB. Cloning and characterization of complementary DNA for human tryptase. J Clin Invest 1989; 84(4):1188–1195.

100. Miller JS, Moxley G, Schwartz LB. Cloning and characterization of a second complementary DNA for human tryptase. J Clin Invest 1990; 86(3):864–870.

101. Pallaoro M, Fejzo MS, Shayesteh L, et al. Characterization of genes encoding known and novel human mast cell tryptases on chromosome 16p13.3. J Biol Chem 1999; 274(6):3355–3362.

102. Min HK, Moxley G, Neale MC, et al. Effect of sex and haplotype on plasma tryptase levels in healthy adults. J Allergy Clin Immunol 2004; 114(1):48–51.

103. Soto D, Malmsten C, Blount JL, et al. Genetic deficiency of human mast cell a-tryptase. Clin Exp Allergy 2002; 32(7):1000–1006.

104. Wang HW, McNeil HP, Husain A, et al. Delta tryptase is expressed in multiple human tissues, and a recombinant form has proteolytic activity. J Immunol 2002; 169(9):5145–5152.

105. Sakai K, Long SD, Pettit DA, et al. Expression and purification of recombinant human tryptase in a baculovirus system. Protein Expr Purif 1996; 7(1):67–73.

106. Schwartz LB, Min HK, Ren S, et al. Tryptase precursors are preferentially and spontaneously released, whereas mature tryptase is retained by HMC-1 cells, Mono-Mac-6 Cells, and human skin-derived mast cells. J Immunol 2003; 170(11):5667–5673.

107. Schwartz LB, Irani AM, Roller K, et al. Quantitation of histamine, tryptase, and chymase in dispersed human T and TC mast cells. J Immunol 1987; 138(8):2611–2615.

108. Alter SC, Kramps JA, Janoff A, et al. Interactions of human mast cell tryptase with biological protease inhibitors. Arch Biochem Biophys 1990; 276(1):26–31.

109. Ren S, Lawson AE, Carr M, et al. Human tryptase fibrinogenolysis is optimal at acidic pH and generates anticoagulant fragments in the presence of the anti-tryptase monoclonal antibody B12. J Immunol 1997; 159(7):3540–3548.

110. Huang C, De Sanctis GT, O'Brien PJ, et al. Evaluation of the substrate specificity of human mast cell tryptase beta I and demonstration of its importance in bacterial infections of the lung. J Biol Chem 2001; 276(28):26276–26284.

111. Schwartz LB. Diagnostic value of tryptase in anaphylaxis and mastocytosis. Immunol Allergy Clin North Am 2006; 26(3):451–463.

112. Schwartz LB, Sakai K, Bradford TR, et al. The a form of human tryptase is the predominant type present in blood at baseline in normal subjects and is elevated in those with systemic mastocytosis. J Clin Invest 1995; 96:2702–2710.

113. Natbony SF, Phillips ME, Elias JM, et al. Histologic studies of chronic idiopathic urticaria. J Allergy Clin Immunol 1983; 71:177–183.

114. Smith CH, Kepley C, Schwartz LB, et al. Mast cell number and phenotype in chronic idiopathic urticaria. J Allergy Clin Immunol 1995; 96:360–364.

115. Schechter NM, Fraki JE, Geesin JC, et al. Human skin chymotryptic proteinase. Isolation and relation to cathepsin g and rat mast cell proteinase I. J Biol Chem 1983; 258(5):2973–2978.

116. Caughey GH, Zerweck EH, Vanderslice P. Structure, chromosomal assignment, and deduced amino acid sequence of a human gene for mast cell chymase. J Biol Chem 1991; 266(20): 12956–12963.

117. Osman IA, Garrett JR, Smith RE. Enzyme histochemical discrimination between tryptase and chymase in mast cells of human gut. J Histochem Cytochem 1989; 37(4):415–421.

118. Xia HZ, Kepley CL, Sakai K, et al. Quantitation of tryptase, chymase, Fc epsilon RI alpha, and Fc epsilon RI gamma mRNAs in human mast cells and basophils by competitive reverse transcription-polymerase chain reaction. J Immunol 1995; 154(10):5472–5480.

119. Pereira PJ, Wang ZM, Rubin H, et al. The 2.2 A crystal structure of human chymase in complex with succinyl-Ala-Ala-Pro-Phe-chloromethylketone: structural explanation for its dipeptidyl carboxypeptidase specificity. J Mol Biol 1999; 286(1):163–173.

120. Murakami M, Karnik SS, Husain A. Human prochymase activation. A novel role for heparin in zymogen processing. J Biol Chem 1995; 270(5):2218–2223.

121. Pejler G, Sadler JE. Mechanism by which heparin proteoglycan modulates mast cell chymase activity. Biochemistry 1999; 38(37):12187–12195.

122. Walter M, Sutton RM, Schechter NM. Highly efficient inhibition of human chymase by alpha (2)-macroglobulin. Arch Biochem Biophys 1999; 368(2):276–284.

123. Omoto Y, Tokime K, Yamanaka K, et al. Human mast cell chymase cleaves pro-IL-18 and generates a novel and biologically active IL-18 fragment. J Immunol 2006; 177(12):8315–8319.

124. Zhao W, Oskeritzian CA, Pozez AL, et al. Cytokine production by skin-derived mast cells: endogenous proteases are responsible for degradation of cytokines. J Immunol 2005; 175(4): 2635–2642.

125. Longley BJ, Tyrrell L, Ma Y, et al. Chymase cleavage of stem cell factor yields a bioactive, soluble product. Proc Natl Acad Sci U S A 1997; 94(17):9017–9021.

126. Hof P, Mayr I, Huber R, et al. The 1.8 A crystal structure of human cathepsin G in complex with Suc-Val-Pro-PheP-(OPh)2: a Janus-faced proteinase with two opposite specificities. EMBO J 1996; 15(20):5481–5491.

127. Schechter NM, Irani AM, Sprows JL, et al. Identification of a cathepsin G-like proteinase in the MCTC type of human mast cell. J Immunol 1990; 145(8):2652–2661.

128. Travis J, Bowen J, Baugh R. Human alpha-1-antichymotrypsin: interaction with chymotrypsin-like proteinases. Biochemistry 1978; 17(26):5651–5656.

129. Korkmaz B, Moreau T, Gauthier F. Neutrophil elastase, proteinase 3 and cathepsin G: physicochemical properties, activity and physiopathological functions. Biochimie 2008; 90(2): 227–242.

130. Sommerhoff CP, Fang KC, Nadel JA, et al. Classical second messengers are not involved in proteinase-induced degranulation of airway gland cells. Am J Physiol 1996; 271(5 Pt 1): L796–L803.

131. Irani AM, Goldstein SM, Wintroub BU, et al. Human mast cell carboxypeptidase. Selective localization to MCTC cells. J Immunol 1991; 147(1):247–253.

132. Goldstein SM, Kaempfer CE, Kealey JT, et al. Human mast cell carboxypeptidase. Purification and characterization. J Clin Invest 1989; 83(5):1630–1636.

133. Feyerabend TB, Hausser H, Tietz A, et al. Loss of histochemical identity in mast cells lacking carboxypeptidase A. Mol Cell Biol 2005; 25(14):6199–6210.

134. Lundequist A, Tchougounova E, Abrink M, et al. Cooperation between mast cell carboxypeptidase A and the chymase mouse mast cell protease 4 in the formation and degradation of angiotensin II. J Biol Chem 2004; 279(31):32339–32344.

135. Metz M, Piliponsky AM, Chen CC, et al. Mast cells can enhance resistance to snake and honeybee venoms. Science 2006; 313(5786):526–530.

136. Schneider LA, Schlenner SM, Feyerabend TB, et al. Molecular mechanism of mast cell mediated innate defense against endothelin and snake venom sarafotoxin. J Exp Med 2007; 204(11):2629–2639.

137. Sillaber C, Baghestanian M, Bevec D, et al. The mast cell as site of tissue-type plasminogen activator expression and fibrinolysis. J Immunol 1999; 162(2):1032–1041.

138. Kanbe N, Tanaka A, Kanbe M, et al. Human mast cells produce matrix metalloproteinase 9. Eur J Immunol 1999; 29(8):2645–2649.

139. Veerappan A, Reid AC, Estephan R, et al. Mast cell renin and a local renin-angiotensin system in the airway: role in bronchoconstriction. Proc Natl Acad Sci U S A 2008; 105(4):1315–1320.

140. Silver RB, Reid AC, Mackins CJ, et al. Mast cells: a unique source of renin. Proc Natl Acad Sci U S A 2004; 101(37):13607–13612.

141. Strik MC, de Koning PJ, Kleijmeer MJ, et al. Human mast cells produce and release the cytotoxic lymphocyte associated protease granzyme B upon activation. Mol Immunol 2007; 44(14):3462–3472.

142. Pardo J, Wallich R, Ebnet K, et al. Granzyme B is expressed in mouse mast cells in vivo and in vitro and causes delayed cell death independent of perforin. Cell Death Differ 2007; 14(10): 1768–1779.

143. Fujishima H, Sanchez Mejia RO, Bingham CO III, et al. Cytosolic phospholipase A2 is essential for both the immediate and the delayed phases of eicosanoid generation in mouse bone marrow-derived mast cells. Proc Natl Acad Sci U S A 1999; 96(9):4803–4807.

144. Tsujimura Y, Obata K, Mukai K, et al. Basophils play a pivotal role in immunoglobulin-G-mediated but not immunoglobulin-E-mediated systemic anaphylaxis. Immunity 2008; 28(4): 581–589.

145. Lynch JM, Henson PM. The intracellular retention of newly synthesized platelet-activating factor. J Immunol 1986; 137(8):2653–2661.

146. Betz SJ, Lotner GZ, Henson PM. Generation and release of platelet activating factor (PAF) from enriched preparations of rabbit basophils: failure of human basophils to release PAF. J Immunol 1980; 125:2749–2755.

147. Triggiani M, Schleimer RP, Warner JA, et al. Differential synthesis of 1-acyl-2-acetyl-sn-glycero-3-phosphocholine and platelet-activating factor by human inflammatory cells. J Immunol 1991; 147(2):660–666.

148. Lynch KR, O'Neill GP, Liu Q, et al. Characterization of the human cysteinyl leukotriene CysLT1 receptor. Nature 1999; 399(6738):789–793.

149. Mita H, Endoh S, Kudoh M, et al. Possible involvement of mast-cell activation in aspirin provocation of aspirin-induced asthma. Allergy 2001; 56(11):1061–1067.

150. Roberts LJ, Sweetman BJ, Lewis RA, et al. Increased production of prostaglandin D2 in patients with systemic mastocytosis. N Engl J Med 1980; 303(24):1400–1404.

151. Jolly PS, Bektas M, Olivera A, et al. Transactivation of sphingosine-1-phosphate receptors by FcepsilonRI triggering is required for normal mast cell degranulation and chemotaxis. J Exp Med 2004; 199(7):959–970.

152. Jolly PS, Bektas M, Watterson KR, et al. Expression of SphK1 impairs degranulation and motility of RBL-2H3 mast cells by desensitizing S1P receptors. Blood 2005; 105(12):4736–4742.

153. Olivera A, Mizugishi K, Tikhonova A, et al. The sphingosine kinase-sphingosine-1-phosphate axis is a determinant of mast cell function and anaphylaxis. Immunity 2007; 26(3):287–297.

154. Xiang Z, Nilsson G. IgE receptor-mediated release of nerve growth factor by mast cells. Clin Exp Allergy 2000; 30(10):1379–1386.

155. Ikeda K, Nakajima H, Suzuki K, et al. Mast cells produce interleukin-25 upon FcεRI-mediated activation. Blood 2003; 101(9):3594–3596.

156. Gibbs BF, Wierecky J, Welker P, et al. Human skin mast cells rapidly release preformed and newly generated TNF- alpha and IL-8 following stimulation with anti-IgE and other secretagogues. Exp Dermatol 2001; 10(5):312–320.

157. Hide M, Francis DM, Grattan CE, et al. Autoantibodies against the high-affinity IgE receptor as a cause of histamine release in chronic urticaria [see comments]. N Engl J Med 1993; 328(22): 1599–1604.

158. Sabroe RA, Fiebiger E, Francis DM, et al. Classification of anti-FcεRI and anti-IgE autoantibodies in chronic idiopathic urticaria and correlation with disease severity. J Allergy Clin Immunol 2002; 110(3):492–499.

159. Ferrer M, Nakazawa K, Kaplan AP. Complement dependence of histamine release in chronic urticaria. J Allergy Clin Immunol 1999; 104(1):169–172.

160. Kikuchi Y, Kaplan AP. A role for C5a in augmenting IgG-dependent histamine release from basophils in chronic urticaria. J Allergy Clin Immunol 2002; 109(1 Pt 1):114–118.

161. Gomez G, Jogie-Brahim S, Shima M, et al. Omalizumab reverses the phenotypic and functional effects of IgE-enhanced FcεRI on human skin mast cells. J Immunol 2007; 179:1353–1361.

162. Spector SL, Tan RA. Effect of omalizumab on patients with chronic urticaria. Ann Allergy Asthma Immunol 2007; 99(2):190–193.

163. Reimers A, Pichler C, Helbling A, et al. Zafirlukast has no beneficial effects in the treatment of chronic urticaria. Clin Exp Allergy 2002; 32(12):1763–1768.

4

Basophils

Donald MacGlashan, Jr. and Sarbjit Saini
Johns Hopkins Asthma and Allergy Center, Baltimore, Maryland, U.S.A.

INTRODUCTION

Basophils are granulocytes that represent only 0.5% to 1.0% of the circulating white blood cells. However, these are the only leukocytes that have histamine-containing granules that can be secreted to initiate blood vessel dilation and modulate local immune responses. A number of substances have been described which can induce histamine release from basophils. These include activation by molecules (e.g., proteins, complex carbohydrates) operating through IgE antibodies bound to the high-affinity IgE receptor and also include molecules binding to innate receptors such as fMLP (formyl Met-Leu-Phe (tripeptide) and C5a (Table 1). In humans, other leukocytes have been reported to express the high-affinity IgE receptor (FcεRI), but there remains some controversy over the functional consequences of this expression. Because of the similar expression of histamine-containing granules and FcεRI on basophils and mast cells, basophils could be viewed as a rapidly mobilized version of the tissue mast cell. There are many more mast cells than basophils in the body, but mast cells are long-lived and basophils have a short lifespan, so that the number of basophils and mast cells being generated at any given moment are about equal. While the two cell types share many characteristics, there are also many distinguishing features that suggest it is not always possible to extrapolate from mast cells to basophils or vice versa.

In the context of urticaria, there are a variety of observations that indicate an involvement of basophils in the expression of this disease, but the causal relationship has yet to be understood. A number of hypotheses have been advanced over the last two decades that implicate FcεRI-mediated activation of basophils and mast cells in chronic urticaria, but perhaps the most interesting recent observation is the remarkable sensitivity of patients with chronic urticaria to treatment with the non-cross-linking anti-IgE antibody, omalizumab (1). This observation implicates participation of IgE in the expression of chronic urticaria, although it remains possible that there is some indirect connection between the immune state mediated by IgE levels and the expression of the disease.

Table 1 Some Characteristics of Human Basophils, Expressed Receptors, Ligands that Activate These Receptors, the Mediators Secreted and Activation Markers that Increase Following Stimulation

	Receptors	Receptors ligands	Secreted substances
Strongly activating receptors	FcεRI C5aR, C3aR, fMLPR	IgE/antigen C5a, C3a, fMLP	Histamine ($1\ \mu g/10^6$) LTC$_4$ (60 pmoles/10^6) IL-4 (1000 pg/10^6)
Modulating or weakly activating receptors	CRTH2 5HPETE CysLT1, LT2 PAFER LTB$_4$ LIR -2, -3, -7 H2, (H3 & H4)* Siglec-8	PGD2 LTD$_4$, LTC$_4$ PAF (weak) LTB$_4$ (chemotaxis) ?? Histamine ??	IL-13 (200 pg/10^6) IL-3 VEGF Tryptase (weak) Activation Markers

Chemokine	CCR1, CCR3, CXCR2,
	  CXCR4, CCR2, CCR4,
	  CCR7, CXCR1
		MCP-2, -3, -4
		Eotaxin-1, -2, -3
		Rantes, TECK, SDF-1α
		MCP-1, HCC-1, MIP-3
		MIP-3β, SLC, 1-309,
		  GCP-2
			CD63 (LAMP-3)
			CD203c
			CD69
			(less characterized)

Adhesion	VLA-4, LFA-1 Mac-1, P150-95 α$_d$β$_2$, α$_4$β$_7$ VLA-6		CD164 CD107a,b (LAMP 1,2) CD13
Cytokine	IL-3, IL-5, GM-CSF NGF IL-1 IFN-γ VEGFR1 SCF	(same as named receptors)	
Toll-like	TLR-2 TLR-4 TLR-9, -10 (mRNA only)	Peptidoglycan LPS (CpG)	

Abbreviations: LT, leukotriene; fMLP, formyl Met-Leu-Phe (tripeptide); GM-CSF, granulocyte-macrophage colony stimulating factor; IL, interleukin; NGF, nerve growth factor; LIR, Leukocyte inhibitory factor (or LILR, leukocyte immunoglobulin-like receptor, e.g., LIR7, LILRA-2; LIR2, LILRB-2; LIR3, LILRB-3); MCP, monocyte chemotactic factor; PGD, prostaglandin; MIP, macrophage inflammatory protein; PAF, platelet activating factor, HCC, human CC; VEGF, vascular endothelial growth factor; LAMP, lysosome-associated membrane protein; CD, cluster of differentiation; SCF, stem cell factor.

It is useful to provide some background on basophil characteristics in order to provide a context for interpreting the various observations that have recently been made regarding basophil behavior before, during, or after the expression of chronic urticaria.

EXPRESSED RECEPTORS

Atopic diseases result from the production of specific IgE antibodies that bind to two types of IgE receptors. The low affinity receptor, FcεRII (CD23), is found on a variety of cell types both in circulation and in tissues, and this receptor appears to have a function on cell surfaces and as a solution phase protein. The biology associated with CD23 seems quite complex, and it remains unclear how this receptor modulates the immune response (2,3). In contrast, the high-affinity IgE receptor, FcεRI, is known to be critical to the expression of atopic disease. This receptor is now found to be expressed by a number of cell types, and this is a situation quite unique to primates. In rodents, where the receptor was first cloned, it was found to be composed of three different subunits expressed in the stoichiometry of αβγ2 (a disulfide-linked dimer of gamma). In rodents, the beta and gamma subunits are obligatory for expression. In humans, the beta subunit is optional for surface expression, although the absence of the beta subunit markedly attenuates expression of the receptor on the cell surface (4). Furthermore, its absence in the receptor complex probably markedly attenuates the kind of signal that is generated when receptor is cross-linked (5). Both the gamma and beta subunits act as chaperones for the alpha subunit that binds IgE antibody, but it appears that the beta subunit is a better chaperone than the gamma subunit. Cells that express the beta subunit, express 10-fold more cell surface FcεRIα. Alternatively, when a cell is capable of expressing FcεRIα, it also acquires an attribute that results in greater synthesis of the alpha subunit leading to higher cell surface expression levels of the mature receptor. Therefore, in humans, cells can express αγ2, and this seems to allow cells other than mast cells and basophils to express low levels of FcεRI on their cell surface. In recent studies where FcεRI was measured simultaneously on plasmacytoid dendritic cells (expressing no beta subunit) and basophils from peripheral blood, basophils expressed approximately 10-fold more receptor (6). In nonatopic subjects, this difference seems to be much greater, although a precise accounting has not been done. One characteristic of receptor expression on basophils is the remarkable densities that can be achieved. A typical cytokine receptor may be expressed at levels less than 1000 molecules per cell, and yet this level is adequate to mediate function. In atopic patients, FcεRI densities have been observed as high as 1 million per cell, and the typical atopic subject has basophils expressing 250,000 per cell. It is interesting to note that at 1 million per cell, the packing fraction on basophils is such that almost all the receptors are close enough to each other (<20 nm) that they can initiate weak signaling. Therefore, even at 250,000 per cell, the density is very high, and spontaneous aggregates of a very transient nature are present for 30% of the receptors. The reason this is important to note is that cytokine and chemokine synthesis by mast cells and basophils is found to occur even with transient signaling of FcεRI. In diseases where subtle shifts in the cytokine environment may mark the expression of the disease versus its quiescence, knowledge about the spontaneous behavior of FcεRI may be relevant. An argument against this possibility is that individuals with very high levels (e.g., helminth infection) do not have clear evidence of a mast cell/basophil disease.

An important attribute of the IgE receptor is that cell surface expression is sensitive to the presence of IgE antibody. Figure 1 shows a cartoon of the current understanding of this behavior. Receptor synthesis is insensitive to the presence or absence of IgE (7,8). Parenthetically, the synthetic rate is sensitive to the presence of various cytokines (7,9–11). Therefore, basophils are steadily synthesizing the receptor, which is placed on their cell surface. However, this unoccupied receptor is sensitive to removal by a mechanism that has yet to be elucidated. In other words, unoccupied receptor is unstable and if IgE does not bind, the receptor is internalized. In the absence of IL-3, the internalized receptor is degraded (12). In the presence of IL-3, some of the internalized receptors can be recycled for another look at the extracellular presence of IgE. Therefore, there is a steady state of surface expression that results from constitutive synthesis balanced by internalization unless IgE binds to the receptor. IgE present in the extracellular environment leads to the accumulation of the receptor and if IgE levels are very high, the receptor rapidly accumulates. Current estimates indicate that basophils that

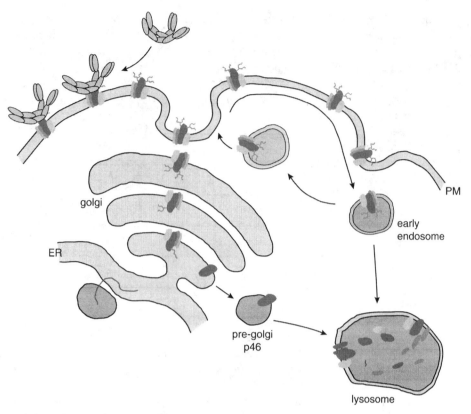

Figure 1 Cartoon of FcεRIα receptor "life-cyle". *Abbreviations:* ER, endoplasmic reticulum; PM, plasma membrane; pre-golgi p46, immature form of FcεRIα before extensive glycosylation in the golgi; MW of ≈ 46 kD, only found internally.

begin expressing receptor in the bone marrow stay there for about six days before entering the circulation (13). This means that they may load 60,000 receptors per day, all of which must be occupied with IgE. But note that because this is a steady state problem, it is possible to express some receptors, about 9000 in human basophils, even in the absence of IgE (or about 25,000, if there is a high IL-3 environment). Consequently, there is a log-linear relationship between serum free IgE and receptor density on basophils. The sensitivity of receptor expression levels to IgE means that local IgE levels may be at least as critical to the mast cell response as circulating IgE levels. This is particularly relevant today because it is becoming better appreciated that there is local IgE production at mucosal surfaces (14–16). This may occur in the near absence of circulating IgE levels, therefore modulating local mast cell FcεRI expression. The basophil would be unlikely to "benefit" from local IgE unless it can migrate into a tissue and remain resident long enough to upregulate receptors, a process that takes days.

One attribute that is very well characterized for human basophils and rarely explored for either mast cells in humans or rodents is the sensitivity of the cells to stimulation through FcεRI. The critical question is how many antigen-specific IgE molecules are required for the cell to achieve 50% of its maximal response. On average, human basophils need about 2000 specific IgE molecules per cell although this number is somewhat sensitive to the nature of the antigen used to aggregate the receptor (17,18). It is interesting that this number varies by about 30-fold in the general population. There are subjects whose basophils can secrete significant quantities of histamine when aggregating only 50 to 100 molecules of antigen-specific IgE. Since a typical basophil expresses about 150,000 receptors (atopics and nonatopics), it means that specific IgE levels need only be about 0.01% of total IgE levels in highly sensitive individuals. For the typical basophil, specific-to-total ratios need to be about 1%. Remarkably, this is the average ratio of antigen-specific to total IgE for a number of antigens (19).

Secretion of mediators in human basophils occurs in response to non-IgE-dependent stimuli (Table 1). There are receptors that appear to use signaling pathways very similar to those used by FcεRI. Currently, it is known that activation of the leukocyte-inhibitory receptor, LILRA-2 (LIR7) and activation of basophils by HrHRF (histamine releasing factor, p23) generate responses similar to anti-IgE Ab (20,21). There are also many 7-transmembrane receptors that markedly induce mediator release. Both the bacterial peptide, fMLP, and the anaphylatoxin, C5a, induce histamine release. However, these receptors do not normally induce secretion of all three classes of mediators (Table 1). Mediators that are preformed and released rapidly during degranulation define one class. A second class of rapidly released mediators are newly synthesized; basophils secrete predominately LTC_4 and no prostaglandins. The third class includes the newly synthesized (for the most part) cytokines and chemokines that require anywhere from 2 to 24 hours to be secreted. While there is still some debate, it appears that between basophils and mast cells, only basophils secrete IL-4. Indeed, it is currently believed that the bulk of IL-4 in the immune response may come from basophils, or at least that the IL-4 that appears rapidly (T-cells requiring longer periods). IL-13 is also well expressed by basophils, although the time course is somewhat slower than the release of IL-4 (22–24). Unpublished studies suggest that IL-13 secretion might be dependent on IgE-mediated secretion of IL-3 by basophils in an autocoid response (25). IL-3 alone can induce IL-13 secretion without IL-4 secretion (24). The various stimuli that induce mediator secretion from basophils do not consistently induce the secretion of all three classes of mediator. IgE-mediated secretion induces release of all mediator classes, fMLP induces secretion of histamine and leukotrienes, while C5a only induces secretion of histamine. Cytokines can alter this profile of secretion. Notably, IL-3 can allow C5a to induce secretion of all three mediator classes (26–28). There is a possible fourth class of mediators. While granules have traditionally been thought to be preformed and fixed in content, recent studies suggest that the cytokine environment can induce the loading of granules in mature basophils with mediators not previously present. The first in this category is granzyme B, which is induced by IL-3 exposure and found in granules after 6 to 18 hours. It can then be rapidly released with other granule contents by any stimulus that induces degranulation (29).

SIGNALING

The IgE receptor activates internal signaling when it is aggregated. There is some debate about this paradigm of secretion, and it is worth exploring this requirement for signaling in some detail because it may have relevance to disease expression.

The paradigm that FcεRI required aggregation to induce signaling was challenged by studies first published in 2001 (30,31). One might argue that it was first challenged by the observations that monomeric IgE could induce expression of its own receptor (32) but, as described above, this has been determined to be a consequence of stabilizing the surface receptor from internalization. Although there is clearly a sensor of the unoccupied state, inhibitors of the normal aggregation-dependent activation cascade demonstrate that these pathways are not required to observe upregulation of FcεRI by IgE (12,33). In contrast, studies using mouse mast cells and RBL cells noted that some monomeric IgE molecules could induce nearly a full expression of the activation cascade previously thought to only result from aggregation. These experiments are difficult to perform without ambiguity because aggregated IgE must be carefully eliminated. However, it has now become clear that there are subtleties that were at first unappreciated that suggest that aggregation is still occurring. Most notably, the first of the monomeric IgE molecules shown to induce secretion was a dinitrophenyl (DNP)-specific IgE (SPE-7) and monovalent DNP-lysine was found to completely inhibit the signaling initiated by adding monomeric SPE-7 to mast cells (30). Subsequent studies found that this particular IgE binds to multiple antigens. Other monoclonal IgE molecules were found to also induce secretion but with considerable variability so the terms "highly-" and "poorly-cytokinergic" were coined (34). It is important to stress that even in these instances of secretion, it almost exclusively results in cytokine secretion. This is a relevant point because activation through FcεRI is thought to be controlled by a process called kinetic-proofreading (35,36). Histamine release is sensitive to kinetic proofreading, while chemokine and cytokine release is not (necessarily) (35). The kinetic-proofreading mechanism is sensitive to the transience of the early signals and as noted above, high densities of receptors generate transient spontaneous "aggregates" (i.e., receptors close enough together so that they could induce a signal). If IgE binds to the receptor and induces even a modest change in the motion of the receptor (e.g., by weak association to each other), the lifetime of the spontaneous "aggregates" is increased significantly. At high densities of receptors using cells developed in high cytokine environments, this may be enough to induce some signaling that is expressed as cytokine/chemokine release. However, even if this is the more appropriate explanation for the monomeric IgE effect, it still raises the possibility that some monomeric IgE antibodies could be particularly adept at inducing signaling in basophils and mast cells under the right conditions. In some individuals, circulating IgE alone could induce mast cell and basophil activation, at least at some level. This possibility will require further study.

The clearly established requirement for aggregation has been studied extensively in rodent mast cells and cell lines, to a lesser extent using human basophils, to an even lesser extent using culture-derived human mast cells, and hardly at all using natural tissue–derived mast cells. It is not surprising that after 30 years of extensive study of signal transduction in a wide variety of cell types that the pathways involved have developed to be quite complex. It goes without saying that secretion must be tightly regulated and that there are many redundant activating and de-activating pathways involved in tuning the response to those conditions where secretion is actually protective and physiologically useful. However, atopic diseases seem to result from a misdirected action of either the IgE axis of the immune response or misdirected behavior of the cells that use IgE antibody. It is possible that imbalance of the signaling pathways creates the conditions necessary for disease expression.

Figure 2 shows a very sparse cartoon of the signaling elements that participate in the FcεRI-mediated reaction. The details for non-FcεRI-dependent secretion are differentiated by the nature of the very earliest steps, and at the current level of understanding, the steps beyond the earliest are often shared amongst all the secretagogues. Therefore, it is the early steps that should be a point of focus for now.

All secretion requires an elevation in cytosolic calcium, the participation of the Erk pathway for free AA generation (LTC$_4$ release), and the activation of NFAT to drive generation of IL-4 (37). Therefore, it is useful to focus on those early events that lead to activation of these pathways.

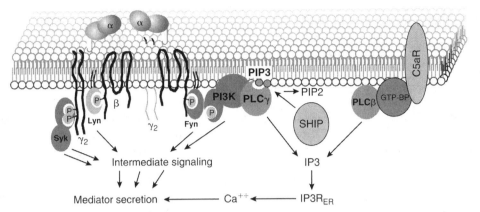

Figure 2 Cartoon of early signaling. A highly simplified diagram that shows both an FcεRI-mediated early reaction and canonical 7-transmembrane receptor-mediated signaling. The α, β, and γ₂ subunits of the IgE receptor are sketched (no IgE is shown). *Abbreviations: L*yn and Fyn, Src-family kinases; Syk, spleen tyrosine kinase; PI3K, phosphatidylinositol 3′ kinase (both p85 and p110 subunits shown); PLCγ and PLCβ, phospholipase C; SHIP, SH2-containing inositol 5′ phosphatase; GTP-BP, GTP binding protein (several possibly family members would serve this role); PIP3, phosphotidylinositol 3,4,5–trisphosphate; PIP2, phosphatidylinositol 3,4 bisphosphate, IP3, inositol 1,4,5 trisphosphate; ER, endoplasmic recticulum; IP3R$_{ER}$, IP3 receptor in the ER; -P, phosphorylated tyrosines on the various proteins.

FcεRI is a receptor without enzymatic activity. It is dependent on the close participation of kinase enzymes that are recruited when aggregation of the receptor occurs. For FcεRI, the primary early enzymatic activities are tyrosine kinases, while for G-protein linked signaling (e.g., fMLP), the early steps are dependent on GTP-switches, phospholipases, and serine/threonine kinases. One of the first steps after aggregation of FcεRI is the phosphorylation of FcεRIβ by an Src-family tyrosine kinase, and this step is rapidly followed by the recruitment of Syk, a tyrosine kinase of the ZAP70 family. Syk is recruited to the phosphorylated gamma subunit (phosphorylated by a Src-family kinase), upon which it becomes active and phosphorylates a wide variety of substrates, including the regulatory subunit of PI3 kinase. In human basophils, the only Class 1a PI3 kinase is PI3 kinase delta (38), and, like Syk, its activity is absolutely required for all three classes of mediator secretion. PI3 kinase generates an important second messenger, PIP3 from membrane PIP2, and PIP3 acts as a site of enzyme recruitment for a variety of other signaling elements needed for secretion. For example, the phospholipase C-gamma enzymes are recruited to the membrane by PIP3 and following phosphorylation by Syk, generate IP3 from PIP2. IP3 is the first second messenger involved in the release of calcium found in the endoplasmic recticulum. IP3 acts on the IP3 receptor to raise cytosolic calcium levels. For G-protein-linked receptors, it is phospholipase C-beta that performs the task of phospholipase C-gamma.

All signaling reactions must have attendant deactivation mechanisms. In recent years, several classes of phosphatases have been implicated in the FcεRI-mediated reaction. Notable among these phosphatases is the 5′ lipid phosphatase, SHIP (SH2-containing 5′ inositol phosphatase). PIP3 levels in cells can be constitutively maintained by another lipid phosphatase, PTEN (39), but it appears that it is SHIP (1 or 2) that controls the amount of PIP3 generated during an ongoing reaction. Domains of SHIP allow it to be recruited to the ongoing reaction complex, and its metabolism of PIP3 slows the activation cascade. Although metabolism of PIP3 is one role for SHIP, its ultimate role may be more complex because it has several domains that might act as adapters (linkers) for activation and for recruiting proteins involved in the downregulation of the Erk pathway. SHIP has received more attention than other signaling elements because studies in SHIP knockout mice showed that mast cell secretory responses without SHIP were highly sensitive to stimulation (40). Indeed, these mast cells may be constitutively active. Consistent with this viewpoint are studies of human basophils obtained from patients who are very sensitive to the cytokine HrHRF. This type of basophil phenotype expresses low levels of SHIP, and this is accompanied by slow metabolism of PIP3 (as evidence by a prolonged phosphorylation of Akt, a phosphorylation that has an obligatory requirement for PIP3) (41). A recent survey of the general population found a weak inverse correlation between SHIP expression and maximal histamine release (more on this below) (18). Therefore, while an explicit causal test for the participation of SHIP in the progress of the FcɛRI-mediated reaction is not available for human basophils, the evidence for its role is suggestive.

This basic sketch of the signaling reaction for FcɛRI leads to questions about the source of biological variability in the general population to stimulation through FcɛRI. It has been known for many years that there is marked variation in responsiveness among subjects' basophils following stimulation by the general aggregating reagent, anti-IgE antibody. Typically a given subjects' basophil response is a stable characteristic, suggesting that it is an intrinsic attribute of the basophil for each individual. Likewise, the cellular sensitivity (discussed above) is a relatively stable characteristic of the basophil. A recent survey of signal element expression (supplemented by yet-to-be-published data) in the general population (which included 20% atopics) shows that of 20 early signaling elements relevant to the IgE-dependent pathway, only expression of Syk shows a strong correlation to histamine release induced by anti-IgE Ab (18). Expression of SHIP was found to be weakly inversely correlated. Notably, the coefficient of variation (standard deviation/mean) for Syk expression matched the CV for histamine release (CV $\approx$ 0.7), while the CV for all other signaling elements is no different than expected from the noise in the Western blot technique used to measure their expression. Indeed, the expression of all the other elements appears to be very tightly controlled. It is remarkable that among the entire leukocyte pool, only basophils show this variability in Syk expression. Even more remarkable, despite Syk being an obligate signaling element, the basophil expresses Syk at levels at least 10-fold below all other leukocytes with the exception of T cells (which have been long known to use ZAP-70 as the TCR tyrosine kinase). Some leukocyte types (pDC and monocytes) express 30-fold more Syk than basophils. Despite these large differences in expression, the other leukocytes very tightly control expression of Syk with a CV for expression that is no different than expected from the noise in the assay. This makes the regulation of Syk expression in basophils unique. The levels of expression range from 6,000 to 60,000 molecules per basophil. Given that basophils typically express 100,000 FcɛRI receptors and that each receptor can bind one Syk molecule, it is clear that the Syk expression level is tuned to be the rate-limiting step. Expression of Lyn kinase, by comparison, is tightly regulated and there appears to be approximately 100,000 molecules of Lyn present. On the other hand, since there is very little variation in Lyn expression levels, these results would suggest that atopic basophils expressing 250,000 to 500,000 receptors would also be limited by the amount of Lyn available. Lyn is but one of the Src-family kinases available in basophils, which also express Fyn, an Src-family kinase member that has been identified as important for signaling in mast cells. But Lyn is thought to participate in both activation and deactivation mechanisms (42–44). So a relative paucity of Lyn, relative to the receptor levels, might lead to unexpected imbalances in stimulation that could result in secretion levels that would not have been easily predicted. This is an area that needs further study. These studies provide a background for the studies of chronic urticaria to be presented below.

CELLULAR DESENSITIZATION

As noted previously, all forms of cellular activation must be accompanied by deactivation mechanisms or runaway stimulation would result. Along with the many activation steps being identified in the mast cell/basophil response, there are deactivation steps. Some of these might be considered homeostatic in that they are constitutively operative and may regulate the set point for responsiveness and/or serve to dampen the constant random noise that occurs in these highly amplified reactions. Other downregulatory mechanisms are explicitly present to turn off a reaction that leads to function. This latter group includes loss of the activating receptor, loss of signaling elements, transitory alterations in signaling elements, recruitment of downregulatory enzymes, and new gene transcription of downregulatory elements. All these methods can be found operative in a standard IgE-mediated activation of basophils. In human basophils, loss of the aggregated receptor occurs but the process is very slow, requiring days for completion (12). A somewhat faster downregulatory step includes the loss of Syk itself. Syk is lost by a mechanism that is universal in eukaryotic cells, the ubiquinylation of a target protein, its recognition by the 26S proteasome, and proteasomal degradation. The attachment of the 8 kD protein, ubiquitin, to another protein is mediated by a family of ligases (so-called E1, E2, E3 ligases). The E3 ligases manage the terminal step; specific E3 ligases couple with their target proteins to attach ubiquitin. The cell uses the ubiquitin to process the target protein; in many cases, poly-ubiquinylation results in degradation but ubiquinylation has other purposes. For Syk, c-Cbl and Cbl-b are the relevant E3 ligases and in human basophils (20,45,46), c-Cbl appears to be the necessary ligase, although definitive proof does not exist. The loss of Syk requires hours and is therefore also slow (47). But it appears to be an integrative process. Very low levels of stimulation that do not result in measurable secretion can continue to result in some loss of Syk. It has been noted that stimulation of basophils through a non-IgE-dependent receptor, also induces some loss of Syk despite this tyrosine kinase not being active during this GTP-binding protein-dependent process. In this instance, fMLP is noted to induce phosphorylation of c-Cbl (20).

There are clearly faster mechanisms of downregulation that serve to mediate the cessation of histamine and leukotriene release. IgE-mediated stimulation of basophils results in both specific and nonspecific desensitization (48). Specific desensitization only serves to shut down the response to the antigen inducing the aggregation of its specific IgE, while nonspecific desensitization serves to attenuate the response of the basophil to non-cross-reacting reactions. In either case, the response of basophils to other non-IgE-dependent stimuli is not altered, indicating that the downregulatory steps following antigenic stimulation have altered only the signaling cascades relevant to FcεRI. The mechanism underlying specific desensitization is not known, but it must occur very early in signaling, probably some form of receptor association, with structures like caveoli. Nonspecific desensitization appears to be associated with the steps that SHIP1 regulates and, in fact, may be due to the activity of SHIP (49,50). Causal testing remains to be done. No form of desensitization is dependent on Syk (51) or PKC activity but all forms are dependent on an Src-family kinase (52).

CYTOKINE-DEPENDENT MODULATION OF SECRETION

Secretion from basophils is modulated by a number of cytokines. IL-3 is notable because it is both required for basophil development and maturation from CD34 progenitors and because it markedly modulates the function of mature basophils in response to all secretatogues. Other cytokines, for example, IL-5, GM-CSF and NGF, IL-1, IFNγ, also modulate function (not always in the same way) but do not appear to be as potent and efficacious as IL-3. IL-3 changes the response of basophils both quantitatively and qualitatively. As noted previously, IL-3 can change the response of basophils to C5a from being restricted to histamine release to one in which all three classes of mediators are secreted. The response to IL-3 occurs in at least three time frames. One or two minutes of exposure to IL-3 will immediately upregulate leukotriene release. This appears to result from two events. One is the synchronizing of the elevation in the cytosolic calcium with the activation of the Erk pathway (which is required for activation of cytosolic PLA2, the generation of free arachidonic acid and therefore the generation of LTC$_4$) and the second is the deactivation of a phosphatase that regulates the Erk pathway. Acute exposure to IL-3 does not alter any earlier FcεRI-dependent signaling step (53). The second time frame for IL-3 effects takes place over a 24-hour period. Following this form of "priming," the cytosolic calcium response that follows stimulation with any secretagogue is greatly enhanced. C5a—without prior exposure to IL-3—induces only a transient elevation of cytosolic calcium that lasts about one minute. A 24-hour exposure to IL-3 (but not acute IL-3) alters the response to include a prolonged influx phase, similar to that observed with fMLP without IL-3 present. The influx phase of the calcium response to other secretagogues (that normally cause a two-phase calcium response) is also markedly enhanced. Preliminary studies indicate that this does not result from changes in iCRAC or STIM1 expression but possibly an increase in a maxi-K channel (large conductance Ca-activated K channel). The third time frame takes place in two to four days (54). At this point, the basophil begins to upregulate a variety of signaling elements (18). Although IL-3 will bring Syk levels in basophils that very poorly express this element to normal levels, it does not have strong effects on "normal" basophils. Instead, expression of many other signaling elements is increased, notably SHIP1 and c-Cbl, both of which are generally considered downregulating elements. As noted above, IL-3 also induces the secretion of IL-13 from basophils. In fact, the IL-13 secretion induced by anti-IgE antibody may be a simple consequence of an autocoid loop that results from the IL-3 secretion induced by anti-IgE antibody. IL-3 alters a host of other basophil responses and since it acts as an anti-apoptotic cytokine, one could conclude that it simply reverses the progressive loss of function associated with apoptosis.

MARKERS OF BASOPHIL FUNCTION AND ACTIVATION

Histamine release was one of the first outcomes to be measured in basophils. Indeed, histamine release from leukocytes was measured long before it was known that basophils were the source. Thus there is an extensive history and context for histamine release studies. Nearly all signaling studies are placed in the context of histamine release (degranulation). As noted above, there are two other classes of mediators to consider, lipid metabolites, cytokines, and chemokines. Each of the pathways to secretion is fairly lengthy and involves very different terminal signaling cascades although they are all dependent on an elevation in cytosolic calcium. "Spontaneous" secretion of any of these mediators could be viewed as a marker of activation although the use of the term spontaneous is placed in quotes because it is possible that there is a ligand bound to its receptor when the basophil is isolated for study in the test tube. Normally, the process of isolation takes so long that it is hard to interpret the biological significance of spontaneous secretion and to separate it from an artifact of cell handling. Stimulated secretion is also a useful method of assessing the status of the basophil although, a priori, one cannot know what kind of secretagogue to use when investigating an unknown disease process like urticaria or angioedema. Indeed, there are ways to activate basophils, for example, stimulation with hyperosmolar solutions, that would not be immediately considered as relevant to in vivo conditions.

In recent years, new markers of basophil activation have been discovered. A variety of tests to assess both the spontaneous or stimulated state of basophil activation in whole blood or quick preparations of enriched basophils have been developed. Most notable of these markers are CD63, CD203c, or CD69. There is very little known about the biological purpose of basophils upregulating the cell surface expression of CD markers, and there is very little known about the signaling cascades that are critical for their expression.

Although CD63 expression (gp53, lysosomal associated membrane protein (LAMP)-3, member of the tetraspanin family that is associated with internal vesicle membranes) has been linked to degranulation because it can be identified in the granules of basophils (55), several lines of evidence clearly dissociate this marker from demonstrable degranulation (56,57). Therefore, like the other markers, it remains a marker of activation rather than a high-fidelity surrogate for measuring degranulation. There may be some contribution of granule-derived CD63 to cell surface expression but it may only be a modest contribution. This marker can be found expressed on purified basophils, so it has its origins with the basophil itself but in studies of whole blood, activated platelets highly express CD63 and activated basophils are known to activate platelets, causing them to adhere to the plasma membrane of basophils. This may result in very bright and skewed fluorescence when samples are analyzed by flow cytometry. One might guess that some of the very non-Gaussian distributions of CD63 expression on basophils observed during flow cytometry might result from the sporadic adherence of activated platelets (this has been observed by microscopy) (56). So studies of CD63 must be interpreted with care. The biological role of CD63 expression is not known except for the possibility that some of its expression reflects granule fusion. There are other ways that CD63 expression can be upregulated that do not depend on activation by known secretagogues (58).

CD203c (E-NPP3) was identified as being expressed only on basophils and mast cells (59,60). Upregulation from a resting level of expression is marked. However, expression of this marker is transient on a time scale that is consistent with the cessation of histamine release or is somewhat longer. CD203c is an ecto-nucleotide pyrophospha-tase/phosphodiesterase whose biological role/function is not known. The tight association with only mast cells or basophils and the marked upregulation make this an attractive candidate for surveying the state of basophil activation in vivo. The signaling mechanisms are not well known and its expression can also be dissociated from degranulation. Some studies have noted that incubation in IL-3 can upregulate CD203c expression (61). Some inhibitory drugs can inhibit CD203c upregulation and histamine release while not altering upregulation of CD63, demonstrating that these endpoints are using signaling pathways that are distinct (57).

CD69 expression has not been explored as extensively. It was first identified as a marker of exposure to IL-3 (58). Indeed, cell surface expression does not increase following stimulation with any secretagogue. So this molecule might be an interesting marker of in vivo priming of basophils with IL-3 or other cytokines.

More recently, additional markers of activation have been identified. These include two additional LAMP family members, CD107a and CD107b (LAMP-1 and 2). CD13 (ecto-enzyme, gp150) and CD164 (transmembrane glycoprotein sialomucin endolyn) are two markers that also appear to be upregulated (62). This is an interesting observation because CD164 and LAMPs may differentiate between two forms of basophil degranulation, so-called piecemeal degranulation (PMD) versus anaphylactic degranulation (AND), respectively, as defined by Dvorak.

There are other readouts that might have some utility. It was noted previously, that IL-3 can induce IL-13 secretion from basophils. A recent study of nasal antigen provocation noted an increase in "spontaneous" IL-13 secretion from basophils isolated 24 hours after nasal challenge. Parenthetically, IL-3 also induces FcεRIβ subunit upregulation (9), and the same nasal provocation induces a modest increase in FcεRIβ in peripheral blood basophils (63). However, this is a difficult marker to assess, and there would be no general baseline on which to compare expression. It would be a relative change before and after an in vivo manipulation that would make it a useful marker of cytokine "priming."

A persistent question that arises in the study of activation of any cell type is whether the single cell response is reflected in the whole population response and whether there are subpopulations of cell responsiveness. A related question is whether cells respond in a graded fashion or display all-or-nothing characteristics. These questions have been asked for basophil responses as well. Although the question has been largely answered during the last two decades (56,64,65), the emergence of flow cytometric techniques to assess basophil responses has raised the issue again. Using flow cytometry and the CD63/CD203c markers, various investigators have noted unusual response distributions and it is reasonable to ask what is occurring. First, studies using purified basophils have clearly demonstrated that the response of basophils is graded and response distributions for a wide variety of signaling endpoints and degranulation are almost always unimodal. Although the responses are always unimodal, they are not always Gaussian. Some very non-Gaussian skewing of the response distributions have been observed for some outcomes. But it is important to distinguish between the studies with purified basophils and studies with impure basophils. This may seem a subtle distinction, but it is possible that during purification of basophils, a subpopulation is selected. More often than not, the purification results in some loss of cells, and it is conceivable that exclusion of a basophil subtype occurs. Therefore in the marker studies where whole blood is used (or a simple leukocyte preparation method), these other subpopulations may become apparent. Bimodal distributions may result, and this would not contradict the conclusion that basophils respond in a graded unimodal fashion but instead suggest that there were subpopulations of phenotypically distinctive basophils similar to the characterization of eosinophils as normo- and hypo-dense that has been noted for many years.

BASOPHIL CHANGES ASSOCIATED WITH DISEASE

Although sporadic, there has been a long history to the study of an association between basophils and expression of chronic urticaria. One good reason is that basophil is the most accessible cell that bears FcεRI and contains histamine. But another reason is that there are notable oddities about basophils obtained from patients with urticaria. This was first noted in the studies of Kern and Lichtenstein (66) and Greaves et al. (67). These studies found consistent basopenia and of the remaining circulating basophils, a considerable reduction in their ability to release histamine in response to stimulation with anti-IgE antibody. These observations have been replicated by several investigators (68,69), although the precise details seem to vary from study to study. However, the hyporesponsiveness through FcεRI may not apply to all basophil secretagogues (70). It is not known today whether these characteristics are a reflection of a role for basophils in the expression of the disease, whether the basophil is an "innocent" bystander to the events occurring in the skin, or whether the response of the basophils that remain in the circulation when there is marked basopenia. A related question is whether the basophil that is isolated from peripheral blood represents the state of the cell before it enters tissues (skin?) or after it has made a passage through tissues and reentered the circulation. No one knows if basophils can survive long enough to both leave the circulation and reenter the circulation, but recent studies in mice make note of the presence of basophils in lymph nodes (71). Perhaps this reflects direct entry into the nodes or migration to the nodes from tissues, but it also raises the possibility that these cells might make their way back to circulation.

The general goal has been to probe the basophils of these patients as a way of deriving clues to the origins of the clinical changes observed in these patients. As noted above, one interesting feature is the reduced responsiveness to activation through the IgE receptor. Indeed, the reduced activation is restricted to FcεRI because responses to non-IgE dependent stimuli appear intact. In recent studies, the reduced activation is restricted to about 50% of patients with chronic urticaria (the nonresponding basophils have been labeled CIU-NR and the responding basophil phenotype, CIU-R) (68), and this attribute of nonresponsiveness was not linked to the presence or absence of autoantibodies to either FcεRI or IgE (see below) (72). Most remarkably, as patients experience a remission in their urticaria, the CIU-NR basophil response returns to a normal state. This apparent linkage to FcεRI functions only provides further evidence that the disease, in general, is linked to IgE. This linkage was made considerably stronger by the observation that patients treated with omalizumab (the non-cross-linking anti-IgE antibody) experienced a rapid reversal of their disease (yet-to-be-published studies by S. Saini). This reversal was accompanied by a return of basophil IgE-mediated function to near normal. This is a remarkable observation because when patients are adequately treated with omalizumab, the levels of free IgE are reduced to such an extent that FcεRI expression on basophils decreases to <15% of the normal density and surface IgE is reduced to less than 5% of the normal density. In a typical atopic patient, such decreases are generally associated with a decrease in the antigen-induced activation and a variable loss in activation by cross-linking anti-IgE antibody (73). However, the ability of omalizumab to reduce free IgE levels and simultaneously reduce receptor expression is limited. As noted above, basophils are exquisitely sensitive to aggregation of the IgE receptor. Less than 5000 receptors/IgE per cell results in amaximal response to anti-IgE Ab. A 95% reduction of free IgE results in 2000 to 5000 IgE per basophil, more than enough to signal strongly. So the increase in the anti-IgE response in these patients' basophils suggests that there is another process at work, a reworking of the cell's signaling apparatus to allow a normally sensitive response.

There have been some improvements in the understanding of the signaling reactions important to IgE-mediated secretion, and as understanding has improved, it has been applied to the problem posed by the behavior of CIU basophils. As noted above, Syk is a critically important early signaling tyrosine kinase whose expression level appears closely tuned to the needs of FcεRI to induce secretion. Results from recent studies have been mixed. In a preliminary comparison, Syk levels were similar between CIU—nonresponding basophils (NR) and normal controls (68). However, a second smaller study noted that there are a greater percentage of patients with CIU-NR basophils that express very low levels of Syk (74). In the general population, 10% to 20% of subjects have basophils that express almost no Syk. In the CIU-NR phenotype, 43% are Syk "negative" and only 17% are Syk negative in the CIU-R phenotype. This is suggestive, but given the profound nature of the suppression in the CIU-NR basophils, Syk expression levels are not a clear marker for the phenotype. A second molecule discussed above that may have some relevance to signaling is SHIP1. Although SHIP1 may have a complex role in signaling, its primary enzymatic activity downregulates the amount of PIP3 that is necessary for activation cascades. It is therefore possible that poorly responding basophils might express high levels of SHIP1 or its close variant, SHIP2. In the Syk study noted above, basophil SHIP1 levels were not increased in the CIU-NR population but SHIP2 levels were (68). In addition, SHIP1 and SHIP2 levels were significantly decreased in CIU-R basophils.

Focusing on the CIU-NR phenotype, these cells tend to have lower Syk expression and higher expression levels of SHIP2. If these observations hold, it is useful to ask how the cells get to this state. Unfortunately, very little is known about the selective regulation of SHIP1 or SHIP2. Selective regulation of Syk has received some study but many questions remain for Syk as well. As noted previously, Syk can be ubiquinylated as it is lost through degradation through the 26S proteasome. Thus, any prior exposure of basophil to stimulation through FcεRI will result in a relative loss of Syk. Recent studies have shown that non-FcεRI receptors that use Syk as well as receptors that phosphorylate c-Cbl (the E3 ligase that is responsible for Syk ubiquinylation) can cause loss of Syk (20). Therefore, there are several ways to envision the loss of Syk in CIU basophils, and at least one of them is compatible with stimulation through the IgE receptor. But since low Syk expression levels is not a general feature of the CIU-NR or CIU-R basophil, this process may not be generally relevant.

Both Syk and SHIP1/2 can be upregulated by exposing basophils to IL-3. Indeed, the expression of several signaling molecules is increased after several days of IL-3 exposure. IL-3 can partially correct the nonreleaser phenotype in the general population by increasing Syk levels, but it remains notable that other signaling species also increase, including those considered to have a downregulatory role (e.g., SHIP and c-Cbl). Thus, IL-3 may have a profound role in determining the basophil phenotype but it does not appear to have the selectivity required to understand the CIU phenotypes.

With the identification of several cell surface markers of basophil activation that are easily measured by flow cytometry, a variety of studies have explored whether circulating basophils show evidence of prior exposure to secretagogues. While these data might be useful, these studies also suffer from being difficult to interpret. All of the markers discussed above can be modulated by cytokines as well as both IgE-dependent and non-IgE-dependent stimuli. Therefore, the source of any variation would be unknown. To date, reports have not been entirely consistent. It is first useful to determine how these markers change under conditions known to induce a systemic biological response. In one study, activation marker changes on basophils that were examined in insect venom-sensitive patients being exposed to avenom challenge (by sting). It was notable that there were increases in CD63, but the changes did not distinguish between individuals with a history of large local and systemic reactions. Both CD69 and CD203c were increased in patients with a history of a systemic reaction (75). The CD69 response was the most evident change, with changes in CD203c being very weak, when compared with what happens during an in vitro challenge of the same basophils. Sting patients responding with only a large local reaction showed no changes. The fact that CD69 showed the most obvious changes and that the CD69 marker is more readily associated with cytokine exposure rather than IgE-mediated stimulation, suggests that the systemic anaphylactic response generated a cytokine environment that altered the basophil phenotype rather than resulting in marked basophil secretion.

This context is useful for interpreting the data obtained from CIU patients. To date, only a few studies of the resting expression of CD63, 69, or 203c have been performed. The results have been mixed, although there remain differences in the methodology and the choice of control subjects. In a recent study by one of the authors, both atopic subjects and CIU subjects showed increased expression of CD63 on resting basophils when compared with nonatopic subjects. Notably, there was no statistical difference in CD203c or CD69 in CIU patients, as compared with nonatopic controls, while CD69 changes were observed in the atopic group (76). The increases, when observed, were small relative to the changes that could be induced by in vitro challenge. Notably, the changes in CD63 expression were not accompanied by changes in CD42 expression, a marker that would indicate the presence of adherent platelets. In a second study, a significant increase in both CD63 and CD203c was observed in the CIU subjects relative to nonatopic controls (61). The authors of this study suggest that the methodology (whole blood analysis) might explain the difference in their results from the former study regarding the expression of CD203c.

BASOPHILS IN A BIOASSAY

A longstanding hypothesis in the study of chronic urticaria has been the presence of autoantibodies in the sera of CIU patients (77–81). Autoantibodies with specificity for either FcεRIα or IgE have been noted. This topic is covered in detail elsewhere in this book, and the assays used to identify the presence of these antibodies are both varied and complex. A critically important bioassay uses the human basophil as a sensor for the presence of functionally relevant antireceptor or anti-IgE antibodies (77–80,82,83). Because the basophil is exquisitely sensitive to stimulation through FcεRI, this can be a very sensitive detector for the presence of these antibodies. Mitigating enthusiasm for this bioassay includes the remarkable variety of ways in which basophils can be activated, and the serum contains many bioactive components. These complications have led to the refinements in the assay and provide more rigorous definitions for what constitutes a positive signal. A related bioassay is the injection of autologous serum into the skin of patients, looking for a rapid wheal and flare-up that would signify the presence of antireceptor or anti-IgE antibodies inducing activation of skin mast cells (84). It is not clear whether the skin test suffers from the fact that the patients' mast cells may have already been exposed, reacted, and desensitized to the circulating antibodies.

From the descriptions of the human basophil above, one can see that a bioassay in which histamine release is an endpoint would be very dependent on the responsiveness of the basophil used as a target that is exposed to the serum being tested. The amount of release obtainable and the cellular sensitivity (see above) would be highly variable. Clearly, one would not want to use a nonreleasing basophil as the biosensor, but to standardize such an assay would also mean a careful and continuing assessment of a stable of basophil donors whose basophils were both highly functional and stable in time. The assay for histamine release is not trivial and cannot be done in a physician's office. The immunoassay for histamine is not very robust and has a poor dynamic range, and an automated fluorometric instrument is too complex for many environments. These problems have led to the recent efforts to shift the outcome measure for the basophil response to the activation markers, notably CD63 or CD203c (8–88). Some recent comparisons have suggested that the specificity and sensitivity of CD203c is somewhat better than CD63 (89), although there remains considerable debate (90). The assay is simplified by being done in whole blood although the flow cytometry instrumentation is expensive, complex, and quality control is a complex issue. Use of whole blood raises the potential problems of cross-talk among cell types when the variety of possible stimuli in the serum can be even larger, when one considers all the possible responses by leukocytes. With CD63 as a measure, platelet activation and adherence to basophils is likely to introduce a new variable into the biosassay. This could be mitigated by simultaneous measurements of CD42. A number of flow cytometric techniques have been used. But, gating on the basis of IgE is not a good choice because the receptor/IgE levels vary by 100-fold, sometimes being quite minimal. And, if the anti-IgE fluorochrome emission is too close to the outcome measure (e.g., a FITC anti-IgE and a CD203c-PE); compensation for the possible 100-fold variation in anti-IgE signal is difficult to set a priori. Perhaps the best approach is to identify basophils with a combination of CD123-PE, BDCA-2-FITC (or HLA(DR)-FITC), and forward scatter/side scatter (FS/SS). CD123 is the IL-3 receptor alpha subunit, and this receptor is only highly expressed on basophils and plasmacytoid dendritic cells (pDC). BDCA-2 or HLA(DR) will allow the cytometer to remove pDCs from the analysis. The use of PE and FITC to gate the basophils allows a second inexpensive infrared laser diode to measure the important outcome variable in a very distinct region of the spectrum. CD203-APC or alexa 647 can therefore be analyzed without any interference from the gating antibodies. Proper FS/SS gating can largely eliminate the pDC without using BDCA-2. This would allow CD42-FITC to be used as an assessment of platelet adherence. This arrangement of reagents would be useful for the biosensor assays as well as general assessment of resting levels of CD63, 69, or 203c. A more complex analysis could be done with more expensive multicolor cytometers.

REFERENCES

1. Gober L, Sterba PM, Eckman JA, et al. Effect of anti-IgE (Omalizumab) in chronic idiopathic urticaria (CIU) patients. J Allergy Clin Immunol 2008; 121:S147.
2. McCloskey N, Hunt J, Beavil RL, et al. Soluble CD23 monomers inhibit and oligomers stimulate IGE synthesis in human B cells. J Biol Chem 2007; 282(33):24083–24091.
3. Aubry JP, Pochon S, Gauchat JF, et al. CD23 interacts with a new functional extracytoplasmic domain involving N-linked oligosaccharides on CD21. J Immunol 1994; 152(12):5806–5813.
4. Donnadieu E, Jouvin MH, Kinet JP. A second amplifier function for the allergy-associated Fc (epsilon)RI-beta subunit. Immunity 2000; 12(5):515–523.
5. Dombrowicz D, Lin S, Flamand V, et al. Allergy-associated FcRbeta is a molecular amplifier of IgE- and IgG-mediated in vivo responses. Immunity 1998; 8(4):517–529.
6. Prussin C, Griffith DT, Boesel KM, et al. Omalizumab treatment downregulates dendritic cell FcepsilonRI expression. J Allergy Clin Immunol 2003; 112(6):1147–1154.
7. MacGlashan DW Jr., Xia HZ, Schwartz LB, et al. IgE-regulated expression of FcɛRI in human basophils: control by regulated loss rather than regulated synthesis. J Leuk Biol 2001; 70: 207–218.
8. Borkowski TA, Jouvin MH, Lin SY, et al. Minimal requirements for IgE-mediated regulation of surface Fc epsilon RI. J Immunol 2001; 167(3):1290–1296.
9. Miura K, Saini SS, Gauvreau G, et al. Differences in functional consequences and signal transduction induced by IL-3, IL-5 and NGF in human basophils. J Immunol 2001; 167:2282–2291.
10. Pawankar R, Okuda M, Yssel H, et al. Nasal mast cells in perennial allergic rhinitics exhibit increased expression of the FcɛRI, CD40L, IL-4 and IL-13 and can induce IgE synthesis in B cells. J Clin Invest 1997; 99:1492–1499.
11. Pawankar R, Ra C. IgE-Fc epsilonRI-mast cell axis in the allergic cycle. Clin Exp Allergy 1998; 28(suppl 3):6–14.
12. MacGlashan DW Jr. Endocytosis, re-cycling and degradation of unoccupied FcɛRI in human basophils. J Leuk Biol 2007; 82:1003–1010.

13. MacGlashan D. Loss of receptors and IgE in vivo during treatment with anti-IgE antibody. J Allergy Clin Immunol 2004; 114(6):1472–1474.
14. Smurthwaite L, Walker SN, Wilson DR, et al. Persistent IgE synthesis in the nasal mucosa of hay fever patients. Eur J Immunol 2001; 31(12):3422–3431.
15. Durham SR, Smurthwaite L, Gould HJ. Local IgE production. Am J Rhinol 2000; 14(5):305–307.
16. Wilson DR, Merrett TG, Varga EM, et al. Increases in allergen-specific IgE in BAL after segmental allergen challenge in atopic asthmatics. Am J Respir Crit Care Med 2002; 165(1): 22–26.
17. MacGlashan DW Jr. Releasability of human basophils: cellular sensitivity and maximal histamine release are independent variables. J Allergy Clin Immunol 1993; 91:605–615.
18. MacGlashan DW Jr. Relationship between Syk and SHIP expression and secretion from human basophils in the general population. J Allergy Clin Immunol 2007; 119:626–633.
19. Erwin EA, Ronmark E, Wickens K, et al. Contribution of dust mite and cat specific IgE to total IgE: relevance to asthma prevalence. J Allergy Clin Immunol 2007; 119(2):359–365.
20. MacGlashan DW Jr., Ishmael S, Macdonald SM, et al. Induced loss of Syk in human basophils by non-IgE-dependent stimuli. J Immunol 2008; 180(6):4208–4217.
21. Vonakis BM, MacGlashan DW Jr., Vilarino N, et al. Distinct characteristics of signal transduction events by histamine releasing factor/translationally controlled tumor protein (HRF/TCTP)-induced priming and activation of human basophils. Blood 2008; 111:1789–1796.
22. Ochensberger B, Daepp GC, Rihs S, et al. Human blood basophils produce interleukin-13 in response to IgE-receptor-dependent and -independent activation. Blood 1996; 88:3028–3032.
23. Redrup AC, Howard BP, MacGlashan DW Jr., et al. Differential regulation of IL-4 and IL-13 secretion by human basophils: their relationship to histamine release in mixed leukocyte cultures. J Immunol 1998; 160:1957–1964.
24. Sin AZ, Roche EM, Togias A, et al. Nerve growth factor or IL-3 induces more IL-13 production from basophils of allergic subjects than from basophils of nonallergic subjects. J Allergy Clin Immunol 2001; 108(3):387–393.
25. Schroeder J. In Vitro Implications of Basophil Phenotypes. Philadelphia: AAAAI Workshop, 2008.
26. Miura K, Hubbard WC, MacGlashan DW Jr. Phosphorylation of cytosolic PLA2 (cPLA2) by Interleukin-3 (IL-3) is associated with increased free arachidonic acid and LTC4 release in human basophils. J Allergy Clin Immunol 1998; 102:512–520.
27. Kurimoto Y, de Weck AL, Dahinden CA. The effect of interleukin 3 upon IgE-dependent and IgE-independent basophil degranulation and leukotriene generation. Eur J Immunol 1991; 21(2): 361–368.
28. Kurimoto Y, de Weck AL, Dahinden CA. Interleukin 3-dependent mediator release in basophils triggered by C5a. J Exp Med 1989; 170(2):467–479.
29. Tschopp CM, Spiegl N, Didichenko S, et al. Granzyme B, a novel mediator of allergic inflammation: its induction and release in blood basophils and human asthma. Blood 2006; 108(7): 2290–2299.
30. Kalesnikoff J, Huber M, Lam V, et al. Monomeric IgE stimulates signaling pathways in mast cells that lead to cytokine production and cell survival. Immunity 2001; 14(6):801–811.
31. Asai K, Kitaura J, Kawakami Y, et al. Regulation of mast cell survival by IgE. Immunity 2001; 14(6):791–800.
32. Hsu C, MacGlashan D J. IgE antibody up-regulates high affinity IgE binding on murine bone marrow derived mast cells. Immunol Lett 1996; 52:129–134.
33. Kitaura J, Xiao W, Maeda-Yamamoto M, et al. Early divergence of Fc epsilon receptor I signals for receptor up-regulation and internalization from degranulation, cytokine production, and survival. J Immunol 2004; 173(7):4317–4323.
34. Kitaura J, Song J, Tsai M, et al. Evidence that IgE molecules mediate a spectrum of effects on mast cell survival and activation via aggregation of the FcepsilonRI. Proc Natl Acad Sci U S A 2003; 100(22):12911–12916.
35. Hlavacek WS, Redondo A, Metzger H, et al. Kinetic proofreading models for cell signaling predict ways to escape kinetic proofreading. Proc Natl Acad Sci U S A 2001; 98(13):7295–7300.

36. Torigoe C, Inman JK, Metzger H. An unusual mechanism for ligand antagonism. Science 1998; 281(5376):568–572.

37. Schroeder JT, Miura K, Kim HH, et al. Selective expression of nuclear factor of activated T cells 2/c1 in human basophils: evidence for involvement in IgE-mediated IL-4 generation. J Allergy Clin Immunol 2002; 109(3):507–513.

38. Miura K, MacGlashan DW Jr. Phosphatidylinositol-3 kinase regulates p21ras activation during IgE-mediated stimulation of human basophils. Blood 2000; 96:2199–2205.

39. Vazquez F, Devreotes P. Regulation of PTEN function as a PIP3 gatekeeper through membrane interaction. Cell Cycle 2006; 5(14):1523–1527.

40. Huber M, Helgason CD, Damen JE, et al. The src homology 2-containing inositol phosphatase (SHIP) is the gatekeeper of mast cell degranulation. Proc Natl Acad Sci U S A 1998; 95(19): 11330–11335.

41. Vonakis BM, Gibbons S Jr., Sora R, et al. Src homology 2 domain-containing inositol 5′ phosphatase is negatively associated with histamine release to human recombinant histamine-releasing factor in human basophils. J Allergy Clin Immunol 2001; 108(5):822–831.

42. Lavens-Phillips SE, MacGlashan DW Jr. Pharmacology of human basophil desensitization. FASEB J 1999; 13:A338.

43. Odom S, Gomez G, Kovarova M, et al. Negative regulation of immunoglobulin E-dependent allergic responses by Lyn kinase. J Exp Med 2004; 199(11):1491–1502.

44. Xiao W, Nishimoto H, Hong H, et al. Positive and negative regulation of mast cell activation by Lyn via the FcepsilonRI. J Immunol 2005; 175(10):6885–6892.

45. Paolini R, Molfetta R, Beitz LO, et al. Activation of Syk tyrosine kinase is required for c-Cbl-mediated ubiquitination of Fcepsilon RI and Syk in RBL cells. J Biol Chem 2002; 277(40): 36940–36947.

46. Zhang J, Chiang YJ, Hodes RJ, et al. Inactivation of c-Cbl or Cbl-b differentially affects signaling from the high affinity IgE receptor. J Immunol 2004; 173(3):1811–1818.

47. MacGlashan D, Miura K. Loss of syk kinase during IgE-mediated stimulation of human basophils. J Allergy Clin Immunol 2004; 114(6):1317–1324.

48. MacGlashan DW Jr., Laven-Phillips S, Katsushi M. IgE-mediated desensitization in human basophils and mast cells. Front Biosci 1998; 3:d746–d756.

49. MacGlashan DW Jr. Two regions of down-regulation in the IgE-mediated signaling pathway in human basophils. J Immunol 2003; 170:4814–4925.

50. MacGlashan DW Jr., Vilarino N. Nonspecific desensitization, functional memory and the characteristics of SHIP phosphorylation following IgE-mediated stimulation of human basophils. J Immunol 2006; 177:1040–1051.

51. MacGlashan DW Jr., Undem BJ. Inducing an anergic state in mast cells and basophils without secretion. J Allergy Clin Immunol 2008; 121(6):1500–1506.

52. Lavens-Phillips SE, Miura K, MacGlashan DW Jr. Pharmacology of IgE-mediated desensitization of human basophils: effects of protein kinase C and Src-family kinase inhibitors. Biochem Pharmacol 2000; 60:1717–1227.

53. Vilarino N, Miura K, MacGlashan DW Jr. Acute IL-3 priming up-regulates the stimulus-induced Raf-1-Mek-Erk cascade independently of IL-3-induced activation of Erk. J Immunol 2005; 175(5):3006–3014.

54. Yamaguchi M, Hirai K, Ohta K, et al. Culturing in the presence of IL-3 converts anti-IgE nonresponding basophils into responding basophils. J All Clin Immunol 1996; 97:1279–1287.

55. Knol EF, Mul FPJ, Jansen H, et al. Monitoring human basophil activation via CD63 monoclonal antibody 435. J All Clin Immunol 1991; 88:328–338.

56. MacGlashan DW Jr. Graded changes in the response of individual human basophils to stimulation: distributional behavior of events temporally coincident with degranulation. J Leukocyte Biology 1995; 58:177–188.

57. Majlesi Y, Samorapoompichit P, Hauswirth AW, et al. Cerivastatin and atorvastatin inhibit IL-3-dependent differentiation and IgE-mediated histamine release in human basophils and downmodulate expression of the basophil-activation antigen CD203c/E-NPP3. J Leukoc Biol 2003; 73(1):107–117.

58. Yoshimura C, Yamaguchi M, Iikura M, et al. Activation markers of human basophils: CD69 expression is strongly and preferentially induced by IL-3. J Allergy Clin Immunol 2002; 109(5): 817–823.

59. Buhring HJ, Simmons PJ, Pudney M, et al. The monoclonal antibody 97A6 defines a novel surface antigen expressed on human basophils and their multipotent and unipotent progenitors. Blood 1999; 94(7):2343–2356.

60. Buhring HJ, Seiffert M, Giesert C, et al. The basophil activation marker defined by antibody 97A6 is identical to the ectonucleotide pyrophosphatase/phosphodiesterase 3. Blood 2001; 97(10): 3303–3305.

61. Lourenco FD, Azor MH, Santos JC, et al. Activated status of basophils in chronic urticaria leads to interleukin-3 hyper-responsiveness and enhancement of histamine release induced by anti-IgE stimulus. Br J Dermatol 2008; 158(5):979–986.

62. Hennersdorf F, Florian S, Jakob A, et al. Identification of CD13, CD107a, and CD164 as novel basophil-activation markers and dissection of two response patterns in time kinetics of IgE-dependent upregulation. Cell Res 2005; 15(5):325–335.

63. Saini S, Bloom DC, Bieneman A, et al. Systemic effects of allergen exposure on blood basophil IL-13 secretion and FcepsilonRIbeta. J Allergy Clin Immunol 2004; 114(4):768–774.

64. MacGlashan DW Jr., Guo CB. Oscillations in free cytosolic calcium during IgE-mediated stimulation distinguish human basophils from human mast cells. J Immunol 1991; 147: 2259–2269.

65. MacGlashan DW Jr., Bochner B, Warner JA. Graded changes in the response of individual human basophils to stimulation: distributional behavior of early activation events. J Leuko Biol 1994; 55:13–23.

66. Kern F, Lichtenstein LM. Defective histamine release in chronic urticaria. J Clin Invest 1976; 57(5):1369–1377.

67. Greaves MW, Plummer VM, McLaughlan P, et al. Serum and cell bound IgE in chronic urticaria. Clin Allergy 1974; 4(3):265–271.

68. Vonakis BM, Vasagar K, Gibbons SP Jr., et al. Basophil FcepsilonRI histamine release parallels expression of Src-homology 2-containing inositol phosphatases in chronic idiopathic urticaria. J Allergy Clin Immunol 2007; 119(2):441–448.

69. Sabroe RA, Francis DM, Barr RM, et al. Anti-Fc(epsilon)RI auto antibodies and basophil histamine releasability in chronic idiopathic urticaria. J Allergy Clin Immunol 1998; 102(4 pt 1): 651–658.

70. Luquin E, Kaplan AP, Ferrer M. Increased responsiveness of basophils of patients with chronic urticaria to sera but hypo-responsiveness to other stimuli. Clin Exp Allergy 2005; 35(4):456–460.

71. Sokol CL, Barton GM, Farr AG, et al. A mechanism for the initiation of allergen-induced T helper type 2 responses. Nat Immunol 2008; 9(3):310–318.

72. Eckman JA, Hamilton RG, Gober LM, et al. Basophil phenotypes in chronic idiopathic urticaria in relation to disease activity and autoantibodies. J Invest Dermatol 2008; 128(8):1956–1963.

73. MacGlashan DW Jr., Bochner BS, Adelman DC, et al. Down-regulation of FceRI expression on human basophils during in vivo treatment of atopic patients with anti-IgE antibody. J Immunol 1997; 158:1438–1445.

74. Vonakis BM, Saini SS. Syk-deficient basophils from donors with chronic idiopathic urticaria exhibit a spectrum of releasability. J Allergy Clin Immunol 2008; 121(1):262–264.

75. Gober LM, Eckman JA, Sterba PM, et al. Expression of activation markers on basophils in a controlled model of anaphylaxis. J Allergy Clin Immunol 2007; 119(5):1181–1188.

76. Vasagar K, Vonakis BM, Gober LM, et al. Evidence of in vivo basophil activation in chronic idiopathic urticaria. Clin Exp Allergy 2006; 36(6):770–776.

77. Hide M, Francis DM, Grattan CE, et al. Autoantibodies against the high-affinity IgE receptor as a cause of histamine release in chronic urticaria. N Engl J Med 1993; 328(22):1599–1604.

78. Hide M, Francis DM, Grattan CE, et al. The pathogenesis of chronic idiopathic urticaria: new evidence suggests an auto-immune basis and implications for treatment. Clin Exp Allergy 1994; 24(7):624–627.

79. Fiebiger E, Maurer D, Holub H, et al. Serum IgG autoantibodies directed against the alpha chain of Fc epsilon RI: a selective marker and pathogenetic factor for a distinct subset of chronic urticaria patients? J Clin Invest 1995; 96(6):2606–2612.

80. Fiebiger E, Hammerschmid F, Stingl G, et al. Anti-FcepsilonRIalpha autoantibodies in autoimmune-mediated disorders. Identification of a structure-function relationship. J Clin Invest 1998; 101(1):243–251.

81. Tong LJ, Balakrishnan G, Kochan JP, et al. Assessment of autoimmunity in patients with chronic urticaria. J Allergy Clin Immunol 1997; 99(4):461–465.

82. Soundararajan S, Kikuchi Y, Joseph K, et al. Functional assessment of pathogenic IgG subclasses in chronic autoimmune urticaria. J Allergy Clin Immunol 2005; 115(4):815–821.

83. Kikuchi Y, Kaplan AP. Mechanisms of autoimmune activation of basophils in chronic urticaria. J Allergy Clin Immunol 2001; 107(6):1056–1062.

84. Sabroe RA, Grattan CE, Francis DM, et al. The autologous serum skin test: a screening test for autoantibodies in chronic idiopathic urticaria. Br J Dermatol 1999; 140(3):446–452.

85. Yasnowsky KM, Dreskin SC, Efaw B, et al. Chronic urticaria sera increase basophil CD203c expression. J Allergy Clin Immunol 2006; 117(6):1430–1434.

86. Gyimesi E, Sipka S, Danko K, et al. Basophil CD63 expression assay on highly sensitized atopic donor leucocytes-a useful method in chronic autoimmune urticaria. Br J Dermatol 2004; 151(2):388–396.

87. Szegedi A, Irinyi B, Gal M, et al. Significant correlation between the CD63 assay and the histamine release assay in chronic urticaria. Br J Dermatol 2006; 155(1):67–75.

88. Frezzolini A, Provini A, Teofoli P, et al. Serum-induced basophil CD63 expression by means of a tricolour flow cytometric method for the in vitro diagnosis of chronic urticaria. Allergy 2006; 61(9):1071–1077.

89. Boumiza R, Monneret G, Forissier MF, et al. Marked improvement of the basophil activation test by detecting CD203c instead of CD63. Clin Exp Allergy 2003; 33(2):259–265.

90. Ocmant A, Peignois Y, Mulier S, et al. Flow cytometry for basophil activation markers: the measurement of CD203c up-regulation is as reliable as CD63 expression in the diagnosis of cat allergy. J Immunol Methods 2007; 320(1–2):40–48.

5

Mechanisms of Bradykinin Formation

Allen P. Kaplan
Department of Medicine, Medical University of South Carolina, Charleston, South Carolina, U.S.A.

INTRODUCTION

The plasma kinin–forming system consists of three essential proteins that interact in a complex fashion once bound to certain negatively charged inorganic surfaces, or to a macromolecular complex formed during an inflammatory response, or bound to proteins along cell surfaces. These are coagulation Factor XII (Hageman factor, HF), prekallikrein, and high molecular weight kininogen (HK). Once Factor XII is activated to Factor XIIa, it converts pre-kallikrein to kallikrein and kallikrein digests HK to liberate bradykinin. Factor XIIa has a second substrate in plasma; namely, coagulation Factor XI and activation of surface-bound Factor XI by Factor XIIa initiates the intrinsic coagulation pathway. Thus the interactions of all four of these proteins are known as contact activation, and the formation of bradykinin is therefore a cleavage product of the initiating step of the cascade (Fig. 1) (1). There is also a tissue pathway (2) by which bradykinin is generated in which there is intracellular conversion of prokallikrein to tissue kallikrein by enzymes that are as yet not well characterized. Tissue kallikrein is secreted into the local milieu where it digests low molecular weight kininogen (LK) to generate Lysyl-bradykinin (kallidin) and an aminopeptidase converts kallidin to bradykinin. The bradykinin that is produced by either pathway is then degraded by plasma enzymes as well as enzymes that are active along the surface of endothelial cells (particularly pulmonary vascular endothelial cells) to lower molecular weight peptides. The major plasma enzyme is carboxypeptidase N (3). This removes the C-terminal arginine from bradykinin to yield an eight amino acid peptide (des-arg-9 bradykinin) (4). The second kininase in plasma is termed "kininase II" and is identical to angiotensin-converting enzyme (5). This latter enzyme predominates along the pulmonary vascular endothelial cell surface. Bradykinin is thereby rapidly degraded within one or two circulation times. This enzyme removes the dipeptide Phe-Arg from the C-terminus of bradykinin to yield a heptapeptide and a second cleavage removes ser-pro to leave a pentapeptide (6). Bradykinin acts on the B2 receptor on the surface of endothelial cells to cause vasodilatation and to increase vascular permeability. Other vasodilators such as nitric oxide are produced secondarily as a result of B2 receptor stimulation (7). Des-Arg-9

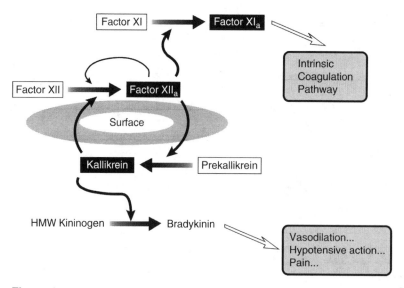

Figure 1 The contact activation pathway leading to bradykinin formation.

bradykinin, the product of carboxypeptidase N, is predominantly active upon B1 receptors (8). These latter receptors, in contrast to B2 receptors, are not constitutively produced but are induced as a result of inflammation due to the presence of cytokines such as interleukin-1 and tumor necrosis factor-α (TNF) (8,9). The heptapeptide and pentapeptide products of kininase II (ACE) are inactive. Additional enzymes that may contribute to bradykinin degradation are encephalinase and aminopeptidase P; any inhibition of these enzymes or polymorphisms that affect their concentration or activity may have a role in angioedema formation due to ACE inhibitors. A schematic diagram of the formation and degradation of bradykinin is shown in Figure 2. Table 1 summarizes some of major physical chemical properties of the various proteins of the contact activation cascade.

Bradykinin Formation

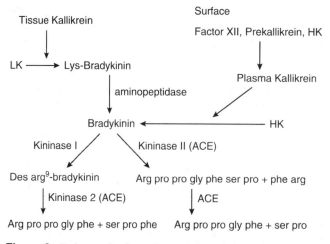

Figure 2 Pathways for formation and degradation of bradykinin.

Table 1 Physiochemical Properties of Proteins of the Contact Activation Cascade

Protein	Factor XII	Prekallikrein	Factor XI	HK
Molecular weight (Da; calculated)	80,427	79,545	140,000	116,643
Carbohydrate (w/w)	16.8%	15%	5%	40%
Isoelectric point	6.3	8.7	8.6	4.7
Extinction coefficient (E1% 280/nm)	14.2	11.7	13.4	7.0
Plasma concentration: g/mL	30–45	35–50	4–6	70–90
nmol/L (average)	400	534	36	686

FACTOR XII

Factor XII circulates as a single chain zymogen that is devoid of enzymatic activity. It has a molecular weight of approximately 80,000 on sodium dodecyl sulfate (SDS) gel electrophoresis, is synthesized in the liver, and circulates in the plasma at a concentration of 30 to 35 µg/mL. Its primary sequence has been deduced from cDNA analysis and from direct protein sequence data (10,11). It has distinct domains analogous to fibronectin, plasminogen, and plasminogen activators at its N-terminal end, whereas the C terminus has the catalytic domain. This latter domain is homologous to serine proteases such as pancreatic trypsin and even more so to the catalytic domain of plasminogen activators. Factor XII is capable of autoactivating once it is bound to initiating surfaces (12) as a result of a conformational change that renders bound Factor XII to become a substrate for Factor XIIa (13). The source of the initiating molecules of Factor XIIa is uncertain; however, it is assumed that trace quantities of Factor XIIa are present and that the amount is far less than the limit of detection. The alternative, that uncleaved native Factor XII possesses some minute amount of enzymatic activity seems less likely. Activation of Factor XII is due to a cleavage at a critical Arg-Val bond contained within a disulfide bridge such that the resultant Factor XIIa is a two-chain disulfide-linked 80 Kd enzyme consisting of a heavy chain of 50 Kd and light of 28 Kd (14). The light chain contains the active site and is located at the C-terminal end, whereas the heavy chain contains the binding site for the surface at the amino-terminal end (15). Further cleavage can occur at the C-terminal end of the heavy chain to produce a series of fragments of activated Factor XII, which retain enzymatic activity (16).

The most prominent of these is a 30-Kd species termed "Factor XIIf" (17). Careful examination of Factor XIIf on SDS gels under nonreducing conditions reveals a doublet in which the higher band at 30 Kd is gradually converted to the lower band, which has a molecular weight of 28.5 Kd (18). Reduced gels demonstrate that these species consist of the light chain of Factor XIIa disulfide linked to small peptides derived from the C-terminus of the heavy chain. These fragments lack the ability to bind to the surface and therefore are unable to convert Factor XI to XIa, (which requires interaction at the surface) but continue to be potent activators of prekallikrein. Thus formation of Factor XIIf allows bradykinin production to continue in the fluid phase until the enzyme is inactivated and the reactions can therefore proceed at sites distant from the initiating surface. This may be important for bradykinin formation in diseases such as C1inhibitor deficiency in which the inhibitor of Factor XIIa and Factor XIIf is absent or dysfunctional. A diagrammatic representation of these various steps in Factor XII activation is shown in Figure 3. Once Factor XIIa interacts with prekallikrein to generate the enzyme kallikrein, there follows an important positive feedback in which kallikrein digests surface bound Factor XII rapidly to form Factor XIIa and then Factor XIIf (19–21). This reaction is far

Bradykinin Formation

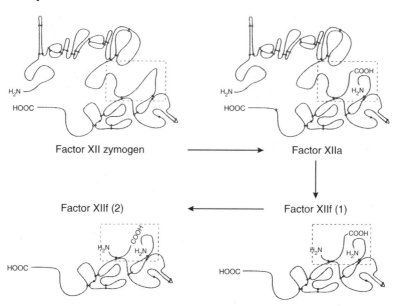

Figure 3 Diagrammatic representation depicting the sequential cleavages occurring in Factor XIIa leading initially to Factor XIIa, followed by cleavages external to the disulfide bridge to form Factor XIIf (1) and Factor XIIf (2). Note on the C-terminal portion of the heavy chain disulfide linked to the light chain.

more rapid than the initiating autoactivation reaction, thus there is a reciprocal reaction involving these two constituents: the initial small amount of Factor XIIa formed by autoactivation converts prekallikrein to kallikrein and kallikrein digests the residual Factor XII to Factor XIIa. The slower activation of this cascade dependent upon autoactivation can be demonstrated in plasma that is congenitally deficient in prekallikrein (Fletcher trait), which cannot generate any kallikrein or bradykinin (20). Coagulation (i.e., conversion of Factor XI to Factor XIa by Factor XIIa) proceeds, although at a much slower rate, and the partial thromboplastin time (PTT) can be shown to shorten progressively, as the time of incubation of the plasma, which the surface is increased prior to recalcification. This appears because of to progressive Factor XIIa autoactivation as the incubation time with the surface is increased. As more and more Factor XIIa forms, the rate of Factor XI activation increases and the PTT approaches normal. The difference in PTT with short incubation times between normal plasma and prekallikrein deficient plasma is due to the absence of the feedback activation of Factor XII by kallikrein.

PREKALLIKREIN

Prekallikrein is also a circulating proenzyme, which requires proteolytic cleavage to generate an active protease. On SDS gels it has two bands at 88 and 85 Kd, and the heterogeneity observed is not reflected in its amino acid sequence (22). Thus it appears likely to be due to two variant glycosylated forms that are present in everyone. It is synthesized with a signal peptide of 19 residues, which is removed prior to secretion. The mature plasma prekallikrein has 619 amino acids with a calculated molecular weight of

69,710, including 15% carbohydrate (23). Activation of prekallikrein by Factor XIIa or Factor XIIf is the result of cleavage of a single Arg-Ile bond within a disulfide bridge such that a heavy chain of 56 Kd is disulfide linked to light chains of either 33 Kd or 36 Kd reflecting the heterogeneity within the two forms of the zymogen. Thus the heterogeneity is reflected in the light chain and the light chain also contains the active site of the enzyme (22). The amino acid sequence of the kallikrein-heavy chain is unusual and homologous only to the corresponding portion of Factor XI. It has four tandem repeats, each of which contains 90 to 91 amino acids (23). The presence of six cysteines per repeat suggests that each repeat contains three disulfide loops. The gene coding for this ancestral structure may have duplicated and then the entire segment duplicated once again to create the four tandem repeats. The light chain containing the active site is homologous to the catalytic domains of many other enzymes of the coagulation cascade.

Prekallikrein circulates in plasma bound to HK in a 1:1 bimolecular complex (24) through a site contained in the heavy chain. The binding is firm with a disassociation constant of 12 to 15 nM, which is unchanged upon conversion of prekallikrein to kallikrein (24,25). It has been shown that 80% to 90% of prekallikrein is normally complexed in this way and it is the prekallikrein/HK complex that binds to surfaces during contact activation. That binding occurs primarily through HK. The disassociation of 10% to 20% of the kallikrein that forms along the surface may serve to propagate the formation of bradykinin in the fluid phase at sites distant from the initiating reaction (26,27).

FACTOR XI

Coagulation Factor XI is an alternative substrate of Factor XIIa; however, it has no role in bradykinin formation. Factor XI is unique among coagulation factors because the circulating zymogen consists of two identical chains linked by disulfide bonds (28,29). This dimer has an apparent molecular weight of 160 Kd on SDS gel electrophoresis and is half that size when reduced. Factor XI activation, like that of prekallikrein, requires a cleavage of a single Arg-Ile bond with a disulfide bridge to yield an amino-terminal heavy chain of 50 Kd and a disulfide-linked light chain of 33 Kd. Since both subunits can be activated, the active enzyme has two active sites, each of which is located on a light chain. Factor XIa is therefore a four-chain protein with two active sites. Its concentration in plasma is only 4–8 ~g/mL, which is among the lowest of the contact activation proteins, and its heavy chain, like that of prekallikrein, binds to the light chain of HK. Thus Factor XI and HK also circulate as a complex (30). The disassociation constant of 70 nM is high enough to ensure that virtually all of Factor XI contained in plasma is complexed to HK. The molar ratio of the complex can consist of one or two molecules of HK per Factor XI because of the dimeric nature of Factor XI. The binding site for HK on Factor XI has been localized to the first of the four tandem repeats contained within the Factor XI heavy chain. The Factor XI/HK complex binds to surfaces by the HK moiety and conversion to Factor XIa occurs as a result of cleavage by Factor XIIa or by thrombin (31,32). Factor XIIf has only 2% to 4% of the activity of Factor XIIa (16), thus Factor XIIf remains a potent activator of prekallikrein but has little impact on the coagulation pathway. The primary function of Factor XIa is to activate Factor IX to Factor IXa, which is the first calcium-dependent reaction in the intrinsic coagulation cascade. The amino acid sequence of Factor XI is closely homologous to that of prekallikrein (33). It also has a 19 amino acid leader peptide, which is cleaved to yield a protein of 607 amino acids contained in each of the two chains of the mature protein. The heavy chain of Factor XIa has four tandem repeats of approximately 90 amino acids, each with 6 cysteines implying 3 double bonds per repeat, as is seen in prekallikrein. However, unpaired cysteines in the first and fourth repeats are postulated to form the interchain disulfide bridges between monomers to produce the homodimer.

HIGH MOLECULAR WEIGHT KININOGEN

HK circulates in plasma as a 115 Kd nonenzymatic glycoprotein with a concentration of 70 to 90 ~g/mL (24,34). Its apparent molecular weight by gel filtration is approximately 200,000, indicating a large partial specific volume resulting from its conformation in solution. It forms non-covalent complexes with both prekallikrein and Factor XI, as indicated above. There is sufficient HK in plasma to theoretically bind both Factor XIIa substrates, leaving about 10% to 20% of circulating HK uncomplexed. The attachment of prekallikrein or Factor XI to HK occurs within the C-terminal region of HK corresponding to the light chain that results after cleavage to release bradykinin (24,25,35,36). The isolated light chain (after reduction and alkylation) derived from cleaved HK possesses the same binding characteristics as the whole molecule. HK therefore functions as a coagulation factor and this activity resides in the light chain (35–37). Within that light chain there is a basic histidine-rich N-terminal domain that binds to initiating surfaces and a carboxy-terminal domain that binds prekallikrein or Factor XI. The single cysteine within the light chain forms the disulfide bridge, which links it to the heavy chain. The kallikrein binding sites maps to residues 194–224 and the Factor XI binding site maps to residues 185–252 (36,38). Since these sites overlap, one molecule of HK can interact with one molecule of prekallikrein or one molecule of Factor XI, but not both. During contact activation, kallikrein cleaves HK at two positions within a disulfide bridge. The first is at a C-terminal Arg-Ser bond followed by cleavage at the N-terminal Lys-Arg bond to release the nonapeptide bradykinin (Arg-Pro-Pro-Gly-Phe-Ser-Pro-Phe-Arg). The two-chain disulfide-linked kinin-free HK results, consists of a heavy chain of 65 Kd disulfide link to a light chain of molecular weight 46 to 49 Kd (37,35–41). It is important to note that tissue kallikrein is immunologically and structurally unrelated to plasma kallikrein. It is secreted by various organs or cells such as salivary glands, kidney, pancreas, prostate, pituitary gland, and neutrophils, and is found in high concentrations of saliva, urine, and prostatic fluid. Its primary substrate is LK but it can release kallidin (Lysl BK) from either HK or LK (42,43). Kallidin is functionally very similar to bradykinin, although slightly less potent. A plasma aminopeptidase removes the N-terminal Lys to convert kallidin to bradykinin.

The very unusual domain structure of HK is shown in Figure 4. Domain 5 of the histadine-rich region at the N-terminal end of the light chain binds to initiating surfaces, while the binding of prekallikrein or Factor XI to the C-terminal domain 6 of the light chain accounts for the cofactor function of HK in intrinsic coagulation and kinin generation. HK has 626 amino acids with a calculated molecular weight of 69,896: an unusually high content of carbohydrate accounts for 40% of its residual molecular weight totaling 115 Kd. The heavy chain of 362 residues is derived from the N terminus. This is followed by the bradykinin sequence (domain 4) and then the light chain of 265 residues. The N-terminal end is blocked with a pyroglutamic acid. The carbohydrate is distributed via three N-linked glycosidic linkages on the HK chain and nine O-linked glycosidic linkages on the light chain. The heavy chain has three contiguous and homologous

Bradykinin Formation

HK Domains

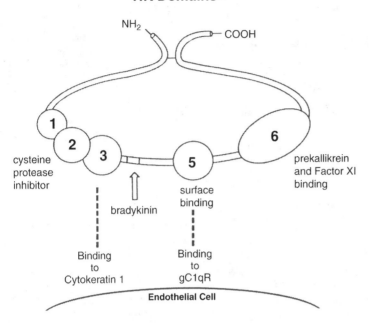

Figure 4 Domain structure of HK depicting attachment to an endothelial cell by domains 3 and 5 interacting with cytokeratin 1 and gC1qR, respectively.

domains consisting of amino acids 1–116, 117–238, and 239–360. There are 17 cysteines, one of which is disulfide linked to the light chain and the others form eight disulfide loops within these domains. The three domains of the heavy chain are homologous to the cystatin family of protease inhibitors. Domains 2 and 3 (but not 1) retain this inhibitory function so that native HK is capable of binding and inactivating two molecules of papain (44–46). Limited proteolysis of the heavy chain can occur at susceptible bonds that separate these domains so that individual domains can be isolated.

Plasma also contains another kininogen known as LK. Its digestion by tissue kallikrein yields Lysyl-bradykinin and a kinin-free two-chain molecule consisting of a 65 Kd heavy-chain disulfide link to a light chain of only 4 Kd. LK is not cleaved by plasma kallikrein. However the heavy chains of the two forms of the kininogen are identical in amino acid sequence starting at the amino terminus through the bradykinin sequence plus the next 12 residues. After that the two sequences diverge. Thus their light chains have no homology to each other. LK does not bind to surfaces nor to prekallikrein or Factor XI. The two forms of kininogen are formed from a single gene thought to have originated by two successive duplications of a primordial cystatin-like gene (47). As represented in Figure 5, there are 11 exons. The first nine code for the heavy chain, thus each of the three domains in this portion of the protein is encoded by three exons. The 10th exon codes for bradykinin and the light chain of HK, whereas the light chain of LK is encoded by exon 11. The mRNAs for HK and LK are produced by alternative splicing at a point 12 amino acids beyond the bradykinin sequence, thus enabling the two proteins to have different light chains (47,48).

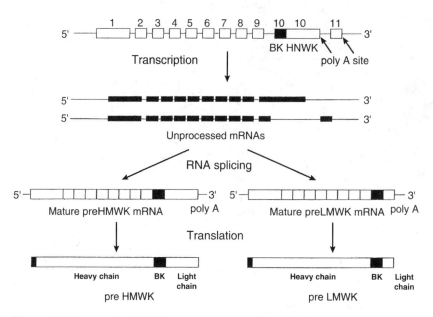

Figure 5 The gene for HK. The mature mRNAs are assembled by alternative splicing events in which the light chain sequences are attached to the 3' end of the 12 amino acid common sequence C-terminal to bradykinin.

MECHANISMS OF BRADYKININ FORMATION (CONTACT ACTIVATION)

Contact activation was initially defined by virtue of the interaction of blood with glass surfaces to initiate coagulation as well as the formation of bradykinin. Subsequently a variety of substances bearing negative charges along the surface were shown to be effective activators of the Factor XII dependent pathways including elagic acid and dextran sulfate. Dextran sulfate is among the few truly soluble activators and is often used to initiate contact activation. High molecular weight preparations of 500 Kd are typically used, but much smaller aggregates have been shown to be effective. Of particular interest is that the rate of Factor XII activation increases markedly with dextran sulfate polymers of 10 Kd or more as a theoretical number of Factor XII molecules capable of binding per particle increases from one to two. This presumably provides a critical intermolecular interaction required for optimal autoactivation. Naturally occurring polysaccharides are effective activators if they are highly sulfated, and these include heparin and condroitin sulfate E (49,50). To a lesser degree, Factor XII autoactivation can be catalyzed by dermatan sulfate, keratin polysulfate, or chondroitin sulfate C. One pathophysiologic substance likely to initiate contact activation in vivo is endotoxin, and there is good reason to believe the contact activation cascade is activated in septic shock and that observed symptoms are due in part to the generation of bradykinin (1). The pooling of fluid outside the vascular tree and the attendant hypotension are examples of abnormalities associated with septic shock that we typically attributed to cytokines but may also be dependent upon the generation of bradykinin.

The various interactions of the constituents required for the formation of bradykinin is shown in Figure 6. The initiating step is a slow autoactivation of Factor XII (12). However once this has occurred and prekallikrein is converted to kallikrein there is a positive feedback in which the kallikrein generated rapidly activates Factor XII to Factor XIIa. This

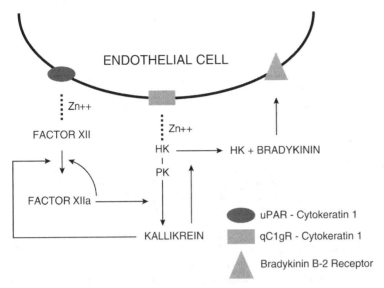

Figure 6 Diagrammatic representation of the binding of Factor XII and the primarily HK-PK complex to endothelial cells indicating that Factor XII binds to the U-PAR-cytokeratin 1 complex, HK binds to the gC1qR-cytokeratin 1 complex, and that activation to produce bradykinin can occur along the cell surface.

reaction is much more rapid than is autoactivation, thus the majority of the Factor XIIa generated is due to kallikrein. The presence of a surface plus this reciprocal interaction leads to a tremendously rapid activation of the cascade. It has been calculated that if one molecule each of Factor XIIa and kallikrein are present per milliliter in a mixture of Factor XII and prekallikrein at plasma concentration, the addition of an initiating surface will lead to a 50% conversion of Factor XII to Factor XIIa in 13 seconds (13). The source of the active enzyme in vivo is unknown but may be formed by other plasma proteases or by endogenous activation along cell surfaces. In fact a very slow turnover of the cascade may always be occurring but is controlled by plasma inhibitors (51). The addition of the cofactor HK (which was not included in the aforementioned kinetic analysis) accelerates these reactions even further. The surface appears to provide a local milieu in the contiguous fluid phase where the local concentrations of reactants are greatly increased (52). In addition, surface-bound Factor XII undergoes a conformational change that renders it more susceptible to cleavage.

The alternative idea–that binding of Factor XII induces a conformational change that exposes an active site–has been disproved, and formation of the active enzyme (Factor XIIa) requires cleavage of the zymogen (Factor XII). Inhibitors such as C1 inhibitor are not bound to the surface; thus the balance between activation and inactivation is lost. The effect of dilution of plasma diminishes the effect of inhibitors far more than slowing of enzymatic reaction rates; thus the net effect is a facilitation of activation. Using dextran sulfate as the initiator, the effect of the surface on Factor XIIa conversion of prekallikrein to kallikrein was 70-fold, whereas the effect on digestion of Factor XII by kallikrein was as much as 3000- to 12,000-fold (13). This latter reaction is about 2000 times more rapid than the rate of Factor XII autoactivation. Because of the predominance of kallikrein as a Factor XII activator, the PTT of prekallikrein-deficient plasma is prolonged but autocorrects if the incubation time with the surface is increased prior to addition of calcium ion. This allows Factor XII activation to occur by the slower autoactivation mechanism. On the other hand, Factor XII deficient plasma has a markedly abnormal PTT that does not autocorrect by increasing the time of incubation with the surface, clearly demonstrating that Factor XII is absolutely requisite for initiation to occur, whereas prekallikrein is not.

In plasma the involvement of HK as a coagulation factor was due to the discovery of persons whose plasma had a very prolonged PTT and who generated no bradykinin upon incubation with initiating surfaces yet were not deficient in Factor XII or prekallikrein. Subsequently HK was identified to be a nonenzymatic cofactor (53,54). It appeared to accelerate activation of both Factor XII and prekallikrein as well as Factor XI (Fig. 6). The discovery that prekallikrein and Factor XI circulate bound to HK provided the mechanistic key to the explanation. One function of HK is to present the substrates of Factor XIIa in a conformation that facilitates their activation (26,53). Thus prekallikrein or Factor XI that is bound directly to the surface in the absence of HK is not readily cleaved and cannot disassociate from the surface. Consistent with this idea is the demonstration that a synthetic peptide containing the HK-binding site for prekallikrein can interfere with contact activation by competitively interrupting the binding of prekallikrein to the HK light chain. A monoclonal antibody to this binding site likewise inhibits contact activation as well as bradykinin formation in plasma. Factor XI activation is almost totally dependent on the formation of a surface-binding complex with HK. More difficult to explain is the effect of HK on the rate of Factor XII activation in plasma since HK does neither interact with Factor XII nor does it augment the activity of kallikrein. This effect seems to be largely indirect. First, HK is required for efficient formation of kallikrein in surface-activated plasma (53,55). Second, since kallikrein can disassociate from surface-bound HK, it can interact with surface-bound Factor XII on an adjacent particle, thereby disseminating the reaction (26,27). As a result the effective kallikrein/ Factor XII ratio is increased in the presence of HK (26). Finally in plasma, HK can displace other adhesive glycoproteins such as fibrinogen from binding to the surface (56). In this sense HK, like Factor XII and prekallikrein, is also a coagulation cofactor because it is required for the generation of kallikrein (a Factor XII activator) as well as the activation of Factor XI. HK-deficient plasma has a profoundly prolonged activated PTT that is almost as abnormal as that of Factor XII deficiency, although persons with congenital HK deficiency have no bleeding diathesis. This is also true of Factor XII deficiency as well as prekallikrein deficiency (57–60). Patients with Factor XI deficiency, however, do have a form of hemophilia, although the magnitude of the abnormality varies greatly among different patients. For homeostasis the tissue factor–dependent pathway clearly predominates, and the role of Factor XI in augmenting coagulation appears to be dependent upon its activation by thrombin when incorporated into a clot (1). Thus the biology of Factor XII, prekallikrein, and HK in physiologic as well as pathologic processes may relate to inflammation, control of the microvasculature, and possibly fibrinolysis, rather than homeostasis or pathologic bleeding. The thrombin-dependent activation of Factor XI has been proposed to explain the absence of bleeding with deficiencies of Factor XII, prekallikrein, or HK; but this assertion has not been proven. Perhaps the capacity to generate bradykinin somehow facilitates bleeding.

CELL SURFACE ASSEMBLY OF THE PLASMA KININ–FORMING CASCADE

All the components of the bradykinin-forming cascade have been demonstrated to bind to endothelial cells. Schmaier et al. and Van Iwaarden et al. first described binding of HK to human umbilical vein endothelial cells (HUVEC) in a zinc-dependent fashion (61,62).

This binding was subsequently demonstrated in situ by immunochemical staining of umbilical cord segments following incubation with HK (63). HK binding to these cells was reversible, dependent upon 25 to 50 ~M zinc, and there were approximately 1 million binding sites per cell with a high affinity (Kd 40–50 nM). Binding is seen with both the heavy and light chain of HK (64) thus a complex interaction with cell membrane constituents is likely. Since prekallikrein binds to HK within the circulation, the complex is brought to the surface of the endothelial cell by virtue of HK binding. There appear to be no separate receptor sites for prekallikrein or Factor XI. When Factor XII interaction with HUVEC was studied, the former was found to bind with characteristics strikingly similar to those seen with HK, including a similar requirement for zinc (65). We subsequently demonstrated that HK and Factor XII could compete for binding at a comparable molar ratio, suggesting that they compete for binding to the same receptor sites. Three endothelial cell-binding sites for HK and for Factor XII have been described thus far. These include gC1qR, (the receptor for the globular heads of the C1q subcomponent of the first component of complement) (66,67), cytokeratin 1 (68,69), and the urokinase plasminogen activator receptor (u-PAR) (70). The binding of Factor XII and HK to each of these proteins is zinc dependent. gC1qR binds specifically to the light chain of HK and not to the heavy chain, and the binding locus is on the C-terminal domain of gC1qR (69). This is in contradistinction to C1q, which binds to the N-terminal domain of gC1qR. Thus C1q does not compete with either HK or Factor XII for binding, and the interaction of C1q with gC1qR is not zinc dependent. Domain 5 of HK located within the N-terminus of the light chain is rich in histidine and arginine residues and contains the site for interaction with gC1qR. A 20 amino acid peptide termed "HKH20" has been shown to be the site of interaction within domain 5, and this peptide can be used to inhibit the interaction of HK with intact endothelial cells (71). The other site for attachment of HK to endothelial cells is found within domain 3, and a peptide containing that binding site has been designated LDC27 (72). The binding affinity of the heavy chain to the cell is approximately 100-fold less than the light chain.

The second endothelial cell-binding site for HK is cytokeratin 1. Like gC1qR, this protein was isolated from cell membrane preparations employing affinity chromatography with HK or LDC27 as ligand. Cytokeratin 1, therefore, represents a major site of interaction for the HK heavy chain; however, it is capable of binding the light chain as well. Thus it does not possess the specificity that gC1qR does. However, light chain binding to gC1qR appears to predominate because of the affinity of the interaction as well as the much larger number of gC1qR-binding sites. u-PAR represents a third cell membrane constituent capable of binding to HK. We were unable to isolate this molecule by HK affinity chromatography; however, it was identified to participate in binding because anti-sera directed to u-PAR can inhibit the cell interaction with HK, and HK can be shown to bind to purified u-PAR in a zinc-dependent fashion. However, affinity chromatography using Factor XII as ligand leads to purification of u-PAR rather selectively, with only trace quantities of cytokeratin 1 or gC1qR present (73). Thus u-PAR may represent an important ligand for interaction with Factor XII, while gC1qR and cytokeratin 1 predominate in terms of HK binding. It had been proposed that gC1qR, cytokeratin 1, and u-PAR may form a trimolecular complex within the cell membrane. However, when we examined this in detail we were able to show that they actually interact as two bi-molecular complexes, with cytokeratin 1 being the common constituent (74). Thus anti-sera to gC1qR can be used to purify both gC1qR and cytokeratin 1, but not u-PAR, whereas antibody to u-PAR can be used to isolate u-PAR and cytokeratin 1, but not gC1qR. It is of interest that none of these three proteins possesses a transmembrane domain; thus its mechanism of attachment within the cell membrane is not clear with the exception of u-PAR. This is known to have a phosphatidyl-inositol linkage within the cell membrane, whereas gC1qR and cytokeratin 1 do not. Nevertheless each of them has been isolated from purified cell membranes and have been demonstrated to exist within the cell membrane by immunoelectronmicroscopy (75) presumably bound to other membrane constituents. In agreement with calculations of numbers of binding sites, gC1qR appears to be predominant within the cell membrane. A summary depicting these interactions is shown in Figure 6.

KININ FORMATION AT THE SURFACE OF ENDOTHELIAL CELLS

We have also demonstrated that Factor XII can slowly autoactivate when bound to endothelial cells (76), and that addition of kallikrein can digest bound HK to liberate bradykinin at a rate proportional to the kallikrein concentration. The final bradykinin level was dependent upon the amount of bound HK. Thus activation of the cascade may occur along the endothelial surface in a fashion analogous to that seen with contact activation of plasma. Bradykinin that is generated can then interact with the endothelial cell B2 receptor to increase vascular permeability (7,77). Bradykinin can also stimulate cultured endothelial cells to secrete tissue plasminogen activator, prostaglandin I_2 (prostacyclin), and thromboxane A2 and thereby modulate platelet function and stimulate local fibrinolysis (78).

An alternative pathway for activating the cascade has recently been demonstrated in which Factor XII is absent from the reaction mixture (79–82). Two different groups have isolated two different proteins, each of which seems to be able to catalyze activation of the HK-prekallikrein complex. One is heat shock protein 90 (83) and the other is a prolylcarboxypeptidase (84). The active site actually responsible for the conversion of prekallikrein to kallikrein is not clear in either case. They have strikingly similar inhibition profiles even though the two proteins are completely different. Heat shock protein 90 has ATPase activity, but no clear peptidase capability, and the prolocarboxypeptidase is an exopeptidase, whereas prekallikrein activation requires an endopeptidase. Neither protein is a direct prekallikrein activator as is Factor XIIa or Factor XIIf, but requires HK to be complexed to the prekallikrein (Fig. 7). The identification of the active

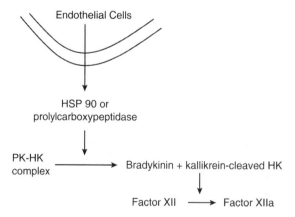

Figure 7   Factor XII – Independent activation of the bradykinin-forming cascade. *Note:* Figures 1, 3, and 5 have been published in Blood, Principles and Practice, Ed. Robert I. Handin, Samuel Lux, and Thomas P. Stossel, in chapter 38, the Contact System and its Disorders, Silverberg, M, Reddigari, SR, and Kaplan, AP., p. 1127–1150, J.B. Lippincott Company, Philadelphia 1995.

site responsible for conversion of prekallikrein to kallikrein has not yet been elucidated, but cleavage of prekallikrein is observed in SDS gels that are indistinguishable from that obtained with Factor XIIf. Nevertheless, each of these appears to make a contribution to Factor XII independent prekallikrein activation, and anti-sera to each protein have been shown to inhibit the process. When whole endothelial cells are incubated with normal plasma or Factor XII deficient plasma, the rate of activation of the deficient plasma is very much slower than that of the normal plasma, the latter being Factor XII dependent (82). Under normal circumstances (with Factor XII present), formation of kallikrein will lead to Factor XIIa formation even if the process was initiated by one of these cell-derived factors.

There are a number of interesting interactions between the proteins of the plasma kinin–forming cascade and the fibrinolytic pathway (85) as well as the renin-angiotensin pathway (86). For example, kallikrein converts plasma prourokinase to urokinase, and prourokinase that is bound to u-PAR is more readily activated (85). Thus kallikrein that has been produced along the cell surface can generate urokinase, which converts plasminogen to the fibrinolytic enzyme plasmin. Kallikrein has also been shown to mediate the acid phase of conversion of prorenin to renin in whole plasma. Renin converts angiotensinogen to angiotensin 1. Angiotensin-converting enzyme cleaves His–Leu from angiotensin 1 to yield angiotensin 2, and it is also a major inactivator of bradykinin (see chapter 22). The aforementioned prolylcarboxypeptidase does the reverse: it degrades angiotensin 2, but leads to bradykinin formation (81). Bradykinin formation relates to a variety of other inflammatory and noninflammatory disorders, including allergic rhinitis, asthma, anaphylaxis (87), pancreatitis, endotoxic shock, hypertension (1,2), coronary artery blood flow, ischemic cardiomyopathy, and Alzheimer's disease (88,89).

REFERENCES

1. Kaplan AP, Silverberg MA. Contact system and its disorders. In: Handin RI, Lux SE, Stossel TP, eds. Blood – Principles Practice of Hematology. 2nd. ed Philadelphia, PA: Lippincott Williams and Wilkins, 1995; 1131–1155.
2. Margolius HS. Tissue kallikreins. Structure, regulation, and participation in mammalian physiology and disease. Clin Rev Allergy Immunol 1998; 16:332–339.
3. Erdos EG, Sloane GM. An enzyme in human plasma that inactivates bradykinin and kallidins. Biochem Pharmacol 1962; 11:585–592.
4. Sheikh IA, Kaplan AP. Studies of the digestion of bradykinin, lysyl bradykinin and kinin degradation products by carboxypeptidases A, B, and N. Biochem Pharmacol 1986; 35:1957–1963.
5. Yang HYT, Erdos EG. Second kininase in human blood plasma. Nature 1967; 215:1402–1403.
6. Sheikh IA, Kaplan AP. Studies of the digestion of bradykinin, lysyl bradykinin and des-arg[9] bradykinin by angiotensin converting enzyme. Biochem Pharmacol 1986; 35:1951–1957.
7. Regoli D, Barabe J. Pharmacology of bradykinin and related kinins. Pharmacol Rev 1980; 32:1–46.
8. Marceau F. Kinin B1 receptors: a review. Immunopharmacology 1995; 30:1–26.
9. Davis AJ, Perkins MN. The involvement of bradykinin B1 and B2 receptor mechanisms in cytokine-induced mechanical hyperalgesia in the rat. Br J Pharmacol 1994; 113:63–68.
10. Cool DE, Edgell CS, Louie GV, et al. Characterization of human bood coagulation factor XII cDNA. J Biol Chem 1985; 25:13666–13676.
11. Que BG, Davie EW. Characterization of a cDNA coding for human factor XII (Hageman factor). Biochemistry 1986; 8:1525–1528.
12. Silverberg M, Dunn JT, Garen L, et al. Autoactivation of human Hageman factor. J Biol Chem 1980; 255:7281–7286.
13. Tankersley DL, Finlayson JS. Kinetics of activation and autoactivation of factor XII. Biochemmistry 1984; 23:273–279.

14. Revak SD, Cochrane CG. The relationship of structure and function in human Hageman factor. The association of enzymatic and binding activities with separate regions of the molecule. J Clin Invest 1976; 57:852–860.

15. McMullen BA, Fujikawa K. Amino acid sequence of the heavy chain of kinin (α factor XIIa (acivated Hageman factor). J Biol Chem 1995; 260:5328–5341.

16. Kaplan AP, Austen KF. A prealbumin activation of prekallikrein II. Derivation of activators of prekallikrein from active Hageman factor by digestion with plasmin. J Exp Med 1971; 133: 696–712.

17. Kaplan, AP, Austen KF. A prealbumin activation of prekallikrein. J Immunol 1970; 105:802–811.

18. Dunn JT, Kaplan AP. Formation and structure of human Hageman factor fragments. J Clin Invest 1982; 70:627–6231.

19. Cochrane CG, Revak SD, Whepper KD. Activation of Hageman factor in solid and fluid phases. A critical role of kallikrein. J Exp Med 1973; 138:1564–1583.

20. Weiss AS, Gallin JI, Kaplan AP. Fletcher factor deficiency. A diminished rate of Hageman factor activation caused by absence of prekallikrein with abnormalities of coagulation, fibrinolysis, chemotactic activity, and kinin generation. J Clin Invest 1974; 53:622–633.

21. Dunn JT, Silverberg M, Kaplan AP. The cleavage and formation of activated Hageman factor by autodigestion and by kallikrein. J Biol Chem 1982; 275:1779–1784.

22. Mandle RJ Jr., Kaplan AP. Hageman Factor substrates II. Human plasma prekallikrein: mechanism of activation by Hageman factor and participation in Hageman factor dependent fibrinolysis. J Biol Chem 1977; 252:6097–6104.

23. Chung DW, Fujikawa K, McMuller BA, et al. Human plasma prekallikrein is a zymogen to a serine protease that contains four tandem repeats. Biochemistry 1986; 25:2410–2417.

24. Mandle RJ, Colman RW, Kaplan AP. Identification of prekallikrein and high molecular weight kininogen as a complex in plasma. Prac Natl Acad Sci 1976; 73:4179–4183.

25. Beck PE, Shore JD, Tans G, et al. Protein-protein interactions in contact activation of blood coagulation. Binding of high molecular weight kininogen and the 5-(iodoacetamido) fluorescein-labeled kininogen light chain to prekallikrein, kallikrein, and the separated kallikrein heavy and light chains. J Biol Chem 1985; 260:12434–12443.

26. Silverberg M, Nicoll JE, Kaplan AP. The mechanism by which the light chain of cleaved HMW kininogen augments the activation of prekallikrein, factor XI, and Hageman factor. Thromb Res 1980; 70:173–189.

27. Cochrane CG, Revak SD. Dissemination of contact activation in plasma by plasma kallikrein. J Exp Med 1980; 152:608–617.

28. Bowma BN, Griffin JH. Human blood coagultion factor SI: purification, properties, and mechanism of activation by factor SII. J Biol Chem 1977; 252:6432–6437.

29. Kurachi K, Davie EW. Activation of human factor XI (partial thromboplastin antecedent) by factor XII (activated Hageman factor). Biochemistry 1977; 16:5831–5839.

30. Thompson RE, Mandle RJ, Kaplan AP. Association of factor XI and high molecular weight kininogen in human plasma. J Clin Invest 1977; 60:1376–1380.

31. Gailani D, Broze GJ. Factor XI activation in a revised model of blood coagulation. Science 1991; 253:909–912.

32. Naito K, Fujikawa K. Activation of human blood coagulation factor XI, independent of factor XII. Factor XI is activated by thrombin and factor XIa in the process of negatively charged surfaces. J Biol Chem 1991; 266:7353–7358.

33. Fujikawa K, Chung DW, Hendrickson LE, et al. Amino acid sequence of human factor XI, a blood coagulation factor with four tandem repeats that are highly homologous with plasma prekallikrein. Biochemistry 1986; 25:2417–2424.

34. Keribiriou DM, Griffin JH. Human high molecular weight kininogen. Studies of structure-function relationships and proteolysis of the molecule occurring during contact activation of plasma. J Biol Chem 1979; 245:12020–12027.

35. Thompson RE, Mandle RJ, Kaplan AP. Studies of the binding of prekallikrein and factor XI to high molecular weight kininogen and its light chain. Proc Natl Acad Sci 1979; 79:4862–4866.

36. Tait J, Fujikawa K. Primary structure requirements for the binding of human high molecular weight kininogen to prekallikrein and factor XI. J Biol Chem 1987; 262:11651–11656.
37. Thompson RE, Mandle RJ, Kaplan AP. Characterization of human high molecular weight kininogen: procoagulant activity associated with the light chain of kinin-free high molecular weight kininogen. J Exp Med 1978; 147:488–499.
38. Tait J, Fujikawa K. Identification of the binding site for plasma prekallikrein in human high molecular kininogen. J Biol Chem 1985; 261:15396–15401.
39. Nakayasu T, Nagasawa S. Studies on human kininogen I. Isolation, characterization, and cleavage by plasma kallikrein of high molecular weight kininogen. J Biochem 1979; 85:249–258.
40. Mori K, Nagasawa S. Studies on human high molecular weight (HMW) kininogen II. Structural change in HMW kininogen by the action of human plasma kallikrein. J Biochem 1981; 89:1465–1473.
41. Reddigari SR, Kaplan AP. Cleavage of high molecular weight kininogen by purified kallikreins and upon contact activation of plasma. Blood 1988; 71:1334–1340.
42. Jacobson S, Kritz M. some data on two purified kininogens from human plasma. Br J Pharmacol 1967; 29:25–36.
43. Mueller-Esterl W, Rauth G, Lottspeich F, et al. Limited proteolysis of human low molecular mass kininogen by tissue kallikrein. Isolation and characterization of the heavy and light chains. Eur J Biochem 1985; 149:15–22.
44. Muller-Esterl W, Fritz H, Machleidt IW, et al. Human plasma kininogens are identical with 2 cystein protease inhibitors. Evidence from immunological, enzymological, and sequence data. FEBS Lett 1985; 182:310–314.
45. Higashiyama S, Ohkubo I, Ishiguro H, et al. Human high molecular weight kininogen as a thiol protease inhibitor: presence of the entire inhibition capacity in the native form of heavy chain. Biocehmistry 1986; 25:1669–1675.
46. Ishiguro H, Higashiyama S, Ohkubo I, et al. Mapping of functional domains of human high molecular weight and low molecular weight kininogens using murine monoclonal antibodies. Biochemistry 1987; 26:7021–7029.
47. Kitamura N, Kitagawa H, Fukushima D, et al. Structural organization of the human kininogen gene and a model for its evolution. J Biol Chem 1985; 260:8610–8617.
48. Takagaki Y, Kitamura N, Nakanishi S. Cloning and sequence analysis of cDNAs for high molecular weight and low molecular weight prekininogen. J Biol Chem 1985; 260:8601–8609.
49. Hojima Y, Cochrane CG, Wiggins RC, et al. In vitro activation of the contact (Hageman factor) system of plasma by heparin and chondroitin sulfate E. Blood 1984; 63:1453–1459.
50. Brunnee T, Reddigari SR, Shibayama Y, et al. Mast cell derived heparin activates the contact system: a link to kinin generation in allergic reactions. Clin Exp Allergy 1997; 27:653–663.
51. Silverberg M, Kaplan, AP. Enzymatic activities of activated and zymogen forms of human Hageman factor (factor XII). Blood 1982; 60:64–70.
52. Griffin JH. Role of surface in surface-dependent activation of Hageman factor (blood coagulation factor XII). Proc Natl Acad Sci 1978; 75:1998–2002.
53. Griffin JH, Cochrane CG. Mechanisms for the involvement of high molecular weight kininogen in surface-dependent reactions of Hageman factor. Proc Natl Acad Sci 1976; 73:2554–2558.
54. Meier HL, Pierce JV, Colman RW, et al. Activation and function of human Hageman factor. The role of high molecular weight kininogen and prekallikrein. J Clin Invest 1977; 60:18–31.
55. Wiggins RC, Bouma BN, Cochraine, CG, et al. Role of high molecular weight kininogen in surface binding and activation of coagulation factor XI and prekallikrein. Proc Natl Acad Sci 1977; 74:4636–4640.
56. Schmaier AH, Silver L, Adams AL, et al. The effects of high molecular weight kininogen on surface-adsorbed fibrinogen. Thromb Res 1984; 33:51–67.
57. Wuepper KD. Prekallikrein deficiency in man. J Exp Med 1973; 138:1564–1583.
58. Colman RW, Bagdasarian A, Talamo RC, et al. Human kininogen deficiency with diminished levels of plasminogen proactivator and prekallikrein associated with abnormalities of the Hageman factor-dependent pathways. J Clin Invest 1975; 56:1650–1662.

59. Wuepper DK, Miller DR, LaCombe MJ. Flaujeac trait; deficiency of human plasma kinongen. J Clin Invest 1975; 56:1663–1672.
60. Donaldson VH, Glueck HI, Miller MA. Kininogen deficiency in Fitzgerald trait: role of high molecular weight kininogen in clotting and fibrinolysis. J Lab Clin Med 1976; 89:327–337.
61. Schmaier AH, Kuo A, Lundberg D, et al. The expression of high molecular weight kininogen on human umbilical vein endothelial cells. J Biol Chem 1988; 263:16327–16333.
62. Van Iwaarden F, de Groot PG, Bouma BN. The binding of high molecular weight kininogen to cultured human endothelial cells. J Biol Chem 1988; 263:4698–4703.
63. Nishikawa K, Kuna P, Calcaterra E, et al. Generation of the vasoactive peptide bradykinin from high molecular weight kininogen bound to human umbilical vein endothelial cells. Blood 1992; 80:1980–1988.
64. Reddigari SR, Kuna P, Miragliotta GF, et al. Human high molecular weight kininogen binds to human umbilical vein endothelial cells via its heavy and light chains. Blood 1993; 81:1306–1311.
65. Reddigari SR, Shibayama Y, Brunnee T, et al. Human Hageman factor 9factor XII) and high molecular weight kininogen compete for the same binding site on human umbilical vein endothelial cells. J Biol Chem 1993; 268:11982–11987.
66. Joseph K, Ghebrehiwet B, Peerschke EIB, et al. Identification of zinc-dependent endothelial cell binding protein for high molecular weight kininogen and factor XII: identity with the receptor that binds to the globular "heads" of C1q (gC1qR). Prac Natl Acad Sci USA 1996; 93: 8552–8557.
67. Herwald H, Dedio J, Kellner R, et al. Isolation and characterization of the kininogen binding protein p33 from endothelial cells. J Biol Chem 1996; 271:13040–13047.
68. Hasan AAK, Zisman T, Schmaier AH. Identification of cytokeratin 1 as a bindgin protein and presentation receptor for kininogens on endothelial cells. Proc Natl Acad Sci USA 1998; 95: 3615–3620.
69. Joseph K, Ghebrehiwet B, Kaplan AP. Cytokeratin 1 and gC1qR mediate high molecular weight kininogen binding to endothelial cells. Clin Immunol 1999; 92:246–255.
70. Colman RW, Pixley RA, Najamunnisa S, et al. Binding of high molecular weight kininogen to human endothelial cells is mediated via a site within domains 2 and 3 of the urokinase receptor. J Clin Invest 1997; 100:1481–1487.
71. Hasan AAK, Cines DB, Herwald H, et al. Mapping the cells binding site on high molecular weight kininogen domain 5. J Biol Chem 1995; 270:19256–19261.
72. Herwald H, Hasan AAK, Godovac-Zimmermann J, et al. Identification of an endothelial cell binding site on kininogen domain D3. J Biol Chem 1995; 270:14634–14642.
73. Joseph K, Kaplan AP. Unpublished observations.
74. Joseph K, Tholanikunnel BG, Ghebrehiwet B, et al. Interaction of high molecular weight kininogen binding proteins on endothelial cells. Int J Thrombosis Haemostasis 2004; 91:61–70.
75. Mahdi F, Shariet-Madur S, Todd RF III, et al. Expression and colocalization of cytokeratin 1 and urokinase plasminogen activator receptor on endothelial cells. Blood 2001; 97:2342–2350.
76. Joseph K, Shibayama Y, Ghebrehiwet B, et al. Factor XII-dependent contact activation on endothelial cells and binding proteins gC1aR and cytokeratin 1. Thromb Haemost 2001; 85: 119–124.
77. Vavrek RJ, Stewart JM. Competitive antagonists of bradykinin. Peptides 1985; 6:161–164.
78. Rojkjaer R, Schmaier AH. Activation of the plasma kallikrein/kinin system on endothelial cells. Proc Assn Am. Physicians 1999; 111:220–227.
79. Motta G, Rojkjaer R, Hasan AAK, et al. High molecular weight kininogen regulates prekallikrein assembly and activation on endothelial cells; a novel mechanism for contact activation. Blood 1998; 91:516–528.
80. Rojkjaer R, Hasan AAK, Motta M, et al. Factor XII does not initiate prekallikrein activation on endothelial cells. Thromb Haemost 1998; 80:74–81.
81. Schamier AH. Contact activation: a revision. Thromb Haemost 1997; 78:101–107.
82. Joseph K, Ghebrehiwet B, Kaplan AP. Activation of the kinin-forming cascade on the surface of endothelial cells. Biol Chem 2001; 382:71–75.

83. Joseph K, Tholanikunnel BG, Kaplan AP. Heat shock protein 90 catalyzes activation of the prekallikrein-kininogen complex in the absence of factor XII. Proc Natl Acad Sci 2001; 99: 896–900.

84. Shariat-Madar Z, Mahdi F, Schmaier AH. Identificationa nd characterization of prolylcarboxypeptidase as an endothelial cell prekallikrein activator. J Biol Chem 2002; 277:17962–17969.

85. Lin YL, Harris RB, Yan W, et al. High molecular weight kininogen peptides inhibit the formation of kallikrein on endothelial cell surfaces and subsequent urokinase-dependent plasmin formation. Blood 1977; 90:690–697.

86. Schmaier AH. The plasma kallikrein-kinin system counterbalances the renin-angiotensin system. J Clin Invest 2002; 109:1007–1009.

87. Kaplan AP, Joseph K, Sliverberg M. Pathways for bradykinin formation of inflammatory disease. J Allergy Clin Immunol 2002; 109:195–209.

88. Shibayama Y, Joseph K, Nakazawa Y, et al. Zinc-dependent activation of the plasma kinin-forming cascade by aggregated β amyloid protein. Clin Immunol 1999; 90:89–99.

89. Maas C, Govers-Riemslag JWP, Bouma B, et al. Misfolded proteins activate Factor X11 in humans, leading to kallikrein formation without initiating coagulation. J Clin Invest 2008; 118:3208–3218.

6

The Complement System: Mechanisms of Activation, Regulation, and Role in Innate and Adaptive Immunity

Berhane Ghebrehiwet
Division of Allergy, Rheumatology, and Clinical Immunology, Department of Medicine, Health Sciences Center, Stony Brook University, Stony Brook, New York, U.S.A.

INTRODUCTION

The complement system[a] is a well-orchestrated, highly complex, and tightly controlled biological system that constitutes a major part of both the innate and adaptive immune systems (1–4). Although its primary function is to recognize and destroy pathogenic microorganisms and therefore has evolved in this capacity a sophisticated mechanism of discrimination between self and nonself, there are situations however, in which complement can turn against the self, thereby causing tissue damage and destruction. Composed of 30 serum and cell surface proteins and three independent activation pathways, the complement system is one of the proteolytic cascade systems of blood plasma (4). In the classical sense, complement is activated primarily when antigen–antibody complexes are formed in either plasma or tissues and, as a consequence, secondary activation peptides are generated that play an important role in many types of immunological reactions and inflammatory processes. Activation of complement requires an initial contact with and recognition of an *activator*. This initial contact is thought to provide the subtle molecular signal that is necessary to trigger a series of protein–protein interactions involving sequentially, the conversion of proteolytic zymogens to active enzymes and the assembly of functionally defined protein complexes on the surface of the activator particle. If the activating agent is a virus, a bacterium, or a tumor cell, activation

---

[a]Terminology used to describe the complement proteins is that agreed on by the World Health Organization (1968). Thus components are named by uppercase letters followed by a number (e.g., C1). Fragments derived from a component are denoted by a lowercase letter after the component from which it was derived (e.g., C3a). A bar over a component or complexes indicates an enzyme (e.g., C1). Only upper case letters designates some alternative pathway components: Factors B, D, H, I, or P (properdin).

of complement will lead to its destruction by causing irreversible structural and functional impairment of its membrane (1–4).

There are three independent pathways of complement activation, each of which culminates in generating the "lytic" macromolecule—a self-assembling, nonenzymatic cascade referred to as the membrane attack complex (MAC) or membrane attack pathway (1–4). The MAC is responsible for the well-known complement-mediated 100 Å lesions seen on biological membranes by electron microscopy (5). The classical pathway (CP) is initiated by immune complexes of the IgG and IgM types and results in the sequential interactions of nine distinct complement components, designated numerically and in their order of participation in the sequence, as C1, C4, C2, C3, C5, C6, C7, C8, and C9 (Table 1). Three of these components—C1r, C1s, and C2—constitute the CP serine proteases. The alternative pathway (AP) on the other hand is activated by IgA antibodies or certain complex polysaccharides of bacterial and microbial cell walls such as bacterial endotoxins, inulin (a polyfructose from plant cell walls), zymosan (an insoluble residue of

Table 1 Plasma Proteins of the Complement Pathways

Components	MW (kDa)	Electrophoretic mobility	Polypeptide chains	Chromosome location conc.	Mean serum conc. (μg/mL)
Classical pathway					
C1q	462	γ_2	18	1p34.1	80
C1r	83	β	2	12p13	50
C1s	83	α	1	12p13	50
C2	102	β_2	1	6p21.3	25
C3[a]	185	β_2	2	19	1600
C4	205	β_1	3	6p21.3	550
MBL or lectin pathway					
MBL	540	—	18	10	1–5
MASP 1	90	—	1	3q27-q28	—
MASP-2	74	—	1	1p36.3-2	—
MASP-3	94	—	1	3q27-q28	—
C2	102	β_2	1	6p21.3	25
C3	185	β_1	2	19	1600
C4	205	β_1	3	6p21.3	550
Alternative pathway					
C3	185	β_2	2	19	1600
Factor B	93	β_2	1	6p21.3	200
Factor D	25	β–γ	1	1	
Factor H	150	β	1	1q	500
Factor I	88	β	—	4q24	35
Properdin	225	γ	4	Xp11.23	25
MAC pathway					
C5	190	β_1	2	9q32-34	75
C6	120	β_2	1	5q	60
C7	110	β_2	1	5q	55
C8[b]	150	γ_1	3 (α,β,γ)	(1p34,1p34,9q)	80
C9	71	γ	1	5p13	60

[a]C3 is the key protein where each pathway converges.
[b]C8 = chromosome location for each of the C8 chains is given in the order shown. *Source*: Modified from Ref. 6.
Abbreviation: MBL, mannan-binding lectin; MASPs, MBL-associated serine proteases, MAC, membrane attack complex.

yeast cell walls), or cobra venom factor (a glycoprotein from cobra venom), which is the cobra equivalent of C3b (1–4). There are six proteins that can be considered components proper of the AP: C3, Factor B, Factor D, Factor H, Factor I, and properdin (P). Of these, Factors B and D belong to the class of serine proteases and represent the AP enzymes, whereas Factor I is an unusual serine enzyme, which is resistant to the classical serine protease inhibitor, such as diisopropylphosphofluoridate, although sequence evidence suggests that it too is a serine protease (6,7). Factor B and perhaps C2 of the CP are examples of a new type of serine protease with catalytic peptide chains of about 60 kDa (8), and Factor D is believed to be the only complement enzyme, which circulates in plasma in its active form. The third pathway of complement activation designated mannan-binding lectin (MBL), or lectin pathway, was discovered only recently (9,10). MBL belongs to group III of a family of Ca^{2+}-dependent carbohydrate-binding lectins, which include the plasma proteins, conglutinin, collectin-43, and two lung surfactant proteins, SP-A and SP-D (11,12). These proteins collectively known as collectins (collagen-containing lectins) have structural similarity with C1q and consist of 12 to 18 polypeptide chains with N-terminal collagen-like regions and carboxyl-terminal (C-terminal) globular "heads" (13). Whereas the globular heads of C1q evolved to recognize IgG or IgM, the globular heads of the collectins contain a unique carbohydrate recognition domain (CRD). The CRD of MBL can therefore recognize and bind to microbial surface structures containing mannose and N-acetylglucosamine thereby triggering a carbohydrate-mediated, antibody-independent activation of complement in a manner that involves a "C1r/C1s-like" serine enzymes designated MASPs (MBL-associated serine proteases). Both genetic evidence and functional similarity suggest that the MASPs and C1r and C1s enzymes may have evolved from a common ancestral gene by duplication or exon reshuffling. Therefore, the regulatory mechanisms that control the C1q-C1r$_2$,C1s$_2$, and the MBL–MASP pathways are likely to be similar. In any event, for a meaningful activation to occur, all three pathways more or less must obey the same sequential steps of molecular organization:

1. An initial contact with, and *recognition* of an activator
2. Initiation of the cascade by *conversion of zymogens* to active enzymes
3. Assembly and *amplification* through newly formed enzyme complexes
4. Generation of *C3/C5 convertases*
5. Nonenzymatic assembly of protein–protein complexes that lead to the *formation of MAC*

Although the significance of complement in health and disease has been recognized almost since its discovery in the latter part of the 19th century (14), a number of critical discoveries made over the past several years, including the recent discovery of the MBL pathway, have collectively underscored the importance of complement in both the innate and adaptive immunity. This chapter will first review the present status of the field by discussing the activation and regulation of the three independent pathways of activation and then provide few examples of the many roles complement plays in host defense and inflammation.

THE CP: ACTIVATION AND REGULATION

Activation of the CP is primarily dependent on the ability of the first component, C1, to recognize and bind polymeric structures of activating substances such as circulating immune complexes, bacteria, viruses, and other activating substances of diverse origin

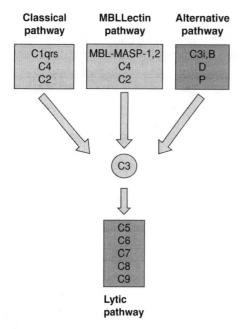

Figure 1 The three pathways of complement activation and the central role of C3. Activation is initiated by immune complexes (classical) or mannose-rich structures on pathogenic microorganisms (MBL) or complex carbohydrate structures (alternative). Each pathway has its own recognition unit, which is responsible for discriminating between self and nonself proteins. All three pathways must first activate C3 and then C5 before the final lytic pathway is activated.

(15) (Fig. 1; Table 1). Although in vivo it is generally agreed that immune complexes of the IgG (IgG$_3$ > IgG$_1$ > IgG$_2$) and IgM isotypes are particularly effective initiators of the classical pathway, activation can, however, proceed without mediation by immunoglobulins (14–17). For example, direct activation of C1 can occur by certain biological particles such as RNA tumor viruses (16), vesicular stomatitis virus (17), complexes of C reactive protein and pneumococcal polysaccharide (18), the lipid A region of certain lipopolysaccharides (19), *Toxoplasma* (20), and plasma enzymes such as kallikrein (21), Hageman factor fragment (HFf, or FXIIf) (22,23), and plasmin (24).

Recognition and Initiation

The first component of complement, C1, (MW 790 kDa) is a 15S to 16S glycoprotein and actually comprises of the recognition unit, C1q (460 kDa), and two modular serine proteases, C1r and C1s (MW 75 and 74 kDa, respectively), associated as a Ca^{2+}-dependent tetramer, C1s-C1r-C1r-C1s, to give a molecular formula of C1qC1r$_2$C1s$_2$ (25–30). However, because C1 in serum is readily dissociable into C1q and the Ca^{2+}-dependent tetrameric structure C1r$_2$C1s$_2$, it may be regarded as a macromolecular assembly of these two weakly interacting proteins (26). During activation of the classical pathway, the C1q molecule, which has no known enzymatic activity, plays a critical role by first recognizing and directly binding to either immune complexes or pathogenic microorganisms and then converting the subtle conformational signals generated as the result of binding into highly specific proteolytic events (29,31). C1q is a collagen-like molecule (29,32) with six flower-like globular heads that constitute the binding sites (33) for the C$_H$2 domain of IgG (34) and C$_H$3 or C$_H$4 domains of IgM (35,36), respectively.

Each globular head contains the C-terminal ends of three highly similar but distinct polypeptide chains A, B, C of MW 28, 25, and 24 kDa respectively, that occur six times in the molecule, forming six structural and functional subunits (37–42). The three chains of C1q are the product of three distinct genes, which are aligned $5' \Rightarrow 3'$ in the same orientation in the order A-C-B on a 24 kb stretch of DNA on human chromosome 1p (41). Each chain has a short N-terminal region involved in the formation of A-B and C-C interchain disulfide bonds and is followed by a collagen-like sequence that gives rise to the formation of six heterotrimeric (A, B, C) collagen-like triple helices, which first associate as a "stalk" and then because of interruptions in the Gly-Xaa-Yaa collagen-like motif, diverge to form six "arms" ultimately merging into a C-terminal globular head region formed by association of the C-termini known as the "C1q modules"(29). The C1q-binding site for C1r$_2$C1s$_2$ resides in the "collagen-like" triple helical segment (37,38). With each globular head capable of binding one IgG molecule, C1q can therefore bind a maximum of six molecules of IgG (33). However, although monomeric IgG can bind C1q, this binding is very weak ($1–5 \times 10^4$ M^{-1}) and unstable and therefore cannot trigger complement activation. On the other hand, the affinity of C1q for clustered IgG, such as those on immune complexes increases more than 1000-fold (5×10^7 M^{-1}), depending on the number of globular heads engaged (4). This type of interaction is thought to induce a series of intramolecular changes within the C1 macromolecule, which eventually leads to the autocatalytic conversion of the single-chain proenzyme C1r to its two-chain proteolytic form. The conversion of C1r to an active protease is the first step in the initiation of the CP (Fig. 2). The mechanism by which this occurs is unclear; however, it has been proposed that complex formation induces a conformational change in the C1q within the C1 macromolecule (43) and that this change exposes a proteolytic site in C1r prior to peptide bond cleavage, converting it to an intermediate form designated "active zymogen" or C1r* (4,40). This form of C1r in turn can catalyze the conversion of C1r $\Rightarrow$ C1r* $\Rightarrow$ fully active C1r (40). Activation occurs through cleavage of a single Arg-Ile bond

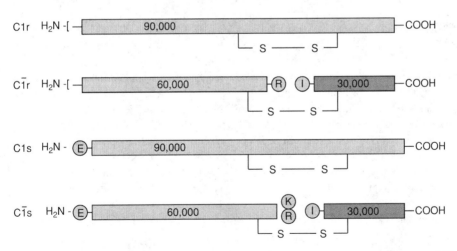

Figure 2 Proteolytic cleavage and activation of C1r and C1s. The activation patterns of C1r and C1s are almost identical. Cleavage of C1r (through autoactivation) occurs at a single site between arginine (R) and isoleucine (I) to give two chains of MW 60 kDa and MW 30 kDa, which remain disulfide-bonded. The smaller fragment contains the catalytic site of the molecule, which converts its substrate C1s to enzymatically active form of C1s by a single peptide bond cleavage between Arg-Ile or Lys-Ile. Again the active site of the C1s molecule resides in the smaller chain at the C-terminal end.

in the single chain C1r, thereby converting it to a two-chain structure in which a heavy chain of 60 kDa is disulfide-linked to a 30-kDa, C-terminal end light chain, which bears the chymotrypsin-like serine protease or catalytic domain (Fig. 2). This site was found to contain three active residues (His, Asp, Ser), which are common to all serine proteases (44). Activated C1r in turn converts C1s to enzymatically active C1s by cleavage of an Arg-Ile bond within a disulfide bridge in a fashion similar to that described for C1r (45) (Fig. 2). Both C1r and C1s are modular serine proteases, exhibiting homologous structural organizations starting sequentially from the N-terminus of CUB module, an epidermal growth factor (EGF)-like module, a second CUB module, two complement control protein (CCP) modules and a C-terminal chymotrypsin-like serine protease domain (29). In spite of their structural and functional similarities, C1r and C1s are two distinct and specific enzymes with entirely different proteins as their substrates. The only natural substrate known for C1r is C1s, whereas both C4 and C2 represent the natural substrates for C1s. Thus, C1s cleaves the fourth (C4) and second (C2) components of complement, each of which is sequentially cleaved into two fragments. For continuity of the cascade, however, cleavage of C4 must precede cleavage of C2 (14). Furthermore, whereas C1s in free solution can cleave free or C4b-bound C2, the cell-bound enzyme does not cleave C2 unless it is bound to C4b (46). C4 consists of three disulfide-linked chains (each of which is a distinct gene product) of differing MWs ($\alpha = 97$ kDa, $\beta = 75$ kDa, and $\gamma = 33$ kDa) in which a single cleavage of the largest chain (termed α) by C1s results in the generation of two fragments: C4a, a 9-kDa fragment and C4b, a larger fragment of 198 kDa. This cleavage not only exposes a labile binding site for cells on the α^1 chain of C4b but also allows firm binding to C2b via the γ chain (6). The active site in the α^1 chain of C4b is a reactive acyl group, which has the capacity to bind covalently to hydroxyl or amino groups on any biological membranes. C4a is one of the three complement-derived anaphylatoxins (47,48), which are important mediators of inflammation as they have the capacity to react with basophils and mast cells, causing them to degranulate (49,50). In this fashion, histamine and other mediators typical of allergic reactions can be released into tissues, resulting in vascular permeability and contraction of smooth muscle. The larger fragment C4b, which results from this digestion (whether cell-bound or in solution) can bind C2 in the presence of Mg^{2+}. If the binding of C2 to C4b occurs in the vicinity of activated C1, then C4b acts as a cofactor for the next enzymatic step of the cascade in which C2 becomes cleaved by C1s to yield two fragments: the C-terminal catalytic fragment C2a (70 kDa) and the noncatalytic, 30 kDa N-terminal piece, C2b (51). The larger fragments, C4b and C2a, form a bimolecular complex (C4b2a) to form the next enzyme in the cascade—the C3 convertase (52). The active site resides on the C2a portion of the molecule (53), and C4b functions as a modulator to facilitate C2 cleavage by C1s (54–57) and stabilize the C2a enzymatic site (55). C4b also possesses a metastable-binding site by which the C4b2a enzyme can attach to target cells. C2 has not been shown to possess any biological activity of its own. It has been proposed, however, that a kinin-like peptide is released as a consequence of C2 cleavage (58,59), which could contribute to the pathogenesis of hereditary angioedema (60–62). However, data obtained during the past decade suggests it is an artifact (see chapter 5).

C3 PLAYS A CENTRAL ROLE IN THE CASCADE

Of the 20+ distinct plasma proteins recognized to date as constituents of the complement system, the third component of complement, C3, is the most abundant (~ 1.6 mg/mL in plasma), versatile, and fulfills a pivotal role in the function of the system (Fig. 3; Table 2).

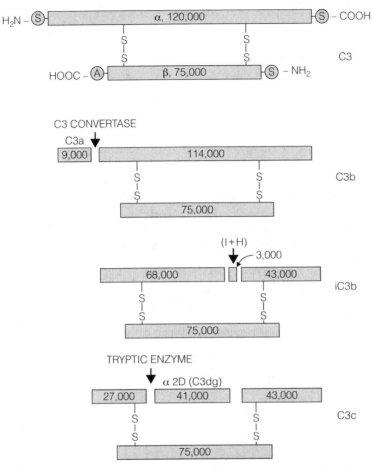

Figure 3 Structure and activation pattern of human C3. The C3 convertase generated by any of the pathways removes a 9-kDa fragment, C3a, by single peptide bond cleavage (Arg-Ser) of the α chain. The α chain of C3b is further cleaved by the regulatory enzyme, Factor I, which in the presence of Factor H makes two cleavages and removes a 3-kDa fragment, leaving 68- and 43-kDa fragments disulfide-bonded to the β chain to give an inactive C3b (iC3b). At this stage, iC3b is susceptible to proteolytic cleavage by tryptic-like enzymes to generate C3c and α2D or C3dg. *Abbreviations*: S, serine; A, alanine.

All three pathways of complement activation merge at the C3 step and continue on to generate the MAC. Therefore, complete deficiency of C3 would have a devastating, but not necessarily fatal, consequence on the individual since the complement-dependent lytic machinery would be impaired, and opsonic fragments that play such a significant role in phagocytosis and immune clearance would not be generated (63). It also functions as a subunit of the initial C3 convertase of the AP. It is no surprise therefore that the structure, molecular biology, and functions of C3 have been the subject of much study during the last two decades (63). The chain structure and cleavage pattern during complement activation have been substantially worked out (Fig. 3). C3 is a 9.5S β-globulin consisting of two non-identical polypeptide chains, α and β, with MWs of 120 kDa and 75 kDa, respectively, that are held together by disulfide bonds and noncovalent forces (64,65). Serine has been found to be the N-terminal amino acid residue of both chains, as well as the C-terminal residue of the α chain, whereas alanine constitutes the C-terminal residue of the β chain (65). C3 is synthesized in the liver (66–68) and by monocytes and macrophages (69,70) as a single polypeptide chain, which after translation, is processed in the cytoplasm to the two-chain molecule that occurs in serum (69,70). Several individuals have been described with a homozygous C3 deficiency, and these individuals have been reported to have numerous episodes of infection caused by pathogenic bacteria, including septicemia and meningococcal meningitis (63,71). In addition, deficiency in C3 results in suppression of complement-mediated functions, e.g., hemolytic and bactericidal activity, opsonization of bacteria, and mobilization of leukocytes in response to chemotactic stimuli.

Native C3 is cleaved by the classical, MBL or AP C3 convertases into two fragments, C3a and C3b by hydrolysis of peptide bond 77 (Arg-Ser) of the α chain (50,65). The activation peptide C3a is a 9-kDa basic peptide, which constitutes one of the three complement-derived anaphylatoxins (C4a and C5a are the others and are derived by a single cleavage of an Arg-X bond in their α chains) and as such, is an important mediator of acute inflammatory responses (Fig. 3; Tables 2 and 3). Doses as low as 1×10^{-12} mol are active, and when compared on a molar basis, C3a is less potent than C5a but more potent than C4a (C5a > C3a > C4a). It causes release of histamine from mast cells,

Table 2 Cleavage Products of C3 and Their Known Biological Activities

Cleavage product	Polypeptide chains	MW kDa	Biological activities
C3a	1	9	Anaphylatoxin
			Release of histamine from mast cells
			Release of enzymes from PMNs
			Smooth muscle contraction
			Suppression of immune responses (T cells)
			Secretion of IL-1 from macrophages
			Stimulation of prostaglandin and thromboxane production (macrophages)
C3b	2	186	Opsonization of biological particles
			Recognition unit of the alternative pathway
			Subunit of C3/C5 convertase of the AP
			Subunit of the C5 convertase of the CP
			Receptor for P and Factor H
			Ligand for CR1 (PMNs, erythrocytes, monocytes, B lymphocytes)
			Potentiation of antibody-dependent cellular cytotoxicity (ADCC)
iC3b	3	177	Ligand for PMN, monocyte, and B lymphocyte receptors (CR3)
			Potentiation of ADCC
			Enhancement of phagocytosis
C3c	3	140	Precursor of C3e
C3d	1	25–35,	Ligand for cellular receptors (CR2)
			Potentiation of ADCC
C3g	1	8	None
C3d-k	1	40	Suppression of T cell functions
			Leukocytosis
C3e	1	10–12	Induction of leukocytosis
			Enhanced vascular permeability
			Release of lysosomal enzymes
			Ligand for PMNs and monocytes

Table 3 Properties of Human Anaphylatoxins

Properties	C3a	C4a	C5a
Electrophoretic mobility	+2.1	+2.1	−1.7
Molecular weight			
Total	9,000	8,650	11,200
Protein	9,000	8,650	8,200
Carbohydrate	0	0	3,000
Amino acid residues	77	77	74
NH-terminus	Serine	Asparagine	Threonine
COOH-terminus	Arginine	Arginine	Arginine
α-Helical structure	50%	54%	45%
Biological activity			
Ileum contraction	1×10^{-8} M	1×10^{-8} M	5×10^{-10} M
Chemotaxis	Selective to eosinophils	None	3×10^{-9} M
Histamine release	1×10^{-6} M	—	1×10^{-6} M
Lethal shock (guinea pig)	1×10^{-8} mol	—	1×10^{-9} mol
Edema and erythema	1×10^{-12} mol	1×10^{-9} mol	1×10^{-15} mol
Immunopotentiation	None	—	10–100 ng/mL
Immunosuppression	100–500 ng/mL	—	None

induces smooth muscle contraction of guinea pigs, causes release of lysosomal enzymes from neutrophils, and upon intracutaneous injection into humans or guinea pigs, enhances vascular permeability (49,50,72). It has been found that C3a suppresses both specific and polyclonal antibody responses by induction of a suppressor T cell population, indicating that C3a may be involved in a nonspecific immunoregulatory network capable of suppressing ongoing immune responses (73).

In vivo, the functions of C3a are controlled by serum carboxypeptidase N (anaphylatoxin inactivator, AI), which removes the essential C-terminal arginyl residue (74). Its structure has been found to be homologous to that of C4a (48) and C5a (75) with a 45% α-helical conformation (76). The large fragment, C3b, like C4b, has a metastable binding site (77–79), and the reactive group appears to be an intramolecular thiolester bond, which in native C3 is inaccessible. However, cleavage and removal of the N-terminal C3a induces a conformational change in the C3b molecule exposing an internal thiolester bond capable of covalently binding with any nucleophile including H_2O and the hydroxyl or amino groups of any biological surfaces (6).

Such interaction converts the thiolester to C3b, which performs several biologically important functions in vivo. First, there are receptors for C3b on numerous cells among which are neutrophils, eosinophils, macrophages, monocytes, and B lymphocytes (80,81). Because neutrophils and macrophages (and to a lesser degree eosinophils) are phagocytic cells, interaction of these cells with immune complexes to which C3b is attached appears to be sufficient to trigger phagocytosis. In this fashion, immune complexes are ingested, and as a consequence of this reaction the secretion of tissue destructive enzymes is initiated. Second, C3b is capable of distinguishing between an activator and a nonactivator of the AP, as reflected by the differential accessibility of bound C3b to the regulator (Factor H) (82) and the C3b inactivator (Factor I), which cleaves the α′ chain at two arginyl-serine peptide bonds removing a 3-kDa fragment designated C3f (83) and two α′ chain fragments, 68 and 43 kDa that remain disulfide-bonded to the β chain (82) (Fig. 3). Such inactivated C3b is termed iC3b and at this stage is extremely susceptible to

Table 4   Properties of Human C3e

Molecular weight	
Gel electrophoresis	12 kDa
Amino acid analysis	10 kDa
Electrophoretic mobility, pH 8.6	-7.5×10^{-5} cm^2 volts^{-1} sec^{-1}
Isoelectric point	4.3
No. of amino acid residues	101
Biological activity	
Induction of leukocytosis (rabbits)	10 µg/kg, intravenously
Increased vascular permeability with leukocyte infiltration	5 µg intradermally
Release of lysosomal enzymes (PMNs)	4–25 µg/mL
Ligand for PMNs	62,000 sites/cell
Ligand for monocytes	43,400 sites/cell

further enzymatic degradation by tryptic-like enzymes. These enzymes cleave the α′ chain in the N-terminal region, removing a 41-kDa piece designated C3dg, which contains the C3d and C3g fragments (84) (Fig. 3; Table 2). C3d contains a particle-binding site and remains bound while C3c is released to the fluid phase. Although the physiologic fragments of C3b, i.e., iC3b, C3dg, and C3d do not participate further in the activation process, they nevertheless, fulfill a diversity of immunoregulatory functions including clearance and solubilization of immune complexes and stimulation of immune responses, by interacting with specific cell surface receptors such as CR2 (for C3dg and C3d) and CR3 (for iC3b). The larger fragment, C3c (140 kDa), is the precursor of a 10-kDa fragment, C3e, which appears to be derived late in the degradation process from the α chain by a yet unidentified plasma, leukocyte, or bacterial derived enzyme (85,86). Although its exact chemical structure has not been elucidated, C3e is of particular interest, as it has been shown to induce leukocytosis in rabbits upon intravenous injection, and when injected intradermally causes increased vascular permeability (85) (Table 4) with cellular infiltration. It has also been postulated that polymorphonuclear neutrophils (PMNs) possess specific receptors for C3e, and upon interaction with the peptide they are induced to release lysosomal enzymes (85), one of which is an enzyme capable of generating a chemotactic activity when incubated with highly purified C5. Another fragment expressing similar biological properties as C3e has also been generated from iC3b by limited proteolytic digestion with kallikrein (87). This fragment, designated C3dK, also induces leukocytosis and is postulated that both C3e and C3dK may share overlapping sequence homology (87). A summary of the physiological split products and functions of C3 is shown Table 2. Another important physiological function of C3b is that it forms a subunit of the C5 converting enzymes of all three pathways (1,6). Formation of C3b in the vicinity of a C4b2a complex confers upon this enzyme the ability to activate and cleave C5, thereby changing its specificity (2). This C4b2a3b enzyme is the CP C5 convertase and releases a 12-kDa peptide from C5, called C5a, and generates C5b, the first protein of the MAC (Fig. 1). C5a possesses two important activities: It shares with C3a and C4a the property of being an anaphylatoxin, and it is a potent chemotactic factor that can attract neutrophils, eosinophils, and monocytes into the vicinity of an inflammatory reaction. Because the predominant cell in the circulation is the neutrophil, it is the most prominent cell seen in C5a-dependent inflammatory reactions. Furthermore, other findings indicate that, in contrast to C3a, which suppresses immune responses, addition of C5a to cultures results in the enhancement of specific and nonspecific humoral responses (73). C5a has been shown to augment antigen- and alloantigen-induced T cell proliferative responses but not mitogen-induced proliferative responses (87–89). In addition, the adjuvant effects exerted by C5a were found to occur within the first 24 hours of culture, with T cells being involved in the C5a-mediated enhancement of humoral immune responses (73). C3a was initially thought to possess the same chemotactic activity as C5a. However, this was shown to be due to contamination by C5a. Subsequently, C3a was shown to have chemotactic activity that was selective for eosinophils (89; Table 3).

Regulation of the Classical Pathway

Regulation of the CP (Tables 5A and B) occurs through a number of mechanisms: (*i*) The intrinsic lability of the activated or assembled proteins, e.g., activated C1 is unstable and the C4b2a enzyme decays in serum with a half-life of only 5 minutes (6). (*ii*) Regulation by serum inhibitors, e.g., C1-INH (or α_2-neuraminoglycoprotein) provides the main control mechanism for activated C1 by binding irreversibly to activated C1r and C1s and dissociating them from the C1 macromolecule (27,90). Furthermore, C1-INH plays a crucial role in the homeostatic regulation of C1 by preventing its dissociation (27), which otherwise results in the autocatalytic activation of C1r (91,92). Genetic deficiency in C1-INH, which is inherited as an autosomal dominant trait, results in a potentially fatal disease called hereditary angioneurotic edema (HANE or HAE). (*iii*) Regulation by proteolytic digestion of certain components such as cleavage of C4b by C4-binding protein (C4-bp) and Factor I and digestion of C3 by Factor I in the presence of Factor H. The C4-bp-like molecule, DAF (decay accelerating factor), has the property of accelerating the dissociation of C4b2a complex and is an essential cofactor for the cleavage of C4b by Factor I (56,93). In this respect, its action is analogous to that of

Table 5A Control Proteins of Complement Activation

Proteins	MW (kDa)	Electrophoretic mobility	Polypeptide chains	Chromosome location	Mean serum conc. (μg/mL)
C1-INH	110	α_2	1	11p11.2	200
C4-bp	500	β_1	?	1q32	250
Factor H	150	β	1	1q	500
Factor I	88	β	2	4q24	35
AI	310	α	multiple	—	50
S-protein[a]	83	α	1	17q11	600
Sp40,40	80	—	1	8p21	50

[a]Also known as vitronectin

Table 5B Membrane Regulators of Complement Activation

Membrane protein	MW (kDa)	Target protein	Chromosome location	Function
DAF	70	C4b2a	1q32	Decay acceleration of C3/C5 convertases
MCP 45–70 (CD46)		C3b,C4b	1q32	Causes breakdown of C3b,C4b
CD59	~19	C5b-8	11p13	Protection of homologous cells from MAC attack
HRF	65	C5b-8	ND	Similar to CD59

Factor H in the AP (see below). In addition, membrane proteins such as CR1 [receptor for C3b and MCP (membrane cofactor protein)] can serve as cofactors for Factor I in the cleavage of C3b and C4b (94).

THE MBL PATHWAY

General Considerations and Background

The MBL pathway of complement activation (9–13,95) is the last of the pathways (Fig. 1; Table 1) to be discovered and therefore, its structure-function relationship at the molecular level has been worked out only recently (96,97). MBL (also known as mannan-binding protein or mannose-binding lectin) belongs to a family of C-type lectins known as collectins (13,98–100). These molecules are structurally similar to C1q in that they are formed from three homologous chains each containing collagen-like sequences contiguous with non-collagen-like stretches that form the "globular heads" (99). Therefore the electron microscopic profile of MBL resembles the bouquet-like structure of C1q, although unlike C1q, MBL can exist in various oligomeric forms including dimers, trimers, tetramers, pentamers, or heaxamers (101,102). Other members of this family of proteins include lung surfactant protein A (SP-A), lung surfactant protein D (SP-D), collectin-43 (CL-43), and bovine conglutinin, (103,104). Their genes characteristically reveal the presence of a small exon encoding a 36-amino acid-long neck region, which links the collagen domain with the globular head containing the CRD. The neck region forms a homotrimeric α-helical coiled-coil, which is essential for orientation of the three 50-Å apart CRDs in a manner as to have the ability to recognize high mannose- and fucose-containing glycoconjugates, which are generally found decorating the surface of microorganisms but *not* on self proteins (105). This unique ability of MBL to recognize patterns of carbohydrate structures on microorganisms and thereby distinguish between self-proteins and nonself components, allows it to play a critical role in innate immunity (96).

The clinical relevance of MBL was recognized when it was discovered that MBL deficiency in children causes frequent infections, with prominent deficiency in opsonic activity (reviewed in 101). This in turn led to the identification of three point mutations in the Gly-Xaa-Yaa repeat of the collagen helix of the wild type or A allotype. The substitution of glycine in codon 54 for an aspartic acid resulted in the B allotype, and a substitution of glycine in codon 57 for glutamic acid gave rise to the C allotype. The D allotype on the other hand resulted from the introduction of a cysteine in the X-position of codon 52 (101).

Initiation, Activation, and Regulation

In plasma, MBL circulates in association with three structurally related serine protease zymogens designated MASP-1 (MBL-associated protein), MASP-2, MASP-3, and a nonenzymatic, truncated version of MASP-2 called MAp-19 (reviewed in 96,97,101). Whereas MASP-1 and MAp-19 form an association with lower molecular weight forms of MBL, MASP-2 and MASP-3 appear to preferentially associate with the higher molecular weight form of MBL (101,105–109). When compared at the molecular level, the domain structure of MASPs is identical to those of C1r and C1s (97). Whereas MASP-1 is strikingly similar to C1r, MASP-2 is similar to C1s, suggesting that MASPs and C1r and C1s genes may have evolved from the same ancestral gene (96,97). MASP-1 and MASP-3 are alternative splice products of a single gene and have identical A chains but have individual B chains encompassing the serine protease domain. MASP-2 and MAp-19, on the other hand are alternative splice products of the MASP-2 gene, with MAp-19 consisting of the first two domains of MASP-2 and additional four amino acid residues (97). Not surprisingly therefore, activation of the MBL pathway is remarkably similar to that of the CP except that initiation does not require the presence of IgG or IgM on the surface of pathogenic microorganisms. Instead, MBL binds directly to microbial carbohydrates—the hydroxyl group of sugar residues found in hexoses—and this in turn induces a conformational change within the MBL-MASP macromolecule resulting in the activation of MASP-2. MBL binds specifically to hexoses found in a broad spectrum of pathogenic microorganisms. However, it does not bind mammalian glycoproteins, which contain mostly sugars in the form of sialic acid and galactose. Therefore MBL has a built in capacity to discriminate between self and non-self (101). What role, if any, MASP-1, MASP-3, and MAp-19 play in the MBL-complex is still unclear. Indeed, although the MASP-1 concentration in plasma is approximately 20-fold more than MASP-2, it is the latter, which is fully responsible for the subsequent cleavage of C4 and C2 in a manner reminiscent of C1s (96). In this manner the C4b2a enzyme (C3 convertase) is generated, and subsequent cleavage of C3 and C5 can proceed to form the lytic molecule, MAC. C1-INH regulates the activities of MASP 1-2, in analogous manner to its inhibition of C1r and C1s.

Another group of lectins, which are structurally similar to MBL are the ficolins, which include L-, M-, and H-ficolins (101). Ficolins are also capable of activating complement by forming complexes with MASPs is the ficolins (101,108,109). Unlike MBL, these lectins do not have typical C-type lectin recognition domains, but instead contain fibrinogen-like domains recognizing specific carbohydrate structures on activating microbial surfaces. Among the ficolins, the L-ficolin and H-ficolin are able to associate with MASPs (109). In fact it is assumed that in vivo, most of the surplus MASP that is not bound to MBL is associated with these proteins.

AP OF COMPLEMENT ACTIVATION

Initiation and Activation

Like the MBL pathway, the AP plays a significant role in innate immunity. It is one of the first lines of host defense capable of neutralizing a variety of potential pathogens in the total absence of antibody (77,110). There are six proteins which are necessary for activation of the AP: C3, Factors B, D, I, and H, and properdin (P) (3) (Fig. 1; Table 1). The most critical and essential component of the AP, however, is surface-bound C3b. By virtue of its discriminatory interaction with biological surface structures, C3b serves as a recognition unit and dictates whether the pathway is triggered or aborted (3). Initiation and activation of this pathway therefore requires the initial deposition of C3b molecules on a biological surface and subsequent recognition of this surface as an activator or nonactivator. However, generation of C3b molecules cannot occur unless C3 is acted on by a C3-converting enzyme. According to the currently accepted theory, a "C3b-like" C3 [C3(H_2O)] arises by nonenzymatic, spontaneous thiolester bond hydrolysis of C3 so that a low, steady-state concentration of the initial C3 convertase (C3iBb) of the AP (6,77–84, 111,112) is generated (Fig. 1). This C3b-like C3 or C3i, which has undergone thiolester hydrolysis without the loss of its C3a fragment, does not have hemolytic activity but behaves functionally like C3b with respect to its ability to bind Factors B and H, its susceptibility to cleavage by Factor I, and most importantly, its ability to form a fluid-phase C3 convertase in the presence of Factors B and D and Mg^{2+}. Thus, in the presence of Mg^{2+}, C3i and Factor B form a loose complex, C3iB, such that the Factor B can now be cleaved by Factor D to generate the initial fluid-phase C3 convertase—C3iBb (113).

The first C3b produced by this enzyme thus sets in motion the C3b-dependent positive-feedback mechanism, provided it binds to an activating surface capable of protecting it from cleavage by Factors H and I (114). The surface-bound C3b is able to form a surface-bound C3bB complex, in which C3b serves as a cofactor (31), for the cleavage of Factor B by Factor D (115). Factor B is cleaved into two fragments: Ab (MW 30 kDa) is released into the medium and has been shown to have some chemotactic activity (116), whereas Bb remains bound to C3b to form the first surface bound C3bBb, which is the C3 convertase of the AP. The larger fragment Bb (MW 93 kDa) bears the active site for C3 cleavage. In addition, Bb has been reported to cause monocytes or macrophages to spread on surfaces (117). Because Factor D is not incorporated into the C3bBb complex, it can thus generate multiple C3 convertases in a short time. However, C3bBb is labile and in the presence of Factor H dissociates to form an inactive Bb (iBb) plus C3bH. This enzyme can be stabilized upon addition of the cofactor properdin (P), which binds reversibly to C3b and forms a more stable PC3bBb enzyme (118,119). This stabilized enzyme then digests C3 to yield C3a and C3b. By analogy with the classical pathway, addition of a second C3b molecule to this complex forms $P(C3b)_2Bb$, which then acts as a C5 convertase (118). The C5 convertases (like the C3 convertases) of both pathways share the same specificity (118,119). There is therefore considerable structural and functional similarity between the enzymes of the alternative and classical and MBL pathways. Factor B is the equivalent of C2, and C3b acts like C4b. However, C2 is cleaved by C1s in solution even in the absence of C4b, but Factor D cleaves Factor B only when it is in complex with its modulator, C3b. The remainder of the cascade, i.e., formation and assembly of the MAC, proceeds exactly in the same manner for all pathways and is described below.

Regulation of the AP

Like the MBL pathway, the AP is a major player in innate immunity (6,112). Initiation of the AP also differs from that of the CP in that the initiating enzyme, Factor D, which has unusual substrate specificity, appears to circulate as an active enzyme, and has no precursor or a proenzyme form (8,120,121). However, unless the substrate of D is assembled "properly" on a surface, activation does not proceed. Although the AP can be activated immunologically, it is by and large, triggered by a variety of nonimmunological agents, e.g., endotoxin (lipopolysaccharide) (122), inulin (polyfructose), zymosan (123), rabbit erythrocytes (123), or certain lymphoblastoid cells (110). In addition, activation can be triggered by immune complexes involving IgA antibody or by IgG antiviral antibody complexed to cells infected with virus. This last reaction has been demonstrated using measles, mumps, influenza, and herpes simplex viruses (124).

Of particular interest is the special function played by two plasma regulators in controlling initiation and amplification of the AP (Tables 5A and B). One protein, Factor H, is a 150-kDa, single-chain molecule that binds to C3b (82) and can therefore dissociate Bb from C3bBb. Once dissociated, Bb is inactive (iBb) and cannot bind, i.e., C3bBb + Factor H → C3bH + iBb, thus disassembling the C3 convertase. Another regulator is Factor I, which in the presence of Factor H can cleave C3b to form iC3b. The latter in turn can no longer interact with Bb to form a viable enzyme (82). However, cleavage of fluid-phase C3b by Factor I is dependent on the presence of Factor H and inactivation of surface-bound C3b is greatly enhanced by Factor H (125). It has been shown that surfaces which initiate the AP have the property of excluding or preventing the reactions involving Factors I and H so that initiation by D proceeds, whereas nonactivating surfaces allow these inhibitors to function and activation is prevented (77,126,127). In one model system, it has been shown that rabbit erythrocytes can initiate the human AP and sheep erythrocytes cannot. Treatment of sheep erythrocytes with neuraminidase to remove sialic acid converts the sheep erythrocytes into an initiator (112,113,127). As predicted, rabbit cells were relatively deficient in sialic acid. It therefore appears that the presence of sialic acid, as well as polyanions such as heparan, favors binding of Factor H to the surface so that initiation of the alternative complement pathway is inhibited. Thus, although a large number of cells are capable of binding C3b, only those that are capable of providing the C3b molecule with a microenvironment protected from the actions of Factors H and I can succeed in promoting a self-destructive event, i.e., activation of complement on their surface. One of the mechanisms by which bystander cells or self-cells are protected against accidental lysis by complement is due to the presence of two types of regulatory proteins with Factor H-like activities that have been isolated from human erythrocytes. The first of these proteins is the 205-kDa glycoprotein, which is the C3b receptor or CR1 (80,128,129) and is present on B cells, PMNs, monocytes, and a certain subpopulation of T cells. It is characterized by its ability to dissociate the C3bBb and C4b2b enzymes, bind C3b, block binding of Factor B to C3b, and modulate C3b and C3bi cleavage by Factor I to form C3c plus C3dg. The second is a 70-kDa glycoprotein, designated decay-accelerating factor (DAF) (130). DAF can efficiently cause the decay dissociation of both the classical and AP C3 converting enzymes (128,131). More recently, another cell surface protein with complement regulatory properties has been identified (132). This molecule named membrane cofactor protein (MCP) can also serve as a cofactor for factor I in the cleavage of C3b and C4b and like DAF has a wide tissue distribution. The biological significance of these regulators was recognized when it was shown that 44% of the red blood cells from a patient with paroxysmal nocturnal hemoglobinuria (PNH), which were susceptible to lysis by acidified complement, were found to be devoid of DAF even though CR1 was present (133). The molecular defect underlying the clinical manifestations of PNH may thus be in part due to the absence of membrane-associated DAF (133). DAF is therefore the critical factor for dissociation of cell-bound C4b2a or C3bBb, although CR1 or fluid-phase C4b-bp and Factor H are capable of doing the same thing. CR1 is also critical as a cofactor for Factor I, a property it shares with C4b-bp and Factor H, but not with DAF. Systemic lupus erythematosus (SLE) patients have been shown to have an inherited partial deficiency in erythrocyte C3b receptors. In addition, some SLE patients with proliferative glomerulonephritis had an absence of glomerular C3b receptors. These deficiencies were postulated to contribute to systemic and organ-specific abnormalities in the clearance of immune complexes and thereby contribute to the pathogenesis of this disease (80).

MEMBRANE ATTACK COMPLEX

Initiation of MAC Pathway

Complement-induced membrane damage and cytolysis is the final step of complement activation regardless of which pathway was initially activated (Fig. 1; Table 1). Membrane damage is caused by the "killer" or "lytic" molecule or MAC. The assembly and formation of MAC is entirely dependent on the initial cleavage of C5 into C5a and C5b and C5b-mediated assembly of four structurally and functionally related proteins: C6, C7, C8, and C9. These proteins have the capacity of undergoing a hydrophilic to amphiphilic transition. The C8 molecule is a heterotrimer composed of α, β, and γ chains, which are the products of three distinct genes and organized in the molecule such that the α and γ subunits are disulfide-linked with each other, while the β subunit is noncovalently associated with the α, γ dimer. A remarkably striking feature of all the members of the MAC with the exception of C8γ is that they contain several structural and functional modules including a thrombospondin (TSR) module, an LDLr module, an EGF module, a MAC-specific domain and a lytic domain which is approximately 200 residues in length (134,135). While the C8α and C8β have an extra TSR module at the C-terminal end, the C8γ, which is not required for hemolytic function, is structurally different from the other members of MAC and therefore does not contain these modules (134–139). The only enzymatic cleavage in the initiation and assembly of MAC is a single peptide bond cleavage in C5 by C5 convertases. This results in the generation of two fragments, C5a and C5b. C5a is one of the most potent complement derived anaphylatoxin, whereas C5b is responsible for the initiation and assembly of the proteins into the supramolecular organization known as MAC (140). Assembly proceeds from formation of the stable bimolecular complex C5b-6 to the reaction of C5b-6 with C7. This results in formation of the intermediate complex C5b-7, which possesses a strong binding site for biological membranes (141). After the three-chain C8 molecule is bound to the C5b-7 via its C5b recognition site on the β chain, the C5b-8 complex reacts with multiple C9 molecules via its α chain leading to the formation of MAC (142). No enzymatic functions has been attributed to C8; however, C6 has been reported to contain a catalytic site, which can hydrolyze acetyl glycyl-lysine-methyl ester and is inactivated by DFP (143); it is assumed that C7 might have similar properties (144). In the fluid phase C8 has a single binding site for C9, and the interaction is reversible (Ka ≈ 10^7 M^{-1} (144,145). However, several C9 molecules are bound to a target cell-bound C5b-8, and this association is virtually irreversible (Ka ≈ 10^{11} M^{-1}) (145). Binding of a molecule of C9 to C5b-8 further facilitates C9–C9 interaction. The energy derived from this interaction effects the unfolding of monomeric C9 (long axis changes from 80 to 160 Å) (145) as it polymerizes to form poly-C9. Poly-C9 is amphiphilic and capable of inserting itself into hydrophobic environments such as lipid bilayers (145). Individually spaced C5b-8 molecules can bind 12 to 16 molecules of C9, and clusters of C5b-8 molecules can bind 6 to 8 molecules. It appears that a larger poly-C9 is generated by an individually spaced C5b-8, and clusters of two C5b-8 form a poly-C9 (146) with fewer molecules.

Assembly of the MAC results in the expression of hydrophobicity by the otherwise hydrophilic proteins. This property seems to be responsible for the insertion of C5b-7 into target membranes (147) and for membrane damage caused by the binding of C8 and C9 to C5b-7 complexes (148,149). Membrane damage and cytolysis caused by MAC has been attributed to lipid bilayer perturbation (150,151) and transmembrane channel (146,152) formation (142,146), followed by osmotic lysis because of ion exchange with the external environment with uptake of water accompanying sodium influx. Each lesion on the target cell membrane actually consists of (C5b-8) poly-C9 and is visualized by electron microscopy as a circular hollow structure ≈ 12 nm above the membrane surface with inner and outer diameters of 10 to 11 nm and 21 nm, respectively (5). Although it is not an essential component of immune hemolysis, C9 markedly increases the rate of lysis of cells bearing C5b-8 [erythrocytes, *Escherichia coli* (153), Raji cells (110), and other nucleated cells]. C9 is also a critical component of the MAC-induced ultrastructural membrane lesions (154,155).

Without C9, the C5b-8 complex possesses a certain degree of membranolytic activity as it can destroy *Neisseria gonorrhoeae* (156), and individuals with homozygous C9 deficiency do not suffer severe infections (157–160). Apparently the phospholipid binding capacity and the ability of the complex to organize and thereby weaken membrane structures are sufficient to impair the normal function of some structures (147,151). It has also been shown that isolated C9 could undergo spontaneous polymerization at 37°C to form circular polymers resembling the ultrastructure of MAC (161). Such poly-C9 can become an integral membrane protein having membranolytic activity and the ultrastructural appearance characteristic of complement-induced membrane lesions (162). Circular poly-C9 forms spontaneously upon prolonged incubation of C9 at 37°C but requires greater activation energy than that mediated by C5b-8. Ultrastructurally, poly-C9 is described as a 160-Å long tubule with an internal diameter of 100 to 110 Å rimmed on one end by a torus with a 210-Å outer diameter terminated on the opposite end by a membrane-binding hydrophobic domain (162). Polymerization is accompanied by a change in secondary structure with doubling of its axis from 80 Å (C9 monomer) to 160 Å and is accompanied by a hydrophilic-amphiphilic transition enabling C9 to insert itself into phospholipid bilayers (162). One unique characteristic of poly-C9 is that it becomes extremely resistant to SDS as well as protease digestion, and it is suggested that this resistance may be a prerequisite for its function as the cytotoxic unit of the MAC complex (145).

Regulation and Control of MAC

The MAC is under control of several plasma (S-protein, SP40,40) or membrane-associated (HRF, CD59) proteins that closely regulate the undesired assembly of MAC on homologous surfaces (Tables 5A and B). The S-protein (vitronectin, 65–80 kDa) binds to C5b-7 complex and prevents C8 from binding and polymerization of C9. Similarly, the apolipoprotein SP40,40, also binds to C5b-7 activity and inhibits membrane insertion. SP40,40 is highly homologous to clusterin (also known as Sertoli cell glycoprotein-2 or SCP-2) is found at high concentrations in seminal fluid, where it is thought to play an important role in protecting spermatozoa from complement attack. On the surface of cell membranes however, the major regulatory proteins are integral membrane proteins such as CD59 (19 kDa) and HRF (homologous restriction factor, MW 65 kDa). Both of these proteins, which are anchored to the membrane by a glycosyl phosphatidylinositol (GPI) anchor, bind to C8 and interfere with the formation of MAC assembly by preventing C9 polymerization. Like DAF, these GPI-anchored proteins are deficient in PNH. Complement-mediated and cytotoxic cell-mediated membrane lesions have striking similarities, which were further confirmed when two types (T1 and T2, 16 and 5 nm in diameter, respectively) of complement-like membrane lesions were observed using cloned mouse natural killer (NK) cells as effectors and rabbit erythrocytes as target cells (163). The lesions apparently arise by membrane insertion of tubular complexes called perforins that are assembled from subunits during the cytolytic action. Perforin, like MAC, has a lytic domain of approximately 200 amino acid residues and is about 25% identical to that of MAC. Unlike MAC however, perforin does not appear to require other proteins for its assembly and lytic function, but does require Ca^{2+} for its function.

COMPLEMENT-DERIVED BIOACTIVE FRAGMENTS

One of the many striking features of the complement system is that its activation results not only in the destruction of a marked target cell, but also in the concomitant generation of several biologically active cleavage products. That such fragments play an important role in various types of immune reactions (e.g., phagocytosis, chemotaxis, anaphylaxis, acute shock, and acute allergic reactions) as well as several other inflammatory responses is well documented (49). It was shown that certain active peptides such as C5a and C3a could interact with the immune system and modulate the immune response (73).

Anaphylatoxins and Inflammation

Activation of the CP leads to the generation of most of the presently well-characterized fragments (Tables 2–4). Enzymatic digestion of C4 by C1s produces two fragments: C4a and C4b. Isolated C4a was found to be spasmogenic (guinea pig ileum at 1 μM), to cause muscle desensitization with respect to C3a but not C5a (i.e., tachyphylaxis at 0.33 μM), and to enhance vascular permeability (human skin, 1 nmol) with immediate erythema and edema formation (48,50). Because the spasmogenic, tachyphylactic, and vascular activities of C4a were abrogated by removal of the C-terminal arginine, a property that is characteristic of C3a and C5a, it was concluded that C4a represents the third complement-derived anaphylatoxin. All three anaphylatoxins, i.e., C3a, C4a, and C5a, are generated by proteolytic cleavage in the course of complement activation and as such share several structural and functional properties. First, all three are regulated by serum carboxypeptidase N or anaphylatoxin inhibitor (AI), which removes the C-terminal arginine residue to generate the "des Arg" forms of the proteins (Table 5A). While the spasmogenic and permeability enhancing functions of the des Arg forms of C3a and C4a are abrogated, C5a still maintains some of its functions notably its vascular permeability and chemotactic activity. Second, partial sequence analysis suggests that there is structural homology between these polypeptides with a helical conformation of 50, 54, and 45% for C3a, C4a, and C5a, respectively (48,50,75) (Table 3). In addition, C3a, C4a, and C5a are capable of inducing histamine release from mast cells and release of hydrolytic enzymes from neutrophils, causing contraction of smooth muscle, and enhancing vascular permeability (49). These activities are mediated by specific anaphylatoxin receptors expressed on these cells. The C5a receptor acts via a GTP-binding protein complex and has approximately 35% sequence identity with the f-Met-Leu-Phe receptor and both mediate similar but not identical responses on monocytes and neutrophils. Contrary to previously held theory that there are two types of anaphylatoxin receptors, one for C5a and the other common to both C3a and C4a, recent studies have suggested that there are in fact two distinct receptors for C3a and C4a at least on monocytes and macrophages. Furthermore, although neither the structure of C3aR nor that of C4aR has been yet elucidated, the structure of C3aR at least is most likely going to be similar to that of C5aR since C3a activates the respiratory burst (164–167) and stimulates Ca^{2+} influx in neutrophils (164,165) via a pertussis toxin sensitive G protein (167).

The C5a receptor (Table 6) is a member of the rhodopsin superfamily of molecules characterized by a seven transmembrane segment and induces transmembrane signals via a guanosine triphosphate (GTP)- and guanosine diphosphate (GDP)-binding intracellular mechanisms (166). Although the mechanism of C3a and C5a-mediated signaling are similar in many ways, C3a does not activate phosphatidylinositol 3-kinase, whereas C5a does. This suggests that overlapping but similar pathways are activated (168). Another unique property of C5a is that it contains in its structure a single oligosaccharide through which it associates with a 60-kDa plasma protein thereby expressing enhanced chemotactic activity. This plasma protein is a vitamin D–binding protein (Gc globulin) designated cochemotaxin (169,170). Furthermore, removal of the oligosaccharide moiety has been shown to restore anaphylatoxin activity to C5a des Arg) demonstrating the functional importance of this site (171). It has also become apparent that these activation peptides can play a role in immune regulation. For example, when cultures of human peripheral blood lymphocytes were incubated with human C3a, the ability of these cells to produce polyclonal antibody was suppressed. Addition of C3a des Arg failed to cause any significant suppression suggesting that the COOH-terminal arginine was required for this activity (88,89). In contrast to C3a, however, highly purified preparations of C5a or C5a

Table 6 Major Cell Surface Receptors/Sites of Complement

Surface protein	MW (kDa)	CD designation	Ligand specificity	Chromosome location
CR1-type D[a]	250	CD35	C3b/C4b	1q32
CR1-type B	220			
CR1-type A	190			
CR1-type C	160			
CR2	145	CD21	C3dg/ C3d	1q32
CR3 (α/β)	$\alpha = 165$	CD11b	iC3b	1q32
	$\beta = 95$	CD18		
CR4 (α/β)[b]	$\alpha = 150$	CD11c	iC3b	1q32
	$\beta = 95$	CD18		
C3a-R	—	—	C3a/C4a	—
C5a-R	45	None	C5a/C5a des Arg	—
cC1q-R/CR[c]	60	None	C1q collagen domain, collectins (MBL, SP-A)	19
gC1q-R/p33	33	None	C1q-globular heads, HK, FXII	17p13.3
C1qRp	126	CD93	MBL, (C1q?)	20

[a]Four structural allotypes
[b]Heterodimer of α and β chains
[c]Identity with calreticulin –CR

des Arg were found to enhance the primary in vitro anti-SRBC responses of both human and mouse lymphocytes (88,89). Concentrations of C5a as low as 10 ng/mL significantly increased the response of mouse spleen cells (88).

Leukocytosis Mobilizing Activity

Another complement-derived fragment capable of exhibiting certain types of immunoregulatory functions is C3d-K, which is a cleavage product derived from iC3b by kallikrein (Table 2) and as such represents a novel peptide with biological functions (88,89). C3d-K was found to inhibit mitogen-antigen- and alloantigen-induced T lymphocyte proliferation (87). Furthermore, this fragment induced leukocytosis when injected intraveneously into mice or rabbits. Because leukocytosis-mobilizing activity was reported to be a property of C3e (85,86), a 10-kDa fragment derived late in the degradation process from C3c, it is postulated that C3d-K possesses some of the functional domains of C3e (87). The C3e fragment, in addition to its ability to induce leukocytosis, causes vascular permeability (Table 4), with cellular infiltration when injected intradermally (85) and causes the release of lysosomal enzymes from PMNs (86). These enzymes can generate chemotactic activity when incubated with highly purified human C5 (86). PMNs and monocytes are also known to bind C3e (86). Because the fragment can be generated from serum by certain types of gram-negative bacteria, e.g., *Pseudomonas aeruginosa* (85), the hypothesis is that it represents a late degradation polypeptide released during bacterial infections and septicemia.

Phagocytosis and Clearance of Immune Complexes

The larger physiologic or activation products also participate in several immunological reactions. The well-known complement-dependent immune adherence reactions, for instance, are mediated largely by the covalently bound complement cleavage products (C3b and C4b), which react with receptors of various types of cells (Table 6). These receptors include CR1 (CD35), which binds both C3b and C4b (172), CR3 (CD11b/CD18 or Mac-1 antigen, $\alpha M\beta 2$), and CR4 (CD11c/CD18 or p150,95), which are specific for iC3b. CR3 and CR4 are members of the integrin family of heterodimeric proteins and play important roles in leukocyte cell adhesion. Another member of the C3 receptor family is CR2, which binds iC3b or C3d and is primarily expressed on B cells. CR2 on B cells is part of a multimolecular complex that includes CD19 and TAPA-1 (target for antiproliferative antibody) (173,174). It is not involved in phagocytosis but plays an important role in the immunoregulatory functions of B cells as evidenced by experiments in which the immune response of animals is impaired upon administration of anti-CR2. It is also now well established that Epstein–Barr virus (EBV) gains access into B cells via CR2 and induces enhanced proliferative response leading cellular immortalization (174).

The C3b in serum or on the surface of activating particles is rapidly cleaved to iC3b by Factor I and its serum or cell surface cofactors (63,131). The subsequent conversion of iC3b to the two physiologic fragments, C3c and C3dg, is however relatively slow. Therefore, the most important receptor in terms of opsonization and phagocytosis is CR3. Receptor-bound C3b (and C4b) is able to opsonize target cells and facilitate phagocytosis. In addition, these molecules are able to induce the release of lysosomal enzymes from a variety of cells (including PMNs, macrophages, and platelets), and potentiate cell-mediated cellular cytotoxicity (173). From studies of the mechanism of phagocytosis (175), it became clear that macrophages possess membrane receptors for Fc and C3b. Ingestion of sensitized erythrocytes depends on the interaction between these receptors and the red blood cell–associated ligands C3b and IgG (176). Furthermore, these receptors have synergistic roles in phagocytosis: C3b receptors mainly promote adherence of the sensitized particles to phagocytes, and the Fc receptors promote ingestion of the particles (176). It appears that C4b reacts with the same receptor and has similar biological effects, though the amount of C4b bound to the complement fixation site is smaller than that of C3b and thus of less significance in vivo. In addition, C3b and C4b have a role in the solubilization of immune complexes. This solubilization apparently results from the intercalation of these proteins into the immune complex lattice (176). Deposition of immune complexes is known to be a major mechanism of tissue injury and inflammation. Thus the interaction of complement-derived peptides with cellular receptors and its contribution to the clearance of immune complexes is of great potential significance (176). The significance of complement receptors in immune complex clearance is well documented especially in immune complex-mediated diseases where complement deficiency is known to perpetuate the inflammatory process. The most abundant cell type in the blood of primates expressing CR1, the receptor for C3b and C4b, is the red cell (platelets on nonprimates), which upon encountering complement bearing immune complexes shuttles them to the liver and spleen. Here, they are dislodged from the erythrocytes and digested by macrophage enzymes while the erythrocyte recirculates into the blood stream.

Other complement receptors (Table 6) that play a role in phagocytosis and immune clearance are those that bind C1q. Binding of C1q to cells is known to elicit a plethora of immunological responses (177–179). These functions include promotion of cell adhesion of fibroblasts, induction of antiproliferative response on B and T cells, stimulation of Ca^{2+} activated K^+ channels and initiation of chemotaxis on mouse fibroblasts and mast cells, and enhancement of phagocytosis by neutrophils (177) and clearance of immune complexes and apoptotic cells (180). Several cell associated molecules referred to as "C1q binding proteins" or "receptors" have been described (177–187) and include gC1q-R (181), cC1q-R, which is identical to calreticulin (177,178,185), C1qRp (179) and most recently, CR1 (182). Whereas the role of CR1 in C3-mediated responses is well established, its role in C1q-mediated responses and indeed whether it binds C1q at all is still debatable. Similarly, although C1qRp, a transmembrane protein, has been shown to enhance the phagocytosis of IgG- or C3b-opsonized particles by monocytes (179) it does not directly bind C1q (183). Therefore, it is postulated that C1q-Rp constitutes a common component activated during a phagocytosis-induced signal (26) regardless of the nature of the extracellular ligand that triggered the process (184). C1q-Rp is an ∼120-kDa O-sialoglycoprotein that is selectively expressed on cells of the myeloid lineage and has been shown recently to be identical to CD93 (184).

INTERACTION BETWEEN THE COMPLEMENT SYSTEM AND THE PLASMA KININ–FORMING SYSTEM

A remarkable similarity exists between the mechanisms involved in the activation of the complement system and those of the Hageman factor (Factor XII)-dependent pathways that lead to blood coagulation, fibrinolysis, and kinin formation. Both systems require initial contact with an activator, which in turn initiates a cascade of reactions involving the sequential activation and conversion of zymogens to their proteolytic form. The inhibitor of C1 (C1-INH), which inactivates C1 by binding to the activated C1r and C1s subcomponents of the molecule, is also a major plasma inhibitor of activated Hageman factor (HFa or XIIa), HFf, FXIIf), Factor XIa, and kallikrein by the formation of stoichiometric complexes. It is also a minor inhibitor of plasmin (24,91,188–191). This inhibitor is known to be functionally absent in patients with hereditary angioedema (58), a disease inherited as an autosomal dominant Mendelian character, which manifests by swelling and recurrent attacks of mucosal edema of the gastrointestinal and upper respiratory tracts. Uninhibited activation of Factor XII may trigger the kinin system by conversion of prekallikrein to kallikrein, which in turn cleaves bradykinin from high-molecular-weight (HK) kininogen. The recent discovery that the endothelial cell surface receptor for both Factor XII and HK is the complement receptor gC1q-R (in association with cytokeratin-1 and uPAR) has made the interrelationship between the CP of the complement system and the contact activation even more intriguing. On the endothelial cell surface therefore, binding of Factor XII and or HK can recruit and assemble the contact pathway proteins, leading thus to the generation of bradykinin (192,193). In the absence of C1-INH any tissue injury that might trigger activation of the kinin-generating cascade would generate large amounts of bradykinin, a potent mediator that causes increased vascular permeability (188). Because the autoactivation of Factor XII, the conversion of prekallikrein to kallikrein, and the effects of kallikrein on Factor XII and HK would be augmented in the absence of C1-INH, it is of particular interest to know that FXIIf (193,194), plasmin (24) and, to a very small degree, Factor XIIa can also activate complement via the classical pathway, whereas kallikrein (188) activates both the classical and alternative pathways. In terms of potency, the major complement activator appears to be Factor XIIf, which directly cleaves and activates C1r (193). The inactivation of bradykinin in plasma is dependent on carboxypeptidase N (kininase I), which cleaves the C-terminal arginine from bradykinin and inactivates it in a manner similar to the inactivation of the anaphylatoxins, C3a, C4a, and C5a (195). Because the anaphylatoxins lead to histamine release from basophils and mast cells, this plasma carboxypeptidase acts to control two types of vasodilators, which have similar phlogistic properties. In contrast, kininase II, which inactivates bradykinin, is also capable of generating the vasoconstrictor angiotensin II from angiotensin I (188), and is better known as angiotensin converting enzyme or ACE.

Interaction of these pathways is also seen in acute gout. In this case monosodium urate crystals are believed to initiate the inflammatory reaction (196,197). In addition to activation of the classical (198) and APs of complement, urate crystals have been shown to activate Factor XII in human plasma and synovial fluid (199). That complement participates in the pathogenesis of gout has been reported previously (59). In view of these findings, it is possible to postulate that activated Factor XII plays a role in the pathogenesis of this disease either through the generation of bradykinin or activation of complement to produce vasoactive peptides. In general, the absence of an inhibitor such as C1-INH may upset homeostatic mechanisms that involve more than one pathway and are more likely to lead to severe disease than is the absence of a proenzyme, particularly if the function of the latter can be bypassed by some other pathway.

ACKNOWLEDGEMENTS

This chapter is dedicated to Larry and Sheila Dalzell whose generosity and encouragement over the years has been simply extraordinary. The time spent writing this chapter was made possible through the support of National Institutes of Health Grant 5R01 AI060866-03.

REFERENCES

1. Müller-Eberhard HJ. Complement: molecular mechanisms, regulation and biologic function. In: Berlin R, Hermann H, Lepow I, et al. (eds). Molecular Basis of Biological Degradative Processes. New York: Academic Press, 1980:65.
2. Müller-Eberhard HJ, Schreiber RD. Molecular biology and chemistry of the alternative pathway of complement. Adv Immunol 1980; 29:1.
3. Cooper NR. Biology of the complement system. In: Gallin JI, Snyderman R, eds. Inflammation: Basic principles and clinical correlates. Philadelphia: Lippincott Williams & Wilkins 1999:281.
4. Lachmann PJ, Hughes-Jones NC. Initiation of complement activation. Springer Semin Immunopathol 1984; 7:143–162.
5. Humphrey JH, Dourmashkin RR. The lesions of cell membranes caused by complement. Adv Immunol 1969; 11:75–115.
6. Law SKA, Reid KBM. Complement. In: Male D, ed. Focus. 2nd ed. Oxford, UK: IRL Press at Oxford Univ Press, 1995.
7. Porter RR. The proteolytic enzymes of the complement system. Methods Enzymol 1981; 80: 3–5.
8. Lesavre PH, Müller-Eberhard HJ. Mechanisms of action of factor D of the alternative complement pathway. J Exp Med 1978; 148:1498.
9. Sastry K, Herman GA, Day L, et al. The human mannose-binding gene. J Exp Med 1989; 10: 1175–1189.
10. Thiel S. Mannan-binding protein, a complement activating animal lectin. Immunopharmacology 1992; 24:91–99.
11. Takada F, Seki N, Masuda Y-I, et al. Localization of the genes for the 100-kDa complement activating components of Ra-reactive factor (CRARF and Crarf) to human 3q27-q28 and mouse 16B2-B3. Genomics 1995; 25:757–759.
12. Matsushita M, Fujita T. Activation of the classical pathway by mannose-binding protein in association with a novel C1s-like serine protease. J Exp Med 1992; 176:1497.

13. Holmskov U, Malhotra R, Sim RB, et al. Collectins: collagenous C-type lectins of the innate immune defense system. Immunol Today 1994; 15:67–74.

14. Ross GD. Immunobiology of the complement system: an introduction for research and clinical medicine.Orlando, Florida: Academic Press, 1986.

15. Cooper NR. Activation and regulation of the first complement component. Fed Proc 1983; 42: 134–138.

16. Cooper NR, Jensen RC, Welsh RM, et al. Lysis of RNA tumor viruses by human serum: direct antibody independent triggering of the classical complement pathway. J Exp Med 1976; 144: 970–984.

17. Mills BJ, Cooper NR. Antibody-independent neutralization of vesicular stomatitis virus by human complement. I. Complement requirements. J Immunol 1978; 121:1549–1557.

18. Volanakis JE, Kaplan MH. Interaction of the C-reactive protein complexes with the complement system. II. Consumption of guinea pig complement by CRP complexes: requirement for C1q. J Immunol 1974; 113:9–17.

19. Cooper NR, Morrison DC. Binding and activation of the first component of human complement by the lipid A region of lipopolysaccharides. J Immunol 1978; 120:1862–1868.

20. Schreiber RD, Feldman HA. Identification of the activation system for antibody to Toxoplasma as the classical complement pathway. J Infect Dis 1980; 141:366–369.

21. Cooper NR, Miles LA, Griffin JH. Effects of plasma kallikrein and plasmin on the first component of complement. J Immunol 1980; 124:1517.

22. Gigli I, Kaplan AP, Austen KF. Modulation of function of the activated first component of complement by a fragment derived from serum: effect on early components of complement. J Exp Med 1971; 134:1466.

23. Ghebrehiwet B, Silverberg M, Kaplan AP. Activation of the classical pathway of complement by Hageman factor fragment. J Exp Med 1981; 153:665–676.

24. Ratnoff OD, Naff GB. The conversion of C1s to C1s by plasmin and trypsin. J Exp Med 1967; 125:337.

25. Medicus RG, Chapuis RM. The first component of complement. I. Purification and properties of native C1. J Immunol 1980; 125:390–395.

26. Ziccardi RJ. The first component of human complement (C1): activation and control. Springer Semin Immunopathol 1983; 6:213–230.

27. Ziccardi RJ, Cooper NR. Active disassembly of the first complement component, C1 by C1-inactivator. J Immunol 1979; 123:788–792.

28. Ziccardi RJ, Cooper NR. The subunit composition and sedimentation properties of human C1. J Immunol 1977; 118:2047–2052.

29. Arlaud, GE, Gaboriaud C, Thielens, NM, et al. Structural biology of C1: dissection of a complex molecular machinery. Immunol Rev 2001; 180:136–145.

30. Arlaud GE, Gaboriaud C, Garnier G, et al. Structure, function and molecular genetics of human murine C1r. Immunobiology 2002; 205:365–382.

31. Müller-Eberhard HJ, Götze O. C3 proactivator convertase and its mode of action. J Exp Med 1972; 135:1003–1008.

32. Calcott MA, Müller-Eberhard HJ. C1q protein of human complement. Biochemistry 1972; 11:3443–3450.

33. Shelton E, Yonemasu K, Stroud RM. Ultrastructure of the human complement component C1q. Proc Natl Acad Sci U S A 1972; 69:65.

34. Kehoe JM, Faugerau M. Immunoglobulin peptide with complement fixing activity. Nature 1969; 224:1212–1213.

35. Hurst MM, Volanakis JE, Hester RB, et al. The structural basis for binding of complement by immunoglobulin M. J Exp Med 1974; 140:1117–1121.

36. Plaut AG, Cohen S, Tomasi TB. Immunoglubulin M: fixation of human complement by the Fc fragment. Science 1972; 176:55–56.

37. Reid KBM, Gagnon J, Frampton J. Completion of the amino acid sequences of the A and B chains subcomponent C1q of the first component of human complement. Biochem J 1982; 203:559.

38. Reid KBM, Porter RR. Subunit composition of subcomponent C1q of the first component of human complement. Biochem J 1976; 155:19.

39. Reid KBM, Sim RB, Faiers AP. Inhibition of the reconstitution of the hemolytic activity of the first component of human complement by a pepsin-derived fragment of subcomponent C1q. Biochem J 1977; 161:239.

40. Porter RR. Structure and activation of the early components of complement. Fed Proc 1977; 36:2191.

41. Sellar GC, Blake DJ, Reid KBM. Characterization and organization of the genes encoding the A-, B-, C- chains of human complement subcomponent C1q. The complete derived amino acid sequence of human C1q. Biochem J 1991; 274:481.

42. Kishore U, Kojouharova Ms, Reid KBM. Recent progress in the understanding of the structure-function relationships of the lobular head regions of C1q. Immunobiol 2002; 205:355.

43. Golan M, Burger R, Loos M. Detection of conformational changes within the C1q molecule with monoclonal anti-C1q antibodies. Mol Immunol 1982; 19:1371.

44. Arlaud GJ, Gagnon J, Porter RR. The catalytic chain of human complement subcomponent C1r. Purification and N-terminal amino acid sequences of the major cyanogen bromide-cleavage fragments. Biochem J 1982; 201:49–59.

45. Valet G, Cooper NR. Isolation and characterization of the proenzyme form of the C1s subunit of the first complement component. J Immunol 1974; 112:339.

46. Vogt W. Substrate modulation as a control mechanism in the activation of plasma multi-enzyme systems. In: Fugii S, Moriya H, Suzuki T, eds. Kinins IIB: Systemic Proteases and Cellular Function. Advances in Experimental Medicine and Biology, vol. 120 B. New York: Plenum, 1979:125.

47. Budzko DB, Müller-Eberhard HJ. Cleavage of the fourth component of human complement (C4) by C1 esterase: isolation and characterization of the low molecular weight product. Immunochemistry 1970; 7:227.

48. Gorski JP, Hugli TE, Müller-Eberhard HJ. C4a; the third anaphylatoxin of the human complement system. Proc Natl Acad Sci U S A 1979; 76:5299–5302.

49. Hugli TE. The structural basis for anaphylatoxin and chemotactic functions of C3a, C4a, C5a. Crit Rev Immunol 1981; 1:321–366.

50. Hugli TE, Müller-Eberhard HJ. Anaphylatoxins: C3a and C5a. Adv Immunol 1978; 26:1–53.

51. Nagasawa S, Stroud RM. Cleavage of C2 by C1s into the antigenically distinct fragments C2a and C2b: demonstration of binding of C2b to C4b. Proc Natl Acad Sci U S A 1977; 74: 2998–3001.

52. Müller-Eberhard HJ, Polley MJ, Calcott MA. Formation and functional significance of a molecular complex derived from the second and the fourth component of human complement. J Exp Med 1967; 125:359–380.

53. Cooper NR. Enzymatic activity of the second component of complement. Biochemistry 1975; 14:4245–4251.

54. Gigli I, Austen KF. Fluid phase destruction of C2^{hu} by C1^{hu}. I. Its enhancement and inhibition by homologous and heterologous C4. J Exp Med 1969; 129:679–696.

55. Gigli I, Austen KF. Fluid phase destruction of C2^{hu} by C1^{hu}. II. Unmasking by C4i^{hu} of C1^{hu} specificity for C2^{hu}. J Exp Med 1969; 130:833–846.

56. Gigli I, Fujita T, Nussenzweig V. Modulation of the classical pathway C3 convertase by plasma proteins C4 binding protein and C3b inactivator. Proc Natl Acad Sci U S A 1979; 76: 6596–6600.

57. Gigli I, Kaplan A, Austen KF. Alteration in complement component utilization following the interaction of C1^{hu} with kallikrein fragment. J Immunol 1971; 107:311.

58. Donaldson VH, Ratnoff OD, DaSilva WD, et al. Permeability increasing activity in hereditary angioneurotic edema plasma. II. Mechanism of formation and partial characterization. J Clin Invest 1969; 48:642–653.

59. Klemperer MR, Donaldson VH, Rosen FS. The vasopermeability response in man to purified C1 esterase. J Clin Invest 1967; 46:1079.

60. Curd JG, Yelvington M, Burridge N, et al. Generation of bradykinin during incubation of hereditary angioedema plasma. Mol Immunol 1982; 19:1365.
61. Fields TR, Ghebrehiwet B, Kaplan AP. Kinin formation in hereditary angioedema plasma: evidence against kinin derivation from C2 and in support of "spontaneous" formation of bradykinin. J Allergy Clin Immunol 1983; 72:54–60.
62. Smith MA, Kerr MA. The kinin activity generated in C1-INH deficient plasma is not derived from C2 and originates from the kallikrein kininogen pathway. Immunobiology 1983; 164:299.
63. Singer L, Colten HR, Wetsel RA. Complement C3 deficiency: Human, animal and experimental models. Pathbiology 1994; 62:14–28.
64. Bokisch VA, Dierich MP, Müller-Eberhard HJ. Third component of complement (C3): structural properties in relation to function. Proc Natl Acad Sci U S A 1975; 72:1989–1993.
65. Tack BF, Morris SC, Prahl JW. Third component of human complement: structural analysis of the polypeptide chains of C3 and C3b. Biochemistry 1979; 18:1497–1503.
66. Alper CA, Johnson AM, Cirtch AG, et al. Human C3: evidence for the liver as the primary site of synthesis. Science 1969; 163:286–288.
67. Brade V, Fries W, Bently C. Identification of properdin, B, D, and C3 as biosynthetic products of guinea pig peritoneal macrophages and influence of culture conditions on their secretion. J Immunol 1978; 120:1766.
68. Colten HR. Ontogeny of the human complement system: in vitro biosynthesis of individual complement components by fetal tissue. J Clin Invest 1972; 51:725–730.
69. Eisenstein LP, Hansen PJ, Ballow M, et al. Biosynthesis of the third component of complement (C3) in vitro by monocytes from both normal and homozygous C3 deficient humans. J Clin Invest 1977; 60:963–969.
70. McClelland DBL, Van Furth R. In vitro synthesis of β_1C/β_1A globulin (the C3 component of complement) by tissues and leukocytes in mice. Immunology 1976; 31:855–861.
71. Lachmann PJ, Rosen FS. Genetic defects of complement in man. Springer Semin Immunopathol 1978; 1:339.
72. Lepow IH, Williams-Kretschmer K, Patrick RA, et al. Cross and ultrastructural observations on lesions produced by intradermal injection of human C3a in man. Am J Pathol 1970; 61:13.
73. Weigle WO, Goodman MG, Morgan EL, et al. Regulation of immune response by components of the complement cascade and their activated fragments. Springer Semin Immunopathol 1983; 6:173–194.
74. Bokisch VA, Müller-Eberhard HJ. Anaphylatoxin inactivator of human plasma: its isolation and characterization as a carboxypeptidase. J Clin Invest 1970; 49:2427.
75. Fernandez HM, Hugli TE. Primary structural analysis of the polypeptide portion of human C5a anaphylatoxin. J Biol Chem 1978; 253:6955–6964.
76. Hugli TE. Human anaphylatoxin (C3a) from the third component of complement: primary structure. J Biol Chem 1975; 250:8293–8301.
77. Pangburn MK, Morrison DC, Schreiber RD, et al. Activation of the alternative pathway: recognition of surface structures on activators by bound C3b. J Immunol 1980; 124:977–982.
78. Pangburn MK, Schreiber RD, Trombold JT, et al. Paroxysmal nocturnal hemoglobinuria: deficiency in factor H-like functions of the abnormal erythrocytes. J Exp Med 1983; 157: 1971–1980.
79. Sahu A, Kozel TR, Pangburn MK. Specificity of the thioester-containing reactive site of human C3 and its significance to complement activation. Biochem J 1994; 302(pt 2):429–436.
80. Fearon DT. Identification of the membrane glycoprotein that is the C3b receptor of the human erythrocyte, polymorphonuclear leukocyte, B lymphocyte, and monocyte. J Exp Med 1980; 152:20–30.
81. Schreiber RD. The chemistry and biology of complement receptors. Springer Semin Immunopathol 1984; 7:221–249.
82. Pangburn MK, Schreiber RD, Müller-Eberhard HJ. Human complement C3b inactivator: isolation, characterization and demonstration of an absolute requirement for the serum protein $\beta1H$ for cleavage of C3b and C4b in solution. J Exp Med 1977; 146:257.

83. Harrison RA, Lachmann PJ. The physiological breakdown of the third component of human complement. Mol Immunol 1980; 17:9–20.

84. Lachmann PJ, Pangburn MK, Oldroyd RG. Breakdown of C3 after complement activation: identification of a new fragment, C3g, using monoclonal antibodies. J Exp Med 1982; 156:205–216.

85. Ghebrehiwet B, Müller-Eberhard HJ. C3e: an acidic fragment of human C3 with leukocytosis inducing activity. J Immunol 1979; 123:616–621.

86. Ghebrehiwet B. The release of lysosomal enzymes from human polymorphonuclear leukocytes by human C3e. Clin Immunol Immunopathol 1984; 30:321–329.

87. Meuth JL, Morgan EL, DiScipio RG, et al. Suppression of T-lymphocyte functions by human C3 fragments: inhibition of human T cell proliferative responses by a kallikrein cleavage fragment of human iC3b. J Immunol 1983; 130:2605.

88. Morgan EL, Thoman ML, Weigle WO, et al. Anaphylatoxin-mediated immune response. II. C5a-mediated enhancement of human humoral and T cell-mediated immune responses. J Immunol 1983; 130:1257–1261.

89. Daffern PJ, Pfeifer PH, Ember JA, et al. C3a is a chemotaxin for human eosinophils but not for neutrophils. I. C3a stimulation of neutrophils is secondary to eosinophil activation. J Exp Med 1995; 181:2119–2127.

90. Laurell AB, Johnson U, Martenson U, et al. Formation of complexes composed of C1r, C1s and C1-inactivator in human serum on activation of C1. Acta Pathol Microbiol Scand [C] 1978; 86C:299–306.

91. Forbes CO, Pensky J, Ratnoff OD. Inhibition of activated Hageman factor and activated plasma thromboplastin antecedent by purified C1 inactivator. J Lab Clin Med 1970; 76: 809–815.

92. Bos IGA, Hack CE, Abrahams JP. Structural and functional aspects of C1-inhibitor. Immunobiol 2002; 205:518–533.

93. Fujita T, Nussenzweig V. The role of C4-binding protein β1H in proteolysis of C4b and C3b. J Exp Med 1979; 150:267.

94. Law SK, Lichsenberg NA, Levine RP. Evidence for an ester linkage between the labile binding site of C3b and receptive surfaces. J Immunol 1979; 123:1388–1394.

95. Ihara I, Harada Y, Ihara S, et al. A new complement-dependent bactericidal factor found in non-immune mouse sera: specific binding to polysaccharide of Ra chemotype Salmonella. J Immunol 1982; 128:1256–1260.

96. Jack DL, Klein NJ, Turner MW. Mannose-binding lectin: targeting the microbial world for complement attack and opsonophagocytosis. Immunol Rev 2001; 180:86–99.

97. Schwaeble W, Dahl MR, Thiel S, et al. The mannan-binding lectin-associated serine proteases (MASPs) and Map19: four components of the lectin pathway activation complex encoded by two genes. Immunobiol 2002; 205:455–466.

98. Drickamer K, Doral MS, Reynolds L. Mannose-binding proteins isolated from rat liver contain carbohydrate-recognition domains linked to collagenous tails. J Biol Chem 1986; 261–1034.

99. Ikeda K, Sannoh T, Kawasaki N, et al. Serum lectin with known structure activates complement through the classical pathway. J Biol Chem 1987; 262:7451–7454.

100. Taylor ME, Brickell PM, Craig RK, et al. Structure and evolutionary origin of the gene encoding a human serum mannose-binding protein. Biochem J 1989; 262:763–771.

101. Holmskov U, Thiel S, Jensenius JC. Collectins and ficolins: humoral lectins of the innate immune defense. Ann Rev Immunol 2003; 21:547–578.

102. Lu J, Thiel S, Wiedman H, et al. Binding of the pentamer/hexamer forms of mannan-binding protein to zymosan activates the proenzyme C1r2C1s2 complex of the classical pathway of complement, without involvement of C1q. J Immunol 1990; 144:2287–2294.

103. Crouch E, Wright JR. Surfacatant proteins A and D and pulmonary host defense. Annu Rev Physiol 2001; 63:521–554.

104. Haagsman HP. Structural and functional aspects of the collectin SP-A. Immunobiology 2002; 205: 476–489.

105. Hoppe H-J, Reid KBM. Trimeric C-type lectin domains in host defence. Structure 1994; 2: 1129–1133.
106. Thiel S, Møller-Kristensen M, Jensen L, et al. Assays for the functional activity of the mannan-binding lectin pathway of complement activation. Immunobiol 2002; 205:446–454.
107. Stover CM, Thiel S, Thelen M, et al. Two constituents of the initiation complex of the mannan-binding lectin activation pathway of complement are encoded by a single structural gene. J Immunol 1999; 162:3481–3490.
108. Matsushita M, Endo Y, Fujita T. Cutting edge: complement activating complex of ficolin and mannose-binding lectin-associated serine protease. J Immunol 2000; 164:2281–2284.
109. Matsushita M, Kuraya M, Hamasaki N, et al. Activation of the lectin complement pathway by H-Ficolin (Hakata antigen). J Immunol 2002; 168:3502–3506.
110. Schreiber RD, Pangburn MK, Medicus RG, et al. Raji cell injury and subsequent lysis by purified cytolytic alternative pathway of human complement. Clin Immunol Immunopathol 1980; 15:384–396.
111. Pangburn MK, Müller-Eberhard HJ. Relation of a putative thioester bond in C3 to activation of the alternative pathway and the binding of C3b to biological targets of complement. J Exp Med 1980; 152:1102–1114.
112. Pangburn MK, Meri S. Molecular mechanism of recognition by the alternative pathway of complement and locations of the restriction and sialic acid sites. Complement Inflamm 1989; 6:383.
113. Fearon DT. Regulation by membrane sialic acid of β1H-dependent decay-dissociation of amplification C3 convertase of the alternative complement pathway. Proc Natl Acad Sci U S A 1978; 75:1971–1975.
114. Götze O, Müller-Eberhard HJ. The C3 activator system in an alternative pathway of complement activation. J Exp Med 1971; 134S:90.
115. Hunsicker LG, Ruddy S, Austen KF. Alternative complement pathway factors involved in cobra venom factor (CoVF) activation of the third component (C3). J Immunol 1973; 110:128.
116. Hamuro J, Hadding V, Bitter-Suermann D. Fragments Ba and Bb derived guinea pig factor B of the properdin system purification: characterization and biological activities. J Immunol 1978; 120:438.
117. Bianco C, Gotze O, Cohn ZA. Regulation of macrophages migration by products of the complement system. Proc Natl Acad Sci U S A 1979; 76:888–891.
118. Fearon DT, Austen KF. Properdin: binding to C3b and stabilization of the C3b-dependent convertase. J Exp Med 1975; 142:856–863.
119. Medicus RG, Götze O, Müller-Eberhard HJ. Alternative pathway of complement: recruitment and precursor properdin by the labile C3/C5 convertase and the potentiation of the pathway. J Exp Med 1976; 144:1076–1093.
120. Volanakis JE, Narayana SVL. Complement factor D. a novel serine protease. Protein Sci 1996; 5:553–564.
121. Xu Y, Narayana SVL, Volanakis JE. Structural Biology of the alternative pathway convertase. Immunol Rev 2001; 180:123–135.
122. Gewurz H, Pickering RJ, Snyderman R, et al. Interactions of the complement system with endotoxic lipopolysaccharides in immunoglobulins deficient sera. J Exp Med 1970; 128: 817–831.
123. Platts-Mills TAI, Ishizaka K. Activation of the alternate pathway of human complement by rabbit cells. J Immunol 1974; 113:348–358.
124. Joseph BS, Cooper NR, Oldstone MBA. Immunologic injury of cultured cells infected with measles virus. I. Role of IgG antibody and the alternative complement pathway. J Exp Med 1975; 141:761–774.
125. Whaley K, Ruddy S. Modulation of the alternative complement pathway by β1H globulin. J Exp Med 1976; 144:1147.
126. Fearon DT, Austen KF. Activation of the alternative complement pathway due to resistance of zymosan-bound amplification convertase to endogenous regulatory mechanisms. Proc Natl Acad Sci U S A 1977; 74:1683–1687.

127. Pangburn MK, Müller-Eberhard HJ. Complement C3 convertase: cell surface restriction of β1H and generation of restriction on neuraminidase-treated cells. Proc Natl Acad Sci U S A 1978; 75:2416–2420.

128. Fearon DT. Regulation of the amplification C3 convertase of human complement by an inhibiting protein isolated from human erythrocyte membrane. Proc Natl Acad Sci U S A 1979; 76:5867.

129. Fearon DT. The human C3b receptor. Springer Semin Immunopathol 1983; 6:159.

130. Nicholson-Weller A, Burge J, Fearon DT, et al. Isolation of human erythrocyte membrane glycoprotein with decay-accelerating activity for C3 convertases of the complement system. J Immunol 1982; 129:184.

131. Medof ME, Lublin DM, Holers VM, et al. Cloning and characterization of cDNAs encoding the complete sequence of decay-accelerating factor of human complement. Proc Natl Acad Sci U S A 1987; 84:2007–2011.

132. Krych-Goldberg M, Atkinson JP. Structure-function relationships of complement receptor type 1. Immunol Rev 2001; 180:112–122.

133. Pangburn MK, Schreiber RD, Müller-Eberhard HJ. Deficiency of an erythrocyte membrane protein with complement regulatory activity in paroxysmal nocturnal hemoglobinuria. Proc Natl Acad Sci U S A 1983; 80:5430–5434.

134. DiScipio RG, Chakravarti DN, Müller-Eberhard HJ, et al. The structure of human complement component C7 and the C5b-7 complex. J Biol Chem 1988; 263:549–560.

135. Rao AG, Howard OMZ, Ng SC, et al. Complementary DNA and derived amino acid sequence of the alpha subunit of human complement C8: evidence for the existence of a separate α subunit messenger RNA. Biochemistry 1987; 26:3556.

136. DiScipio RG, Hugli TE. The molecular architecture of human complement C6. J Biol Chem 1989; 264:16197–16206.

137. Haefliger JA, Tscopp J, Vial N, et al. Complete primary structure and functional characterization of the sixth component of the human complement system. J Biol Chem 1989; 264:18041–18051.

138. Haefliger JA, Tscopp J, Naedlli D, et al. Complementary DNA cloning of complement C8γ and its sequence homology to C9. Biochemistry 1987; 26:3551.

139. Howard OMZ, Rao AG, Sodetz JM. Complementary DNA and derived amino acid sequence of the β subunit of the human complement protein C8: identification of a close structural and ancestral relationship to the α subunit and C9. Biochemistry 1987; 26:3565.

140. Kolb WP, Müller-Eberhard HJ. The membrane attack mechanism of complement: verification of a stable C5b-9 complex in free solution. J Exp Med 1973; 138:438.

141. Podack ER, Biesecker G, Kolb WP, et al. The C5b-6 complex: reaction with C7, C8, C9. J Immunol 1978; 121:484.

142. Tranum-Jensen J, Bhakdi S, Bhakadi-Lehnen B, et al. Complement lysis: the ultrastructure and orientation of the C5b-9 complex on target sheep erythroctye membranes. Scand J Immunol 1978; 7:45–46.

143. Kolb WP, Kolb LM, Savary JR. Biochemical characterization of the sixth component (C6) of human complement. Biochemistry 1982; 21:294–301.

144. Scibek JJ, Plumb ME, Sodetz JM. Binding of human complement C8 to C9: role of the N-terminal modules in the C8α subunit. Biochemistry 2002; 41:14546–14551.

145. Podack ER, Tschopp J, Müller-Eberhard HJ. Molecular organization of C9 within the membrane attack complex of complement: induction of circular C9 polymerization by the C5b-8 assembly. J Exp Med 1982; 156:268–282.

146. Podack ER, Müller-Eberhard HJ, Horst H, et al. Membrane attack complex of complement (MAC): three dimensional analysis of MAC-phospholipid vesicle recombinants. J Immunol 1982; 128:2353–2357.

147. Podack ER, Müller-Eberhard HJ. Binding of desoxycholate, phosphatidylcholine vesicles, lipoprotein and of the S protein to complexes of terminal complement components. J Immunol 1978; 121:1025.

148. Podack ER, Stoffel W, Esser AF, et al. Membrane attack complex of complement: distribution of subunits between hydrocarbon phase of target membranes and water. Proc Natl Acad Sci U S A 1981; 78:4544–4548.

149. Hu VW, Esser AF, Podack ER, et al. The membrane attack of complement: photolabeling reveals insertion of terminal proteins into target membranes. J Immunol 1981; 127:380.

150. Esser AF, Kolb WP, Podak ER, et al. Molecular reorganization of lipid bilayers by complement: a possible mechanism for membranolysis. Proc Natl Acad Sci U S A 1979; 76:1410–1414.

151. Podack ER, Biesecker G, Müller-Eberhard HJ. Membrane attack complex of complement: generation of high affinity phospholipid binding sites by the fusion of six hydrophilic, plasma proteins. Proc Natl Acad Sci U S A 1979; 76:897.

152. Mayer MM. Mechanisms of cytolysis by complement. Proc Natl Acad Sci U S A 1972; 69: 2954.

153. Schreiber RD, Morrison DC, Podack ER, et al. Bactericidal activity of the alternative complement pathway generated from eleven isolated plasma proteins. J Exp Med 1979; 149: 870.

154. Podack ER, Esser AF, Biesecker G, et al. Membrane attack complex of complement: a structural analysis of its assembly. J Exp Med 1980; 151:301–313.

155. Dourmashkin RR. The structural events associated with the attachment of complement components to cell membranes in reactive lysis. Immunology 1978; 35:205–212.

156. Harriman GR, Esser AF, Podack ER, et al. The role of C9 in complement-mediated killing of Neisseria. J Immunol 1981; 127:2386–2390.

157. Haeney MR, Thompson RA, Faulkner J, et al. Recurrent bacterial meningitis in patients with genetic defects of terminal complement components. Clin Exp Immunol 1980; 40:16–24.

158. Lee TJ, Schmoyer A, Snyderman R, et al. Familial deficiencies of the sixth and seventh components of complement associated with bacteremic Neisserial infections. In: Brooks GF, Gotschlich EC, Holmes KK, et al. eds. Immunology of Neisseria Gonorrhoeae. Washington, D.C.: American Society for Microbiology, 1978:204–206.

159. Lee TJ, Utsinger PD, Snyderman R, et al. Familial deficiency of the seventh component of complement associated with recurrent bacteremic infections due to Neisseria. J Infect Dis 1978; 138:359–368.

160. Snyderman R, Durack DT, McCarty GA, et al. Deficiency of the fifth component of complement in human subjects. Am J Med 1979; 67:638–645.

161. Tschopp J, Müller-Eberhard HJ, Podack ER. Formation of transmembrane tubules by spontaneous polymerization of the hydrophilic complement protein C9. Nature 1982; 298: 534–538.

162. Podack ER, Tschopp J. Polymerization of the ninth component of complement (C9): formation of poly (C9) with a tubular ultrastructure resembling the membrane attack complex of complement. Proc Natl Acad Sci U S A 1982; 79:574.

163. Podack ER, Dennert G. Assembly of two types of tubules with putative cytolytic function by cloned natural killer cells. Nature 1983; 302:442–445.

164. Elsner J, Oppermann M, Czech W, et al. C3a activates the respiratory burst in human polymorphonuclear neutrophilic leukocytes via pertussis toxin-sensitive G-proteins. Blood 1994; 83:3324–3331.

165. Elsner J, Oppermann M, Czech W, et al. C3a activates reactive oxygen radical species production and intracellular calcium transients in human eosinophils. Eur J Immunol 1994; 24:518–522.

166. Gerard C, Gerard NP. C5a anaphylatoxin and its seven transmembrane-segment receptor. Annu Rev Immunol 1994; 12:775–808.

167. Gerard C, Gerard NP. The pro-inflammatory seven transmembrane segment receptors of the leukocyte. Curr Opin Immunol 1994; 6:140–145.

168. Murakami Y, Imamachi T, Nagasawa S. Characterization of C3a anaphylatoxin receptor on guinea- pig macrophages. Immunology 1993; 79:633–638.

169. Kew RR, Webster RO. Gc-globulin (vitamin D-binding protein) enhances the neutrophil chemotactic activity of C5a and C5a des Arg. J Clin Invest 1988; 82:364–369.

170. Perez HD, Kelly E, Chenoweth DE, et al. Identification of the C5a des Arg cochemotaxin: identity with vitamin D-binding protein (group specific component globulin). J Clin Invest 1988; 82:360–363.

171. Gerard C, Hugli TE. Identification of classical anaphylatoxin as the des Arg form of the C5a molecule: evidence of a modulator role for the oligosaccharaide unit in human des-Arg 74 C5a. Proc Natl Acad Sci U S A 1981; 78:1833–1837.

172. Ahearn JM, Fearon DT. Structure and function of the complement receptors, CR1 (CD35) and CR2 (CD21). Adv Immunol 1989; 46:183–219.

173. Fearon DT, Carter RH. The CD19/CR2/TAPA-1 complex of B lymphocytes: linking natural to acquired immunity. Ann Rev Immunol 1995; 13:127–149.

174. Nemerow G, Luxembourg A, Cooper N. CD21/CR2: its role in EBV infection and immune function. Epstein Barr Rep 1994; 1:59–64.

175. Ehlenberger AG, Nussenzweig V. The role of membrane receptors for C3b and C3d in phagocytosis. J Exp Med 1977; 145:357–371.

176. Nussenzweig V. Interaction between complement and immune complexes: role of complement in containing immune complex damage. In: Fougerau M, Dausset J, eds. Progress in Immunology. New York: Academic, 1980.

177. Ghebrehiwet B, Lim B-L, Kumar R, et al. Structure and function of gC1q-R: a multiligand binding cellular protein. Immunobiol 1998; 199:225–238.

178. Sim RB, Moestrup SK, Stuart GR, et al. Interaction of C1q and the collectins with the potential receptors calreticulin (cC1q-R/collectin receptor) and megalin. Immunobiol 1998; 199: 208–224.

179. Tenner AJ. C1q receptors: regulating specific functions of phagocytic cells. Immunobiol 1998; 199:250–264.

180. Ogden CA, de Cathelineau A, Hoffmann PR, et al. C1q and mannose binding lectin engagement of cell surface calreticulin and CD91 initiates macropinocytosis and uptake of apoptotic cells. J Exp Med 2001; 194:781–795.

181. Ghebrehiwet B, Lim B-L, Peerschke EIB, et al. Isolation, cDNA cloning and overexpression of a 33 kDa cell surface glycoprotein which binds to the globular "heads" of C1q (gC1q-R). J Exp Med 1994; 179:1809–1821.

182. Klickstein L, Barbashov S, Liu T, et al. Complement receptor type 1(CR1,CD35) is a receptor for C1q. Immunity 1997; 7:345–355.

183. McGreal EP, Ikewaki N, Akatsu H, et al. Human C1qRp is identical with CD93 and the mNI-11 antigen but does not bind C1q. J Immunol 2002; 168:5222–5232.

184. Steinberger P, Szekeres A, Willie S, et al. Identification of human CD93 as the phagocytic C1q receptor (C1qRp) by expression cloning. J Leuk Biol 2002; 71:133–140.

185. Sontheimer RD, Nguyen TQ, Cheng S-T, et al. The unveiling of calreticulin: a linically relevant tour of modern biology. J Investig Med 1995; 43:362–370.

186. Jianzhong J, Zhang Y, Krainer A, et al. Crystal structure of p32, a doughnut shaped acidic mitochondrial matrix protein. Proc Natl Acad Sci U S A 1999; 96:3572–3577.

187. Ghebrehiwet B, Lim, B-L, Kumar R, et al. gC1q-R, a member of a new class of multifunctional and multicompartmental cellular proteins, is involved in inflammation and infection. Immunol Rev 2001; 180:65–77.

188. Kaplan AP, Joseph, K, Shibayama Y, et al. The intrinsic coagulation/kinin-forming cascade: assembly in plasma and cell surfaces in inflammation. Adv Immunol 1997; 66:225–272.

189. Harpel PD, Cooper NR. Studies on human plasma C1 inactivator-enzyme interactions. I. Mechanisms of interaction with C1s, plasmin and trypsin. J Clin Invest 1975; 55:593–604.

190. Ratnoff OD, Pensky D, Ogston D, et al. The inhibition of plasmin, plasma kallikrein, plasma permeability factor and the C1r subcomponent of the first component of complement by serum C1 esterase inhibitor. J Exp Med 1969; 129:315.

191. Schreiber AD, Kaplan AP, Austen KF. Inhibition by C1-INH of Hageman factor fragment activation of coagulation, fibrinolysis and kinin-generation. J Clin Invest 1973; 52:1401.

192. Joseph K, Ghebrehiwet B, Peerschke EIB, et al. Identification of the zinc-dependent endothelial cell binding protein for high molecular weight kininogen and factor Xii: identity with the receptor which binds the globular heads of C1q (gC1q-R). Proc Natl Acad Sci U S A 1996; 93:8552–8557.

193. Joseph K, Ghebrehiwet B, Kaplan AP. Cytokeratin 1 and gC1q-R mediate high molecular weight kininogen and factor XII binding to endothelial cells. Clin Immunol 1999; 92:246–255.

194. Ghebrehiwet B, Randazzo BP, Dunn JT, et al. Mechanisms of activation of the classical pathway of complement by Hageman factor fragment. J Clin Invest 1983; 71:1450–1456.

195. Erdos EG, Sloane EM. An enzyme in human blood plasma that inactivates bradykinin and kallidins. Biochem Pharmacol 1962; 11:585–592.

196. Giclas PC, Ginsberg MH, Cooper NR. Immunoglobulin G independent activation of the classical pathway by monosodium urate crystals. J Clin Invest 1979; 63:759–764.

197. Fields TR, Abramson SB, Weissmann G, et al. Activation of the alternative pathway of complement by monosodium urate crystals. Clin Immunol Immunopathol 1983; 26:249–257.

198. Naff GB, Byers PH. Complement as a mediator of inflammation in acute gouty arthritis. I. Studies on the reaction between human serum complement and sodium urate crystals. J Lab Clin Med 1973; 81:747.

199. Ginsberg MH, Jaques B, Cochrane CG, et al. Urate crystal-dependent cleavage of Hageman factor in human plasma and synovial fluid. J Lab Clin Med 1980; 95:497–506.

7

The IgE-Mediated Cutaneous Late-Phase Reaction

Lori Wagner, Kristin M. Leiferman, and Gerald J. Gleich
Departments of Dermatology and Medicine, The University of Utah Health Sciences Center, University of Utah, Salt Lake City, Utah, U.S.A.

HISTORY

Antigen exposure with production of an immediate wheal and flare in allergic individuals may lead to a prolonged inflammatory response known as the late-phase reaction (LPR) and also referred to as the dual-phase response. The LPR was described in 1873 by Blackley who was allergic to grass pollen and underwent a bout of sneezing and coryza lasting six to eight hours after grass pollen inhalation (1). On a different occasion, he accidentally inhaled a considerable quantity of pollen and developed nasal and systemic symptoms that lasted for many hours and prevented him from working for two days. In 1922, Cooke described a wheal and flare skin reaction after exposure to horse dander, followed by erythema and edema continuing into the next day (2). In 1924, Vaughn observed persistent inflammation at the site of skin tests (3). In 1952, Herxheimer stressed that the "late bronchial response" was "of great practical importance," and was associated with more severe asthma than the asthma in patients without late reactions (4). Prausnitz and Küstner observed that the cutaneous inflammation associated with passive transfer of sensitivity lasted at least a day (5). This persistent inflammation was termed the late-phase response or LPR.

The LPR is an IgE-mediated immune response. During the 1960s, Pepys and his colleagues called attention to dual skin reactions in patients with allergic aspergillosis and showed dermal deposition of IgG, IgM, and C3 (6) as well as marked tissue infiltration by neutrophils, suggesting an Arthus reaction (Gell and Coombs type III hypersensitivity) as the mechanism for prolonged inflammation. However, late reactions also occurred after skin testing with grass pollen extract (6), in which precipitating antibodies are uncommon, suggesting this was not a type III reaction. A key observation was that of Dolovich and his colleagues who showed that the LPR occurred after injection of specific antibody to IgE (7,8), suggesting that IgE played a central role in provocation of the LPR. Subsequently, Solley et al. (9) reported that the LPR could be passively transferred by purified IgE antibodies, and that a reaction similar to the LPR could be stimulated by mast cell activators. Their observations implicated IgE and the mast cell as essential components for initiation of the cutaneous LPR.

The skin is a useful model for studying the LPR because it is easily accessible for testing. Recent studies have concentrated on identification of the mediators involved in the LPR and pharmacologic agents that block the reaction with the goal of providing insights into the pathogenesis of allergic diseases. Although the LPR has been investigated extensively in the skin, it is likely representative of the pathogenesis of chronic allergic disease in other epithelial organs, especially the respiratory tract, including nasal mucosa and bronchial tissues. The LPR has been reviewed previously (10), and the reader is directed to this literature for discussions of the role of the LPR in chronic allergic diseases (11–16).

CHARACTERISTICS

The cutaneous LPR usually follows injection of a known allergen in a sensitized individual, although the reaction has also been triggered by intradermal injection of an activating anti-IgE or by passive sensitization with specific IgE antibody and subsequent allergen challenge (7–9,17). Theoretically, the LPR can be induced by any antigen that elicits a wheal and flare, and it is more likely to occur with higher concentrations of antigen. However, the LPR does not always follow an immediate reaction; for example, the wheal and flare reaction stimulated by cold exposure in patients with cold urticaria does not usually evolve into an LPR. Typically, the immediate IgE-mediated cutaneous reaction peaks at 15 to 30 minutes following antigen exposure (Fig. 1). Over the next 30 minutes, the involved area becomes increasingly edematous and erythematous with loss of a distinct wheal. Symptoms remain minimal over the following two to three hours, but then the recurrence of pruritus heralds an increase of inflammation peaking at 6 to 12 hours after the initial antigen exposure. The peak LPR lesion is characterized by intense erythema, edema, tenderness, pruritus, and warmth. It is more diffuse and less defined than the immediate wheal and flare reaction and encompasses a larger area of the skin. The LPR nearly always follows a wheal and flare if stimulated by sufficient allergen. It appears that an immediate wheal of at least eight to nine millimeters consistently stimulates a clinically observable LPR. For example, Dolovich et al. initially observed that a wheal of at least eight millimeters is required to induce an LPR (8), and Solley et al. later noted that a wheal of 15 millimeters or greater reproducibly induces the LPR (9). The duration of the LPR is usually 24 to 48 hours, and residual petechiae may remain for days. Shaikh et al. showed that the skin develops a relatively refractory state with repeated antigen stimulation producing a less intense response (18).

Histologically, the LPR is characterized by progressive edema and infiltration of inflammatory cells (9,19). There may also be significant vascular damage with hyalinization, fibrin deposition, hemorrhage, or necrosis. The composition of the inflammatory infiltrate varies with the progression of the reaction. Initially, there is perivascular infiltration primarily of eosinophils, neutrophils, and mononuclear cells. At the peak of the LPR, a more diffuse infiltration of leukocytes is present consisting of mononuclear cells, neutrophils, and eosinophils. Studies using immunohistochemical staining demonstrate the significant presence of other inflammatory cells, such as mast cells and basophils, which may not be readily apparent during histological examination due to degranulation or loss of characteristic staining properties due to the effects of fixation (20). Although most physical urticarias do not show LPRs, delayed pressure urticaria histologically shows strong similarities to the LPR (21). Also, the pathology of the autologous serum skin test in chronic urticaria resembles an IgE-mediated LPR (22).

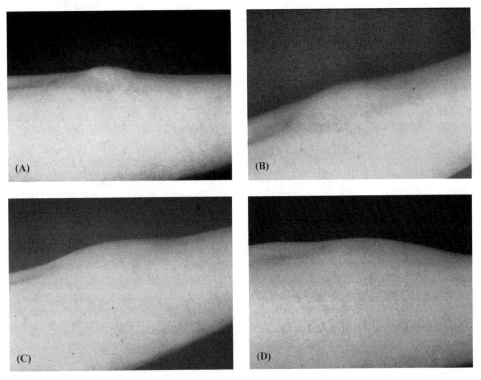

Figure 1 The IgE-mediated Late Cutaneous Reaction: A. Result at 15 minutes. Note the small scar just to the left of the ring of erythema that serves as a landmark for the development of inflammation. The antecubital fossae are on the left. B. Result at 90 minutes. Note that the edema has almost extended to the scar and the margins of the wheal are less distinct than at 15 minutes. C. Result at five hours. The edema has extended to and beyond the scar, and down the forearm. D. Result at eight hours. The spreading edema has now enveloped the landmark small scar and has also extended down the forearm. A reticulated erythema covers the reaction area. *Source*: From Ref. 9.

DEPENDENCE ON IGE

In 1968, Pepys et al. studied the LPR in patients with allergic bronchopulmonary aspergillosis (6). Using immunofluorescence studies of biopsy tissue, they found deposition of IgG, IgM, and C3, and designated the LPR as a type III (Arthus) immune response dependent on complement activation. Later studies pointed to IgE as the major immunoglobulin involved in the reaction. Some of the strongest evidence for IgE involvement is that of Dolovich et al., who found that the LPR is stimulated by injection of sheep anti-IgE or its F(ab)$_2$ fragments and not by normal sheep serum or IgG F(ab)$_2$ fragments (7,23). In the LPRs of atopic individual sensitized with *Bacillus subtilis,* Dolovich and his colleagues found no evidence of IgA, IgM, IgG, or complement, supporting another mechanism, such as an IgE-mediated reaction, as the major immune response in the LPR.

Additional significant support for the role of IgE came from the work of Solley et al. using the passive transfer (or Prausnitz-Küstner) model (9). Although the passive transfer of allergic serum produced a less intense and shorter-lived LPR, it served as a useful model for studying the role of IgE due to its ability to manipulate IgE contained within the sensitizing serum. First, sera from allergic donors were heated at 56°C for four hours in order to denature IgE (radioimmunoassay showed that IgE was depleted by 97–99%); the

Table 1 Competitive Inhibition of Immediate and Late-Phase Responses by IgE Myeloma P.S.

| Solution Number | Composition of sensitizing material | | | |
	IgE myeloma P.S.	M.C. serum[a] (mL)	0.9% NaCl	P.S. IgE:M.C. IgE
1	0.1 (5 mg/mL)	0.1	–	1,000:1
2	0.1 (0.5 mg/mL)	0.1	–	100:1
3	0.1 (0.05 mg/mL)	0.1	–	10:1
4	0.1 (5 mg/mL)	–	0.1	–
5	–	0.1	0.1	–
6[b]	–	–	–	–

| | Average diameter of edema (mm)[c] at stated time interval | | | | | |
	½ h	1 h	2 ½ h	5 h	8 h	12 h
1	7	–	–	–	–	–
2	12	10	–	–	–	–
3	15.5	11.5	39	30	44	40
4	–	–	–	–	–	–
5	20	19	33.5	37.5	50	54
6	–	–	–	–	–	–

[a]Allergic serum from patient M.C., IgE protein 5,000 ng/mL.
[b]Site not sensitized before allergenic challenge.
[c]After challenge of sensitized site with ragweed antigen.
Source: Adapted from Ref. 9.

heated serum lost its ability to passively transfer the immediate reaction and the LPR. Second, removal of 99.7% IgE by an anti-IgE solid-phase immunoabsorbent abolished the ability of the serum to transfer both the immediate and late-phase response. Third, when the IgE was recovered from the anti-IgE solid-phase immunoabsorbent by acid elution, the capacity for passive transfer of both immediate and late-phase responses was also recovered. Finally, as shown in Table 1, a mixture of myeloma IgE in excess of the serum IgE resulted in an inhibition of the dual-phase response, suggesting competition between myeloma IgE and the sensitizing IgE required to initiate the response. The use of passive sensitization and injection of anti-IgE have both reliably reproduced the LPR in numerous later studies, although the former is no longer utilized because of the concern for transmission of blood-borne diseases.

DEPENDENCE ON INFLAMMATORY CELLS AND THEIR MEDIATORS

The histological observations demonstrating progressive infiltration of various inflammatory cells throughout the LPR suggest that these cells interact during the development of the LPR. However, enumeration of infiltrating cells by routine histology can be misleading because degranulated cells are often unrecognizable (20). To reveal the contribution of cells, immunohistochemical staining is necessary, especially for the presence of granulated cells such as basophils, mast cells, neutrophils, and eosinophils. Ying et al. stained biopsies of cutaneous allergen-induced LPRs to sequentially delineate infiltration of various inflammatory cells, using a series of monoclonal antibodies specific for eosinophils, CD3 lymphocytes, mast cells, neutrophils, macrophages, and basophils (24). The staining results of LPR biopsies from six hours to seven days are shown in Table 2.

Table 2 Infiltration of Inflammatory Cells in Allergen-Induced Skin LPR

	Diluent	6 h	24 h	48 h	72 h	7 days
Elastase[+] neutrophils	4.2 (0.0–38.2)	101.4 (11.8–153.4)	59.3 (14.7–122.9)	48.5 (1.5–116.6)	41.6 (30.4–80.1)	7.1 (1.9–11.4)
EGD2[+] eosinophils	0.0 (0.0–2.5)	78.9 (44.8–161.7)	66.1 (19.6–160.2)	42.1 (10.5–94.2)	40.3 (21.5–64.9)	7.8 (4.3–45.9)
BB-1[+] basophils	0.4 (0.0–2.9)	17.7 (0.1–40.4)	33.1 (12.1–61.9)	5.6 (0.8–36.9)	3.5 (0.3–3.8)	1.7 (0.0–3.7)
Tryptase[+] mast cells	83.3 (35.8–100.4)	37.7 (14.7–58.8)	53.2 (4.9–85.3)	49.5 (19.6–84.3)	53.9 (38.2–71.8)	58.8 (46.7–60.9)
CD3[+] T cells	74.2 (46.2–107.9)	92.6 (59.9–130.8)	181.1 (86.4–290.1)	172.7 (47.0–214.6)	69.4 (45.1–71.9)	67.1 (39.6–75.6)
CD68[+] macrophages	52.3 (11.8–151.9)	54.2 (14.7–214.5)	117.9 (15.7–328.3)	116.9 (18.6–301.4)	163.3 (158.3–208.7)	102.3 (95.6–130.9)

Results are expressed as median and range of positive cells per mm^2 of skin biopsies.
Source: Modified from Ref. 24.

These results indicate a dynamic flux of infiltrating cells as the LPR proceeds with a predominance of neutrophils at 6 hours, a predominance of CD3 lymphocytes at 24 hours, and a predominance of macrophages at 48 hours, 72 hours, and 7 days. Resident mast cell numbers decreased at six hours, suggestive of mast cell degranulation early in the reaction. At 24 hours, T-cell numbers peaked, and the numbers of neutrophils and eosinophils decreased. At this time point, mast cell counts increased, likely due to regranulation and recovery.

Other studies have shown similar results regarding degranulation (25–28). To illustrate the extent of eosinophil and neutrophil degranulation, Leiferman et al. used immunofluorescence for localization of neutrophil elastase, eosinophil-derived neurotoxin (EDN), and eosinophil major basic protein (MBP) in biopsy specimens taken from allergen-induced and passively transferred LPRs (20). The deposition of these proteins peaked at 8 hours, decreased by 24 hours, and persisted at 56 hours. The deposition of these granule proteins was out of proportion to the numbers of eosinophils and neutrophils seen on hematoxylin and eosin staining, suggesting degranulation had occurred. Further support for degranulation was obtained by electron microscopy that showed the presence of degenerating eosinophils as well as free eosinophil granules in the tissue. Ying made similar observations to Leiferman et al. (20), who found a significant decrease in the numbers of mast cells in the first eight hours of the reaction with recovery of cell numbers at 56 hours (28).

Reactions that were passively transferred to nonatopic subjects showed a comparable response, but with less intensity in all aspects. In passively sensitized subjects, as in atopic subjects challenged with antigen, deposition of eosinophil and neutrophil granule proteins was dependent on the presence of IgE antibodies and was out of proportion to the number of infiltrating cells (20). Overall, these results indicate that the flux of infiltrating cells shown in Table 2 must be viewed with the knowledge that, at least for eosinophils and neutrophils, simple enumeration of the numbers of cells underestimates their participation in the LPR. Thus, the findings in Table 2 may misrepresent neutrophil and eosinophil involvement because these cells are known to degranulate and lose their morphologic integrity. A thorough analysis of the LPR should not only enumerate the numbers and kinds of infiltrating cells but also quantitatively describe the degree of cell degranulation.

The Mast Cell

Evidence points to a central role for the mast cell in the cutaneous LPR. This conclusion is based on the knowledge that IgE is the major immunoglobulin stimulating the LPR, that the mast cell is the predominant tissue dwelling cell possessing a high-affinity receptor for IgE, that the LPR is preceded by mast cell degranulation in the immediate reaction, and that mast cells contain mediators, such as histamine, capable of initiating inflammation. Thus, mast cells are activated early in the response to injected allergen and play a critical role in the LPR evolution. The FcεRI receptor (high-affinity IgE receptor) is present on the mast cell surface and is cross-linked when bound IgE interacts with multivalent allergen, leading to activation and degranulation (29,30). Additional evidence for the centrality of the mast cell comes from experiments using nonspecific mast cell activators; for example, injection of Compound 48/80, a potent mast cell–activating substance (31), provokes a reaction similar to the LPR (9). Furthermore, injection of anaphylatoxin and complement-fixing immune complexes induce the LPR (32). Finally, injection of mast cell granules or purified granule proteins also may produce the LPR (33,34). Mast cells degranulate early in the allergic reaction, and their numbers are correspondingly decreased on histological specimens as described above. Leiferman et al. observed morphologic changes in mast cells with large granules in contact with the extracellular space on electron microscopy three hours after allergen challenge (Leiferman KM, unpublished observations). Additionally, mast cell–deficient mice show a blunted cutaneous LPR (35).

The mechanisms by which mast cells contribute to the intense inflammation found in the LPR remain a subject of investigation. Although the immediate reaction is clearly dependent on the release of mediators, such as histamine and leukotrienes, the mast cell mediators for the LPR are still being defined (see below). Studies on rat mast cells established that an LPR could be produced by injection of granules (33,34,36–40) and that the neutrophil is the predominant infiltrating cell. Characterization of the granule factors responsible for neutrophil infiltration revealed the existence of biologically active high- and low-molecular-weight moieties (40); the high-molecular-weight inflammation-producing activity could be separated from chymase and heparin. Because of the centrality of the mast cell in the LPR, the experimental approach adopted in these investigations, namely characterization of the mast cell granule–derived proteins, appears valid, but it has not yet been used for studies of factors from human mast cell granules. This approach also assumes that preformed proteins in the mast cell granule have the ability to transfer the LPR, and as will be discussed below, the possibility exists that the mast cell de novo synthesizes molecules essential for the LPR.

The mast cell contains many factors that may be active in the LPR, and several thought to be pertinent to the LPR are discussed below (12,41,42). Histamine is a preformed mediator released by mast cell granules and is an important contributor to the immediate hypersensitivity response (43). During the development of the LPR, histamine tissue levels typically increase in the first hour following antigen exposure, and then sharply decline (42). A second, small histamine peak occurs around eight hours and is correlated with basophil infiltration and activation (12). Injection of histamine, while stimulating an intense immediate reaction, does not stimulate the LPR nor do classic H1 blockers robustly inhibit the LPR, as they do the immediate reaction (44), although certain reports have shown a modest inhibitory effect of antihistamines on the cutaneous LPR (45,46).

Tryptase and chymase are proteases released from mast cells. Tryptase makes up the majority of mast cell protein, and antibody to tryptase (labeled with a suitable tag) is a useful mast cell stain. In the LPR, tryptase levels lag slightly behind those of histamine (47). Four classes of tryptase inhibitors have been devised and tested in the airways and skin of allergic sheep (48) and in the skin of mice (49) with results supporting a role for tryptase in the LPR. Aerosol administration of these inhibitors has abolished late-phase bronchoconstriction and airway hyperresponsiveness in a dose-dependent manner (49). A test of one of these, APC-366, a peptidic inhibitor, significantly reduced the LPR to allergen inhalation in atopic asthmatics without affecting bronchial hyperreactivity (50).

Newly formed lipid mediators derived from the arachidonic acid pathway such as prostaglandin-D2 (PGD_2) and leukotreine-C4 (LTC_4) are able to stimulate a wheal-and-flare response when injected intradermally (51,52). These mediators have actions similar to those of histamine and potentiate effects such as vasodilatation, increased vascular permeability, and smooth muscle contraction. Leukotrienes also have chemoattractant properties, particularly for neutrophils and eosinophils. PGD_2 levels rise early in the LPR and remain elevated throughout its peak (51). LTC_4 levels are increased at four to six hours following antigen exposure, near the peak of the LPR (53). Although H1 antihistamines do not inhibit the LPR, the combination of a potent antihistamine, loratidine, and a leukotriene receptor antagonist, zafirlukast, markedly inhibited allergen-induced early- and late-phase airway obstruction, approximately 75% (54). Another potentially active lipid mediator is platelet-activating factor (PAF) (55). PAF produces prolonged pulmonary inflammation following inhalation and, for a time, was believed to be an important mediator of the LPR in asthma. However, trials with PAF inhibitors discourage belief that PAF is critical for the LPR in the lung (56).

Mast cell derived cytokines include tumor necrosis factor- α (TNF-α), interleukin (IL)-4, IL-5, IL-6, and IL-8. Cytokines that likely play a role in the LPR will be discussed below, but it is pertinent to note that mast cell production of IL-4 and IL-5 implies a role for the mast cell in promoting a Th2 environment (57). IL-8 is a potent neutrophil chemoattractant. Chemokines released from mast cells include macrophage inflammatory protein-1α (MIP-1α), monocyte chemotactic protein-1 (MCP-1), "regulated on activation, normal T cell expressed and secreted" (RANTES), and eotaxin (58).

The Basophil

The basophil is similar to the mast cell, including its high-affinity IgE receptor and its histamine content. However, it must migrate into the tissue to participate in the inflammatory response. The peak of basophil infiltration in the LPR is six to eight hours after antigen exposure, and basophil numbers continue to increase for 24 hours before diminishing (24). Basophil chemoattractants include C5a as well as the chemokines, RANTES, and MCP-1, which are secreted by cells involved in the LPR (59,60). Basophils are often difficult to recognize on hematoxylin and eosin–stained specimens, so immunohistochemical staining with BB1 or 2D7 antibasophil monoclonal antibodies has been useful (26,27). Another monoclonal antibody, J175-7D4, recognizes the proform of the MBP, and also appears specifically to stain basophils (61).

Many of the mediators released by activated basophils are similar to those described for mast cells, including histamine, tryptase (basophils contain only 1% of the tryptase in mast cell granules), arachidonic acid metabolites, and PAF. Basophils also have some features in common with eosinophils in that they contain molecules such as MBP, although this is likely the MBP proform, and the Charcot-Leyden crystal protein (61,62). Cytokines and chemokines released by basophils include IL-4, IL-8, IL-13, and MIP-1α (63,64).

The Eosinophil

The eosinophil begins to infiltrate the perivascular region of tissues involved in the cutaneous LPR within the first hour following antigen exposure. Significant degranulation also begins at this time and continues with a peak correlating roughly with the peak of the LPR (20). As noted above, this degranulation results in difficulty visualizing intact cells on histological examination; therefore, immunohistochemical staining with EG2 monoclonal antibody, reactive with EDN and eosinophil cationic protein (ECP) (65), or with antibodies to MBP, EDN, or ECP have been useful to evaluate degranulated eosinophils (20,24). Eosinophil infiltration in the LPR is dependent on IgE as discussed earlier. Recent data show that omalizumab inhibits the LPR and eosinophilia in the LPR (66,67).

Eosinophils are attracted into the tissue by several mediators released from mast cells and T lymphocytes, including LTB$_4$ and PAF as well as various cytokines and chemokines, especially eotaxin. Eotaxin is released from skin cells, including fibroblasts and keratinocytes stimulated by IL-4 and TNF-α, and potently attracts eosinophils (68–71). During in vitro studies, PAF potently attracts eosinophils as well as induces degranulation and production of free radicals and lipid mediators (72,73). Cytokines found in the LPR, such as IL-5 and IL-9, promote eosinophil maturation and enhance survival (74). Although some reports have claimed that the eosinophil, like the mast cell and basophil, expresses a high-affinity IgE receptor; other reports have failed to confirm this claim (75,76). Eosinophils, however, do possess low-affinity IgE receptors (72). These receptors may be important in the eosinophil's role in parasite immunity, but their role in the allergic response remains unclear.

The principal granule proteins in the eosinophil are MBP1 and 2, EDN, ECP, and eosinophil peroxidase (72,77). These proteins are cytotoxic and are bactericidal and helminthotoxic, but they also have other inflammatory properties as well. MBP1, in particular, activates neutrophils and stimulates histamine release from mast cells and basophils. Both MBP1 and EDN induce an immediate wheal and flare when injected intradermally (78,79). Activated eosinophils also release lipid mediators including PAF, destructive enzymes, and oxygen free radicals. Numerous cytokines and chemokines are liberated from eosinophils (80); those that may influence the LPR include IL-1, IL-4, IL-5, IL-6, IL-8, RANTES, and MIP-1α.

The role of eotaxin in the LPR has been increasingly analyzed. Injection of timothy grass pollen stimulates an immediate and a late-phase cutaneous reaction and causes an increase in eotaxin-1, as well as eotaxin-2, MCP-3, MCP-4, and RANTES mRNA and protein, suggesting their roles in the LPR (59). Direct eotaxin injection causes an immediate reaction and an LPR. However, cutaneous mast cells express CCR3, the eotaxin receptor, and a plausible explanation for eotaxin's ability to stimulate the immediate and late reaction is through the activation of mast cells (81). Injection of MCP-1α/CCL2 and MIP1/CCL3 stimulates both an immediate reaction and an LPR, but this ability may also be due to their ability to activate mast cells (82). Cells that are positive for eotaxin (in this case, eotaxin-1) after six hours include macrophages, endothelial cells, T cells, eosinophils and, to a lesser extent, mast cells, basophils, and neutrophils (59). Eotaxin-2 and eotaxin-3 are also expressed 48 hours after allergen challenge in the bronchial mucosa (83), and eotaxin-3 is expressed in lung epithelial cells and in dermal fibroblasts stimulated with IL-4 (84). The importance of the eotaxin pathway is shown by experiments demonstrating that CCR3 (eotaxin receptor) knockout mice lack skin eosinophilia in an ovalbumin sensitization model (85). Overall, these results suggest that eotaxin activity is likely essential for eosinophil infiltration in skin following an IgE-mediated stimulus.

The experiments of Ying and his colleagues show that eotaxin is not present either as mRNA or as protein before allergen injection, and that injection of allergen (into the skin of an allergic subject) stimulates eotaxin production (28). Eotaxin production appears to be stimulated by IL-4, TNF-α, and IL-13 production, and both mast cells and T lymphocytes are able to produce these molecules. IL-4 induces eotaxin mRNA in human dermal fibroblasts (69,70). IL-4 and TNF-α stimulate eotaxin-1 and eotaxin-3 protein production in human dermal fibroblasts and keratinocytes (68,71). Remarkably, IL-4 transgenic mice spontaneously develop a pruritic inflammatory disease similar to atopic dermatitis, including eosinophilia, and expression of IgE and IgG1 (86). In contrast, IL-4 deficient mice (IL-4$^{-/-}$) show a reduction in eosinophils in an experimental murine model of atopic dermatitis (87). IL-13 induces eotaxin protein in human lung fibroblasts, especially in synergy with TGF-β (88). In addition, levels of eotaxin-3 are high in patients with atopic dermatitis (89). Finally, it is likely that eotaxin production and eosinophil infiltration are mast cell and T cell dependent. For example, both mast cell deficient and anti-CD4 treated mice have reduced intensity of the LPR and also reduced eosinophil skin infiltration (35,90). Thus, these results suggest that both mast cells and T lymphocytes participate in the pathophysiology of the LPR by the production of the cytokines that are able to stimulate eotaxin production.

The Neutrophil

Neutrophils infiltrate early, and are one of the predominant cells throughout the LPR. Neutrophils are recruited to tissue by numerous chemotactic factors that are known to be involved in the LPR, such as IL-8 and LTB4. IL-8 is a member of the C-X-C chemokine family and appears to be the most potent neutrophil chemotactic factor. IL-8 is also involved in neutrophil degranulation, respiratory burst, and adherence to endothelial cells (91). IL-8 increases progressively in LPR blister fluid during the first six hours following antigen exposure and correlates with increasing infiltration of neutrophils (42).

Although the exact role of the neutrophil in allergic inflammation is unclear, neutrophil degranulation is known to produce tissue damage correlating with pathologic changes in the LPR (92). The azurophilic or primary neutrophilic granules contain elastase, which is deposited diffusely throughout LPR biopsy specimens (20). Activation of neutrophils also results in the liberation of numerous enzymes, oxygen free radicals, and lipid mediators, specifically LTB_4, PAF, and thromboxane A_2 (TXA_2).

The Lymphocyte

Lymphocytes infiltrating the LPR are primarily $CD45RO^+$ memory T-lymphocytes, which peak in numbers at 24 hours following antigen exposure (T cells may switch into the Th2 subtype in the environment of Th2 cytokines such as IL-4 and IL-5). In the LPR, Th2 cytokines are released by mast cells, eosinophils, and T cells (57). Not only do IL-4 and IL-5 serve to perpetuate the Th2 environment, they also stimulate B-cell antibody class switching to IgE and participate in eosinophil recruitment and survival. Other cytokines produced by Th2 lymphocytes in the LPR include IL-1, IL-6, IL-9, IL-10, and IL-13. The role of these and other cytokines are discussed further below.

CYTOKINES AND CHEMOKINES IN THE LPR

Cytokines

Cytokines are a diverse class of signaling proteins involved in virtually all types of inflammation. They are secreted by many cell types and have numerous and overlapping functions. Several cytokines have been identified as important mediators in the LPR. IL-1 and IL-6 are proinflammatory cytokines functioning as lymphocyte activators (91), and they also stimulate enhancement of IL-2 production and IL-2 receptor expression. These cytokines have been found in the LPR with both an early and a late peak (93,94). B cells are also stimulated to proliferate and increase immunoglobulin synthesis.

IL-4 and IL-5, as mentioned above, are important in supporting a Th2 environment, enhancing IgE production, and recruiting eosinophils (57). TNF-α, GM-CSF, and IL-3 are also eosinophil chemotactic factors, although they, along with IL-5, appear less potent than eotaxin (95). In situ hybridization analysis of mRNA for IL-4 and IL-5 in LPR biopsy specimens demonstrated colocalization and a significant increase in the production of these cytokines in the first six hours following antigen exposure, and they continued to increase for 24 hours paralleling the clinical LPR (57). In this study, immunohisto-chemistry was employed to show colocalization of IL-4 and IL-5 mRNA with T cells, EG2-staining (anti-EDN) eosinophils, and tryptase-staining mast cells, supporting the role of each of these cells in potentiating the Th2 environment.

IL-9 is another T-cell derived cytokine that is found in the LPR (96). IL-9 potentiates IL-4 and IL-5 functioning to stimulate IgE production by the development of B cells and eosinophils (97,98). IL-9 also increases IL-5 receptor expression. Analysis of

IL-9 mRNA using in situ hybridization demonstrated a progressive increase with a peak at 48 hours after antigen exposure in the skin of atopic patients (96). The rise in IL-9 mRNA production correlated with the rise of Congo red–staining eosinophils in these specimens as well. IL-10, usually thought to be an inhibitory cytokine, may be involved in allergic inflammation, as IL-10$^{-/-}$ mice have lessened eosinophil infiltration and decreased IL-4, IL-5, and eotaxin secretion (99).

IL-13, another T-cell derived cytokine, likely contributes to the LPR along with IL-4 and IL-5. IL-13 is genetically linked to the gene cluster on chromosome 5, containing IL-4, IL-5, as well as granulocyte-monocyte colony stimulating factor (GM-CSF) (100–102). IL-13 is functionally similar to IL-4 in its ability to activate B-cell proliferation and IgE production. It is also a cofactor with IL-4 in the induction of vascular cell adhesion molecule-1 (VCAM-1) expression. VCAM-1 is an adhesion molecule that binds the integrin $\alpha_4\beta_1$ on the surface of inflammatory cells and is important in the recruitment of lymphocytes, monocytes, eosinophils, basophils, and mast cells in the LPR (103). IL-4 and IL-13 mRNA and protein products are present in cutaneous LPR specimens, and measurements of IL-4 and IL-13 are correlated with the progression of the LPR with a peak at 24 hours (103). Inhibition of IL-13 function by injection of the competitive soluble IL-13 receptor in mice reduced the LPR in a model of allergic rhinitis, and IL-13 deficient mice also had a diminished LPR (104). In a murine LPR model, treatment with antibodies to ICAM-1, VCAM-1, and VLA-4 reduced eosinophil infiltration by 66.2%, 61%, and 54%, respectively, emphasizing the importance of these molecules for eosinophil infiltration (105).

Chemokines

Chemokines are chemotactic proteins that typically mediate cellular locomotion. They, like other cytokines, derive from various cell sources and have overlapping functions. Chemokines are divided into families based on the structure of the first cysteine residues. C-C indicates adjacent cysteines, and C-X-C indicates a single amino acid separating the cysteines. Most of the chemokines that appear to be important in the LPR are C-C chemokines such as the eotaxins, RANTES, MIP-1α, MCP-1, MCP-3, and MCP-4 (14,106).

Eotaxin-1, -2, and -3 bind to the CCR3 receptor, which is expressed on the surfaces of eosinophils, basophils, and mast cells. The effect of eotaxin on eosinophil infiltration appears to be dependent on IL-5; IL-5 administration increases the peripheral blood pool of eosinophils that are attracted by eotaxin (95). IL-5 had little eosinophilotactic activity in its own right. Expression of eotaxin mRNA and protein peaks at six hours following introduction of antigen into the skin of sensitized subjects, suggesting that eotaxin regulates eosinophil infiltration at this time point (59). At 24 hours, eosinophil infiltration and expression of eotaxin-2 and MCP-4 mRNA are correlated (59). Expression of eotaxin mRNA was paralleled by the occurrence of the eotaxin receptor, CCR3, on 83% of the eosinophils. A CCR3 receptor antagonist inhibits both early- and late-phase allergic inflammation in the conjunctiva (107). Other chemokines such as RANTES, MCP-3, and MCP-4 bind to the CCR3 receptor leading to eosinophil and basophil chemotaxis, but they also bind to the CCR1 receptor located on neutrophils, eosinophils, monocytes, T cells, and basophils. Peak expression of MCP-3 occurs at six hours in the LPR; MCP-4 and RANTES peak later, at 24 hours (28). Curiously, no significant correlations were observed between basophil infiltration, as detected by BB1 basophil-specific antibody staining, peaking at 24 hours, and expression of eotaxin, eotaxin-2, RANTES, MCP-3, and MCP-4. Overall these results suggest that eotaxin has a role in the early six-hour recruitment of eosinophils, whereas eotaxin-2 and MCP-4 are involved in the later 24-hour infiltration of eosinophils.

In a different study, Ying and his colleagues described the activity of another chemokine that acts on the CCR1 receptor, MIP-1α (24).This chemokine also stimulates histamine release from mast cells and basophils, in addition to the stimulation of cellular motility. Peak expression of MIP-1α occurs at six hours after antigen challenge with continued elevation for 24 hours. At six hours, MIP-1α mRNA colocalized to neutrophils and basophils, and at 24 hours, colocalization was with macrophages. The expression of the CCR1 receptor also correlates with the presence of MIP-1α.

The effects of intradermal allergen challenge and histamine injection on eotaxin mRNA and protein generation in atopics have been examined more closely with respect to endothelial production of eotaxin (108). Sixty minutes after allergen challenge, there is a prompt increase in degranulating cutaneous mast cells with a simultaneous increase in eosinophils. The number of eotaxin-positive cells in tissues increases and peaks three hours post challenge. In vitro, endothelial cells produce dose- and time-dependent eotaxin mRNA and protein after incubation with histamine. Preincubation of endothelial cells with histamine induces a significant increase in eosinophil adherence, which is inhibited by eotaxin-blocking monoclonal antibody (108). Thus, antigen-induced eotaxin expression by endothelial cells, and adherence and migration of eosinophils from microvasculature to tissues, occur rapidly and are influenced by histamine from mast cells.

PHARMACOLOGIC INTERVENTION

The cutaneous LPR serves as a useful tool for the investigation of pharmacologic agents that may be treatments for chronic allergic diseases in the skin, nose, and lung. Most drugs that inhibit the immediate hypersensitivity response do not inhibit the LPR and vice versa. For example, H1 antagonists significantly attenuate the immediate wheal and flare, but they have minimal effect on the LPR (109). Cetirizine, an H1 antihistamine, however, has been found to have some effect on the size and symptoms of the LPR with a decrease in inflammatory cell infiltration but without a change in the mediator profile; this indicates an antiinflammatory mechanism for cetirizine other than histamine blockade (46). Glucocorticoids remain the most effective agents for the inhibition of the LPR. When given prior to antigen exposure or injection of IgE, a wheal and flare is produced without a subsequent LPR (110). Minimal or variable inhibition of the LPR has been observed with cyclooxygenase inhibitors, 5-lipoxygenase inhibitors, and beta-adrenergic agonists (15). Mepolizumab, anti-IL-5 therapy, did not improve the cutaneous LPR although intact eosinophils were decreased (111). The authors suggested that eosinophils do not contribute to the late phase of the IgE-mediated allergic reaction because their depletion did not reduce the magnitude of the reaction. However, because eosinophil granule proteins may be important mediators of the late-phase inflammation, it is important to know whether the deposition of these granule proteins was also reduced.

MECHANISMS RESPONSIBLE FOR THE CUTANEOUS LPR

As noted earlier, the mast cell is central to the LPR, particularly its surface high-affinity IgE receptor. Although early studies showed the importance of IgE by stimulating the LPR through the use of anti-IgE and by passive transfer of IgE antibodies, essentially all of the recent analyses have stimulated the LPR by injection of allergens into allergic subjects. While this is eminently reasonable and a safe way to proceed in view of the dangers of transmitting blood-borne diseases, this approach may obfuscate investigations of the LPR because the allergens have the ability to stimulate both the LPR and the immune response. For example, the striking evidence for lymphocyte participation in the LPR (Table 2) may be part of a more complicated immune response to the antigen, not just a component of the LPR. Ideally, one would prefer to dissect the LPR using tools to activate only the mast cell. Thus, a comparison of the LPR stimulated by allergen injection in a sensitive subject and the LPR stimulated by only mast cell activation might yield valuable information about the mechanisms important for the instigation of the LPR that are not a part of the overall immune response to the allergen. In this regard, experiments performed on mast cell and CD4-positive lymphocyte deficient mice are relevant. Mast cell-deficient mice injected with antigen have no immediate response and a diminished, yet definitely present, LPR in comparison with controls. Eosinophil infiltration at 24 hours is still increased over baseline in these mice, yet not as substantially as in wild-type mice (35). Mice rendered CD4 lymphocyte deficient by injection of CD4 antibody also showed decreases in edema and eosinophil infiltration in the LPR (90). Thus, these results point to a role for both mast cells and T cells in orchestrating cellular infiltration of the murine LPR. However, these findings are subject to the criticism that the murine LPR may not faithfully reproduce the mechanisms of the IgE-mediated human LPR.

SUMMARY

The cutaneous LPR is a complex inflammatory reaction that is not the product of a single cell or mediator. It requires the production of IgE in a Th2 environment. Although the LPR itself is a transient event, its mechanism may correlate with the pathogenesis of chronic allergic disease. The LPR is easily induced in the skin with the use of intradermal allergen or activating anti-IgE, and these models are accessible for study using biopsy specimens or skin blister chamber fluid. Alternatively, the absence of an LPR in physically induced urticarias, such as cold urticaria or dermographism, may point to a requirement for persisting antigen or at least a persisting stimulus for mast cell activation. With increased knowledge of the LPR pathophysiology, more directed therapy may be developed for the treatment of chronic allergic diseases with focus on immunomodulatory effects.

REFERENCES

1. Blackley C. Experimental researches on the causes and nature of Catarrhus Aestivus (hay fever or hay asthma). Bailliere, Tindell and Cox, reprinted at London: Dawson's of Pall Mall, 1959; 1873:77–81.
2. Cooke R. Studies in specific hypersensitiveness. IX. On the phenomenon of hyopsensitization (the clinically lessened sensitiveness of allergy). J Immunol 1922; 7:219.
3. Vaughn W. A study of eczema as an allergic phenomenon. South Med J 1924; 17:749.
4. Herxheimer H. The late bronchial reaction in induced asthma. Int Arch Allergy Appl Immunol 1952; 3:323.
5. Prausnitz C, Küstner H. Studien uber Uberempfindlichkeit. Centralbl Bakteriol Abt I Orig 1921; 86:160.
6. Pepys JT-WM, Dawson PL, Hinson KFW. Arthus (type III) skin test reactions in man. Excerpta Medica International Congress Series, Allergology, Proceedings of the Sixth Congress of the International Association of Allergology, 1968; 162:221.
7. Dolovich JLD. Correlates of skin test reactions to Bacillus subtilis enzyme preparations. J Allergy Clin Immunol 1972; 49:43.

8. Dolovich J, Hargreave FE, Chalmers R, et al. Late cutaneous allergic responses in isolated IgE-dependent reactions. J Allergy Clin Immunol 1973; 52:38–46.

9. Solley GO, Gleich GJ, Jordon RE, et al. The late phase of the immediate wheal and flare skin reaction. Its dependence upon IgE antibodies. J Clin Invest 1976; 58:408–420.

10. Dorsch W, ed. Late phase allergic reactions. Boca Raton: CRC Press, 1990.

11. Gleich G. The late phase of the immunoglobulin E-mediated reaction: a link between anaphylaxis and common allergic disease?. J Allergy Clin Immunol 1982; 70:160–169.

12. Charlesworth EN, Hood AF, Soter NA, et al. Cutaneous late-phase response to allergen. Mediator release and inflammatory cell infiltration. J Clin Invest 1989; 83:1519–1526.

13. Zweiman B, Atkins PC, Moskovitz A, et al. Cellular inflammatory responses during immediate, developing, and established late-phase allergic cutaneous reactions: effects of cetirizine. J Allergy Clin Immunol 1997; 100:341–347.

14. Zweiman B, Kaplan AP, Tong L, et al. Cytokine levels and inflammatory responses in developing late-phase allergic reactions in the skin. J Allergy Clin Immunol 1997; 100:104–109.

15. Peters SPZJ, Fish JE. Late phase allergic reactions. In: Middleton E Jr., Reed CE, Ellis EF, Atkinson NF Jr., Busse WW, Yuninger JW, eds. Allergy, Principles and Practice. St Louis: Mosby 5th ed., 1998:342–355.

16. Gelfand EW. Inflammatory mediators in allergic rhinitis. J Allergy Clin Immunol 2004; 114: S135–S138.

17. Zetterstrom O. Dual skin test reactions and serum antibodies to subtilisin and Aspergillus fumigatus extracts. Clin Allergy 1978; 8:77–91.

18. Shaikh W, Umemoto L, Poothullil J, et al. Relative refractory state for late cutaneous allergic responses. J Allergy Clin Immunol 1977; 60:242–246.

19. Atkins P, Green GR, Zweiman B. Histologic studies of human skin test responses to ragweed, compound 48–80, and histamine. J Allergy Clin Immunol 1973; 51:263–273.

20. Leiferman KM, Fujisawa T, Gray BH, et al. Extracellular deposition of eosinophil and neutrophil granule proteins in the IgE-mediated cutaneous late phase reaction. Lab Invest 1990; 62:579–589.

21. Mekori YA, Dobozin BS, Schocket AL, et al. Delayed pressure urticaria histologically resembles cutaneous late-phase reactions. Arch Dermatol 1988; 124:230–235.

22. Grattan CE, Boon AP, Eady RA, et al. The pathology of the autologous serum skin test response in chronic urticaria resembles IgE-mediated late-phase reactions. Int Arch Allergy Appl Immunol 1990; 93:198–204.

23. Dolovich J HF, Chalmers R, Shier KJ, et al. Late cutaneous allergic responses in isolated IgE-dependent reactions. J Allergy Clin Immunol 1973; 52:38.

24. Ying S, Meng Q, Barata LT, et al. Macrophage inflammatory protein-1alpha and C-C chemokine receptor-1 in allergen-induced skin late-phase reactions: relationship to macrophages, neutrophils, basophils, eosinophils and T lymphocytes. Clin Exp Allergy 2001; 31: 1724–1731.

25. Frew AJ, Kay AB. The relationship between infiltrating CD4+ lymphocytes, activated eosinophils, and the magnitude of the allergen-induced late phase cutaneous reaction in man. J Immunol 1988; 141:4158–4164.

26. Irani AM, Huang C, Xia HZ, et al. Immunohistochemical detection of human basophils in late-phase skin reactions. J Allergy Clin Immunol 1998; 101:354–362.

27. Macfarlane AJ, Kon OM, Smith SJ, et al. Basophils, eosinophils, and mast cells in atopic and nonatopic asthma and in late-phase allergic reactions in the lung and skin. J Allergy Clin Immunol 2000; 105:99–107.

28. Ying S, Robinson DS, Meng Q, et al. C-C chemokines in allergen-induced late-phase cutaneous responses in atopic subjects: association of eotaxin with early 6-hour eosinophils, and of eotaxin-2 and monocyte chemoattractant protein-4 with the later 24-hour tissue eosinophilia, and relationship to basophils and other C-C chemokines (monocyte chemoattractant protein-3 and RANTES). J Immunol 1999; 163:3976–3984.

29. Kinet JP. The high-affinity IgE receptor (Fc epsilon RI): from physiology to pathology. Annu Rev Immunol 1999; 17:931–972.

30. Segal DM, Taurog JD, Metzger H. Dimeric immunoglobulin E serves as a unit signal for mast cell degranulation. Proc Natl Acad Sci U S A 1977; 74:2993–2997.

31. Paton WD. Compound 48/80: a potent histamine liberator. Br J Pharmacol Chemother 1951; 6: 499–508.

32. Stalenheim G, Zetterstrom O. Late cutaneous allergic reactions without the participation of IgE. Monogr Allergy 1979; 14:264–267.

33. Tannenbaum S, Oertel H, Henderson W, et al. The biologic activity of mast cell granules. I. Elicitation of inflammatory responses in rat skin. J Immunol 1980; 125:325–335.

34. Oertel HL, Kaliner M. The biologic activity of mast cell granules. III. Purification of inflammatory factors of anaphylaxis (IF-A) responsible for causing latephase reactions. J Immunol 1981; 127:1398–1402.

35. Togawa M, Kiniwa M, Nagai H. The roles of IL-4, IL-5 and mast cells in the accumulation of eosinophils during allergic cutaneous late phase reaction in mice. Life Sci 2001; 69:699–705.

36. Oertel H, Kaliner M. The biologic activity of mast cell granules in rat skin: effects of adrenocorticosteroids on late-phase inflammatory responses induced by mast cell granules. J Allergy Clin Immunol 1981; 68:238–245.

37. Lemanske RF Jr., Joiner K, Kaliner M. The biologic activity of mast cell granules. IV. The effect of complement depletion on rat cutaneous late phase reactions. J Immunol 1983; 130: 1881–1884.

38. Lemanske RF Jr., Guthman DA, Oertel H, et al. The biologic activity of mast cell granules. VI. The effect of vinblastine-induced neutropenia on rat cutaneous late phase reactions. J Immunol 1983; 130:2837–2842.

39. Lemanske RF Jr., Guthman DA, Kaliner M. The biologic activity of mast cell granules. VII. The effect of anti-neutrophil antibody-induced neutropenia on rat cutaneous late phase reactions. J Immunol 1983; 131:929–933.

40. Lemanske RF Jr., Esser B, Kopp D, et al. The biologic activity of mast cell granules. VIII. In vivo and in vitro characterization of mast cell granule-derived inflammatory factors involved in rat late-phase reactions. J Allergy Clin Immunol 1987; 79:32–39.

41. Naclerio RM, Proud D, Togias AG, et al. Inflammatory mediators in late antigen-induced rhinitis. N Engl J Med 1985; 313:65–70.

42. Zweiman B, Von Allmen C. Temporal patterns of mediator release during developing cutaneous late-phase reactions. Clin Exp Allergy 2000; 30:856–862.

43. Lorenz W, Doenicke A. Histamine release in clinical conditions. Mt Sinai J Med 1978; 45: 357–386.

44. Juhlin L, Michaelsson G. Cutaneous reactions to kallikrein, bradykinin and histamine in healthy subjects and in patients with urticaria. Acta Derm Venereol 1969; 49:26–36.

45. de Weck AL, Derer T, Bischoff SC, et al. The effect of terfenadine on the immediate and late-phase reactions mediated by immunoglobulin E. Int Arch Allergy Immunol 1993; 101: 326–332.

46. Nielsen PN, Skov PS, Poulsen LK, et al. Cetirizine inhibits skin reactions but not mediator release in immediate and developing late-phase allergic cutaneous reactions. A double-blind, placebo-controlled study. Clin Exp Allergy 2001; 31:1378–1384.

47. Schwartz LB, Atkins PC, Bradford TR, et al. Release of tryptase together with histamine during the immediate cutaneous response to allergen. J Allergy Clin Immunol 1987; 80:850–855.

48. Rice KD, Tanaka RD, Katz BA, et al. Inhibitors of tryptase for the treatment of mast cell-mediated diseases. Curr Pharm Des 1998; 4:381–396.

49. Oh SW, Pae CI, Lee DK, et al. Tryptase inhibition blocks airway inflammation in a mouse asthma model. J Immunol 2002; 168:1992–2000.

50. Krishna MT, Chauhan A, Little L, et al. Inhibition of mast cell tryptase by inhaled APC 366 attenuates allergen-induced late-phase airway obstruction in asthma. J Allergy Clin Immunol 2001; 107:1039–1045.

51. Pienkowski MM, Adkinson NF Jr., Plaut M, et al. Prostaglandin D2 and histamine during the immediate and the late-phase components of allergic cutaneous responses. J Allergy Clin Immunol 1988; 82:95–100.

52. Soter NA, Lewis RA, Corey EJ, et al. Local effects of synthetic leukotrienes (LTC4, LTD4, LTE4, and LTB4) in human skin. J Invest Dermatol 1983; 80:115–119.

53. Dorsch W, Ring J, Weber PC, et al. Detection of immunoreactive leukotrienes LTC4/D4 in skin-blister fluid after allergen testing in patients with late cutaneous reactions (LCR). Arch Dermatol Res 1985; 277:400–401.

54. Roquet A, Dahlen B, Kumlin M, et al. Combined antagonism of leukotrienes and histamine produces predominant inhibition of allergen-induced early and late phase airway obstruction in asthmatics. Am J Respir Crit Care Med 1997; 155:1856–1863.

55. Henderson WR Jr. Eicosanoids and platelet-activating factor in allergic respiratory diseases. Am Rev Respir Dis 1991; 143:S86–S90.

56. Henig NR, Aitken ML, Liu MC, et al. Effect of recombinant human platelet-activating factor-acetylhydrolase on allergen-induced asthmatic responses. Am J Respir Crit Care Med 2000; 162:523–527.

57. Barata LT, Ying S, Meng Q, et al. IL-4- and IL-5-positive T lymphocytes, eosinophils, and mast cells in allergen-induced late-phase cutaneous reactions in atopic subjects. J Allergy Clin Immunol 1998; 101:222–230.

58. Kimura Y, Pawankar R, Aoki M, et al. Mast cells and T cells in Kimura's disease express increased levels of interleukin-4, interleukin-5, eotaxin and RANTES. Clin Exp Allergy 2002; 32:1787–1793.

59. Ying S, Meng Q, Zeibecoglou K, et al. Eosinophil chemotactic chemokines (eotaxin, eotaxin-2, RANTES, monocyte chemoattractant protein-3 (MCP-3), and MCP-4), and C-C chemokine receptor 3 expression in bronchial biopsies from atopic and nonatopic (Intrinsic) asthmatics. J Immunol 1999; 163:6321–6329.

60. Alam R, Grant JA. The chemokines and the histamine-releasing factors: modulation of function of basophils, mast cells and eosinophils. Chem Immunol 1995; 61:148–160.

61. Plager DA, Weiss EA, Kephart GM, et al. Identification of basophils by a mAb directed against pro-major basic protein 1. J Allergy Clin Immunol 2006; 117:626–634.

62. Ackerman SJ, Weil GJ, Gleich GJ. Formation of Charcot-Leyden crystals by human basophils. J Exp Med 1982; 155:1597–1609.

63. Gilmartin L, Tarleton CA, Schuyler M, et al. A comparison of inflammatory mediators released by basophils of asthmatic and control subjects in response to high-affinity IgE receptor aggregation. Int Arch Allergy Immunol 2008; 145:182–192.

64. Dahinden CA, Rihs S, Ochsensberger B. Regulation of cytokine expression by human blood basophils. Int Arch Allergy Immunol 1997; 113:134–137.

65. Nakajima H, Loegering DA, Kita H, et al. Reactivity of monoclonal antibodies EG1 and EG2 with eosinophils and their granule proteins. J Leukoc Biol 1999; 66:447–454.

66. Ong YE, Menzies-Gow A, Barkans J, et al. Anti-IgE (omalizumab) inhibits late-phase reactions and inflammatory cells after repeat skin allergen challenge. J Allergy Clin Immunol 2005; 116:558–564.

67. D'Amato G. Role of anti-IgE monoclonal antibody (omalizumab) in the treatment of bronchial asthma and allergic respiratory diseases. Eur J Pharmacol 2006; 533:302–307.

68. Dulkys Y, Schramm G, Kimmig D, et al. Detection of mRNA for eotaxin-2 and eotaxin-3 in human dermal fibroblasts and their distinct activation profile on human eosinophils. J Invest Dermatol 2001; 116:498–505.

69. Mochizuki M, Bartels J, Mallet AI, et al. IL-4 induces eotaxin: a possible mechanism of selective eosinophil recruitment in helminth infection and atopy. J Immunol 1998; 160:60–68.

70. Mochizuki M, Schroder J, Christophers E, et al. IL-4 induces eotaxin in human dermal fibroblasts. Int Arch Allergy Immunol 1999; 120(suppl 1):19–23.

71. Igawa K, Satoh T, Hirashima M, et al. Regulatory mechanisms of galectin-9 and eotaxin-3 synthesis in epidermal keratinocytes: possible involvement of galectin-9 in dermal eosinophilia of Th1-polarized skin inflammation. Allergy 2006; 61:1385–1391.

72. Kita HGG. The eosinophil structure and functions. In: Kaplan AP, ed. The Immune System and Inflammation. 2nd ed. Philadelphia: Saunders, 1997:148–177.

73. Sur SAC, Gleich GJ. Eosinophils: biochemical and cellular aspects. In: Middleton E Jr., Reed CE, Ellis EF, Adkinson NF, Yunginger JW, Busse WW, eds. Allergy: Principles and Practice. 4th ed. St Louis: Mosby, 1993, vol 1.

74. Gounni AS, Nutku E, Koussih L, et al. IL-9 expression by human eosinophils: regulation by IL-1beta and TNF-alpha. J Allergy Clin Immunol 2000; 106:460–466.

75. Seminario MC, Saini SS, MacGlashan DW Jr., et al. Intracellular expression and release of Fc epsilon RI alpha by human eosinophils. J Immunol 1999; 162:6893–6900.

76. Kita H, Kaneko M, Bartemes KR, et al. Does IgE bind to and activate eosinophils from patients with allergy? J Immunol 1999; 162:6901–6911.

77. Gleich GJ. Mechanisms of eosinophil-associated inflammation. J Allergy Clin Immunol 2000; 105:651–663.

78. Gleich GJ, Schroeter AL, Marcoux JP, et al. Episodic angioedema associated with eosinophilia. Trans Assoc Am Physicians 1984; 97:25–32.

79. Leiferman KM LD, Gleich GJ. Production of wheal-and-flare skin reactions by eosinophil granule proteins. Clin Res 1984; 32:598A.

80. Kita H. The eosinophil: a cytokine-producing cell? J Allergy Clin Immunol 1996; 97:889–892.

81. Menzies-Gow A, Ying S, Sabroe I, et al. Eotaxin (CCL11) and eotaxin-2 (CCL24) induce recruitment of eosinophils, basophils, neutrophils, and macrophages as well as features of early- and late-phase allergic reactions following cutaneous injection in human atopic and nonatopic volunteers. J Immunol 2002; 169:2712–2718.

82. Gaga M, Ong YE, Benyahia F, et al. Skin reactivity and local cell recruitment in human atopic and nonatopic subjects by CCL2/MCP-1 and CCL3/MIP-1alpha. Allergy 2008; 63:703–711.

83. Ravensberg AJ, Ricciardolo FL, van Schadewijk A, et al. Eotaxin-2 and eotaxin-3 expression is associated with persistent eosinophilic bronchial inflammation in patients with asthma after allergen challenge. J Allergy Clin Immunol 2005; 115:779–785.

84. Banwell ME, Tolley NS, Williams TJ, et al. Regulation of human eotaxin-3/CCL26 expression: modulation by cytokines and glucocorticoids. Cytokine 2002; 17:317–323.

85. Ma W, Bryce PJ, Humbles AA, et al. CCR3 is essential for skin eosinophilia and airway hyperresponsiveness in a murine model of allergic skin inflammation. J Clin Invest 2002; 109:621–628.

86. Chan LS, Robinson N, Xu L. Expression of interleukin-4 in the epidermis of transgenic mice results in a pruritic inflammatory skin disease: an experimental animal model to study atopic dermatitis. J Invest Dermatol 2001; 117:977–983.

87. Spergel JM, Mizoguchi E, Oettgen H, et al. Roles of TH1 and TH2 cytokines in a murine model of allergic dermatitis. J Clin Invest 1999; 103:1103–1111.

88. Wenzel SE, Trudeau JB, Barnes S, et al. TGF-beta and IL-13 synergistically increase eotaxin-1 production in human airway fibroblasts. J Immunol 2002; 169:4613–4619.

89. Kagami S, Kakinuma T, Saeki H, et al. Significant elevation of serum levels of eotaxin-3/CCL26, but not of eotaxin-2/CCL24, in patients with atopic dermatitis: serum eotaxin-3/CCL26 levels reflect the disease activity of atopic dermatitis. Clin Exp Immunol 2003; 134:309–313.

90. Sengoku T, Sato S, Sakuma S, et al. Characterization of Ascaris-induced biphasic skin allergic reaction model in mice: possible roles of mast cells in early-phase and CD4-positive T cells in late-phase reactions. Pharmacology 2001; 63:82–89.

91. Borish L RL. Cytokines in Allergic Inflammation. In: Middleton E Jr., Reed CE, Ellis EF, Adkinson NF, Yunginger JW, Busse WW, eds. Allergy: Principles and Practice. 5th ed. St Louis: Mosby, 1998:108–119, vol. 1.

92. Shalit M, von Allmen C, Atkins PC, et al. Increased expression of CR3 (C3bi receptor) on neutrophils in human inflammatory skin reactions. J Clin Immunol 1987; 7:456–462.

93. Bochner BS, Charlesworth EN, Lichtenstein LM, et al. Interleukin-1 is released at sites of human cutaneous allergic reactions. J Allergy Clin Immunol 1990; 86:830–839.

94. Lee CE, Neuland ME, Teaford HG, et al. Interleukin-6 is released in the cutaneous response to allergen challenge in atopic individuals. J Allergy Clin Immunol 1992; 89:1010–1020.

95. Collins PD, Marleau S, Griffiths-Johnson DA, et al. Cooperation between interleukin-5 and the chemokine eotaxin to induce eosinophil accumulation in vivo. J Exp Med 1995; 182:1169–1174.

96. Ying S, Meng Q, Kay AB, et al. Elevated expression of interleukin-9 mRNA in the bronchial mucosa of atopic asthmatics and allergen-induced cutaneous late-phase reaction: relationships to eosinophils, mast cells and T lymphocytes. Clin Exp Allergy 2002; 32:866–871.

97. Fawaz LM, Sharif-Askari E, Hajoui O, et al. Expression of IL-9 receptor alpha chain on human germinal center B cells modulates IgE secretion. J Allergy Clin Immunol 2007; 120: 1208–1215.

98. Gounni AS, Gregory B, Nutku E, et al. Interleukin-9 enhances interleukin-5 receptor expression, differentiation, and survival of human eosinophils. Blood 2000; 96:2163–2171.

99. Laouini D, Alenius H, Bryce P, et al. IL-10 is critical for Th2 responses in a murine model of allergic dermatitis. J Clin Invest 2003; 112:1058–1066.

100. McKenzie AN, Culpepper JA, de Waal Malefyt R, et al. Interleukin 13, a T-cell-derived cytokine that regulates human monocyte and B-cell function. Proc Natl Acad Sci U S A 1993; 90: 3735–3739.

101. Minty A, Chalon P, Derocq JM, et al. Interleukin-13 is a new human lymphokine regulating inflammatory and immune responses. Nature 1993; 362:248–250.

102. Bochner BS, Klunk DA, Sterbinsky SA, et al. IL-13 selectively induces vascular cell adhesion molecule-1 expression in human endothelial cells. J Immunol 1995; 154:799–803.

103. Ying S, Meng Q, Barata LT, et al. Associations between IL-13 and IL-4 (mRNA and protein), vascular cell adhesion molecule-1 expression, and the infiltration of eosinophils, macrophages, and T cells in allergen-induced late-phase cutaneous reactions in atopic subjects. J Immunol 1997; 158:5050–5057.

104. Miyahara S, Miyahara N, Matsubara S, et al. IL-13 is essential to the late-phase response in allergic rhinitis. J Allergy Clin Immunol 2006; 118:1110–1116.

105. Hakugawa J, Bae SJ, Tanaka Y, et al. The inhibitory effect of anti-adhesion molecule antibodies on eosinophil infiltration in cutaneous late phase response in Balb/c mice sensitized with ovalbumin (OVA). J Dermatol 1997; 24:73–79.

106. Benson M, Langston MA, Adner M, et al. A network-based analysis of the late-phase reaction of the skin. J Allergy Clin Immunol 2006; 118:220–225.

107. Nakamura T, Ohbayashi M, Toda M, et al. A specific CCR3 chemokine receptor antagonist inhibits both early and late phase allergic inflammation in the conjunctiva. Immunol Res 2005; 33: 213–221.

108. Menzies-Gow A, Ying S, Phipps S, et al. Interactions between eotaxin, histamine and mast cells in early microvascular events associated with eosinophil recruitment to the site of allergic skin reactions in humans. Clin Exp Allergy 2004; 34:1276–1282.

109. Massey WA. Pathogenesis and pharmacologic modulation of the cutaneous late-phase reaction. Ann Allergy 1993; 71:578–584.

110. Gronneberg R, Strandberg K, Stalenheim G, et al. Effect in man of anti-allergic drugs on the immediate and late phase cutaneous allergic reactions induced by anti-IgE. Allergy 1981; 36: 201–208.

111. Phipps S, Flood-Page P, Menzies-Gow A, et al. Intravenous anti-IL-5 monoclonal antibody reduces eosinophils and tenascin deposition in allergen-challenged human atopic skin. J Invest Dermatol 2004; 122:1406–1412.

8

Diagnostic Techniques for Urticaria and Angioedema

Malcolm W. Greaves
St. John's Institute of Dermatology, St. Thomas' Hospital, London, U.K.

Allen P. Kaplan
Department of Medicine, Medical University of South Carolina, Charleston, South Carolina, U.S.A.

Clive Grattan
*Dermatology Centre, Norfolk and Norwich University Hospital, and
St. John's Institute of Dermatology, St. Thomas' Hospital, London, U.K.*

INTRODUCTION

This chapter attempts to guide the reader on the art and science of history-taking and clinical examination in patients with urticaria and angioedema. It also advises on which tests should (and should not) be done—and why—in these patients, and their interpretation. In this chapter the term "urticaria" should be taken to include the deeper lesions of associated angioedema. Details of the different forms of urticaria and angioedema referred to can be found in the corresponding chapters.

URTICARIA

History and Examination

Relapses punctuated by remissions are the hallmark of most forms of urticaria. Inevitably the patient is often symptom-free at the time of presentation in the clinic. Accordingly a painstaking history is vital in the evaluation of the patient.

Does the patient actually have urticaria? In some cases it is quite hard to be sure. Urticaria is characterized by the presence of one or more wheals. A wheal has four features: a central pale swelling, surrounding redness, sometimes with a peripheral patchy bright red axon reflex flare, itching, and most importantly a duration of less than 24 hours in most patients. Unfortunately many patients are unsure of the duration of individual wheals so it is often necessary to get the patient or care-giver to make this measurement on a random sample of wheals using a ballpoint pen. Urticaria look-alikes in which the duration of the wheal is greater than 24 hours include urticarial vasculitis, urticarial dermatitis, delayed pressure urticaria, and lesions of some virus and drug exanthems. The individual wheals of physical urticarias have a duration of less than one hour, except for delayed pressure urticaria, which is much more persistent.

In the classification of urticaria the total duration of the urticaria is important. By long tradition, and more recently by consensus in the European Guidelines (1) chronic urticaria is defined as occurrence of daily or almost daily wheals for more than six weeks. The corresponding definition of acute urticaria requires a total duration of less than six weeks. In reality, most patients with acute urticaria rarely experience symptoms for longer than hours or a few days at the most. Some patients have recurrent episodes of acute urticaria (intermittent urticaria). These definitions are manifestly arbitrary, but they have been found useful as a guide to planning investigations and treatment.

Many patients with chronic urticaria turn out to have a physical urticaria either as a stand-alone diagnosis or associated with "ordinary" chronic idiopathic urticaria. It is important to elicit a history of delayed provocation of wheals by pressure, e.g., tight clothes or footwear, gripping implements (delayed pressure urticaria), scratching or rubbing (symptomatic dermographism), exercise, heat, or emotion (cholinergic urticaria) cold contact (cold urticaria), sunlight exposure (solar urticaria) or, rarely wetting the skin with water (aquagenic urticaria), and contact heat urticaria.

Most patients believe, or have been led to believe, that ingestion of certain food items is responsible for their urticaria. While food ingestion is an important cause of acute urticaria, in which case the reaction to the culprit food will occur within minutes or an hour of intake, it is highly controversial as a cause of chronic urticaria. Reaction to food items occurs occasionally in the general population and the frequency of this occurrence is no higher in patients with chronic urticaria; withdrawal of these items does not help patients with chronic urticaria. "Pseudoallergens" (azo dyes, food preservatives) have been incriminated by some authors (1,2). Possibly "pseudoallergens" may merely exacerbate pre-existing urticaria rather than being the prime cause. Postulated involvement of pseudoallergens in an individual patient must be backed up by results of placebo-controlled double blind challenge (3,4). One rare type of urticaria in which food ingestion unarguably precipitates attacks is food- and exercise-induced urticaria. In this condition, food alone and exercise alone are harmless, but if food ingestion precedes exercise, then urticaria, often with prominent angioedema, ensues, and occasionally anaphylaxis may develop. There are two subtypes. In type one attacks follow ingestion of any food, followed by exercise (non – specific); in type 2, the reaction only occurs with specific foods, and is IgE-mediated (5).

Drugs may also cause urticaria. Nonsteroid anti-inflammatory drugs (NSAIDs) such as aspirin and indomethacin are well recognized nonallergic (idiosyncratic) causes of acute urticaria, and, additionally, can aggravate preexisting urticaria (6). Acute urticaria can be triggered by almost any drug as well as vaccines and radiocontrast media, but antibiotics and NSAIDs are the commonest culprits. Drug-induced urticaria has recently been reviewed (7). Angiotensin convertase enzyme (ACE) inhibitors are the commonest cause of acute life-threatening angioedema in the emergency room, and unlike other causes of drug-evoked angioedema its onset may be many weeks after commencing therapy (8). However, like hereditary angioedema (HAE), ACE inhibitors hardly ever cause urticaria. HAE is a dominantly inherited disorder. It is clearly important to take a detailed and comprehensive drug history in patients with urticaria and angioedema and family history in patients with angioedema (no urticaria). However, this is not always easy in patients with angioedema. It is essential to establish whether he or she has airway involvement (usually glossal, pharyngeal, or laryngeal involvement). Tell-tale signs include a hoarse croaky voice or dysarthria. Patients with oropharyngeal

Table 1 Conditions Mimicking Urticaria and Angioedema

Mimic urticaria	Mimic angioedema[b]
Maculopapular exanthema	Cellulitis
Erythema multiforme	Acute allergic contact dermatitis
Urticarial dermatitis (9)	Crohns disease
Pre-pemphigoid	Melkersson–Rosenthal syndrome
Sweet's syndrome (acute febrile neutrophilic dermatosis)	Tumid lupus erythematosus
Erythropoietic protoporphyria (10)[a]	Superior vena cava syndrome
Still's disease (11)	Ascher syndrome (12)

[a]Mimics solar urticaria.
[b]Especially face or lips.

or glossal angioedema are often panic-stricken and unable to give a history. With severe glossal angioedema, speech may be impossible and a history will have to be sought from a care-giver or accompanying friend.

Apart from determining the severity of the urticaria, duration of individual wheals, and the sites of predilection of the wheals (e.g., wheals localized to the waist, or under the brassiere strap would suggest symptomatic dermographism or delayed pressure urticaria), physical examination of the urticaria patient is often uninformative as to the cause. Certain patterns of urticaria are however characteristic. The urticarial rash of cholinergic urticaria is symmetrical, characteristically affecting the neck, forearms, wrists, lower legs, and thighs. Individual wheals are small, maculopapular, and monomorphic in size and shape, although they can become confluent. Patients with symptomatic dermographism present with linear wheals in accessible areas and at sites of local pressure such as under the belt. The junction between covered and exposed involved skin may be sharply demarcated in solar urticaria. Although the morphology of wheals of chronic urticaria is variable (e.g., annular or serpiginous), this has no bearing on the etiology.

Some of the conditions that mimic urticaria are listed in Table 1.

Clinical Tests

Physical Urticaria

It is important to exclude a physical urticaria in all patients with a diagnosis of chronic urticaria. A physical urticaria may be the only manifestation of urticaria or it may be concurrent with another type of chronic urticaria—in which case it is important to establish from the history its relative importance as a source of handicap to the patient. Physical urticaria challenge testing is described in detail in chapter 11, and the tests for the commoner types are summarized here in Table 2.

Food Allergy and Skin Prick Tests

These are appropriate in investigation of acute urticaria if a food allergen is suspected. They are also indicated in food- and exercise-evoked urticaria and anaphylaxis (type 2, *vide supra*). They are rarely, if ever, indicated in chronic urticaria. As in challenge-testing for physical urticarias, patients should be advised to desist from taking any H1 antihistamine for at least 48 hours prior to carrying out the test to avoid false negative results. Skin prick tests are carried out in duplicate on the flexor surface of the forearms, including saline (negative) and histamine (positive) controls. In exceptionally rare cases of chronic urticaria

Table 2 Challenge Test for Physical Urticarias

Physical urticaria[a]	Clinical test[b]
Symptomatic dermograpism	Firm stroking of skin causes rapid wheal and flare with itch (13)
Delayed pressure urticaria	Application of pressure perpendicular to the skin causes a delayed (2–6 hr) indurated wheal (14)
Cholinergic urticaria	Raising body temperature (warm bath; exercise) causes rapid onset of punctate or maculopapular pruritic symmetrical eruption. Intracutaneous methacholine injection can also be used, but the sensitivity of this test is low (15)
Cold contact urticaria	Application of ice cube to skin for 15 min causes local wheal and itch (16)
Heat contact urticaria	Application of a beaker of water at 45°C for 5 min causes local wheal and itch (17)
Solar urticaria	Exposure to natural sunlight or a solar simulator causes local wheal and itch (18)
Aquagenic urticaria	Wetting the skin with water at any temperature causes local wheal and itch (19)

[a]Different physical urticarias may coexist concurrently.
[b]For details see chapter 11.

where food additives such as tartrazine, sodium benzoate, azo dyes are suspected, identification of the culprit requires double blind, placebo-controlled oral challenge-testing.

The Autologous Serum Skin Test

The autologous serum skin test (ASST) has been widely adopted internationally as a clinical marker of circulating endogenous vasoactive factors in patients with the ordinary presentation of chronic urticaria since it was first described in 1986 (20). It is a test for autoreactivity rather than a specific investigation for functional autoantibodies. This was highlighted by two studies that showed retention of autoreactivity in the low molecular weight fractions (21) and IgG-depleted sera (22) in CU patients with positive ASSTs. Autoreactivity is characterized by a wheal and flare response to vasoactive factors in autologous serum, acting indirectly through the release of mediators from mast cells or directly on the cutaneous microvasculature. About 50% of patients with autoreactivity also have a positive basophil histamine release assay using healthy donor basophils. The proportion of CU patients with autoreactivity on skin testing together with histamine-releasing activity on basophils and mast cells and anti-IgE or anti-FcεRI autoantibodies is around 25% (23). Despite having modest sensitivity or specificity compared to basophil histamine release (24) and a number of practical disadvantages, including lack of standardization, the ASST remains a simple low-cost test that provides a convincing demonstration of the endogenous nature of chronic urticaria for patients and may be of limited value in predicting both the course and management of the disease for clinicians.

Venous blood is collected into sterile glass tubes without accelerator or anticoagulant [e.g., separation (450–500 g for 10 min)]. Fresh serum should be used whenever possible for immediate skin testing to minimize risk of sample contamination, although storage of serum between −20°C and −70°C does not appear to influence the outcome of testing. Fifty microlitres of undiluted serum are introduced with a 27 to 29 G needle by superficial intradermal injection into the volar forearm skin to raise a palpable "bleb" within the papillary dermis. Impalpable skin tests should be repeated. The timing of venesection and skin testing in relation to daily activity of continuous urticaria does not appear to influence the test result (20). Physiological (normal) saline (50 µL) is used for an adjacent negative control test. The ASST response should be validated by performing a positive histamine control either by skin prick testing (10 mg/mL) or intradermal injection (0.5–1 µg histamine in 50 µL). H1 antihistamines should be discontinued at least two days before skin testing, allowing more time for long-acting antihistamines (e.g., 6 days for desloratidine and 2 weeks for doxepin). No published information exists on the potential inhibitory effects of leukotriene receptor antagonists or oral corticosteroids, but prior use of high-dose systemic steroids or application of potent topical steroids at the site of testing should be avoided. Skin testing with autologous serum on the day of finishing cyclosporin did not inhibit the autoreactive response to stored serum (25).

A 30-minute reading for the ASST has become standard practice, but a weal and flare response is usually apparent within 10 minute. A positive ASST will enlarge with redness and a surrounding flare over 30 minutes as a result of inflammatory edema, whereas the noninflammatory saline control will usually become flatter and remain pale. Perpendicular diameters of the red wheal response should be recorded and the mean value compared with the negative control. Late-onset wheals should be documented.

Different criteria have been used to define a positive response by comparing it against the negative or positive control skin tests. For routine clinical purposes, the ASST can be interpreted as positive if a red wheal response is present at 30 minute (usually with a surrounding flare) in the absence of a reaction to the negative control skin test. If the serum wheal response is pale rather than uniformly red, the test is negative. The ASST should be considered as uninterpretable and the test repeated if a red wheal develops at the saline skin test or the histamine skin prick test is negative due to previous antihistamine use or other reasons. A minimum difference of 2 mm between the serum wheal diameter and any residual noninflammatory edema at the negative control site should be used to define a positive response.

Autoreactivity appears to be (almost) specific for the ordinary presentation of spontaneous CU. Between 30% and 60% of CU patients have a positive ASST response. By contrast, healthy subjects are negative in most reported series and in the experience of the authors, as are patients with symptomatic dermographism and cholinergic urticaria (23). Autoreactivity has been reported in patients presenting with acute urticaria after nonsteroidal anti-inflammatories (NSAIDs) (26) or antibiotics (27), and sera from some of these patients evoked histamine release in vitro, suggesting that they may belong to a similar population as CU.

An association between thyroid autoimmunity and autoreactive CU supports an autoimmune etiology for this group of patients (28). Other authors found that the ASST remained positive in most patients with thyroid antibodies after disease remission but not in those without (29). The reason for this observation is uncertain since histamine-releasing autoantibodies were not assayed and other measures of skin mast cell releasability (e.g., intradermal codeine injection) were not tested. HLA-DR4 was strongly associated with autoreactive CU, especially in patients with in vitro evidence of basophil histamine–releasing activity (30), illustrating the potential importance of genotype in CU etiopathogenesis. There was no difference in the frequency of immediate autoreactivity (within 30 min) between CU patients with and without intolerance to single or multiple NSAIDs, but delayed skin reactions (after 30 min) were seen in the majority of NSAID-intolerant patients (31), suggesting that delayed onset reactions might be a marker for this group of patients. No correlation was found between *Helicobacter pylori* infection in CU patients and autoreactivity (32).

The clinical characteristics of autoreactive CU patients are similar to those without autoreactivity although patients with a positive ASST have a longer disease duration

(33,34) and may be less likely to give a history of delayed pressure urticaria (20). They also require more H1-antihistamines (34). Autoreactivity did not predict a good response to ciclosporin (35), but patients with a positive ASST and positive basophil histamine–releasing activity were more likely to do well with ciclosporin than autoreactive patients without in vitro evidence of functional autoantibodies (25). Similarly there was no obvious difference in response to IVIG infusions in a small series of CU patients with and without autoreactivity and a history of delayed pressure urticaria (36), but a high proportion of patients with both autoreactivity and basophil histamine–releasing activity responded in a different open series (37).

In routine practice, management decisions are generally based on disease severity and clinical need rather than the outcome of the ASST, which should not therefore be regarded as an essential part of a clinical assessment. The main strength of a positive ASST is to illustrate to the patient that circulating endogenous vasoactive factors may be important in the causation of their condition, rather than avoidable exogenous influences including food allergy and intolerance reactions to food additives. A positive result may, in some cases, provide additional support for moving beyond treatment with H1-antihistamines to a trial of immunotherapies when in vitro assays of serum histamine–releasing autoantibodies are not available.

Blood Tests in Urticaria

The erythrocyte sedimentation rate (ESR) should be routinely determined; patients with urticaria with or without angioedema may have an underlying vasculitis, and an elevated ESR should prompt consideration of this possibility including a skin biopsy. A total and differential white blood cell count can also be justified on the basis that parasite infestation, a recognized cause of acute urticaria in less developed parts of the world, is associated with a blood eosinophilia, and a normal eosinophil count should effectively rule this diagnosis out.

Although often sought by patients, RAST serum testing or CAP FEIA (fluoroenzyme immunoassay) for food or drug allergy is rarely necessary in acute urticaria and essentially never justifiable in chronic urticaria. A negative result in a patient with a suggestive history of penicillin reactivity is unlikely to be reassuring to patient or physician alike. RAST testing is available for certain food items for which no prick test allergen product is available.

Autoimmune thyroiditis is a recognized association with chronic idiopathic urticaria, and, though less strong, there is also a positive association between hyperthyroidism and chronic urticaria (38,39). If patients with chronic urticaria are segregated according to the presence or absence of anti-FcεRI or anti-IgE autoantibodies, then antithyroid autoantibodies (anti-microsomal and anti-thyroglobulin autoantibodies) cosegregate with those patients with evidence of autoimmune urticaria (28). Thus in patients with chronic urticaria and angioedema, it is reasonable to test the patient's serum for presence of thyroid autoantibodies; confirmation of their presence should prompt consideration of the possibility that the patient has autoimmune urticaria.

Immunoassays [Western blot; Elisa (enzyme-linked immunosorbent assay)] have a low specificity (23) and are not recommended for the diagnosis of autoimmune urticaria. A diagnosis of autoimmune urticaria and/or angioedema should therefore be confirmed by demonstrating the capacity of the patient's serum to release histamine (or other reactant) in vitro from donor basophils or a basophil leukemia cell line (40,41). This test is now commercially available, and since the relevant IgG autoantibodies are stable, the patient's serum can safely be dispatched. It is important to establish this diagnosis because it has implications for prognosis (42) and, in selected patients, for treatment (25). Serum protein investigations relevant to patients presenting with angioedema but without urticaria are discussed separately below.

Skin Biopsy for Histological Examination

This is not recommended as a routine procedure in the investigation of urticaria. However, if the history (including poor response to antihistamines), clinical examination (including prolonged duration of wheals, residual staining of affected skin, arthritis), and routine laboratory investigations (raised ESR) are suggestive of vasculitis and/or associated systemic disease then a skin biopsy should be performed. The finding of histological evidence of leucocytoclastic vasculitis (post capillary venular endothelial cell swelling, nuclear dust, fibrin deposition, erythrocyte diapedesis) confirms a diagnosis of urticarial vasculitis and should then prompt thorough investigation for causes and consequences of vasculitis (*vide infra*). Besides urticarial vasculitis, a skin biopsy may be necessary to exclude "pseudourticaria" (Table 1), especially that due to urticarial dermatitis (9).

Investigation of Urticarial Vasculitis

Urticarial vasculitis is generally considered to be rare, occurring in 1% to 3% of patients referred with chronic urticaria. However it is the authors' view that this diagnosis is often missed, as the classical presentation outlined above may not be present and the clinical features may be essentially indistinguishable from "ordinary" chronic idiopathic urticaria. The clinical and laboratory features of urticarial vasculitis have been reviewed (43). This diagnosis should not be deemed confirmed unless supported by histological changes in a skin biopsy, as there are important implications for prognosis, investigation, and treatment. The most important investigations are listed in Table 3. Investigations for systemic involvement should also be carried out for chronic interstitial or obstructive pulmonary disease and glomerulnephritis.

ANGIOEDEMA WITHOUT URTICARIA

Angioedema without urticaria may be hereditary or acquired. In the latter case, it is important to exclude ACE (angiotensin convertase enzyme) inhibitor angioedema, which is rarely accompanied by urticaria. Both acute (especially that due to NSAIDs) and

Table 3 Investigation of Urticarial Vasculitis[a]

Causation	Investigation
Connective tissue disease	Serum antinuclear factor
Infection	Hepatitis B/C serology
Inflammatory bowel disease	Endoscopy
Paraproteinaemia	Serum protein electrophoresis, cryoglobulins
	Serum C4, C1q binding assay for circulating immune complexes, CH50
	Urine microscopy, protein
	Chest X ray
	Pulmonary function testing

[a]Diagnosis must first be confirmed by skin biopsy.

chronic acquired angioedema can also occur without urticaria, but this is rare. B cell lymphoma and autoimmune connective tissue disorders can cause angioedema with C1 esterase inhibitor deficiency due to increased consumption of the latter, and IgG autoantibodies directed against C1 inhibitor itself can cause acquired angioedema. These disorders are dealt with in detail in chapter 16.

History and Examination

Patients with angioedema, which characteristically affects mucous membranes as well as skin, frequently have glossal or laryngeal swelling and may be incapable of giving a history, so in acute presentations reliance may have to be placed on accounts from carers or accompanying friends. Abdominal pain due to bowel mucosal angioedema is also a common presentation in the emergency room. Patients with ACE inhibitor angioedema may have taken the drug for several weeks or months before a onset of angioedema.

HAE is inherited in an autosomal-dominant fashion, and onset often occurs at school age. Eighty-five percent of patients have a quantitative deficiency of C1 inhibitor protein (type 1) and 15% a dysfunctional C1 inhibitor protein (type 2) (44). Trauma either accidental (as in physical contact sports) or deliberate (as in dental or surgical maneuvres) is a frequent triggering event. Recently a third (type 3) form of HAE has been described (45) occurring primarily in women, attacks being precipitated by pregnancy and the contraceptive pill. These patients have no C1 esterase inhibitor protein deficiency. However a mutation in a gene encoding for Factor XII (Hageman factor) has been identified in some patients with type 3 HAE, leading to a gain of function (46).

Examination reveals skin-colored non-pruritic swellings with a predilection for the head and neck and genitalia. The mucous membranes are frequently involved and the tongue may protrude from the mouth. There may be multiple abdominal scars suggestive of previous episodes of bowel angioedema in patients with HAE. Although there is hardly ever any urticaria in angioedema due to C1 esterase inhibitor deficiency (hereditary or acquired) or in angioedema due to ACE inhibitors, a prodromal rash has been reported to precede onset of angioedema (47) in occasional patients with HAE.

Serological Tests

No serological tests are indicated in ACE inhibitor–induced angioedema; the diagnosis is based on history and clinical examination alone. In all cases of C1 esterase inhibitor deficiency, the complement C4 level is invariably reduced in the presence of angioedema. In remission, C4 is reduced in 95% of cases. Therefore, in patients in whom there is a strong clinical suspicion, the C1 esterase level, quantitative and functional should be determined despite a normal C4 in between attacks. In type 1 HAE, immunoreactive C1 esterase inhibitor levels are reduced below 50%, but they are normal or raised in type 2 hereditary angioesema. Functional C1 esterase inhibitor is low in both type 1 and type 2. In infants less than one year old, complement measurements are inaccurate, and for confirmation of HAE in this age group recourse must be made to genetic studies.

The C′4 level is also reduced in acquired C′1 inhibitor deficiency (due to overconsumption), but the complement profile is normal in HAE type 3. Nonhereditary (acquired) C1 esterase inhibitor deficiency is distinguished from HAE by determining the serum C1q level, which is low in acquired C1 esterase inhibitor deficiency, but not in HAE. The laboratory diagnosis of angioedema (44) is discussed in detail in chapter 16 and is summarized in Table 4.

Table 4 Investigation of Angioedema (no Urticaria)

Type	Association	Mechanism	C1 INH protein	C1 INH function	C4 (relapse)	C4 (remission)	C1q
HAE type 1			<50%	<50%	low	Low in 95%[a]	normal
HAE type 2			Normal or raised	<50%	low	Low in 95%[a]	normal
Acquired type 1	B cell lymphoma, autoimmune connective tissue disease	Increased consumption of C1 INH	<50%	<50%	low	Usually low	low
Acquired type 2	Autoantibodies against C1 INH	Increased consumption of C1 INH	<50%	<50%	low	Usually low	low

[a]If clinical suspicion is strong, check C1 INH level even if the C4 is normal.

Diagnosis of Rare Urticarial Syndromes

Schnitzler's Syndrome (48)
This is a rare chronic often non-pruritic urticaria, which should be considered in any adult with chronic urticaria resistant to H1 antihistamines and with systemic symptoms. The appearance of the lesions closely mimics those of chronic idiopathic urticaria. Systemic symptoms are common, including fever and bone pain. Lymphadenopathy is present in about 40% of cases and a peripheral neuropathy in 5% to 10%. Histologically, a skin biopsy characteristically shows neutrophilic urticaria, although occasionally vasculitis may be present, and often the histological features are nonspecific. Direct immunofluorescent examination of a skin biopsy may show monoclonal IgM deposition along the basement membrane or in vessel walls (49). Radiologically, long bones show osteosclerosis, and occasionally lytic lesions. The majority of patients have a high ESR and a monoclonal IgM gammopathy with a κ-light chain. However cases with a IgG paraprotein have also been reported (50).

Autoinflammatory Syndromes
Recently a group of systemic inflammatory disorders in which no infectious or autoimmune basis could be identified has been defined (51). These include familial Mediterranean fever, hyperimmunoglobulin D syndrome with periodic fever, and TRAPS (tumor necrosis factor receptor associated periodic syndrome). Others are also associated with urticaria or urticaria-like eruptions: familial cold autoinflammatory syndrome (FCAS), Muckle-Wells syndrome (MWS), and chronic infantile neurological cutaneous articular syndrome (CINCA). These disorders share the common underlying feature of a mutation in the CIAS1 gene, and are together termed cryopyrin-associated syndromes. Pathophysiologically, these syndromes also collectively feature hyperactive neutrophils and macrophages and abnormal innate immune signaling. Autoinflammatory syndrome should be suspected in any infant with onset of chronic urticaria at or soon after birth. FCAS used to be called familial cold urticaria. Patients with FCAS present with cold urticaria at birth, associated with fever and other systemic symptoms. MWS patients suffer chronic urticaria from birth with sensorineural deafness, and eventually, renal amyloidosis. CINCA infants have a triad of urticaria, arthritis,

and CNS disorders. Elevated plasma levels of interleukin-1 are found in these syndromes, which may respond to the anti-interleukin-1 drug anakinra (52,53). Although a tentative diagnosis can be made from the history of persistent urticaria since birth accompanied by fever and systemic symptoms and signs, confirmation of the diagnosis relies on genetic studies leading to identification of a mutation in the CIAS1 gene. This group of hereditary urticarial disorders with systemic features is dealt with in detail in chapter 15.

REFERENCES

1. Michaelsson G, Juhlin L. Urticaria induced by preservatives and dye additives in food and drugs. Br J Dermatol 1973; 88:525–532.
2. Henz BM, Zuberbier T. Causes of urticaria. In: Henz B, Zuberbier T, Grabbe J, Monroe E, eds. Urticaria: Clinical Diagnostic and Therapeutic Aspects. Berlin, Heidelberg: Springer Verlag, 1998:19.
3. Mathews KP. Urticaria and angioedema. J Allergy Clin Immunol 1983; 72:1–14.
4. Greaves MW. Food intolerance in urticaria and angioedema and urticarial vasculitis. In: Brostoff J, Challacombe S, eds. Food Allergy and Intolerance 2nd ed. Philadelphia: WB Saunders, 2002:623–629.
5. Chong S-U, Worm M, Zuberbier T. Role of adverse reactions to food in urticaria and exercise – induced anaphylaxis. Int Arch Allergy Immunol 2002; 129:19–26.
6. Grattan CEH. Aspirin sensitivity and urticaria. Clin Exp Dermatol 2003; 28:123–27.
7. Greaves MW, Hussein SH. Drug induced urticaria and angioedema. Pathomechanisms and frequency in a developing country, and in developed countries. Int Archs Allergy Immunol 2002; 128:1–7.
8. Slater EE, Merrill DD, Guess HA, et al. Clinical profile of angioedema associated with angiotensin converting enzyme inhibition. J Amer Med Assoc 1988; 260:967–970.
9. Kossard S, Hamann I, Wilkinson B. Defining urticarial dermatitis. A subset of dermal hypersensitivity reaction. Arch Dermatol 2006; 142:29–34.
10. Magnus IA, Jarrett A, Prankerd TAJ, et al. Erythropioetic protoporphyria. Lancet 1961; ii: 448–452.
11. Setterfield JF, Hughes GVR, Black AK. Urticaria as a presentation of adult onset Still's disease. Br J Dermatol 1998; 118:904–927.
12. Sanchez MR, Lee M, Moy JA, et al. Ascher Syndrome: a mimicker of acquired angioedema. J Amer Acad Dermatol 1993; 29:650–651.
13. Kaur S, Greaves MW, Eftekari N. Factitious urticaria (dermographism): treatment by cimetidine and chlorpheniramine in a randomised double –blind study. Br J Dermatol 1981; 104:185–100.
14. Sussman GL, Harvey RP, Schocket AL. Delayed Pressure urticaria. J Allergy Clin Immunol 1982; 70:337–342.
15. Commens CA, Greaves MW. Tests to establish the diagnosis in cholinergic urticaria. Br J Dermatol 1978; 98:47–51.
16. Kobza Black A, Lawlor F, Greaves MW. Consensus meeting on the definition of physical urticarias and urticarial vasculitis. Clin Exp Dermatol 1996; 21:424–446.
17. Koro O, Dover JS, Francis DM, et al. Release of prostaglandin D2 and histamine in a case of localised heat urticaria, and effects of treatments. Br J Dermatol 1986; 115:721–728.
18. Ramsay CA. Solar urticaria. Int J Dermatol 1980; 19:233–236.
19. Sibbald RG, Kobza Black A, Eady RAJ, et al. Aquagenic urticaria. Evidence of a cholinergic and histaminergic basis. Br J Dermatol 1981; 105:297–302.
20. Grattan CEH, Wallington TB, Warin RP, et al. A serological mediator in chronic idiopathic urticaria – a clinical immunological and histological evaluation. Br J Dermatol 1986; 114: 583–590.
21. Grattan CEH, Hamono CGB, Cowan MA, et al. Preliminary identification of a low molecular weight serological mediator in chronic idiopathic urticaria. Br J Dematol 1988; 119:179–184.

22. Fagiolo U, Kricek F, Ruf C, et al. Effects of complement inactivation and IgG depletion on skin reactivity to autologous serum in chronic idiopathic urticaria. J Allergy Clin Immunol 2000; 106: 567–572.

23. Sabroe RA, Fiebiger E, Francis DM, et al. Classification of anti-FcεR1 and anti-IgE autoantibodies in chronic idiopathic urticaria and correlation with disease activity. J Allergy Clin Immunol 2002; 110:492–499.

24. Sabroe RA, Grattan CEH, Francis DM, et al. The autologous serum skin test: a screening test for autoantibodies in chronic idiopathic urticaria. Br J Dermatol 1999; 140:446–452.

25. Grattan CEH, O'Donnell BF, Francis DM, et al. Randomised double blind study of cyclosporin in chronic idiopathic urticaria. Br J Dermatol 2000; 143:365–372.

26. Asero R, Tedeschi A, Lorini M. Autoreactivity is highly prevalent in patients with multipleintolerances to NSAIDS. Ann Allergy Asthma Immunol 2002; 88:468–472.

27. Asero R, Tedeschi A, Lorini M, et al. Sera from patients with multiple drug allergy syndrome contain circulating histamine releasing factors. Int Archs Allergy Immunol 2003; 131:195–200.

28. Kikuchi Y, Fann T, Kaplan AP. Antithyroid antibodies segregate with anti-receptor antibodies in chronic urticaia and angioedema. J Allergy Clin Immunol 2003; 112:218–223.

29. Fusari A, Colangelo C, Bonifazi F, et al. The autologous serum skin test in the follow up of patients with chronic urticaria. Allergy 2005; 60:256–258.

30. O'Donnell BF, O'Neill CM, Francis DM, et al. Human leucocyte antigen class 11 association in chronic idiopathic urticaria. Br J Dermatol 1999; 140:853–858.

31. Erbagci Z. Multiple NSAID intolerance in chronic idiopathic urticaria is correlated with delayed, pronounced and prolonged autoreactivity. J Dermatol 2004; 31:376–382.

32. Baskan EB, Turker T, Gulten M, et al. Lack of correlation between *Helicobacter pylori* infection and autologous serum skin test in chronic idiopathic urticaria. Int J Dermatol 2005; 44:993–995.

33. Toubi E, Kessel A, Avshovich N, et al. Clinical and Laboratory parameters in predicting chronic urticaria: a prospective study of 139 patients. Allergy 2004; 59:869–873.

34. Staubach P, Onnen K, Vonend A, et al. Autologous whole blood injections to patients with chronic urticaria and a positive autologous skin test: a placebo – controlled trial. Dermatology 2006; 212:150–159.

35. Tobi E, Blant A, Kessel A, et al. Low dose cyclosporine A in the treatment of severe chronic idiopathic urticaria. Allergy 1997; 52:312–316.

36. Dawn G, Urcelay M, Ah Weng A, et al. Effect of high dose intravenous immunoglobulin in delayed pressure urticaria. Br J Dermatol 2003; 149:836–840.

37. O'Donnell BF, Barr RM, Kobza Black AK, et al. Intravenous immunoglobulin in autoimmune chronic urticaria. Br J Dermatol 1998; 138:101–106.

38. Leznoff A, Sussman GL. Syndrome of idiopathic chronic urticaria and angioedema with thyroid autoimmunity: a study of 90 patients. J Allergy Clin Immunol 1989; 84:66–71.

39. Kaplan AP. Urticaria and angioedema. Pathogenic mechanisms and treatment. J Allergy Clin Immunol 2004; 114:415–424.

40. Nimii N, Francis DM, Kermani F, et al. Dermal mast cell activation by autoantibodies against the high affinity IgE receptor in chronic urticaria. J Invest Dermatol 1996; 106:1001–1006.

41. Sabroe RA, Greaves MW. Chronic idiopathic urticaria with functional antibodies: 12 years on. Brit J Dermatol 2006; 154:813–819.

42. Sabroe RA, Seed PT, Francis DM, et al. Chronic idiopathic urticaria: comparison of clinical features of patients with and without anti-FcεR1 or anti – IgE autoantibodies. J Amer Acad Dermatol 1999; 40:443–450.

43. O'Donnell BF, Black AK. Urticarial vasculitis. Int Angiol 1995; 14:166–174.

44. Kaplan AP, Greaves MW. Angioedema J Amer Acad Dermatol 2005; 53:373–388.

45. Bork K, Barnstedt SE, Koch P, et al. Hereditary angioedema with normal C1-inhibitor activity in women. Lancet 2000; 356:213–217.

46. Bouillet L, Ponard D, Rousset H, et al. A case of hereditary angioedema type 111 presenting with C1 – inhibitor cleavage and a missense mutation in the F12 gene. Br J Dermatol 2007; 156: 1063–1065.

47. Agostoni A, Aygoren – Pursen E, Binkley KE, et al. Hereditary and acquired angioedema: problems and progress: proceedings of third C1 esterase inhibitor deficiency workshop and beyond. J Allergy Clin Immunol 2004; 114:S51–S131.

48. Schnitzler L. Lesion urticariennes chroniques permanents (erythema petaloide?) Case cliniques n. 46B. Journee Dermatologique d Angers 1972; 28th Abstr. 46.

49. Lipsker D, Veran Y, Grunenberger F, et al. The Schnitzler syndrome. Four new cases and a review of the literature. Medicine 2001; 80:37–44.

50. Nashan D, Sunderkotter C, Bonsmann G, et al. Chronic urticaria, arthralgia, raised erythrocyte sedimentation rate and IgG4 paraproteinaemia: a variant of Schnitzler syndrome? Br J Dermatol 1995; 133:132–134.

51. Galon J, Aksentijevich I, Mc Dermot MF, et al. TNFRSF1A mutations and autoinflammatory syndromes. Curr Opin Immunol 2000; 12:479–486.

52. Hoffman HM, Rosengren S, Boyle BL, et al. Prevention of cold – associated acute inflammation in familial cold autoinflammatory syndrome by interleukin – 1 – receptor antagonist. Lancet 2004; 364:1779–1785.

53. Hawkins PN, Lachmann HJ, Aganna E, et al. Spectrum of clinical features in Muckle – Wells syndrome and response to anakinra. Arthritis and Rheum 2004; 50:607–612.

9

Acute Urticaria

Ruth A. Sabroe

Department of Dermatology, Barnsley Hospital NHS Foundation Trust, Sheffield, U.K.

INTRODUCTION

Acute urticaria is usually defined as the occurrence of spontaneous transient red itchy raised wheals that occur daily or almost daily for short periods (1). If the disease persists for longer than six weeks, it is then classified instead as chronic urticaria (1).

Acute urticaria is thought to be the most common type of urticaria, but, since it is short-lived and may not be severe, it often does not come to the attention of doctors, and patients are only infrequently referred to a hospital department. Perhaps this explains the relatively small number of publications describing large cohorts of patients with acute urticaria (2–4), although there are multiple case reports. Additionally, descriptive reports of collections of patients with all types of urticaria often do not separate patients with acute urticaria from those with chronic urticaria when documenting details such as symptoms, associated angioedema, causes, and response to treatment (5–8). A similar problem afflicts publications describing urticaria in childhood (9–14), with few articles addressing acute urticaria specifically (12).

The following chapter will detail what is known about the clinical features of acute urticaria. It will exclude acute angioedema without wheals, contact urticaria, and only briefly mention urticaria in childhood, since these topics are covered elsewhere.

EPIDEMIOLOGY

Urticaria as a whole is thought to affect 12% to 22% of the population at some time in their lives (15–17). In one study, the prevalence of urticaria in the general population was 0.11% to 0.14%, and about one-third of sufferers had acute urticaria (18). The numbers of patients seen in hospital clinics with acute urticaria may depend on the population studied, local referral patterns, and on the special interests of the hospital department to which they are referred, for example, Accident and Emergency, Allergy, Dermatology, or Immunology. In one hospital department in India, 1.7% of referred patients had urticaria, and, of these, 56% had acute urticaria (8). In most other studies, a much lower proportion of patients referred with urticaria had acute urticaria, for example, 10% of 215 patients (7), 16% of 390 patients (6), and 7.6% of 562 patients with urticaria (5). Acute urticaria, however, was reported as the most commonly observed skin disorder (35%) presenting to an emergency department, with 676 cases seen over a six-year period (4).

In most studies about 60% of patients are female (2–4), although in the report from India 60% of patients referred with acute urticaria were male (8).

Acute urticaria is more common in younger people, but the age range is wide. One study identified 50 patients with acute urticaria aged between 3 months and 88 years, with an average age of 24.7 years (2), and other groups reported very similar findings (3,4).

The majority of very young children with urticaria appear to have acute and not chronic disease. A report describing urticaria in 40 children under the age of two years found that 85% had acute urticaria, and that all children under the age of six months had this type of urticaria (10). In older children, the proportion of the total number of patients with urticaria having the acute form appears to resemble more closely that in adults (9,11,14).

CLINICAL FEATURES

The patient usually presents with spontaneous transient red raised wheals, which are generally extremely itchy (3,8). Wheals usually last only for a few hours, and at most 24 hours (1). The number and size of wheals varies, but the attack may be severe with involvement of more than 50% of the body surface area (3). In one study the rash was described as generalized in 48% of patients (4). Angioedema may coexist, and was present in 31% of patients in one report (4). In children under the age of three years angioedema may be more commonly associated, occurring in about 60% of cases (10,12), and hemorrhagic lesions may also occur (10,12).

The majority of patients present with cutaneous involvement only, but if the attack is severe, systemic symptoms may occur. In one study, 7.3% of patients reported mild breathlessness, 2.7% dizziness, 1.8% headache, 1.8% nausea, and 0.9% diarrhea (3). In a second report, 7.4% of patients had a fever, 5.8% respiratory symptoms such as rhinorrhoea, cough, or bronchospasm, 3.9% gastrointestinal symptoms including vomiting, abdominal pain, or diarrhea, 1.9% hypotension or a tachycardia, 1.6% joint pains, 1.3% conjunctivitis, and 0.6% headache (4). Anaphylaxis may present as acute urticaria with systemic symptoms, and there is probably a disease continuum between the two (19).

ETIOLOGY

It is more common to find a cause for acute urticaria than for chronic disease (8), but acute urticaria is still thought to be idiopathic in approximately 30% to 50% of cases (2–4) (Table 1). There is quite a wide variation between reports in the proportion of patients in which a cause can be identified, and in which causes are thought to be important. Where a cause can be identified, most reports find infections to be the most common culprit (2,3),

Table 1 Causes of Acute Urticaria

Idiopathic

Infections, particularly viral upper respiratory tract infections.

Drugs, e.g., antibiotics, NSAIDs, ACE inhibitors, "biologicals" such as infliximab, transfusion products, and radiocontrast media.

Type 1 hypersensitivity reactions to food (e.g., nuts, milk, fruit, fish), latex, and insect stings or bites.

Other illnesses, e.g., systemic lupus erythematosus.

Abbreviations: NSAIDs, nonsteroidal anti-inflammatory drugs; ACE, angiotensin-converting enzyme.

but in one study no infective cause was mentioned (4). The proportion may depend partly on the age of the population studied, since in one study a cause could be identified in just over 50% of patients aged less than 50 years old, but in almost 80% of older patients (4). This was because the urticaria was more commonly drug-induced, especially due to nonsteroidal anti-inflammatory drugs (NSAIDs), in the older group (4). If a pediatric population is studied, infection is usually reported as the most common cause, with or without drug treatment, it being difficult to separate the two (9,10,12,14). However, in children under the age of six months, the urticaria appeared due to cows' milk allergy in 75% of the cases (10).

In studies reporting infection as a cause of urticaria, upper respiratory tract infections appear to be a common precipitant, accounting for 39.5% of attacks in one study (3). In another report, 64% of 50 patients had had symptoms that might be suggestive of acute bacterial or viral infections, although many of the respiratory and gastrointestinal symptoms described may have been attributable to the urticaria itself rather than to an infection, and seven (14%) had taken anti-inflammatory drugs or antibiotics as well (2). There are multiple case reports implicating a large range of infective organisms, including recently *Mycoplasma pneumoniae* (20) and parvovirus B19 infection (21), and urticaria is also one of the preicteric symptoms of viral hepatitis, A, B, or C (22).

Drugs are another common causative factor accounting for 9.2% of cases in one study (3) and 27% in another (4). Antibiotics and NSAIDs are the most common culprits (3,4). NSAIDs may be a problem in older adults more often than in young adults and children (4), but since drugs are often given for infective episodes, it can be difficult to know which is the cause (10,12). Antibiotics such as penicillins, cephalosporins, sulfonamides, or macrolides are thought to cause urticaria via a type 1 hypersensitivity reaction, but aspirin and other NSAIDs, opiates and ACE inhibitors, precipitate urticaria by other mechanisms (2,3,5,23,24). Multiple reports implicating other drugs have been published, such as bupropion (25), or rarely isotretinoin (26), the use of blood products (27,28), intravenous immunogobulins (29), biologicals such as infliximab (30), and vaccines (4) such as those for *Haemophilus influenzae b* (31) or hepatitis B (32). Radiocontrast media and gadolinium-based contrast media for magnetic resonance imaging may also precipitate acute urticaria (4,33).

It was previously thought that type 1 hypersensitivity reactions to foods were a fairly common cause of acute urticaria (34), accounting for urticaria in 12 of 21 patients in one study (7). In more recent reports, however, the proportion of food-induced urticaria varies from 0% to 18% (2–4), except in those under six months old where cow's milk allergy may be more important (10). Foods implicated most commonly are fish and seafood, nuts, tomatoes and other vegetables and fruit, eggs, and dairy products (4,5,9,10,35).

Acute urticaria may occur as part of a type I hypersensitivity reaction to latex (5,12), insect stings or bites (2–4,7), and after contact with hedgehog spines (36). Ingestion of the fish nematode anisakis simplex has also been associated with acute urticaria (37), and acute urticaria has even been reported after the use of a "gomutra" (cows' urine) gargle (38). Rarely acute urticaria may be the presenting clinical feature of underlying systemic disease, such as systemic lupus erythematosus (35).

DIFFERENTIAL DIAGNOSIS

Acute urticaria should be easy to distinguish from other forms of urticaria since it is the only type that persists for less than six weeks (1). However, this may not be clear initially. The presence of small wheals with a large surrounding flare, linear wheals, or irregularly shaped wheals in pressure sites, might raise the suspicion of the early onset of cholinergic urticaria, dermographism, or delayed pressure urticaria, respectively (1). A careful history should exclude these and other physical urticarias, such as cold or solar urticaria (1). Challenge tests for physical urticarias are occasionally helpful and should be performed according to defined protocols by experienced observers usually under hospital supervision (see chap. 11). Wheals of long duration may be confused with those of delayed pressure urticaria or urticarial vasculitis. The latter can present in episodic form and would warrant more detailed investigations, including a skin biopsy (1). Urticaria is also one of the possible presenting symptoms of anaphylaxis, and there is probably a spectrum of disease connecting the two (19).

Some reactive maculopapular or morbilliform rashes, such as drug eruptions, may produce urticated lesions, and the lesions of erythema multiforme may be confused with annular urticarial wheals. However, in both of these other rashes, lesions remain fixed in the same place for several days, which usually distinguishes them from urticaria (35). Bullous pemphigoid may have a prodromal phase in which lesions appear urticarial or urticated (35). Urticaria can also occur as a manifestation of systemic lupus erythematosus (35).

INVESTIGATIONS

As in all forms of urticaria, there is no substitute for excellent history taking. In straightforward acute urticaria it may not be necessary to do any other investigations at all, since the disease is self-limiting and generally benign (3,39). However, if a type I hypersensitivity reaction is suspected, it may be helpful to confirm a potential allergen by doing skin prick tests or measuring serum allergen-specific IgE. These tests should not be done as routine screening, as false positives and negatives occur which may be misleading (39). For prick tests, the observer should have appropriate experience and training, and, although very rarely required, treatment for anaphylaxis should be available. In some patients it may be helpful to check a full blood count and erythrocyte sedimentation rate, to exclude an eosinophilia (potential IgE-mediated disease, drug reaction, or nematode infestation) or neutrophilia (potential infective or inflammatory cause), but it is generally felt that investigations in acute urticaria are unnecessary and should be kept to a minimum (39,40).

MANAGEMENT

Treatment is aimed at symptom control, and those patients with mild short-lived disease may not require treatment. The avoidance of known allergens and triggering drugs is important. Menthol (1% to 2%) in aqueous cream may provide transient relief from itching (41).

There are very few studies of the use of H1 antagonists in acute urticaria, however, orally, as for all other forms of urticaria, they are usually the treatment of first choice (39,40). They should be taken regularly during an attack, and the patient may wish to keep a small supply in case of accidental exposure to a known precipitant at a later date. Low-sedating antihistamines, such as loratadine (3), are most suitable for daytime symptoms. Sedating antihistamines, such as hydroxyzine, can also be helpful (2,42).

Sometimes a short (3–5 day) course of prednisolone is needed for a severe attack. In one study, the disease went into remission within three days in 93.8% of patients after a three-day course of prednisolone 50 mg daily compared with 65.9% of patients instead taking loratadine 10 mg daily (3). In a second report, the addition of prednisolone 20 mg twice daily for four days to hydroxyzine led to a more rapid reduction in itch scores and to a greater improvement in rash (42).

Although two studies have shown intramuscular H2 antagonists, cimetidine (43) or famotidine (44), to be helpful in patients with acute urticaria, intramuscular treatment is generally felt to be unnecessary and the use of H2 antagonists is controversial in other forms of urticaria. This treatment is not recommended in the guidelines for the treatment of acute urticaria (39).

If the urticaria is associated with severe systemic symptoms or if there is associated angioedema of the airway, then intramuscular epinephrine may be required. Indeed, if there is a possibility of anaphylaxis then full emergency resuscitation will be required, and the guidelines for anaphylaxis should be followed (19,39). The patient is likely to require hospital admission for treatment and careful observation in any of these circumstances.

PROGNOSIS

By definition acute urticaria is short-lived, and if it persists for more than six weeks it is then reclassified as chronic urticaria instead (1). In one study all patients treated with either prednisolone or loratadine had gone into remission within three weeks, and none of the 109 patients included went on to develop chronic disease, although the length of follow-up is not recorded (3). In another study 43 of 50 patients given antihistamines were free of urticaria after 2 weeks, 5 went into remission in 3 months, and 2 patients had disease for over a year (2). Of interest, 12% of 109 patients were reported as having had a brief episode of acute urticaria 6 months to 10 years before the presenting episode (3), and so one might expect some patients to develop more episodes at a later date. Similarly, after an attack of acute urticaria in childhood, one group reported that 20% to 30% of patients had another episode or developed chronic disease within two years (12), although in another study, this proportion was much lower, and only 3.5% to 5% developed further urticaria, usually short-lived, over an eight year follow-up period (13).

SUMMARY

Acute urticaria is a short-lived attack of spontaneous raised itchy transient wheals, which may, if severe, be associated with angioedema and/or systemic symptoms. It is most commonly idiopathic, but many causes have been reported, particularly infections and drugs. Investigations are often unnecessary, and if treatment is required antihistamines and/or a short course of prednisolone are usually sufficient. However, acute urticaria can be a presenting symptom of anaphylaxis, in which case full resuscitation and hospital admission will be required. By definition attacks last for less than six weeks, but in practice, most attacks last for less than three weeks. A small proportion of patients may have another attack at a later date.

REFERENCES

1. Zuberbier T, Greaves MW, Juhlin L, et al. Definition, classification, and routine diagnosis of urticaria: a consensus report. J Invest Dermatol Symp Proc 2001; 6:123–127.
2. Aoki T, Kojima M, Horiko T. Acute urticaria: history and natural course of 50 cases. J Dermatol 1994; 21:73–77.
3. Zuberbier T, Iffländer J, Semmler C, et al. Acute urticaria: clinical aspects and therapeutic responsiveness. Acta Derm Venereol (Stockh) 1996; 76:295–297.

4. Simonart T, Askenasi R, Lheureux P. Particularities of urticaria seen in the emergency department. Eur J Emerg Med 1994; 1:80–82.

5. Nettis E, Pannofino A, D'Aprile C, et al. Clinical and aetiological aspects in urticaria and angio-oedema. Br J Dermatol 2003; 148:501–506.

6. Humphreys F, Hunter JAA. The characteristics of urticaria in 390 patients. Br J Dermatol 1998; 138:635–638.

7. Nizami RM, Baboo MT. Office management of patients with urticaria: an analysis of 215 patients. Ann Allergy 1974; 33:78–85.

8. Sehgal VN, Rege VL. An interrogative study of 158 urticaria patients. Ann Allergy 1973; 31:279–283.

9. Kauppinen K, Juntunen K, Lanki H. Urticaria in children. Retrospective evaluation and follow-up. Allergy 1984; 39:469–472.

10. Legrain V, Taieb A, Sage T, et al. Urticaria in infants: a study of forty patients. Pediatr Dermatol 1990; 7:101–107.

11. Ghosh S, Kanwar AJ, Kaur S. Urticaria in children. Pediatr Dermatol 1993; 10:107–110.

12. Mortureux P, Leaute-Labreze C, Legrain-Lifermann V, et al. Acute urticaria in infancy and early childhood: a prospective study. Arch Dermatol 1998; 134:319–323.

13. Haas N, Birkle-Berlinger W, Henz BM. Prognosis of acute urticaria in children. Acta Derm Venereol 2005; 85:74–75.

14. Sackesen C, Sekerel BE, Orhan F, et al. The etiology of different forms of urticaria in childhood. Pediatr Dermatol 2004; 21:102–108.

15. McKee WD. The incidence and familial occurrence of allergy. J Allergy 1966; 38:226–235.

16. Sheldon JM, Mathews KP, Lovell RG. The vexing urticaria problem: present concepts of etiology and management. J Allergy 1954; 25:525–560.

17. Swinny B. The atopic factor in urticaria. South Med J 1941; 34:855–887.

18. Hellgren L. The prevalence of urticaria in the total population. Acta Allerologica 1972; 27:236–240.

19. (UK) PTotRC. Emergency medical treatment of anaphylactic reactions. Project Team of The Resuscitation Council (UK). Resuscitation 1999; 41:93–99.

20. Kano Y, Mitsuyama Y, Hirahara K, et al. Mycoplasma pneumoniae infection-induced erythema nodosum, anaphylactoid purpura, and acute urticaria in 3 people in a single family. J Am Acad Dermatol 2007; 57:S33–S35.

21. Lipsker D, Boeckler P. Acute urticaria and dry cough with interstitial pneumonia: a clue for the diagnosis of primary parvovirus B19 infection. Clin Exp Dermatol 2006; 31:473–474.

22. Cribier B. Urticaria and hepatitis. Clin Rev Allergy Immunol 2006; 30:25–29.

23. Huston DP, Bressler RB. Urticaria and angioedema. Med Clin North Am 1992; 76:805–840.

24. Inman WHW, Rawson NSB, Wilton LV, et al. Postmarketing surveillance of enalapril. I:Results of prescription-event monitering. Br Med J 1988; 297:826–829.

25. Fays S, Trechot P, Schmutz JL, et al. Bupropion and generalized acute urticaria: eight cases. Br J Dermatol 2003; 148:177–178.

26. Saray Y, Seckin D. Angioedema and urticaria due to isotretinoin therapy. J Eur Acad Dermatol Venereol 2006; 20:118–120.

27. Henderson RA, Pinder L. Acute transfusion reactions. N Z Med J 1990; 103:509–511.

28. Shemin D, Briggs D, Greenan M. Complications of therapeutic plasma exchange: a prospective study of 1,727 procedures. J Clin Apher 2007; 22:270–276.

29. Hamrock DJ. Adverse events associated with intravenous immunoglobulin therapy. Int Immunopharmacol 2006; 6:535–542.

30. Lequerre T, Vittecoq O, Klemmer N, et al. Management of infusion reactions to infliximab in patients with rheumatoid arthritis or spondyloarthritis: experience from an immunotherapy unit of rheumatology. J Rheumatol 2006; 33:1307–1314.

31. Humphreys F. Acute urticaria and angio-oedema following Haemophilus influenzae b vaccination. Br J Dermatol 1994; 131:582–583.

32. Barbaud A, Trechot P, Reichert-Penetrat S, et al. Allergic mechanisms and urticaria/angioedema after hepatitis B immunization. Br J Dermatol 1998; 139:925–926.

33. Li A, Wong CS, Wong MK, et al. Acute adverse reactions to magnetic resonance contrast media – gadolinium chelates. Br J Radiol 2006; 79:368–371.
34. Monroe EW, Jones HE. Urticaria. An updated review. Arch Dermatol 1977; 113:80–90.
35. Cooper KD. Urticaria and angioedema: diagnosis and evaluation. J Am Acad Dermatol 1991; 25: 166–176.
36. Fairley JA, Suchniak J, Paller AS. Hedgehog hives. Arch Dermatol 1999; 135:561–563.
37. Del Pozo MD, Audícana M, Diez JM, et al. *Anisakis simplex*, a relevant etiologic factor in acute urticaria. Allergy 1997; 52:576–579.
38. Bhalla M, Thami GP. Acute urticaria following 'gomutra' (cow's urine) gargles. Clin Exp Dermatol 2005; 30:722–723.
39. Grattan CE, Humphreys F. Guidelines for evaluation and management of urticaria in adults and children. Br J Dermatol 2007; 157:1116–1123.
40. Zuberbier T, Greaves MW, Juhlin L, et al. Management of urticaria: a consensus report. J Investig Dermatol Symp Proc 2001; 6:128–131.
41. Bromm B, Scharein E, Darsow U, et al. Effects of menthol and cold on histamine-induced itch and skin reactions in man. Neurosci Lett 1995; 187:157–160.
42. Pollack CV Jr., Romano TJ. Outpatient management of acute urticaria: the role of prednisone. Ann Emerg Med 1995; 26:547–551.
43. Moscati RM, Moore GP. Comparison of cimetidine and diphenhydramine in the treatment of acute urticaria. Ann Emerg Med 1990; 19:12–15.
44. Watson NT, Weiss EL, Harter PM. Famotidine in the treatment of acute urticaria. Clin Exp Dermatol 2000; 25:186–189.

10

Contact Urticaria

Heidi P. Chan, Esther Kim, and Howard I. Maibach
Department of Dermatology, UCSF School of Medicine, San Francisco, California, U.S.A.

INTRODUCTION

Maibach and Johnson defined the contact urticaria syndrome as a biological entity in 1975 (1). Contact urticaria is an immediate contact reaction that appears on the skin within minutes to an hour after an eliciting substance has been in contact with the skin. The prototype reaction of contact urticaria is a local wheal and flare, although other reactions such as nonspecific symptoms (itching, tingling, burning), generalized urticaria, and anaphylaxis occur (Table 1) (2).

Many substances cause contact urticaria; therefore, a detailed history and the need to have a specialist with a broad knowledge of the allergens and its clinical relevance to the patient are essential to establish the etiology (3).

Contact urticaria symptoms usually appear within an hour after contact with the eliciting substance, and the patient may be able to attribute these symptoms to a specific exposure. The extent of extracutaneous involvement should be obtained. The patient may be able to identify exactly what he or she was doing at the onset of the symptoms, allowing the physician to narrow down the possibilities. Details of a patient's employment should be ascertained since many of the causes of contact urticaria are occupation related. A personal or family history of atopy should always be ascertained as part of the history, as well as a history of previous anaphylaxis when applicable. Signs on physical exam may be variable depending on when the patient presents, since contact urticaria lesions disappear by definition within 24 hours of onset.

The prevalence of contact urticaria in the general population is unknown because much of the epidemiological data is from occupational settings. Kanerva gathered statistical data on occupational contact urticaria in Finland; the most affected occupations were (in decreasing order) farmers, domestic animal attendants, bakers, nurses, chefs, and dental assistants (4). Elpern studied the relationship between race, gender, and age in Hawaii and found no difference in racial predisposition, slight increase incidence in female patients, and constant incidence from the second to the eighth decade (5). Contact urticaria syndrome can be categorized into two broad categories by mechanism of action: (*i*) nonimmunological contact urticaria (NICU) and (*ii*) immunological contact urticaria (ICU).

Table 1 Staging of Contact Urticaria Syndrome

Stage 1	Cutaneous (skin) reactions only
	Localized urticaria (redness and swelling)
	Dermatitis (after repeated exposures)
	Nonspecific symptoms (itching, tingling, burning)
Stage 2	Generalized urticaria
Stage 3	Extracutaneous reactions
	Bronchial asthma (wheezing)
	Rhinitis, conjunctivitis (runny nose, watery eyes)
	Orolaryngeal symptoms (lip swelling, hoarseness, difficulty swallowing)
Stage 4	Anaphylactoid reactions (shock)

Source: Adapted from Ref. 2.

NONIMMUNOLOGIC URTICARIA

NICU is the most common type of immediate contact reaction and occurs without prior sensitization. The NICU reactions usually appear within minutes to an hour, and the edema disappears within one hour, but redness may last for six hours after contact with the eliciting substance (6). The symptoms vary depending on the substance, concentration, site of exposure, vehicle, and the mode of exposure. The symptoms usually appear and remain in the contact area (1). Generalized urticaria is rare after contact with a NICU substance and is usually seen in ICU. Different anatomic sites show marked variation in susceptibility to NICU agents, with the most sensitive area being the face, (in decreasing order) antecubital fossa, upper back, upper arm, volar forearm, and lower back (7).

The guinea pig ear-swelling test has been used as an animal model to screen for putative agents and to clarify the mechanisms (8). Substances are applied to the earlobes and a positive reaction comprises erythema and edema. The increase in thickness is measured, with a maximal response being a 100% increase. The swelling response in the guinea pig depends on the concentration of the substance, which is similar to the human skin.

The guinea pig also demonstrates the tachypylaxis phenomenon, which is a decrease in reactivity to NICU agents after repeated application of the eliciting substance. The refractory period for the following substances are 4 days for methyl nicotinate, 8 days for diethyl fumarate and cinnamic aldehyde, and 16 days for benzoic acid, cinnamic acid, and dimethyl sulfoxide (2).

Mechanism of NICU

The mechanism of NICU is incompletely understood. It was previously assumed that the reaction was a result of nonspecific histamine release from mast cells in response to exposure to an eliciting susbtance. However, antihistamines do not inhibit reactions to common NICU agents such as dimethyl sulfoxide, benzoic acid, cinnamic acid, cinnamic aldehyde, or methyl nicotinate (9). However, these common NICU agents can be inhibited by acetylsalicylic acid (ASA) and nonsteroidal anti-inflammatory drugs (NSAIDs) both orally and topically suggesting the role of prostaglandins (10–12).

The duration of inhibition by ASA taken orally may be up to four days (13). There is a release of prostaglandin D_2 without concomitant histamine release following topical application of sorbic acid, benzoic acid, and cinnamic aldehyde (14–16).

UVA and UVB irradiation inhibits the NICU reaction for at least two weeks. This inhibition also includes areas of the skin that was sheltered from irradiation suggesting a systemic effect (17). Psoralen + UVA (PUVA) treatment also has an inhibitory effect on NICU reaction (18).

These results suggest that prostaglandin rather than histamine is the main mediator of NICU reactions and that the source of prostaglandins is in the epidermis, although the cells that produce prostaglandins in the skin remain to be identified. The systemic effect of UV irradiation suggests that some other substances are also involved in the reaction.

The role of cutaneous nerves has been studied using capsaicin, which release substance P and other active peptides from the axons of unmyelinated C-fibers of sensory nerves (19). Capsaicin pretreatment does not impair NICU from benzoic acid and methyl nicotinate but does inhibit the flare of histamine prick tests (19,20). Local anesthesia has shown a slight inhibitory effect on the NICU reaction (19).

The molecular structure of a NICU substance is important, since a minor change in the structure can greatly alter its capacity to produce a reaction. Pyridine carboxaldehyde has three isomers: 2-, 3-, and 4-PCA (polychloroalkanes). Among the three isomers of PCA, 3-PCA was the strongest in both the human skin and in the guinea pig ear-swelling test and 2-PCA was the weakest (21).

IMMUNOLOGIC URTICARIA

ICU, a type I hypersensitivity immunologic reaction, is mediated by allergen-specific IgE in a previously sensitized individual (22). Sensitization can be at the cutaneous level, but can also be through the mucous membranes, the respiratory, and gastrointestinal (GI) tracts. The radioallergoabsorbent test (RAST) is an assay used to detect the specific IgE antibodies in the serum. ICU is mediated primarily by histamine, although other mediators such as prostaglandins, leukotrienes, and kinins are involved (2). The reaction usually appears within 5 to 15 minutes after contact with the eliciting substance, and a reaction of medium intensity usually disappears in 20 to 30 minutes. The severity of the reaction varies from mild symptoms, such as a local itch and erythema, to widespread generalized urticaria and anaphylactic shock (6).

Anaphylactic reaction is a clinical syndrome in which the predominant clinical feature is cardiovascular collapse along with other manifestations such as bronchospasm, airway impairment, and pulmonary edema. Anaphylactic reactions are immediate, allergic, and IgE-mediated. Complications of contact urticaria in the form of anaphylaxis are rare; however, it is a serious concern since it can be lethal. Contact urticaria and anaphylaxis is most commonly observed with latex allergy (23). However, contact urticaria with anaphylactic reactions is caused by numerous substances such as oxybenzone (24), formaldehyde (25), rifamycin (26), bacitracin and polysporin ointment (27), raw potato (28), codfish (29), chestnut (30), cornstarch glove powder (31), and benzophenone (32), to name a few.

A common cause of ICU is natural rubber latex, and it is frequently seen in health workers (3). The route of exposure to natural rubber latex includes direct contact with intact or inflamed skin as well as mucosal exposure such as inhalation of powder from the latex gloves (33,34). The majority of cases involve reaction to natural rubber gloves although reactions to nonmedical natural rubber latex such as balloons, condoms, and toys occur (35). In the case of glove-related reactions to natural rubber latex, diagnosis can often be confounded by the presentation of ICU from cornstarch glove powder, which adsorbs the protein (31,36). The number of reported cases has increased more than any other agent and as a result has become a major medical, occupational health, medicolegal, and financial problem for health care workers and glove-wearing occupations (37,38).

Murine models have been used to investigate the role of route of exposure on the development of latex allergy to provide a mechanism for the evaluation of new technologies aimed at reducing the allergenicity of latex products (39,40).

Numerous reasons have been documented as causing ICU (Table 9), with newly reported cases discussed later in the chapter.

Mechanism of ICU

The mechanism of ICU is a type I hypersensitivity immunologic reaction that requires that the persons be previously "sensitized", which means that they have already been exposed to the causative agent and therefore has produced specific IgE antibodies. In immediate allergy, sensitization most usually takes place in the airways. The specific IgE reacts with high affinity IgE receptors on mast cells, basophils, eosinophils, langerhans cells, and numerous other cells. An allergen molecule reacts with two adjacent IgE molecules that are bound to the cell membrane of mast cells, leading to the release of histamine, neutral proteases, exoglyosidases, and proteoglycans. The allergen-IgE reaction also leads to a synthesis of leukotrienes, prostaglandins, and platelet-activating factor in the cell membranes of the activated mast cells. This results in a wheal-and-flare reaction on the skin and sometimes can lead to anaphylaxis if massive amounts of these active substances are released (2,6). Nitric oxide has been shown to be involved in immediate immunological reactions. The nitric oxide synthase inhibitor, NG-nitro-L-arginine (L-NAME) was injected intracutaneously prior to provocation tests and was shown to augment immediate immunological reactions (prick test) (41).

Cross-allergy is often seen in many ICU reactions. The patient may be sensitized to one protein and react to other proteins that contain the same or a chemically related allergenic molecule. One of the largest cross-allergy families are between birch pollen, fruits, and vegetables and was found in the 1970s (42), followed by observations of pollen and spice allergies (43). One of the main causes of cross-allergy between pollens and fruits and vegetables was a pan-botanical protein, profilin (44). The cross-reactivity of IgE antibodies with these allergens was demonstrated in vitro (45). Many latex allergy patients experience symptoms from banana, chestnut, and avocado (46–48). Hevein is one of the panallergens among latex and related foods and patients with latex allergy would be recommended to avoid fruits such as chestnuts because of a high risk of contact urticaria and even anaphylaxis, as recent cases have been reported (30). Another recent case demonstrated cross-reactivity of shrimps and scallops with the primary cross-reactive allergen being the muscle topomyposin seen in both phyla (49).

TESTING

The diagnosis of contact urticaria is based on both a detailed history and skin testing. Commonly used in vivo skin testing for both immunological and nonimmunological urticaria are the open test, the prick test, the scratch test, the scratch-chamber test, and the use test. In any of the above tests, it is important to perform positive (histamine, 1 mg/mL) and negative (normal saline) controls. In addition to in vivo methods, the diagnosis of ICU can be done using in vitro RAST. This method detects antigen-specific IgE molecules from the patient's serum and is seldom needed for ICU diagnosis, although it may be beneficial in determining cross-allergenity. NSAIDs, antihistamines, and exposure to UV light can cause false negative results, as can tachyphylaxis. In testing for ICU in patients with a history of extracutaneous involvement, particular care must be taken to use low concentrations of test substances, beginning with very dilute allergen concentrations and using serial dilutions if required, to avoid reproducing systemic reactions. Resuscitation equipment should be immediately available (2,50). It is generally recommended that suspected agents be tested in the following manner (51):

1. Open test application to normal skin.
2. If negative, open test application to previously affected, yet normal appearing, skin.
3. If testing on eczematous skin, test on an area showing only slight erythema so that urticaria responses can occur.
4. If all of the above are negative, then occluded patch tests on normal or previously affected skin.
5. If still negative, then perform prick testing. Scratch and scratch-chamber are more likely to produce false-positive responses.

- In the open test, 0.1 mL of the test substance in a vehicle (petrolatum, ethanol, water) is spread over a 3×3 cm area on the desired site. Alcoholic vehicles are suggested, since the addition of propylene glycol to a vehicle enhances the sensitivity of the test compared with previously used petrolatum and water vehicles. The test should first be performed on nondiseased skin and if negative, then on previously or currently affected skin because there is a marked difference between skin sites in their capacity to elicit contact urticaria typically in NICU but also seen in ICU (52,53). The test sites are usually read at 20, 40, and 60 minutes, in order to see the maximal response. ICU reactions typically appear within 15 to 20 minutes, while NICU reactions can be delayed up to 45 to 60 minutes following application (2) (Table 2).
- The prick test is often the method of choice for testing if the open test is negative. The allergen in vehicle is applied to the volar aspect of forearms and the site pierced with a lancet to introduce the allergen into the skin. Prick testing theoretically runs the lowest risk of anaphylaxis, as only minute amounts of allergen are introduced into the skin. The test sites are usually read within 30 minutes (Table 3).
- The scratch test is a less standardized method than the prick test, but it is useful for nonstandardized allergens. It is important to have at least > 10 people as control test to avoid false interpretation of results. The allergen in vehicle is applied to the skin site and the area is scratched using needles. The test sites are usually read within 30 minutes (Table 4).
- The chamber test is an occlusive method of applying the substance to be tested. The substances to be tested are applied in small aluminum containers and

Table 2 Open Test

Materials	1. Allergen in vehicle (petrolatum, ethanol, water)
	2. Vehicle
	3. Cotton-tipped applicators or other devices to spread the preparations.
Method	Allergen and vehicle are applied to skin.
Reading time	Up to 1 h.
Interpretation	Urticarial reaction is positive
Precautions	General anaphylaxis not very likely because of the small amount of allergen introduced, but a physician should always be available for such occurrences. The patient should not leave the premises during the first 30 minutes after the test.
Controls	Required to aid in discriminating ICU from NICU; in NICU the reaction will be noted in most controls.

Source: Adapted from Ref. 50.

Table 3 Prick Test

Materials	1. Allergens in vehicles 2. Vehicle (negative control) 3. Histamine in 0.9% NaCl (positive control) 4. Prick lancets
Method	One drop of each test allergen, vehicle, and histamine control is applied to the volar aspects of forearms. The test site is pierced with a lancet to introduce the allergen into the skin.
Reading time	15–30 min
Interpretation	An edematous reaction (wheal) of at least 3 mm in diameter and at least half the size of the histamine control is considered positive in the absence of such reaction in the vehicle control.
Precautions	See Table 2
Controls	Required

Source: Adapted from Ref. 50.

Table 4 Scratch Test

Materials	1. Allergens in vehicles 2. Vehicle (negative control) 3. Histamine in 0.9% NaCL (positive control) 4. Needles
Method	A drop of each test allergen, vehicle, and histamine control is applied to the volar aspects of forearms or back, and needles are used to scratch the skin slightly at these areas.
Reading time	Up to 30 min
Interpretation	Difficult because of unstandardized procedure. Edematous reaction at least as wide as the histamine control is considered positive in the absence of such reaction in the vehicle control.
Precautions	See Table 2
Controls	Required

Source: Adapted from Ref. 50.

Table 5 Scratch-Chamber Test

Materials	1. Scratch test materials (Table 4) 2. Chambers
Method	As with scratch test, but scratch sites are covered with aluminum chambers for 15 min
Reading time	30 min
Interpretation	See Table 4
Precautions	See Table 2
Controls	Required

Source: Adapted from Ref. 50.

attached to the skin via a porous tape for 15 minutes, and the results read at 20, 40, and 60 minutes. The advantages of this method are that occlusion enhances percutaneous penetration and, therefore, the sensitivity of the test is probably higher and a smaller area of the skin is required than in an open test (Table 5).

Table 6 Scale to Score Erythema

Score	Description
1+	Slight erythema, either spotty or diffuse
2+	Moderate uniform erythema
3+	Intense redness
4+	Fiery redness with edema

Source: Adapted from Ref. 54.

Table 7 Scale to Score Edema

Score	Description
1	Slight edema, barely visible or palpable
2	Unmistakable wheal, easily palpable
3	Solid, tense wheal
4	Tense wheal, extending beyond the test area

Source: Adapted from Ref. 7.

- The use test is a method in which a subject known to be affected uses the causative substance in the same way as when the symptoms first appeared; for example, wearing surgical gloves on wet hands provokes latex ICU.

In all of the above test methods, contact urticaria can be graded visually by degree of erythema and edema on an ordinal scale (Tables 6 and 7) (7,54).

Recently, the basophil activation test by flow cytometry was suggested as a standardized tool for in vitro diagnosis of immediate hypersensitivity (55). This test is based on the appearance of a membrane protein marker as a consequence of exposure to allergens; further, this method may be helpful in dealing with rare allergens wherein specific IgE antibodies are not available (22).

AGENTS CAUSING CONTACT URTICARIA

NICU Substances

Table 8 (adapted from Warner et al.) (51) lists many substances identified as nonimmunolgic causes of contact urticaria, including chrysanthemum (56).

A 34-year-old gardener and horticultural worker developed local urticaria on the hands and forearms, with no systemic symptoms after contact with chrysanthemum flowers. The patient was symptom-free on holidays and symptoms decreased on the weekends. Patch tests and RAST were negative to chrysanthemum. A positive rub test with chrysanthemum blossoms and a positive cellular antigen stimulation test (CAST) confirmed the skin reaction. The complement activated (C5a) CAST stimulates isolated leukocytes of the patient with interleukin-2 and detects sulfidoleukotrienes when sensitization with tested agent is present. The CAST was negative for control persons. These results favor a non-IgE-mediated reaction classified as a NICU response (56).

Table 8 List of Agents Causing NICU

Foods	Jellyfish
Fish	Moths
Cayenne pepper (capsicum)	Roe Deer (*Capreolus capreolus*)[a]
Thyme	Stinging insects
Fragrance and flavoring	**Plants**
Balsam of Peru	Coral
Benzaldehyde	Nettles
Cassia (cinnamon) oil	Sea anemone
Cinnamic acid	Chrystanthemum[a]
Menthol	Preservatives and germicidals
Vanilla	Benzoic acid
Medicaments	Formaldehyde
Alcohols	Chlorocresol
Benzocaine	Sodium benzoate
Camphor	Sorbic acid
Cantahrides	**Miscellaneous**
Capsaicin	Acetic acid
Chloroform	Ammonium persulfate
Dimethylsulfoxide	Benzophenone
Friar's balsam	Butyric acid
Methyl salicylate	Cobalt chloride
Mustard (black)	Naphtha 21/99
Myrrh	Pine oil
Nicotinic acid esters	Sulfur
Tar extracts	Resorcinol
Tincture of benzoin	Turpentine
Thyme oil	
Witch hazel	
Animals	
Arthropods	
Caterpillars	

[a]Agents discussed in this chapter.
Source: Adapted from Ref. 51.

ICU Substances

Table 9 (adapted from Warner et al. and Amin) (2,51) lists many of the substances that have been identified as immunologic causes of contact urticaria. Recent additions to the list are discussed below.

A 55-year-old male professional hunter with no other past or present allergic diseases experienced contact urticaria and rhinitis after exposure to roe deer. Roe deer is one of the most common game animals in Europe, and although occupational allergies to roe deer seem to be rare, the possibility should always be considered among people having contact with these animals. There is no specific deer dander allergen for specific IgE and skin tests, and therefore the relationship had to be confirmed using a rub test with the roe deer's fur. There was a clear positive urticaria reaction on the patient's skin as well as nasal itch, sneezing, and rhinorrhea following skin exposure to the fur. No reaction was noted in the control person (57).

Potassium persulfate is a common ingredient in hair dyes. A 37-year-old housewife developed itch and erythema of the ears, neck, forehead, and hands after application of a hair dye. Prick tests were performed with isolated booster components that were found in

Table 9 List of Agents Causing ICU

Animal products
  Amnion fluid
  Blood
  Brucella abortus
  Cercariae
  Cheyletus malaccensis
  Chironomidae, Chironomus thummi[a]
  Cockroaches
  Dander
  Dermestes maculates
  Gelatine
  Gut
  Hair
    Giraffe hair[a]
  Listrophorus gibbus
  Liver
  Locust
  Mealworm
  Placenta
  Roe deer[a]
  Saliva
  Serum
  Silk
  Spider mite
  Wool

Food
  Dairy
    Cheese
    Egg
    Milk
  Fruits
    Apple
    Apricot
    Apricot Stone
    Banana
    Kiwi
    Litchi
    Lime
    Mango
    Orange
    Peach
    Plum
    Strawberry
    Watermelon
  Grains
    Buckwheat
    Maize
    Malt
    Rice
    Wheat
    Wheat bran
    Lupine flour[a]

  Honey
  Nuts
    Peanuts
    Peanut butter
    Sesame seed
    Sunflower seed
  Meats
    Beef
    Chicken
    Lamb
    Liver
    Pork
    Sausage
    Turkey
  Salami casing mold
  Seafood
    Cod
    Crab
    Fish
    Oysters
    Prawns
    Shrimp
  Vegetables
    Beans
    Cabbage
    Carrot
    Castor bean
    Celery
    Chives
    Cucumber
    Cucumber pickle
    Endive
    Garlic
    Lettuce
    Onion
    Parsley
    Parsnip
    Potato
    Rutabaga
    Tomato
    Soybean
    Winged bean

Fragrances and flavorings
  Balsam of Peru
  Benzoic acid
  Cinnamic aldehyde
  Menthol
  Vanillin
Hair care products
  Basic Blue 99
  Henna
  Hydrolyzed animal proteins

(Continued)

Table 9 List of Agents Causing ICU (*Continued*)

Paraphenylenediamine
Potassium persulfate[a]

Medicaments
Acetylsalicylic acid
Antibiotics
    Ampicillin
    Bacitracin
    Cephalosporins
    Chloramphenicaol
    Gentamycin
    Iodochlorhydroxyquin
    Mezlocillin
    Neomycin
    Penicillin
    Rifamycin
    Streptomycin
Benzocaine
Benzoyl peroxide
Clobetasol 17-propionate
Dinitrochlorobenzene
Diphenylcyclopropene
Etophenamate
Fumaric acid derivatives
Hydrocortisone[a]
Lindane
Mechlorethamine
Mexiletine hydrochloride
Phenothiazines
    Chlorpromazine
    Levomepromazine
    Promethazine
Pyrazolones
    Aminophenazone
    Methamizole
    Propylphenazone
Tocopherol

Metals
Cobalt
Copper
Gold
Iridium
Mercury
Nickel
Palladium
Platinum
Rhodium
Rutherium
Tin
Zinc

Plant products
Abietic acid
Algae

Birch
Bishop's weed (*Ammi majus*)[a]
Bougainvillea
Camomile
Chrysanthemum
Cinchona
Colophony
Cornstarch
Cotoneaster
Elm tree
Emetin
Eruca sativa
Eucalyptus
Fennel
Ficus benjamina[a]
Garlic
Grevillea juniperina
Hakea suaveolens
Hawthorn, *Crataegus monogyna*
Henna
Hops (*Humulus lupulus*)[a]
Latex rubber
Lichens
Lily
Limba
Limonium tatricum
Mahogany
Mulberry
Mustard
Obeche
Papain
Perfumes
Phaseolus multiflorus
Rose
Rouge
Semecarpus anacardium
Spathe flower (*Spathiphyllum wallisii*)[a]
Spices
Teak
Tobacco
Tulip
Yucca[a]

Preservatives and disinfectants
Ammonia
Benzoic acid
Benzyl alcohol
Butylated hydroxytoluene
Chlorhexidine
Chloramine
Chlorocresol
Chlorohexidine
1,3-Diiodo-2-hydroxypropane

Table 9 List of Agents Causing ICU (*Continued*)

Formaldehyde	Diethyltoluamide
Gentian violet	Ethylenediamine
Hexamidine[a]	Epoxy resin
Hexantriol	Formaldehyde resin
para-Hydrozxybenzoic acid	HBTU[a]
Parabens	Hypochlorite
Phenylmercuric propionate	Lanolin alcohols
Phenylmercuric acetate	Methyl ethyl ketone
ortho-Phenylphenate	Methylhexaphydropthalic and
Polysorbates	Methyltetrahydropthalic anhydrides
Sodium hypochlorite	Monoamylamine
Sorbitan monolaurate	Morpholinylmercaptobenzothiaole
Sorbitan sesquioleate	Naphtha
Tropicamide	Naphthylacetic acid
Enzymes	Nylon
α-Amylase	Oleylamide
Cellulases	Patent blue dye
Xylanases	Perlon
Miscellaneous	Phosphorus sesquisulfide
Acetyl acetone	Phthalic anhydride[a]
Acrylic acid	Plastic
Acrylic monomer	Polypropylene
Alcohols (amyl, butyl, ethyl, isopropyl)	Polyethylene[a]
Aliphatic polyamide	Polyethylene glycol
p-Aminodiphenylamine	Potassium ferricyanide
Ammonia	Seminal fluid
Ammonium persulfate	Sodium silicate
Ammonium chloride	Sodium sulfide
Bacillus-subtilis-derived detergent protease[a]	Sulfur dioxide
Benzophenone	Terpinyl acetate
Benzophenone-3[a]	Tinofix S
Carbonless copy paper	1,1,1-Trichloroethane
Chlorothalomil	Textile finish
Chlorothanil	Tobacco
Citraconic anhydride	Vinyl pyridine
Cu(II)-acetyl acetonate	Xylene
Cyclopentolate hydrochloride[a]	Zinc diethyldithicarbamate
Dentanium benzoate	Zinc pentamethylenedithiocarbamate
Dicyanidiamide	Zinc dibutyldithiocarbamate

[a]Agents discussed in this chapter.
Source: Adapted from Refs. 2, 51.

the hair dye. All ingredients were negative except for potassium persulfate. Four controls were negative to this agent (58).

Recent case reports two atopic patients who developed contact urticaria from a hydrocortisone injection or infusion. Patient 1 was positive on skin prick tests to hydrocortisone, prednisolone, and methylprednisolone. Patient 2 had a positive intradermal test reaction to prenisolone. Eleven control persons were negative when tested with the same corticosteroids. Both patients had elevated IgE values (patient 1: 286, patient 2: 488 kU/I) and patient 2 had IgE antibodies to hydrocortisone and methylprednisolone conjugated with human serum albumin (59).

An atopic 31-year-old worked as a florist for five years, and for the last two years, she suffered severe rhinitis and urticaria lesions on her hands after contact with bishop's weed. Skin prick test was performed using the flower proper, which was positive in the patient but negative in the four atopic and six nonatopic controls. The patient had elevation of bishop-weed-specific IgE level of 9.7 PRU/mL in the serum by RAST (60).

Occupational contact urticaria from plants is often reported, but it is less often attributed to decorative houseplants. A 22-year-old atopic gardener and caretaker of plants developed contact urticaria when exposed to decorative houseplants. Contact with weeping fig, spathe flower, and yucca leaves caused immediate skin symptoms, and the patient subsequently underwent allergologic investigation. Strong allergic prick test reactions were noted to yucca leaves, spathe flower (leaves and pollen), and weeping fig. Control testing of the three plants was done on 20 unexposed persons, and the result was negative. Specific IgE antibodies were elevated to birch, spathe flower, and weeping fig by RAST. Total IgE was 169 kU/l (61).

Humulus lupulus is a perennial vine that grows female flowers resembling cones that mature in late summer. These ripe dried cones are called hops, and they are used in breweries and in herbal therapy. A 29-year-old man, who had also suffered urticaria-angioedema after intake of peanut, chestnut, and banana, complained of urticaria on both hands while handling ripe dried hops. Prick testing was positive and total IgE was 64 IU/mL to ripe dried hops (62).

A 27-year-old atopic man who worked at a chemical enzyme factory developed contact urticaria after contact with liquid proteases and amylases. Prick tests were performed with *Bacilus subtilus*–derived detergent protease (BSDDP), which provoked a strong test reaction. Twenty controls were negative when prick tested with BSDDP. RAST to BSDDP were also elevated (63).

Benzophenone-3 is a common sunscreen ingredient and is known variously as oxybenzone. The occurrence of contact urticaria with benzophenone-3 is rare. However, a recent case reports a patient who developed contact urticaria reaction to the agent. The patient is a 40-year-old child care assistant who developed urticaria and anaphylaxis after applying a sunscreen to her daughter's skin in May. She also developed contact urticaria to certain lipsticks and shampoos that were later found to contain benzophene-3. Patch testing was positive for benzophenone-3 with five controls being negative (32).

Among the most common mydriatic eyedrops is cyclopentolate hydrochloride, and a recent case reports contact urticaria to cyclopentolate hydrochloride eyedrops, with tolerance to other eyedrops. A 72-year-old man developed erythema, edema, itching, and burning in his right eye, with an urticarial rash on his right cheek following the path of drug-containing tears after administration of several drugs in his right eye: Colircusi Tropicamida®, 1% cyclopentolate hydrochloride, and 10% phenylephrine. Patch testing was positive for cyclopentolate hydrochloride, but negative for all other eyedrops. Eight healthy controls were negative for cyclopentolate hydrochloride. Tests are not available to ascertain the presence of IgE against cyclopentolate to confirm an immunologic mechanism, although this is the most probable mechanism, since negative results in all controls challenge the concept of a NICU mechanism (64).

A 46-year-old cook had had chronic urticaria since 1985 and had been treated at many hospitals, which had prescribed him antihistamine and antiallergenic drugs, with no improvement. After a detailed interview, it was established that his condition worsened when he put on polyethylene gloves at work. Prick and scratch tests with a solution extracted from his gloves showed a wheal-and-flare reaction at 15 minutes. Control testing on three healthy persons was negative to the extracts (65).

A 19-year-old zookeeper volunteer experienced hives on her forearms following contact with giraffe fur, which resolved spontaneously after one to two hours. Skin contact with other animals such as zebra, goat, and elephant did not elicit any wheals as it did with giraffe exposure. Skin prick testing of the common aeroallergens were positive for pollens. The patient was also skin-pricked with extracts of giraffe hair from two giraffe species (prepared accordingly) and showed positive results, but not in the control subjects. Using the basophil activation test, expression of the activation marker CD63 was induced by extract on giraffe hair on the cells from the patient, but not on those unaffected controls (66).

Since the 1990s, lupine flour has been used as a substitute for flours and as additives to other flours in Europe. Lupine seeds are roasted in Mediterranean countries and eaten as snack food. A 52-year-old woman, known to have peanut intolerance, developed facial and mucosal edema, dizziness, and shortness of breath a few minutes after ingesting a nut croissant, requiring emergency medical treatment. Diagnostic evaluations for allergy showed a highly elevated concentration of IgE specific to lupine seed (42.9 kU/L) and birch pollen (2.57 kU/L); skin prick test with the native lupine flour yielded a strong positive reaction (4+). Birch pollen and lupine flour are known to cross-react with nuts. Cross-reactivity could be detected by immunoblotting techniques, which in this case, was negative (67).

Chironimus larvae, also known as red grubs, are used as fish food. Commercially available as freezed dried or deep frozen, *Chironimus* larvae are potent allergens, as skin testing alone may cause anaphylactic shock. A 14-year-old girl experienced urticaria, angioedema, and wheezing while in contact with the red grubs. Skin prick tests were initially performed to common fishes, mollusks, and crustaceans. Slightly positive results were obtained from tuna, trout, and oyster. On the next appointment, skin test with red grubs was carried out, and almost immediately, the patient complained of generalized pruritus. She was given 50 mg PO diphenhydramine and 10 mg PO of cetirizine. Fifteen minutes later, the patient complained of dizziness and was immediately administered 0.3 mg of subcutaneous adrenaline with rapid resolution of her symptoms. The skin test to red grubs was positive of 8 mm wheal (dilution 1:20) (68).

Hexamidine is an aromatic diamine antiseptic. With broad antibacterial and antifungal properties, this chemical is topically used in skin and corneal infections. A seven-year-old atopic boy, with no history of food and drug hypersensitivity, experienced generalized urticaria and facial edema within one hour of eating a peanut-containing slice. His father recalled applying a topical antiseptic [Medi Crème® (Pharmacare)] to the abrasion on his right elbow at about the same time. There were no respiratory or cardiovascular symptoms, and the urticaria and swelling resolved within two hours. Six months later, the same cream was applied to the abrasion over his chest, and it resulted in a localized 15-cm urticarial swelling. He was skin prick tested to the ingredients of Medi Crème (hexamidine isothionate, chlorhexidine aceate, cetrimide, and lignocaine hydrochloride) with the help of the manufacturer. After 15 minutes, only hexamidine isothionate resulted in a 5-mm pruritic wheal, while reaction to the rest of the active and inert ingredients was negative. The patient also underwent skin prick tests to relevant foods including peanut, Brazil nut, cashewnut, pecan, walnut, sunflower seed, and sesame seed, which were negative (69).

Phthalic anhydride is an industrially produced low-molecular-weight compound used for plasticizing agents, alkyd resins, and unsaturated polyester resins. Like most anhydrides, it covalently bonds to proteins, thus acting like haptens in an immune response. A 43-year-old man who had worked in a refinery of petrochemical products for four years presented with a seven- to eight-month history of generalized urticaria and pruritus with an onset of a few minutes after beginning his working day at the refinery. He sometimes also experienced ocular pruritus, rhinorrhea, dry cough, wheezing, and tightness of the chest. Pertinent physical examination revealed pale nasal mucosa, hyperemic ocular mucosa, and isolated rhonchus on lung auscultation. Skin prick test with a battery of common inhaled allergens (using antihistamine as the positive control) showed weakly positive for *Dermatophagoides pteronyssinus*. Skin prick test with 1% phthalic anhydride resulted to a 4 × 4 mm papule; skin prick test with the same material was negative in the control group. Total IgE concentration was 350 IU/mL, and analysis of specific IgE for phthalic anhydride showed greater than 100 IU/mL and 20.2 IU/mL for maleic anhydride (70).

HBTU (o-(bezotriazol-1-yl)-N,N,N′,N′-tetramethyluronium hexafluorophosphate) is a chemical widely used for solid and solution-phase peptide synthesis. A 28-year-old male laboratory worker for three years synthesized peptides using various chemicals such as f-moc amino acids and HBTU. The patient did not wear a respiratory mask when handling the chemicals in powder forms. One year prior to being seen, the patient experienced redness and a burning sensation on his face associated with dyspnea, faintness, as well as skin erythema. Oral antihistamine that controlled his symptoms was given. Thereafter, he worked in a fume hood where he had to handle these chemicals. Six months later, the patient experienced the previous symptoms accompanied by breathing difficulty. The patient felt faint and was given intramuscular corticosteroid and peroral antihistamine; he was sent to a university hospital emergency room and observed until his symptoms subsided. Skin prick test with "occupational" allergens revealed positivity to HBTU (71).

MEDICAL CARE

Contact urticaria is treated by prevention, which re-emphasizes the importance of clinical testing to identify the causative substance. The patient should then be advised to avoid that substance or products containing that substance, to prevent recurrence. Patient education is critical to prevention and patients need to be well informed about the nature of their reaction. Patients with ICU should be advised to carry a medic alert tag, listing their allergen as well as potential cross-reacting substances and should also carry antihistamines and self-administered subcutaneous epinephrine. Other than avoiding the specific eliciting substance, there is no need to observe specific dietary guidelines nor is there any restriction on physical activity.

In a 2007 review article, Sheikh identified and compared international guidelines for the emergency medical management of anaphylaxis in terms of the posture of the patient (supine/left lateral/recumbent), the use of oxygen supplement, the use and administration of adrenaline, antihistamines, and corticosteroids. Data were collected mainly from the PubMed database, Internet search engines, the World Allergy Organization, and anaphylaxis support group in the United States, Canada, the Netherlands, Germany, Italy, Australia, New Zealand, and Japan through the U.K.-based Anaphylaxis Campaign to ascertain if they were aware of any guidelines being used in their own countries. All searches were conducted during June to September 2006. The comparison of the key international guidelines is listed in Table 10 (72).

In another review article, Sheikh et al. endeavored to establish an evidence-based management using H_1 antihistamines for the treatment of anaphylaxis by searching randomized and controlled trials utilizing information gathered from (*i*) the Cochrane Central Register of Controlled Trials (CENTRAL, *The Cochrane Library*), (*ii*) MEDLINE (1966 to June 2006), (*iii*) EMBASE (1966 to June 2006), (*iv*) Cumulative Index to Nursing & Allied Health Literature (CINAHL) (1982 to June 2006), and (*v*) Inter-Services Intelligence (ISI) Web of Science. They found no high quality of evidence either for or against the use of H_1 antihistamines in anaphylaxis because this drug is not expected to relieve airway obstruction,

Table 10 Brief Summary of Recommendations of the Key International Guidelines for the Emergency Medical Management of Anaphylaxis

Country (Yr. of publication) (reference)	Posture	Supplemental oxygen	Adrenaline	Antihistamine	Corticosteroids
Australia (2006) (73)	Supine or left lateral; elevate legs if possible	Yes High flow O_2	0.01 mg/kg; (max. 0.5 mg); I.M. at lateral thigh; (1:1000 solution)	Not recommended	Not recommended
Canada (2003) (74)	Not Stated	Yes	(1:1000 solution, IM) Child: 0.01mg/kg (max. 0.3 mL) Adult: 0.3–0.5 mL (1:1000 solution, I.M.)	Diphenhydramine (IV, IM, or PO) Adult: 25–50 mg Child: 1.25 mg/kg +Ranitidine (IV or PO) Adult: 50mg IV or 150 mg PO Child: 1.25 mg/kg IV or 2 mg/kg PO	IV Methyl-prednisolone or Prednisolone PO Adult: 125 mg IV or 50 mg PO Child: 1 mg/kg IV or 1mg/kg PO
Russia (2004) (75)	Supine, chin upwards, head turned to the left side	Yes O_2 + ethanol as an antifroth agent	(1:1000 solution); Adult: 0.3–0.5 mL (0.3–0.5) (1:1000 solution, IM or SC) Child: 0.01 mg/kg	Diphenhydramine Adult: 25–50 mg Child: 1–2 mg/kg (IV or IM) Promethazine 2.5% to 2–4 mL IV or IM Chorpheniramine 2% to 2–4 mL IV or IM	Prednisolone 1–2 mg/kg IV Hydrocortisone 100–300 mg IM or IV Dexamethasone 4–20 mg IV

(Continued)

Table 10 Brief Summary of Recommendations of the Key International Guidelines for the Emergency Medical Management of Anaphylaxis (*Continued*)

Country (Yr. of publication) (reference)	Posture	Supplemental oxygen	Adrenaline	Antihistamine	Corticosteroids
United Kingdom (1999) (76)	Supine with legs elevated (unless in respiratory distress)	Yes High flow O$_2$ (10–15 L/min)	(1:1000 solution) Adult: 0.5 mL (0.5mg) IM Child: > 12 yr up to 0.5 mg IM 6–12 yr 0.25 IM > 6 mo–6 yr: 0.12 mg IM < 6 mo: 0.05 mg IM	Chlorpheniramine > 12 yr: 10–20 mg IM or slow IV 6–12 yr: 5–10 mg IM 1–6 yr: 2.5 mg IM	Hydrocortisone 12 yr >100–500 mg IM or slow IV 6–12 yr: 100 mg IM 1–6 yr: 50 mg IM
Ukraine (2002) (77)	Supine	Yes O$_2$ + ethanol as an antifroth agent	1:1000 solution SC or IM Adult: 0.3–0.5 mL (0.3–0.5 mg) Child: 0.01 mg/kg	Diphenhydramine Adult: 25–50 mg Child: 1–2 mg/kg IV or IM or Promethazine 2.5% to 2–4 mL IV or IM	Prednisolone 1–2 mg/kg IV Hydrocortisone 100–300 mg IM or IV Dexamethasone 4–20 mg IV
U.S.A. (2005) (78)	Recumbent with legs raised	Yes 6–8 L/min guided by arterial blood gasses or oxymetry	(1:1000 solution) 0.2–0.5 mL Child: 0.01 mg/kg (max. 0.3 mg) IM or SC lateral thigh	Diphenhydramine Adult: 25–50 mg IV Child: 1 mg/kg up to 50 mg. Oral may be sufficient for mild attacks + Ranitidine Adult: 1 mg/kg Child: 12.5 mg infused over 10–15 min	Not recommended

Source: Adapted from Ref. 72.

GI symptoms, shock, and prevent the release of other release of mediators from mast cells and basophils. The authors hypothesize that the foremost reason why there are no randomized and controlled trials is simply the fact that anaphylaxis is a medical emergency and as such, will raise ethical questions (79).

PROGNOSIS

Prognosis is entirely dependent on the ubiquity of the eliciting substance and the patient's ability to avoid contact with it. The prognosis is usually quite good in patients who take an active role in avoiding the substance as well as controlling their environment.

CONCLUSION

Contact urticaria is the whealing of skin when it comes into contact with certain substances. The urticarial lesions disappear by definition within 24 hours of onset. Contact urticaria can be categororized into two NICU and ICU, with nonimmunologic being more common than immunologic.

NICU does not require pre-sensitization of the patient's immune system to an allergen. The mechanism of NICU is incompletely understood. However, there is evidence that NICU may be primarily mediated by prostaglandins rather than histamine, since the NICU reaction is inhibited by ASA and NSAIDs both orally and topically.

Immunologic contact urticaria is a Type I hypersensitivity reaction mediated by IgE antibodies and is less frequent in clinical practice than nonimmunologic contact urticaria. Prior immune (IgE) sensitization is required to the eliciting substance. Sensitization may be via the skin, mucus membranes, and respiratory or GI tracts. Atopics are predisposed towards ICU. Establishing a diagnosis of ICU is important because ICU reactions may spread beyond the site of contact and progress to generalized urticaria, or may lead to anaphylactic shock, which can potentially be life threatening.

Both types can be identified by using skin-testing methods. ICU agents are confirmed by positive RAST to specific agents and by negative skin tests on control subjects. NICU agents elicit a positive reaction in previously unexposed subjects, therefore control subjects test positive.

Numerous substances that are commonly encountered in daily life may cause contact urticaria. The list of agents causing contact urticaria is large and dynamic. Numerous case reports of contact urticaria caused by a variety of compounds continue to be reported.

It is important to identify the eliciting substance, since contact urticaria is treated primarily by prevention. Prognosis is usually good in patients who avoid the eliciting substance.

REFERENCES

1. Maibach HI, Johnson HI. Contact urticaria syndrome: contact urticaria to diethyltoluamide (immediate type hypersensitivity). Arch Dermatol 1975; 111:726–730.
2. Amin S, Maibach HI. Introduction, Chapter 1: Nonimmunologic contact urticaria, and Chapter 2: Immunologic contact urticaria definition. In: Amin S, Lahti A, Maibach HI, eds. Contact Urticaria Syndrome. Boca Raton: CRC Press, 1997.
3. Usmani N, Wilkinson SM. Allergic skin disease: investigation of both immediate- and delayed-type hypersensitivity is essential. Clin Exp Allergy 2007; 37(10):1541–1546.

4. Kanerva L, Toikkanen J, Jolanki R. Statistical data on occupational contact urticaria. Contact Dermatitis 1996; 35(4):229–233.
5. Elpern DJ. The syndrome of immediate reactivities (contact urticaria syndrome). An historical study from a dermatology practice. I. Age, sex, race, and putative susbstances. Hawaii Med J 1985; 44:426–439.
6. Hannuksela M. Mechanisms in contact urticaria. Clin Dermatol 1997; 15:619–622.
7. Gollhausen R, Kligman AM. Human assay for identifying substances which induce non-allergic contact urticaria: the NICU test. Contact Dermatitis 1985; 13:98–106.
8. Lahti A, Maibach HI. Long refractory period after one application of nonimmunologic contact urticaria agents to the guinea pig ear. J Am Acad Dermatol 1985; 13(4):585–589.
9. Lahti A. Terfenadine (H1-antagonist) does not inhibit nonimmunologic contact urticaria. Contact Dermatitis 1987; 16:220.
10. Lahti A, Oikarinen A, Viinkka L, et al. Prostaglandins in contact urticaria induced by benzoic acid. Acta Dermatol Venereol (stockh) 1983; 63:425–427.
11. Lahti A, Vaananen A, Kokkonen E-L, et al. Acetylsalicylic acid inhibits non-immunologic contact urticaria. Contact Dermatitis 1987; 16:133–135.
12. Johansson J, Lahti A. topical non-steroidal anti-inflammatory drugs inhibit non-immunologic immediate contact reactions. Contact Dermatitis 1988; 19:161–165.
13. Kujala T, Lahti A. Duration of inhibition of non-immunologic contact reactions of acetylsalicylic acid. Contact Dermatitis 1989; 21:60–61.
14. Morrow JD, Minton TA, Awad JA, et al. Release of markedly increased quantities of prostaglandin D2 from the skin in vivo in humans following the application of sorbic acid. Arch Dermatol 1994; 130:1408–1412.
15. Downard CD, Roberts LJ, Morrow JD. Topical benzoic acid induces the increased synthesis of prostaglandin D2 in human skin in vivo. Clin Pharmacol Ther 1995; 74:441–445.
16. VanderEnde D, Morrow J. Release of markedly increased quantities of prostaglandin D2 from the skin in vivo in humans after the application of cinnamic aldehyde. J Am Acad Dermatol 2001; 45:61–67.
17. Larmi E. Systemic effect of ultraviolet irradiation on nonimmunologic immediate contact reactions to benzoic acid and methyl nicotinate. Acta Derm Venereol (Stockh) 1989; 69:296–301.
18. Larmi E. PUVA treatment inhibits nonimmunologic immediate contact reactions to benzoic acid and methyl nicotinate. Int J Derm 1989; 28:609–611.
19. Larmi E, Lahti A, Hannuksela M. Effects of capsaicin and topical anesthesia on nonimmunologic immediate contact reactions to benzoic acid and methyl nicotinate. In: Frosch PJ, Dooms-Goossens A, Lachapelle J-M, et al., eds. Current Topics in Contact Dermatitis. Berlin Heidelberg: Springer-Verlag, 1989:441–447.
20. Bernstein JE, Swift, RM, Keyoumars S, et al. Inhibition of axon vasodilation by topicaly applied capsaicin. J Invest Dermatol 1981; 76:394.
21. Hannuksela A, Lahti A, Hannuksela M. Nonimmunologic immediate contact reactions to three isomers of pyridine carboxaldehyde. In: Frosch PJ, Dooms-Goosses A, Lachaplelle JM, et al., eds. Current Topics in Contact Dermatitis. Berlin Heidelberg: Springer-Verlag, 1989:448–452.
22. Amaro C, Goossens A. Immunological occupational contact urticaria and contact dermatitis from proteins: a review. Contact Dermatitis 2008; 58(2):67–75.
23. Nettis E, Dambra P, Traetta M, et al. Systemic reactions on SPT to latex. Allergy 2001; 56:355–356.
24. Emonet S, Pasche-Koo F, Perin-Minsini MJ, et al. Anaphylaxis to oxybeonzone, a frequent constituent of sunscreens. J Allergy Clin Immunol 2001; 107(3):556–557.
25. Moder B, Kranke B. Anaphylactic reaction to formaldehyde. Allergy 2001; 56:263–264.
26. Mancuso G, Masara N. Contact urticaria and severe anaphylaxis from rifamycin SV. Contact Dermatitis 1992; 27(2):124–125.
27. Knowles S, Shear N. Anaphylaxis from bacitracin and polymixin B (polysporin) ointment. Int J Dermatol 1995; 34(8):572–573.
28. Beausoleil JL, Spergel JM, Pawlowski NA. Anaphylaxis to raw potato. Ann Allergy Asthma Immunol 2001; 86(1):68–70.

29. Kalogeromitros D, Armenaka M, Katsarou A. Contact urticaria and systemic anaphylaxis from codfish. Contact Dermatitis 1999; 41(3):170–171.

30. Tomitaka A, Matsunaga K, Akita H, et al. Four cases with latex allergy followed by anaphylaxis to chestnut. Arerugi 2000; 49(4):327–334.

31. Fisher AA. Contact Urticaria and anaphylactoid reaction due to corn starch surgical glove powder. Contact Dermatitis 1987; 16:224–225.

32. Yesudian PD, King CM. Severe contact urticaria and anaphylaxis from benzophenone-3 (2-hydroxy 4-methoxy benzophenone). Contact Dermatitis 2002; 46(1):55–56.

33. Palczynski C, Walusiak J, Wittczak T, et al. Natural history of occupational allergy to latex in health care workers. Med Pr 2001; 52(2):79–85.

34. Roy DR. Latex glove allergy–dilemma for health care workers. An overview. AAOHN J. 2000; 48(6):267–277.

35. Murphy R, Gawkrodger DJ. Occupational latex contact urticaria in non-health-care occupations. Contact Dermatitis 2000; 43(2):111.

36. Assalve D, Cicioni C, Perno P, et al. Contact urticaria and anaphylactoid response from cornstarch surgical glove powder. Contact Dermatitis 1988; 19:61.

37. Wakelin SH, White IR. Latex allergy. Clin Exp Dermatol 1999; 24:245–248.

38. Estlander, T, Jolanki, R, Kanerva, L. Contact Urticaria from rubber gloves: a detailed description of four cases. Acta Der Venereol Suppl (Stockh) 1987; 134:98–102.

39. Hostynek JJ, Lauerma AI, Magee PS, et al. A local lymph-node assay validation study of a structure-activity relationship model for contact allergens. Arch Dermatol Res 1995; 287(6): 567–571.

40. Meade J, Woolhiser M. Murine models for natural rubber latex allergy assessment. Methods 2002; 27:63–68.

41. Wallengre J, Larsson B. Nitric oxide participates in prick test and irritant patch test reactions in human skin. Arch Dermatol Res 2001; 293(3):121–125.

42. Hannuksela M, Lahti A. Immediate reactions to fruits and vegetables. Contact Dermatitis 1977; 3:79–84.

43. Niinimaki A, Hannuksela M. Immediate skin test reactions to spices. Allergy 1981; 26:487–493.

44. Ebner C, Hirschwehr R, Bauer L, et al. Identification of allergens in fruits and vegetables: IgE cross-reactivities with the important birch pollen allergens Bet v 1 and Bet v 2 (birch profiling). J Allergy Clin Immunol 1995; 95:962–969.

45. Halmepuro L, Vuontela K, Kalimo K, et al. Cross-reactivity of IgE antibodies with allergens in birch pollen, fruits and vegetables. Int Arch Allergy Appl Immunol 1984; 74:235–240.

46. Rodriguez M, Vega F, Carcia MT, et al. Hypersensitivity to latex, chestnut, and banana. Ann Allergy 1993; 70:31–34.

47. Makinen-Kiljunen S. Banana allergy in patients with immediate-type hypersensitivity to natural rubber latex: characterization of cross-reacting antibodies and allergens. J Allergy Clin Immunol 1994; 93:990–996.

48. Lavaud F, Prevost A, Cossart C, et al. Allergy to latex, avocado pear, and banana: evidence for a 30 kd antigen in immunoblotting. J Allergy Clin Immunol 1995; 95:557–564.

49. Goetz DW, Whisman BA. Occupational asthma in a seafood restaurant worker: cross-reactivity of shrimp and scallops. Ann Allergy Asthma Immunol 2000; 85(6 Pt 1):461–466.

50. Amin S, Lauerma A, Maibach HI. Diagnostic tests in dermatology. In: Maibach HI, ed. Toxicology of Skin, Philadelphia: Taylor and Francis, 2001:389–399.

51. Warner MR, Taylor JS, Leow Y. Agents causing contact urticaria. Clin Dermatol 1997; 15: 623–635.

52. Lahti A, Maibach HI. Immediate contact reactions (contact urticaria syndrome). In: Maibach HI, ed. Occupational and Industrial Dermatology, 2nd ed. Chicago: Year Book Medical, 1986: 32–44.

53. Maibach HI. Regional variation in elicitation of contact urticaria syndrome (immediate hypersensitivity syndrome): Shrimp. Contact Dermatitis 1986; 15:100.

54. Frosch PJ, Kligman AM. The soap chamber test. A new method for assessing the irritancy of soaps. J Am Acad Dermatol 1979; 1(1):35–41.

55. Boumiza R, Debard AL, Monneret G. The basophil activation test by flow cytometry: recent developments in clinical studies, standardization and emerging perspectives. Clin Mol Allergy 2005; 3:9–16.
56. Fischer TW, Bauer A, Hipler UC, et al. Non-immunologic contact urticaria from chrysanthemum confirmed by the CAST method. Complement-activated (C5a) cellular antigen stimulation test. Contact Dermatitis 1999; 41(5):293–295.
57. Spiewak R, Dutkiewicz J. Allergic contact urticaria and rhinitis to roe deer (Capreolus capreolus) in a hunter. Ann Agric Environ Med 2002; 9(1):115–116.
58. Estrada Rodriguez JL, Gozalo Reques F, Cechini Fernandez C, et al. Contact urticaria due to potassium persulfate. Contact Dermatitis. 2001; 45(3):177.
59. Rasanen L, Tarvainen K, Makinen-Kiljunen S. Urticaria to hydrocortisone. Allergy 2001; 56:352–353.
60. Kiistala R, Makinen-Kiljunen S, Heikkinen K, et al. Occupational allergic rhinitis and contact urticaria caused by bishop's weed (Ammi majus). Allergy 1999; 54(6):635–639.
61. Kanerva L, Estlander T, Petman L, et al. Occupational allergic contact urticaria to yucca (Yucca aloifolia), weeping fig (Ficus benjamina), and spathe flower (Spathiphyllum wallisii). Allergy 2001; 56(10):1008–1011.
62. Estrada JL, Gozalo F, Cecchini C, et al. Contact urticaria from hops (Humulus lupulus) in a patient with previous urticaria-angioedema from peanut, chestnut and banana. Contact Dermatitis 2002; 46(2):127.
63. Kanerva L, Vanhanen M. Occupational allergic contact urticaria and rhinoconjunctivitis from a detergent protease. Contact Dermatitis 2001; 45(1):49–51.
64. Munoz-Bellido FJ, Beltran A, Bellido J. Contact urticaria due to cyclopentolate hydrochloride. Allergy 2000; 55(2):198–199.
65. Sugiura K, Sugiura M, Shiraki R, et al. Contact urticaria due to polyethylene gloves. Contact Dermatitis 2002; 46(5):262–266.
66. Herzinger T, Scharrer E, Placzek M, et al. Contact urticaria to giraffe hair. Int Arch Allergy Immunol 2005; 138(4):324–327.
67. Brennecke S, Becker WM, Lepp U, et al. Anaphylactic reaction to lupine flour. J Dtsch Dermatol Ges 2007; 5(9):774–776.
68. Nguyen M, Paradis L, Des Roches A, et al. Adverse reactions resulting from skin testing in the diagnosis of red grubs (Chiromides) allergy. Allergy 2007; 62(12):1470–1471.
69. Mullins RJ. Systemic allergy to topical hexamidine. Med J Aust 2006; 185(3):177.
70. Gutiérrez-Fernández D, Fuentes-Vallejo MS, Rueda-Ygueravides MD, et al. Contact urticaria to phthalic anhydride. J Invest Allergol Clin Immunol 2007; 17(6):422–423.
71. Hannu T, Alanko K, Keskinen H. Anaphylaxis and allergic contact urticaria from occupational airborne exposure to HBTU. Occup Med (Lond) 2006; 56(6):430–433.
72. Alrasbi M, Sheikh A. Comparison of international guidelines for the emergency medical management of anaphylaxis. Allergy 2007; 62(8):838–841.
73. Brown SGA, Mullins RJ, Gold MS. Anaphylaxis: diagnosis and management. MJA 2006; 185:283–289.
74. Ellis AK, Day JH. Diagnosis and management of anaphylaxis. CMAJ 2003; 169:307–312.
75. Dadikina AB, Duhanina IB, Namazova LC, et al. Pre-hospital management in acute allergic reactions: theory and practice. National scientific practice society of emergency medicine. Guidelines for immediate management of anaphylactic reactions. http://www.doktor.ru, 2004; accessed 17 May 2007.
76. Resuscitation Council (UK). The emergency medical treatment of anaphylactic reactions for first medical responders and for community nurses. http://www.resus.org/pages/reaction.htm, 2005; accessed 3 April 2007.
77. Soloshenko EH. Drug induced anaphylaxis shock. Medicus Amicus 2002; 1:8–9.
78. Lieberman P, Kemp SF, Oppenheimer J, et al. (eds). The diagnosis and management of anaphylaxis: an updated practice parameter. J Allergy Clin Immunol 2005; 115:S483–S523.
79. Simons FE, Sheikh A. Evidence-based management of anaphylaxis. Allergy 2007; 62(8): 827–829.

11

Physical and Cholinergic Urticarias

Anne Kobza Black

St. John's Institute of Dermatology, St. Thomas' Hospital, London, U.K.

PHYSICAL AND CHOLINERGIC URTICARIAS

The physical urticarias are a distinct subgroup of urticarias in which a specific physical stimulus induces reproducible whealing (1–3). They are classified according to the eliciting stimulus (4,5) (Table 1). Cholinergic urticaria (CU) occurs in response to stimulation of sweating, such as caused by general overheating compared with local heat application. Although it is not strictly a physical urticaria, as it also may be triggered by stimulation of emotional and gustatory sweating, it is frequently included in the physical urticaria group for convenience. Aquagenic and adrenergic urticaria, which morphologically resemble cholinergic urtiaria, are also included.

Wheals induced by physical stimuli usually occur in minutes at the site of contact with the skin and resolve within two hours (immediate contact type). However, sometimes a physical stimulus needs to induce a generalized body challenge to induce a reflex type. For example, cooling the body core temperature can induce reflex cold urticaria and raising core body temperature can induce CU. In these urticarias, multiple wheals occur on widespread areas of the body. In a few forms of physical urticaria [e.g., delayed pressure urticaria (DPU), delayed dermographism] a delay, often of several hours, occurs from the stimulus to the onset of whealing, which can persist for 24 hours or longer. Combination of a physical urticaria with other physical urticarias or with ordinary urticaria in the same person is not uncommon. The quality of life of patients with physical urticarias can be markedly reduced, in particular cholinergic and DPU (6).

The frequency of physical urticarias in the general population is unknown. However, of all urticaria cases seen in a dermatology clinic 19% were physical urticarias (7), but 30% in a more recent series (8). In patients with chronic urticaria the physical urticarias accounted for 31% (9) and 33% (10). In children, the reported frequency of physical urticarias among chronic urticaria patients varies between 6.2% (11) and 25.5% (12), with cold urticaria predominating in many series.

The pathogenesis of physical urticarias is not well defined. A working hypothesis for immediate contact urticarias is that the physical stimulus induces a neoantigen. This

Table 1 Classification of Physical and Cholinergic Urticarias

I. Due to mechanical trauma
   Dermograhism
      Immediate dermographism
         Simple
         Symptomatic
      Localized
      Delayed—occurring after a delay of 30 min
      Variants
         Red dermographism
         Cholinergic dermographism
         Associated with mastocytosis
   Immediate pressure urticaria
   Delayed pressure urticaria
   Vibratory angioedema
      Inherited
      Acquired
II. Temperature changes
   Heat
      Cholinergic urticaria
         Variants
            Cholinergic pruritus
            Cholinergic erythema
            Cholinergic dermographisn
            Exercise-induced anaphylaxis (some)
      Localized heat contact urticaria
   Cold
      Typical positive cold contact stimulation test
         Primary
         Secondary—cryoglobulins, cryofibrinogen, cold hemolysins
      Atypical cold stimulation tests
         Acquired Contact
            Delayed cold urticaria
            Localized cold urticaria
            Cold-induced dermographism
            Cold erythema
            Localized reflex
            Cold-induced vasculitis
         Systemic
            Familial
            Reflex cold urticaria
            Cold-induced cholinergic
III. Exercise-induced anaphylaxis
   Pure
   Food-dependent exercise-induced anaphylaxis
      Specific
      Nonspecifc
   Cold-dependent exercise-induced anaphylaxis
IV. Adrenergic Urticaria
 V. Solar Urticaria
VI. Aquagenic Urticaria

Combinations of different types of physical urticarias are common.

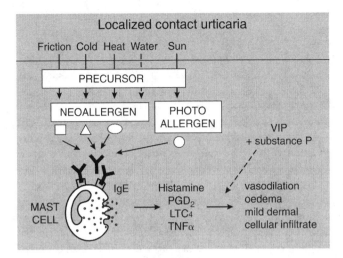

Figure 1 Proposed mechanisms of localized contact urticarias.

stimulates production of an IgE antibody, which binds to the mast cells. On further challenge a type I allergic response ensues with liberation of mast cell mediators, inducing a whealing response (Fig. 1).

It is important to establish the diagnosis of physical urticarias, by appropriate history and challenge tests, to prevent unnecessary investigation such as for food allergies and to institute correct therapy.

URTICARIA DUE TO MECHANICAL FORCES

Dermographism

Dermographism (13,14) literally means skin writing. The commoner forms are simple dermographism and immediate symptomatic dermographism (factitious urticaria).

Firm stroking of the skin of normal people can induce some erythema and whealing at the site, but in 5% of normal young people the whealing response is conspicuous enough to warrant the term *simple dermographism* (15). There is no associated itching, and this response can be regarded as an exaggerated physiological response. The people are aware of their condition and no treatment is necessary.

In *immediate symptomatic dermographism* (factitious urticaria) erythema and whealing occurs in response to minor stroking of the skin, and is accompanied by itching. The response is maximal in 5 to 10 minutes and subsides within 30 to 60 minutes (15).

The prevalence of symptomatic dermographism in the community is not well defined and varies, but in one study an incidence of 4.2% in the population was found if a stroking pressure of 49.0 g/mm^2 was used (16). In some dermatology departments 9% urticaria patients had predominant dermographism (7–9), but 17% in an other series (10), and is the commonest physical urticaria. There is a report of a family with dermographism in an autosomal-dominant inheritance (17) and in identical twins (18).

In symptomatic dermographism there is no evidence for increased mast cells in the skin (19,20). However, mast cell degranulation and an associated rise in plasma histamine levels (20) occurs in dermographic skin, and mast cells are necessary to induce dermographism (21). Mast cell activation may have an immunological basis. Dermographism has been successfully transferred with IgE (22) and occasionally IgM

(23) when patients' sera have been injected into normal recipients' skin. It is also possible to transfer the whealing response from the serum of patients with severe dermographism to monkeys (24). It is postulated that an antigen induced by mechanical stimulation of the skin induces specific antibodies (usually IgE) directed against it. When the antigen reacts with these antibodies bound to mast cells, activation and mediator release occurs. Substance P and VIP may potentiate histamine in the wheal formation (25).

Symptomatic dermographism can occur at any age, but the greatest incidence is in young adults (13), with 29% occurring among those below 19 years (16). Patients complain of itching, which is often disproportionately severe compared with visible signs. The itching is worse with heat, alcohol, and stress and often is most severe at night (13). It can occur on the scalp, palms, and soles and may be a cause of genital pruritus and vulvodynia (26). Erythema and whealing occur at sites of friction, e.g., at collar and cuff lines and at sites of scratching. The eliciting stimulus determines the shape of the wheals, but these are often linear at scratch sites. The erythema and wheals usually subside within 30 to 60 minutes. It is unusual for mucosal surfaces to be affected. There is no association with systemic disease or food allergy or an increased incidence in chronic urticaria (13). Dermographism is usually idiopathic. Occasionally it occurs transiently after medication such as penicillin (27) and famotidine (28), after DNCB sensitization (29), and after infestations such as scabies (30) and trauma from a coral reef (31). Intolerance to topical applications may be due to the physical rubbing of the product onto the skin of patients with dermographism rather than contact dermatitis or contact urticaria from the product (32).

Dermographism may last for months or years with an average course of 20 months in one study (30) and 5 years in another (13), though it can persist for 10 years or longer, or be present intermittently.

Symptomatic dermographism is most precisely diagnosed by using a calibrated instrument, the dermographometer (33). This pen-like instrument has a spring-loaded stylus, the pressure application of which can be adjusted to a predetermined setting (Fig. 2). Stroking the skin at a pressure on the skin of less than 36 g/mm^2 on the upper back (13) induces a linear itching wheal within 10 minutes (Fig. 3). One such instrument can be bought from Hook & Tucker Zenyx Ltd, Vulcan Way, New Addington, Croydon CRO 9UG, U.K., but it then needs to be calibrated. Using a dermographometer set at 49 g/mm^2, the volar forearm, upper back, and abdomen were equally sensitive areas in inducing dermographism in approximately 70% of people with clinical dermographism (34). Weighted knitting needles have been used alternatively for objective testing (35). If these are not available, moderate friction with a blunt instrument such as a spatula can be used with practice.

Treatment of symptomatic immediate dermographism with low-sedating H_1 antihistamines is often effective, sometimes in low doses. For the more severely affected, higher than the recommended doses may be necessary, but there is no clinical benefit in combining H_2 antagonists with H_1 antagonists (36). Some improvement of itching may be obtained with broadband ultraviolet B (UVB) (37), but psoralen and UVA (PUVA) provides only temporary relief of itching (38).

Localized dermographism may occur rarely on areas with prior skin condition such as site of previous patch tests (33), fixed drug eruption (39), or tattoos.

Red dermographism is different in that repeated rubbing (rather than a simple stroke to the skin) is necessary to induce erythematous areas studded with small wheals (40).

Cholinergic dermographism is seen in some patients with CU whose dermographic response consists of an erythematous line studded with punctate wheals characteristic of cholinergic wheals (41) (Fig. 4 A, B).

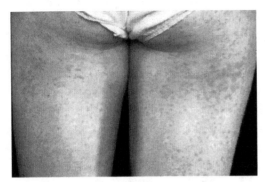

Figure 1.1 Cholinergic urticaria in a 12-year-old female. The prominent blanching surrounding the wheals is due to a vascular "steal" effect (see text) (*see page 3*).

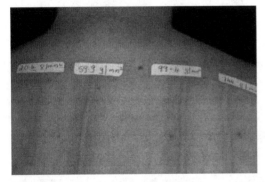

Figure 11.3 Itchy linear wheals with surrounding flare, appeared 10 minutes after stroking the dermographometer (Fig. 2) perpendicular to the back at the settings shown. There is a large wheal and flare even at the lowest setting (*see page 185*).

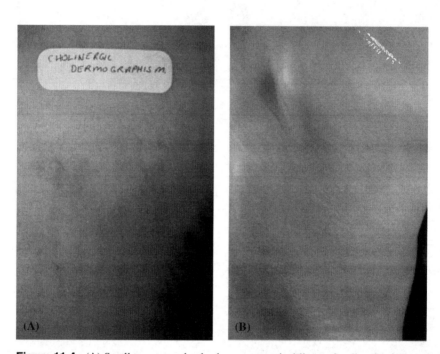

Figure 11.4 (**A**) Small punctate wheals along two vertical lines, after linear stroking of the back, being most marked on the right-hand side. (**B**) Small punctate linear wheals in a patient with cholinergic urticaria and dermographism, appearing within minutes of scratching his back. Some of the wheals had coalesced (*see page 186*).

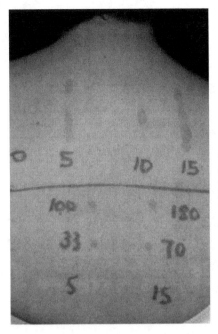

Figure 11.5 Upper part. Firm wide linear wheals, seen 6 hours after the stroking the back of a patient with a dermographometer at the settings shown, in the patient with delayed pressure urticaria. Lower part shows firm papules appearing on the back of the patient with delayed pressure urticaria. The derographometer set at 100 g/mm^2 was applied perpendicular to the back, and held there for 5 to 180 seconds. The required application time at the above pressure for the diagnosis of delayed pressure is 70 seconds. This patient also developed papules even after 5 second application (*see page 186*).

Figure 11.7 A firm red tender wheal, at the site of a brassiere strap. This occurred several hours after wearing it, and the wheal lasted for many hours. She did not have immediate symptomatic dermographism (*see page 188*).

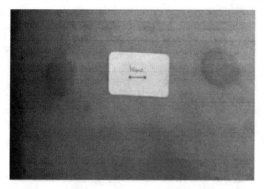

Figure 11.8B The test areas on the thighs are examined at six hours later for development of rounded tender plaques six hours later (*see page 189*).

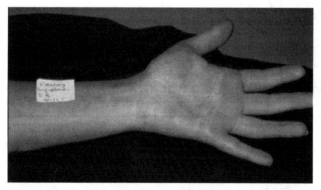

Figure 11.9B The patient developed itchy red swelling of the lower forearm from transmitted vibration from the rod, which did not touch the forearm (under label) within minutes after vibration. The patient also had mild dermographism and the erythema of the palms could have been due to this or vibratory angioedema (*see page 191*).

Figure 11.11 Itchy small wheals (2–3 mm in diameter) with a surrounding flare developing on the trunk within minutes of moderate exercise in a patient with cholinergic uticaria (*see page 192*).

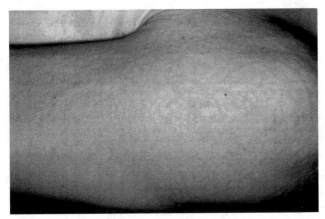

Figure 11.12 Severely affected patient with cholinergic urticaria. A typical small wheal is seen on his chest, but on his arms they had enlarged and coalesced (*see page 193*).

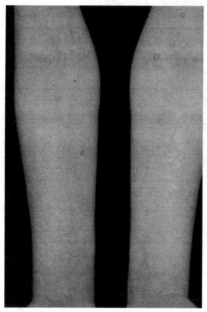

Figure 11.13 Typical small erythemaous macules of cholinergic erythema, usually 2 to 4 mm in diameter distributed symmetrically on the forearms. If individual macules are marked as in diagram, they will be seen to disappear in 40 to 60 minutes, with others appearing elsewhere (*see page 194*).

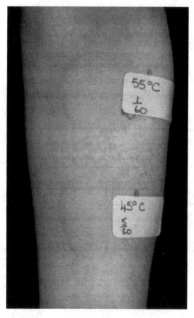

Figure 11.14 Wheals appearing in a patient with localized heat contact urticaria, within one minute of application of a beaker at 55°C, and within five minutes of application at 45°C (*see page 195*).

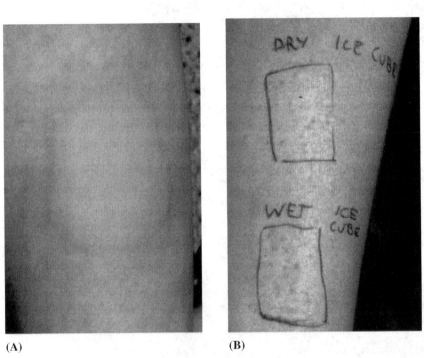

(A)   **(B)**

Figure 11.15 (**A**) Circumscribed confluent wheal appearing at the site of application of an ice cube in a plastic cover, for 10 minutes on the forearm of a patient with contact cold urticaria. (**B**) Small wheals localized to cold application of a wet and covered ice cube in a patient with a not uncommon combination of contact cold and cholinergic urticaria. However, this morphology is unusual in a positive ice cube test (*see page 197*).

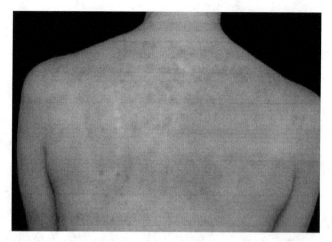

Figure 11.16 Wheals localized to areas on the back exposed to the sun, and sparing covered areas in a patient with solar urticaria (*see page 201*).

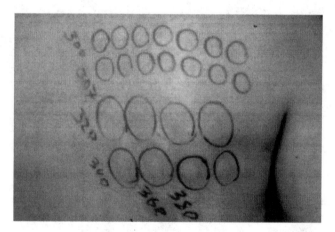

Figure 11.17 Wheals appearing at test sites with a monochromator at 320, 340, 360 nm, but not at 300 and 307 nm, in a patient with solar urticaria (*see page 201*).

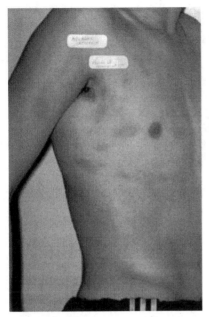

Figure 11.18 Aquagenic urticaria with small sparse wheals, resembling cholinergic urticaria, within minutes of bathing in water for 15 minutes at skin temperature (*see page 203*).

Figure 11.19 The appearance described for adrenergic urticaria. Small wheals 3 to 4 mm in diameter resembling cholinergic urticaria, surrounded by areas of blanching (*see page 204*).

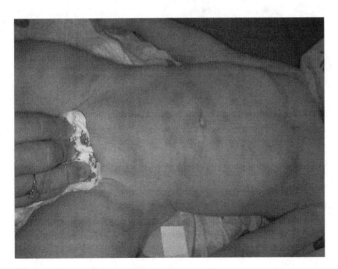

Figure 12.1 Young child with acute urticaria following a viral infection (*see page 219*).

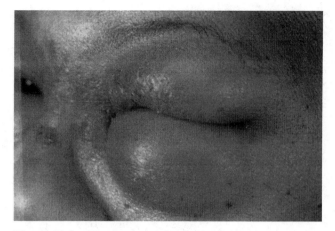

Figure 14.1 Allergic contact dermatitis—LATEX. (*see page 252*).

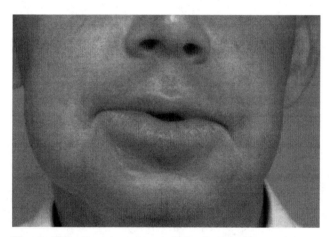

Figure 14.2 Granulomatous cheilitis: Crohn's disease. (*see page 253*).

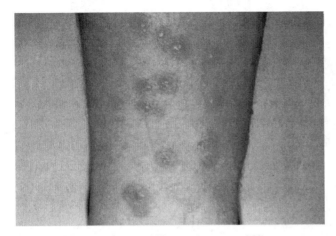

Figure 14.3 Erythema multiforme. (*see page 253*).

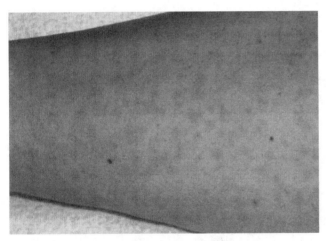

Figure 15.2 Photograph of the lower leg of a patient with FCAS. The leg was not directly exposed to cold prior to onset of rash (*see page 266*).

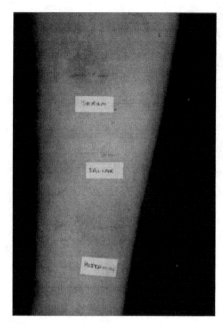

Figure 17.3 Autologous serum skin test (*see page 305*).

ADDITIONAL PHOTOGRAPHS

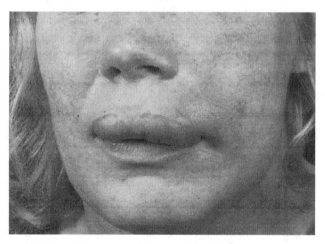

Angioedema appeared within 15 min of a dose of ampicillin.

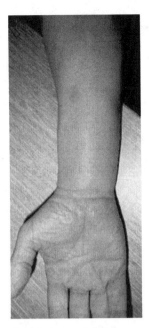

Aspirin-induced AE.

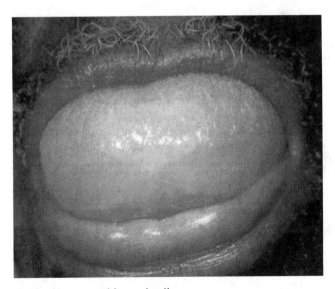

Angioedema caused by enalapril.

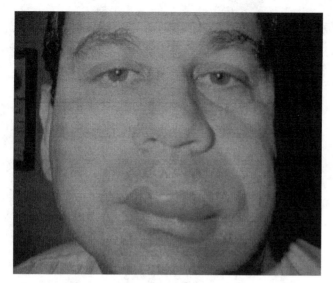

Idiopathic AE of upper lip with urticaria.

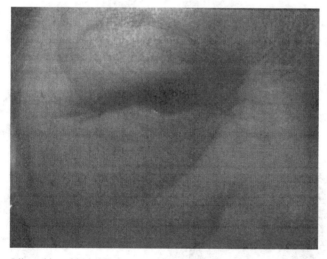

Idiopathi corbital AE.

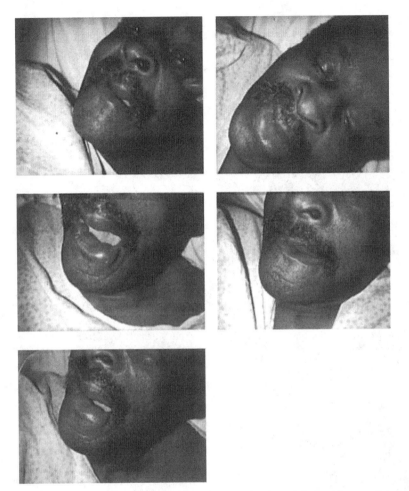

A 62-year-old African-American man (in a nursing home) had a history of recurrent AE without urticaria of 2 years' duration. Episodes lasted from 96 to 108 h, unresponsive to epinephrine, hydroxyzine, and methylprednisone, occurring every 2–6 weeks. *Upper left.* Episode of AE first noted at 7 am and patient was given zileuton 600 mg and doxepin 25 mg. *Middle left.* At 8 am, lower lip edema was noted to be progressing. *Bottom left.* At 9 am, lower lip and upper chin became more edematous. *Upper right.* At 11 am, entire lower lip and chin were markedly swollen. Second dose of zileuton 600 mg advised. *Middle right.* At 12 noon, before dose was administered AE had resolved. Patient was given zileuton 600 mg every 6 h for that day and every 12–24 h thereafter. Each time the zileuton was discontinued, the AE recurred with in 5–7 days.

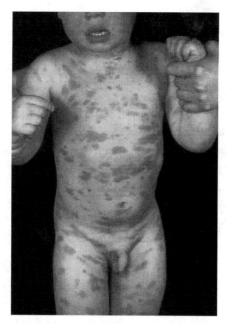

A child with systemic mastocytosis shows lesions of urticaria pigmentosa, a facial flush, and Darier's sign (midabdomen).

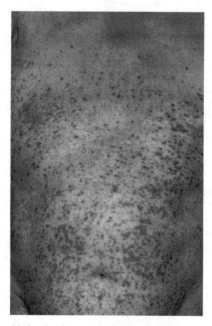

Urticaria pigmentosa in an adult with systemic mastocytosis.

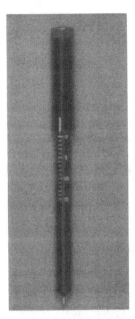

Figure 2 A dermographometer, a pen-like instrument containing a spring. The markings can be calibrated, with the settings of this instrument being $0 = 20.4$ g/mm^2, $5 = 59.9$ g/mm^2, $10 = 99.4$ g/mm^2, and $15 = 1144$ g/mm^2.

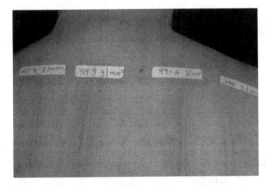

Figure 3 (*See color insert*) Itchy linear wheals with surrounding flare, appeared 10 minutes after stroking the dermographometer (Fig. 2) perpendicular to the back at the settings shown. There is a large wheal and flare even at the lowest setting.

Pure delayed dermographism is rare. After a normal fading of the triple response or an immediate dermographic response, a wheal returns in the same site but is usually tender and persists up to 48 hour (42,43). The mechanism is unknown but is closely related to pressure urticaria where a delayed dermatographic response may occur in 55% of patients (44) (Fig. 5).

The presence of whealing following friction (Darier's sign) is characteristic of the lesions of urticaria pigmentosa where mast cells are increased and may be a presenting sign of systemic mastocytosis (45).

Not all forms of dermographism are urticarial. *White dermographism* (due to capillary vasoconstriction following light stroking of the skin) occurs normally and is

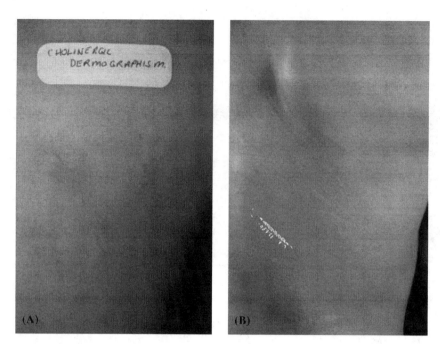

Figure 4 (*See color insert*) (**A**) Small punctate wheals along two vertical lines, after linear stroking of the back, being most marked on the right-hand side. (**B**) Small punctate linear wheals in a patient with cholinergic urticaria and dermographism, appearing within minutes of scratching his back. Some of the wheals had coalesced.

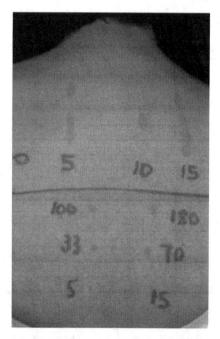

Figure 5 (*See color insert*) Upper part. Firm wide linear wheals, seen 6 hours after the stroking the back of a patient with a dermographometer at the settings shown, in the patient with delayed pressure urticaria. Lower part shows firm papules appearing on the back of the patient with delayed pressure urticaria. The derographometer set at 100 g/mm^2 was applied perpendicular to the back, and held there for 5 to 180 seconds. The required application time at the above pressure for the diagnosis of delayed pressure is 70 seconds. This patient also developed papules even after 5 second application.

particularly pronounced in atopics. *Black dermographism* is discoloration of the skin after pressure from a metallic object.

Immediate Pressure Urticaria

Immediate pressure urticaria is when whealing occurs within minutes of applying perpendicular pressure stimulus to the skin. Histology of the lesions shows dermal edema with a mild perivascular infiltrate (46). Patients develop itchy wheals within minutes after leaning against furniture, crossing legs, or handling a steering wheel (46). These may persist for 30 minutes to a few hours. There is no evidence of dermographism from stroking the skin. Immediate pressure urticaria may occur in association with the hypereosinophilic syndrome (47) or with DPU (46). Antihistamines are helpful.

Delayed Pressure Urticaria

DPU (44,48–50) is characterized by development of swellings, which occur at sites of sustained pressure on the skin after a delay of at least 30 minutes. These can persist for several days.

DPU as the predominant or only problem is uncommon, accounting for 1% to 2% of urticarias (7–9). However it occurs to some degree in up to 37% of patients with chronic ordinary urticaria, although they may not be aware of this unless directly questioned or tested (51).

The underlying mechanism for DPU is unclear. On histological examination of DPU wheals, there are decreased numbers of stainable mast cells (52) suggesting previous activation. Release of chemo-attractant factors could account for the lesional dermal leukocyte infiltrate (53), which has been likened to a late-phase cutaneous reaction (54), but no allergen can usually be identified. Neutrophils are present in the majority of early lesions (< 9 hours) and the minority of late lesions (> 24 hours), and eosinophils are found in early and especially in late wheals (53). These cellular changes correlated with upregulation of vascular adhesion molecules E-selectin and VCAM (53). Increased levels of IL-6 (55) and TNF-α and IL-3 expression derived from mast cells or the inflammatory cell infiltrate (56) in lesions may amplify and perpetuate the process. A proposed scheme is shown in Figure 6.

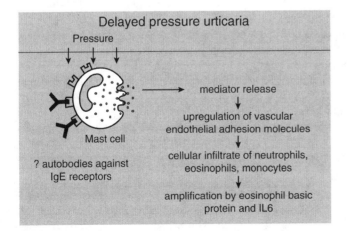

Figure 6 Proposed mechanisms for delayed pressure urticaria. The possibility of involvement of autoantibodies directed against the IgE receptor is included, as over 30% of patients with ordinary urticaria have these autoantibodies, and 40% of these patients have delayed pressure uricaria. However any involvement is conjectural.

Figure 7 A firm red tender wheal, at the site of a brassiere strap. This occurred several hours after wearing it, and the wheal lasted for many hours. She did not have immediate symptomatic dermographism.

The swellings of DPU occur within 30 minutes to 12 hours after pressure application, are usually red, often itchy and painful, and persist for 12 to 72 hours (44) and very occasionally can blister (57). In one such case histological examination showed epidermal bullae with eosinophils accompanied by a dense predominantly eosinophilic infiltrate in the dermis (58). Lesions appear at sites of tight clothes (Fig. 7), e.g., at the waistline, on hands after manual work, on buttocks after sitting on hard surfaces, and on soles after prolonged walking or standing, especially up ladders. Locally it may cause problems after dental treatment (59), sexual intercourse (60), and even cause urinary obstruction (61). DPU may be associated with flu-like symptoms, leukocytosis, myalgia, and arthralgia (44), sometimes of sufficient severity that patients present initially to a rheumatologist. DPU may also be mistaken for urticarial vasculitis, where some wheals also can appear at pressure sites (62). There is no good evidence for associated atopy or food allergy. Generally DPU may severely affect the quality of life (6), and can cause loss of manual occupations. Patients with DPU nearly always have associated chronic ordinary urticaria (49,63) and sometimes angioedema. Other physical urticarias such as delayed dermographism (55%), symptomatic immediate dermographism, and cold urticaria may also be associated (44).

The diagnosis of DPU is confirmed by objective testing, when after application of standardized weights to defined areas for specified times, red palpable wheals result at the application sites two to eight hours later. One method is to apply weighted rods, modified from Illig (64), with a convex end diameter of 1.5 cm to the thighs and back. Weights of 2.5 kg or 4.5 kg applied for 20 minutes and 15 minutes, respectively, in patients with DPU, result in an indurated wheal occurring six hours later at the application site (Fig. 8 A, B). Using this response as a gold standard for the diagnosis of DPU, pressing a dermographometer, set at 100 g/mm^2 at right angle on the back for various times, a

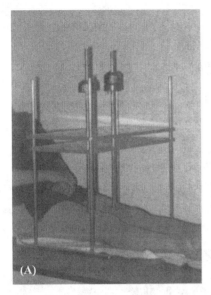
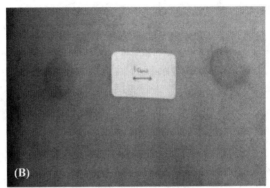

Figure 8 (**A**) An instrument where two Perspex platforms are supported firmly at the corners with fixed supporting rods. Rods with varying weights attached can be slotted into circular holes in the Perspex platforms to rest on the thighs for varying times. (**B**) (*See color insert*) The test areas on the thighs are examined at six hours later for development of rounded tender plaques six hours later.

whealing response at the 70 second site, six hours later gave the best combination of sensitivity and specificity (51,65) (Fig. 5). Less precise methods include hanging a weight (15 lb) on a wide strap for 15 minutes over the shoulder (48,49) or strapping a marble onto the forearm for 5 minutes (66,67) to induce wheals after several hours. Areas of DPU may be refractory to further pressure-induced lesions for up to 48 hours (68). Histological examination of a pressure-induced wheal would exclude urticarial vasculitis. In the latter, in addition to a dermal cellular infiltrate, leukocytoclasia and less frequently fibrinoid necrosis would also be evident.

Treatment of DPU is difficult, and only a few controlled trials exist. Usually DPU responds poorly to antihistamine therapy (44,49), which, however, may help the ordinary associated urticaria. Cetirizine in high doses (10 mg tid) has been advocated as it also inhibits eosinophils (69), but in clinical practice it has been generally disappointing. Although nonsteroidal anti-inflammatory drugs may be helpful for the pressure-induced wheals (51), they may exacerbate the ordinary urticaria. Anti-inflammatory drugs such as dapsone, 50 mg daily (70), and sulfasalazine (71), chloroquine 200 mg/day (72), the leukotriene receptor antagonist, montelukast 10 mg daily (73), and also tranexamic acid, usually used for hereditary angioedema (74), have been reported to be beneficial in isolated case reports. A randomized placebo-controlled study in 36 patients with DPU showed that although there was some improvement of the dermographometer-induced DPU lesions with desloratadine 5 mg daily, the combination with montelukast 10 mg daily was more efficacious (75). A controlled trial of nimesulide 100 mg daily for two weeks, then combined with ketotifen 1 mg bid for three weeks, then ceasing nimesulide, at seven weeks showed there was improvement (76), but this needs confirmation. In one open study theophylline 200 mg bid as an add-on therapy to cetirizine 10 mg daily was more effective than cetirizine alone (77). Systemic steroids can provide symptomatic relief but in doses that are usually unjustifiable for long-term therapy, usually over 30 mg of prednisolone per day (44,49). However, they can be used short term for severe exacerbations, e.g., difficulty walking due to gross foot swelling. Topical steroids such as clobetasol proprionate under occlusion (78) or applied as a foam twice a day (79) may be helpful in pretreating frequently affected localized areas. Oral cyclosporine at a dose of 4 mg/kg/day is helpful in chronic urticaria associated with DPU and may help where pressure urticaria is the predominant symptom. Other newer treatments include high-dose intravenous immuno-globulin where in an open study three of eight DPU patients treated achieved remission, two after one and one after three infusions (80). There is a report of successful treatment of a patient with DPU, who had anti-TNF-α treatment for his coexistent psoriasis (81).

The prognosis is variable with symptoms fluctuating in severity. In a series of 44 patients, the mean duration was three to nine years (44), but it can persist for longer.

Vibratory Angioedema

Vibratory angioedema is a very rare physical urticaria, which was first described in its familial autosomal-dominant form (82) and also in another family (83). Any vibratory stimulus such as jogging, vigorous toweling, or using lawn mowers induces a localized, red, itchy swelling within minutes lasting less than a few hours.

Increased levels of circulating histamine have been found in the familial vibration-induced swellings, and may play an important role (84,85). If the stimulus is severe, generalized erythema and headache may occur.

Occasionally, an *acquired vibratory angioedema* occurs (86,87). This is usually milder, and can be associated with other physical urticarias such as DPU and immediate dermographism (88). A recommended screening test is application of a laboratory vortex-resting on the forearm or finger for one to five minutes to induce angioedema. However a positive response is not uncommon in patients with CU (85) and in normal people (89). The diagnosis is best made by a calibrated vibration-inducing machine, where frequency and amplitude can be adjusted (88) (Fig. 9 A, B). Avoidance of the precipitating stimuli enables patients to lead normal lives.

A rare *delayed form* also occurs within one to two hours of the vibratory stimulus, peaking in four to six hours (90). In this, patient trauma produced by vibration, but not by static pressure, resulted in angioedema.

TEMPERATURE CHANGES

Heat Urticaria

Cholinergic Urticaria
CU is a very distinctive type in which characteristic small wheals appear because of stimulation of sweating, whether induced by a rise in core temperature or emotional stress (91,92). Sometimes it occurs in response to gustatory stimuli such as to peppery and sour foods and to alcohol (93).

CU is not uncommon, with a prevalence of 11% in young adults (94). In one family there were several cases reported (95).

The pathogenesis is still not clear. It is thought to be related to stimulation of the cholinergic postganglionic sympathetic nerve supply to the sweat glands (96). The abnormality at the nerve-ending receptor level is unclear. There is a report of impaired cholinesterase with likely accumulation of acetylcholine (97). A temporary increase in acetylcholine receptors has been described in one patient (98). There is not a generalized disturbance of autonomic function (99). Increased histamine levels have been detected in

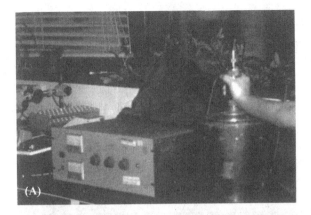

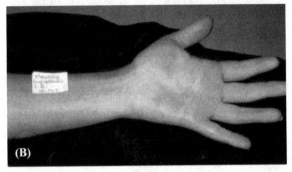

Figure 9 (**A**) A machine where the vibration amplitude and frequency can be altered to the vertical rod held by the patient. (**B**) (*See color insert*) The patient developed itchy red swelling of the lower forearm from transmitted vibration from the rod, which did not touch the forearm (under label) within minutes after vibration. The patient also had mild dermographism and the erythema of the palms could have been due to this or vibratory angioedema.

the blood of patients with CU (85). It was originally postulated that acetylcholine can release histamine, perhaps in an indirect way (96), but such a mechanism is conjectural. Passive transfer tests with serum of affected individuals are sometimes positive, probably due to an immunoglobulin (100). Such an antibody may prime the mast cell for activation. Recently the involvement of the physical process of sweating in the pathogenesis of CU has been postulated. Patients with CU demonstrated an immediate-type wheal reaction to intradermal injections of autologous sweat (101). On the basis of observations including that the CU in two patients was exacerbated in the winter and also associated with hypohidrosis because of to superficial obstruction of the acrosyringium, a concept that CU was due interference of the delivery of sweat to the skin surface was suggested (102). A similar observation of the high association of CU with hypohidrosis was made in a group of 644 subjects (103). Now it has been proposed that CU can be divided into two subsets on the basis of their whealing responses to intradermal injections of autologous sweat and serum (104). The first subtype had non-follicular wheals clinically, showed strong reactions to autologous sweat and negative reactions to autologous serum, and satellite wheals to intradermal injections acetylcholine. The second subtype showed follicular wheals, and on intradermal injections a weak reaction to sweat, a positive reaction to autologous serum, and no satellite wheals to acetylcholine. The pathogenesis of both types suggested hypersensitivity or autoimmunity of varying degrees to sweat that leaks from the sweat duct into the dermis. The positivity to the autologous skin test in CU was in contradistinction to the findings of Sabroe et al. (105), where only 1/10 patients with CU had a positive reaction to autologous serum. The usefulness of the separation of CU into two subtypes needs further elucidation.

Decreased levels of the protease inhibitor, antichymotrypsin, have been detected in the serum of some patients (106). For proposed mechanisms see Figure 10.

The disease typically occurs in adolescents of either sex and may be worse in the winter months (102,107). The patient complains of itching wheals that appear within minutes of exertion, when hot, or after sudden emotional disturbances, or even eating spicy food. The wheals characteristically are small, 1 to 3 mm across, with or without a well-marked flare (Fig. 11). Sometimes, the erythematous component is more pronounced, especially in the blush areas, and is confluent and studded with wheals. Oblique lighting is helpful to observe the wheals, especially in dark skin. Sometimes the

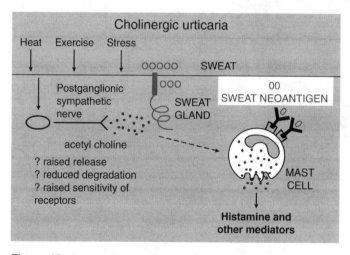

Figure 10 Proposed mechanisms for cholinergic urticaria.

Figure 11 (*See color insert*) Itchy small wheals (2–3 mm in diameter) with a surrounding flare developing on the trunk within minutes of moderate exercise in a patient with cholinergic uticaria.

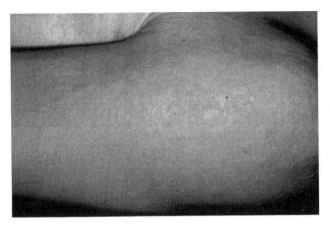

Figure 12 (*See color insert*) Severely affected patient with cholinergic urticaria. A typical small wheal is seen on his chest, but on his arms they had enlarged and coalesced.

wheals become large and coalesce to form large areas of wheals (Fig. 12), and angioedema of face and limbs may occur (92,108). The lesions persist for a few minutes to an hour or two. Ordinary "idiopathic" urticaria as well as other physical urticarias coexist in some CU patients. The dermographis response may be small wheals at sites of friction (cholinergic dermographism) (41). There is an increased incidence of atopy (92). In some patients CU is mild (92,94), but in others systemic symptoms such as flushing, faintness, palpitations (109), headache, abdominal pain, salivation, or wheezing may occur (110,111).

Exercise-induced anaphylaxis (EIA) may occur as part of the CU spectrum after severe exercise (112). However, EIA in others does not appear to be associated with CU and often occurs in patients sporadically and unpredictably, and appears to be a distinct entity (113). It is possible that some are examples of unrecognized food and EIA.

CU tends to improve gradually, but in a series of 35 patients, 60% had it for more than five years, and 30% for more than 10 years (92).

The diagnosis of CU is best confirmed by provoking typical wheals after warming, e.g., in a hot bath at 42°C for 15 minutes to raise the core temperature by 0.7°C to 1°C or by exercise in a hot environment (114). Intradermal injections of cholinergic drugs such as acetylcholine or methacholine may produce satellite wheals round the injection site, but this test is unreliable (114).

Some patients get partial relief from antihistamines, generally low sedating ones, used either regularly or before they predict attacks, but most have to modify their lifestyle by reducing exercise. Ketotifen, an antihistamine with mast-cell stabilizing properties, may be more helpful in some patients than other antihistamines (115). A few patients find that they can bring on a severe attack by suitable exertion, and afterward can achieve freedom for up to 24 hours. One report suggested that the addition of montelukast, a leukotriene receptor antagonist is useful for exercise-induced CU (116). There is a report that β-adrenergic blockers may improve CU, but should not be given if patients have asthma (117). For selected severely affected patients not responding to antihistamines, the attenuated androgen, danazol improved whealing in a controlled trial (106). Usefulness is limited by its side effects, but in suitable patients could be used short term, e.g., in summer months for a few years.

In the hypohidrotic CUs due to superficial acrosyringial obstruction occurring especially in winter, it has been suggested that topical antikeratolytic agents to the

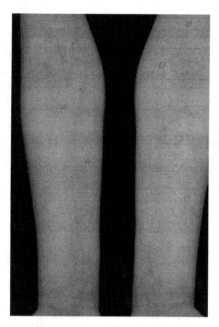

Figure 13 (*See color insert*) Typical small erythemaous macules of cholinergic erythema, usually 2 to 4 mm in diameter distributed symmetrically on the forearms. If individual macules are marked as in diagram, they will be seen to disappear in 40 to 60 minutes, with others appearing elsewhere.

affected areas may be helpful (103). Topical and systemic anticholinergic agents should in theory be useful if the side effects are acceptable and oral atropine sulfate 1 mg/day appeared to be effective in one patient (102) and oral scopolamine butylbromide, 10 mg tid, in another patient (118).

Cholinergic itching without wheals has been described (119,120). Here heat, exercise, and emotion can induce itching, which may be burning and intolerable. The condition may progress to CU (120). Antihistamines have not been helpful (120,121) nor UVB therapy in the author's patients. One patient responded to stanozolol (120).

In persistent cholinergic erythema multiple, small erythematous macules are distributed symmetrically on trunk and limbs (Fig. 13), increasing in number after exercise. Individual macules are short lived (45 minutes to an hour) but appearing at different sites over a prolonged period, sometimes continuously, giving the overall impression of a persisting rash (122).

In cold-induced cholinergic urticaria only exercise in the cold induced whealing resembling CU (123).

Localized Heat Urticaria

Here warmth applied to the skin induces whealing restricted to the warmed area (124,125). This is one of the rarest forms of physical urticaria, with less than 50 cases described. It usually affects female adults (126), but it has been described in a child (127). The pathomechanism is variable with reported histamine release in some (128–130) with eosinophil degranulation (131), prostaglandin D_2 release (130), and complement activation in some (132,133) but not in others (129,134). In one woman, localized heat urticaria was associated with a whealing reaction to intradermal injections of heated autologous serum (135).

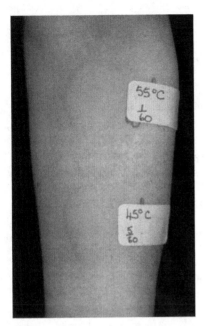

Figure 14 (*See color insert*) Wheals appearing in a patient with localized heat contact urticaria, within one minute of application of a beaker at 55°C, and within five minutes of application at 45°C.

Patients develop whealing within minutes of contact with heat, e.g., on hands after washing up in warm water, in areas in contact with radiant heat such as a radiator and on skin exposed to warm sunshine. It must be distinguished from CU and also solar urticaria (136). Systemic symptoms such as flushing, syncope (137) headache, nausea, wheezing, and abdominal pain have been described. Localized heat urticaria may be associated with cold urticaria (138). Diagnosis is made by applying heated objects such as a heated cylinder at 39°C to 56°C for 2 to 5 minutes onto the skin. Whealing occurs within minutes at the test site lasting 1 hour (Fig. 14). Treatment with H1 antihistamines, combination of H1 and H2 antihistamine (129), may be helpful. In one patient addition on montelukast to doxepin failed to improve her symptoms (139). Induction of tolerance by repeated heat exposure can be helpful (130,137,140,141).

A family with a delayed heat urticaria has been described (142).

Cold Urticaria

Cold urticaria encompasses a variety of syndromes where cold induces urticaria (143–147). Idiopathic cold contact urticaria is the most common, comprising 95% of a series of cold urticaria patients (145), while others are rare.

The incidence in the population is unknown, but cold urticaria was 2% of urticaria patients in some studies (7–9). It is common in young adults and occurs in children (148).

Histamine released from cutaneous mast cell activation has been recovered from venous blood (149), and tissue fluid draining whealed areas induced by cold (150,151) and plays a partial role in cold urticaria (152). Histological changes are mild, but electron microscopy shows some evidence of mast cell degranulation with evidence of edema in epidermis and dermis (153). In some patients with idiopathic cold contact urticaria, their serum can passively transfer the cold urticarial response to normal recipients (154), monkeys (155), and guinea pigs (156). This autoantibody is usually IgE-like (144), but IgM has been recorded (157). In vitro histamine release occurred from skin challenged with cold (154). The antigen may be either a protein produced normally by cold exposure or, less likely, an abnormal protein. Wanderer believes that IgG and IgM anti-IgE antibodies are probably immune complex cryoproteins, but the concentrations are so low that they are not routinely detected (158). The immunological change may in some cases be triggered by infection. HIV infection may predispose to cold and aquagenic urticaria. The mechanism may be due to the HIV-I gp 120 acting as a superantigen and interacting with the VH3 region of IgE, to induce histamine release from FcεRI-bearing cells such as mast cells (159).

Elevated antibodies to measles, CMV, HSV, and Mycoplasma pneumonia in patients with cold urticaria were considered to be a sign of disordered immunity (160).

The contribution of other mediators detected, such as neutrophil (161) and eosinophil chemotactic factors (162), PGD_2 (163), leukotriene E4 (164), Leukotriene C4 (165), platelet-activating factor (166), and TNF-α (167) remains to be elucidated. Reduced serum α-1 anti-trypsin was found in some studies (168), but this was unrelated to disease activity.

Cold Urticarias with a Typical Cold Stimulation Test

Idiopathic immediate cold urticaria (without an underlying cause). This is by far the commonest form, occurring at any age but most frequently in young adults. It is twice as common in females (169). It may be preceded or associated with nonspecific upper respiratory viral infections, steptococcal throat infections (145), infectious mononucleosus (170,171), dental infections (172), and HIV (173,174) or after wasp (175), bee (176), or jelly fish stings. Itching and whealing of the skin occur on cold exposure within minutes and last up to one hour. Patients also may have problems washing up in cold water or taking food out of the freezer. Cold winds and cold rain are particularly effective stimuli. Cold urticaria, however, may occur in the tropics (177,178). Sometimes, the mouth and pharynx may swell after drinking cold liquids (179). Systemic symptoms include flushing, palpitations, headache, wheezing, and loss of consciousness. Thirty percent of patients have other associated urticarias, both physical and ordinary (145). The mean duration of cold urticaria was six years in one series (145), but it may persist for many years (179).

Diagnosis is made by application of an ice cube in a thin plastic bag for 20 minutes onto the skin, and whealing occurs within 15 minutes at the test site, on rewarming the skin (145) (Fig. 15 A, B). The vast majority are positive to the ice cube test, and the severity can be partially judged by the time of application of the ice cube needed (varying from 1 second to 20 minutes) to induce wheals. Negative results from this test may occur very rarely even in cold contact urticaria (180). In a few patients, temperatures at 7°C to 15°C may be necessary or be more effective than ice to induce whealing (180). If cold urticaria is mild and ice cube test is negative, sometimes, a more extensive local challenge such as placing a hand and forearm into cold water at 10°C for five minutes, or iced water for two minutes, may induce whealing. More recently an improved method has been devised to perform and standardize the cold challenge test using a Peltier-effect-based electronic device, and it is available commercially (147). It allows exposure of the skin to defined temperatures to assess both stimulation temperatures and times. It is very rare to find a cryoprotein in typical cold contact urticaria, but cryoglobulins (clotted blood must be kept warm until tested in the laboratory) should be looked for. In addition, in older patients if indicated, evidence for a myeloma or leukemia, with a blood count and serum immunoglobulins and serum protein electrophoresis should be sought.

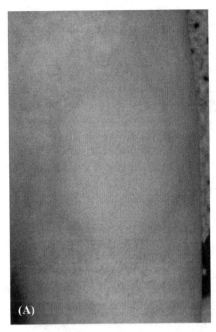
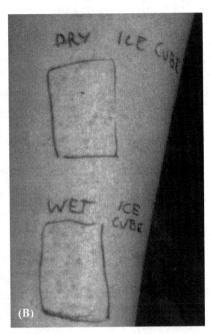

Figure 15 (*See color insert*) (**A**) Circumscribed confluent wheal appearing at the site of application of an ice cube in a plastic cover, for 10 minutes on the forearm of a patient with contact cold urticaria. (**B**) Small wheals localized to cold application of a wet and covered ice cube in a patient with a not uncommon combination of contact cold and cholinergic urticaria. However, this morphology is unusual in a positive ice cube test.

Patients should avoid cold exposure as much as possible, but it may have an impact on occupation (181). It is important to warn against cold-water bathing due to risk of anaphylaxis and potentially of drowning from cold water bathing. This is particularly important for those who have associated oropharyngeal angioedema after ingesting cold foods/liquids, as they may be more at risk of anaphylaxis (182). For the most severely affected in special situations where there is a risk of falling into cold water, epinephrine injections should be available for administration. Prior to an operation, medical attendants should be informed so that they are aware of the condition in order to prevent misdiagnoses of adverse drug reactions (183) and so that special precautions can be taken (184,185). Treatments with low-sedation antihistamine are variably effective (145,186–189), but they are at least as effective as the previously favoured cyproheptadine, with fewer side effects (190). In one study, a combination of terbutaline 2.5 mg and aminophylline 150 mg each given tid was helpful (172). One patient is reported to have improved with montelukast, a leukotriene receptor antagonist (191). A combination of cetrizine 10 mg daily and zafirkulast 20 mg bid in two patients was superior subjectively and by objective evaluation with ice cube tests, than either alone (192). Induction of tolerance by repeated graduated exposures to cold can be helpful for selected patients (147,187,193) but it is time consuming, taking one to two weeks, preferably in hospital. The procedure is not always effective, and some patients cannot continue taking a cold shower or bath daily (194). Tolerance is lost within a few days if regular cold exposure is discontinued. The mechanism of induction of tolerance in unknown but is not due to mast cell mediator depletion or tachyphylaxis of cutaneous vasculature (195). In one series, high doses of antibiotics (e.g., penicillin 1.2 megaunits equivalent to 750 mg penicillin V daily or tetracycline 2 g)

(158) daily were given for three weeks. The reported improvement was not reproduced in the author's experience.

Systemic steroids do not appear to be effective (152). Cyclosporin and IVIG treatment in a few of our patients was not useful, but the role of immunomodulation needs further eleucidation. More recently there are case reports of successful treatment of cold urticaria with cyclosporine (196) and anti-igE in a child (197).

Cold urticaria secondary to serum cryoproteins. This is rare and was found in only 1% of one series (145). It is associated with other manifestations such as Raynaud's phenomenon, purpura, and skin necrosis. Cryogobulinemia may be idiopathic or occur in collagen vascular disease, chronic lymphatic leukemia, myeloma, and in infectious diseases including infectious mononucleosis. Cold urticaria is said to occur in only 3% of people with cryoglobulinemia (198). Treatment is directed against the underlying condition. Cryofibrinogen occurred in the blood of 3.4% of a large hospital population (199) and in 3% of patients in cold urticaria (200). Its significance in relationship to cold urticaria remains to be determined. Cold agglutinins are not usually associated with cold urticaria (201). Cold hemolysins usually associated with syphilis have not been detected in recent series.

Cold Urticaria with Atypical Stimulation Tests

Acquired contact.
In delayed contact cold urticaria where whealing occurs after a delay of hours after cold contact is very rare (202,203). The delay may be up to 24 hours and persist for 48 hours. A single patient whose immediate wheal persisted for seven days has been described (204). A familial form has been reported (205). A persistent ice cube test may suggest the presence of cold urticaria with vasculitis (206).

In localized cold contact urticaria, cold-induced whealing occurs on restricted areas of the body only. It is very rare (207–209). Onset has been reported at sites of ragweed immunotherapy, pollen immunotherpy (210), after insect stings. An obvious cause may not be present (208,209). In localized reflex cold urticaria, a patient developed small wheals in the vicinity of, but not in the area of, contact with an ice cube (211). Cold precipitated dermographism occurred in a person with ordinary contact cold urticaria, but in addition she developed dermographism only in areas that had been exposed to cold (212). A patient with systemic cold urticaria, and dermographism exaggerated by cold has also been described (213). Acquired cold contact erythema occurred as painful erythema without whealing occurred in response to cold (214), but in other patients it may be a forme fruste of immediate cold contact urticaria.

Systemic.
Familial cold urticaria. This rare form is inherited as an autosomal-dominant trait. Here the cold-induced wheals occur as a result of generalized cooling and are widespread. They are persistent and associated with fever, arthralgia, and leukocytosis and sometimes associated with amyloidosis. The ice cube test is negative. It is caused by mutations of the same gene CIAS1 on 1q44 as for the Muckle-Wells syndrome (215,216). CIAS1 encodes for cryopyrin. Cryopyrin interacts with ASC (an intercellular adaptor protein that is involved in IL-1 release). This interaction leads to activation of caspase and subsequent release of IL-1 as well as activation of nuclear factor κB (NF-κB), which results in release of many cytokines (217). Familial cold urticaria has been renamed as familial cold autoinflammatory syndrome (FCAS) and classified into the group of familial periodic fever syndromes (215,218). In one family with familial cold urticaria there was a good clinical response to

the oral anabolic steroid stanozolol (219). More recently a good response has been demonstrated to IL-1 receptor antagonist anankira (217).

In generalized reflex cold urticaria, widespread wheals, often more marked on elbows, knees, and buttocks occur in response to cooling of core body temperature (213,220,221). The ice cube test is negative. Placing the patient in a cold room at 4°C for 30 minutes in light clothes induces the lesions. As this test is not usually performed, the incidence may be underestimated. In cold-induced CU, additional exercise is necessary in the cold room to induce wheals (123,222).

EXERCISE-INDUCED ANAPHYLAXIS (EIA)

EIA is a syndrome where anaphylactic symptoms occur in response to exercise (223–225). Severe CU, which is associated with typical small cholinergic wheals on exercise, and symptoms occur in response to passive heating without exercise (112,226). This should not strictly be included in the syndrome of exercise-induced anaphylactic syndromes (227,228). In true EIA, anaphylaxis occurs only after exercise. In some patients this is not related to prior food ingestion (224,228). However in the majority (224), symptoms occur only if exercise is taken within four hours after food ingestion. The meal may not contain a specific constituent (nonspecific food-dependent EIA). Sometimes it may occur only after ingestion of single or multiple specific foods followed by exercise (specific food-dependent EIA). The incidence is unknown. It is more common in the young adult females, but can occur in children (229). It can be familial (230).

EAI is associated with mast cell degranulation (228). In those with specific food sensitivity, the mechanism is partly IgE-dependent as prick and/or specific IgE test to these foods are positive (224,231–234). A lower mast cell threshold for mediator release has been demonstrated after exercise (228,231,232). The most common precipitants of EIA are jogging and active sport, where it can be a major problem (235). Often the first symptom is itching, followed by urticaria and often angioedema, which tends to persist during an episode that lasts 30 minutes to four hours. Systemic symptoms that may follow include nausea, vomiting, abdominal colic, stridor, and collapse. There may be reduced pulmonary function (236). Atopy is more common in individual with EIA (223,231). In specific food-dependent EAI common foods or combination of foods involved (236) include shellfish (231,234), wheat (231,234,237), and vegetables such as celery (238). Involvement of fruits such as grapes (231), apples, tomatoes, and also nuts have been described. The induction and severity of food-dependent EIA also may depend on other factors such as the amount of food allergen ingested (233), prior ingestion of aspirin (234), and other nonsteroidal anti-inflamatory medication and alcohol (234). One patient developed EIA only if exercising in the cold (239). An ice cube test was positive, so it could be distinguished from cold-induced CU (221).

Diagnosis is suspected from history. If food-associated EIA is suspected, prick tests for specific IgE substances commonly causing specific food-dependent EIA can be undertaken. Confirmation can be made by reproducing clinical induction of lesions, under close supervision. A hot bath should be undertaken to exclude CU.

Treatment is as for any other anapylaxis. Prevention is to restrict exercise in EIA and to have self-injectable epinephrine available, as sometimes the occurrence and severity is unpredictable. In food-dependent EIA, exercise should be avoided within four hours of food, alcohol, and aspirin, and if known eliminating the specific food/s. Although prick tests may be positive to a number of foods, and symptoms appear to occur only after ingestion of one of them, it is best to avoid all prick test–positive substances before exercise (224). There is a report that oral disodium cromoglycate taken before exercise may be helpful (237).

SOLAR URTICARIA

In solar urticaria (240–243) itching erythema and wheals develop within minutes at sites of sun exposure, with lesions usually fading within two hours. By convention, the name is applied to the urticarial response from the ultraviolet and visible parts of the electromagnetic spectrum from any source (280–700 nm wavelengths), though solar urticaria due to infrared radiation of wavelengths 700–2,5000 nm (without detectable heat urticaria) has been recorded (244).

Passive and reverse passive transfer of solar urticaria has been demonstrated since 1942. It now postulated that a chromophore in the skin or circulation on absorption of radiation of an appropriate wavelength induces a neoallergen–a photoallergen. This induces a specific IgE autoantibody that binds to mast cells. On reexposure to the appropriate wavelengths, mast cells degranulate, releasing histamine, and other mediators. So far, chromophores have been detected in the serum of some patients who wheal on intradermal injections of their serum irradiated by wavelengths that induce clinical whealing (action spectrum). The serum photoallergens have not been identified, but some have molecular weights ranging from 25 to 45 Kd and from 300 to 1000 Kd (245). The action spectrums in solar urticarias are variable, so it is probable that a number of chromophores are responsible. Most patients develop urticarial wheals at the site of autologous serum, which has been irradiated with the wavelength of the action spectrum (79% in a Japanese cohort) (243). In solar urticarial lesions there is evidence of mast cell degranulation (246,247). At two to four hours the site shows infiltration with neutrophils and eosinophils without visible lesions (248). Increased histamine in venous effluent from urticated areas (246,248,249) has been detected as well as neutrophil and eosinophil chemotactic factors (250), but the relative importance of all these factors is not known.

Solar urticaria is rare. It can occur in all races, but appears to be less frequent in American-Africans than Caucasians (251). Most cases of solar urticaria occur in patients in their 20s and 30s (241,243,252,253), though the median age of onset of solar urticaria alone was 41 years (242). It can occur in children (254,255).

The onset of the first episode may be sudden and dramatic (256). Erythema, itching, burning, and wheals occur in some exposed areas within minutes (Fig. 16). Areas commonly affected are the V of the chest and shoulders and arms, less so the face and back of hands, possibly due to tolerance from repeated exposure (257). Patients may be affected through window glass (if wavelengths are greater than 320 nm), through thin clothing, and from artificial radiation sources such as sunbeds, halogen, and fluorescent bulbs. Widespread exposure can cause flushing, headache, or collapse (243) and also pure angioedema of the eyelid and lips (258). The severity of solar uticaria will depend on the sensitivity and time of exposure.

Rarely, solar urticaria may occur in erythropoietic protoporphyria and porphria cutanea tarda (259) (though solar urticaria is not observed in the vast majority of patients with porphyria), in systemic lupus erythematosus, and following drugs such as chlorpromazine (252), tetracycline (260), and repirinast (261) and progesterone compounds in oral contraceptives (262). However, usually no cause can be identified. Only a few studies suggest that there is an increased incidence of atopy (253,257). In the series from Scotland of 87 patients with solar urticaria, 23% had associated polymorphic light

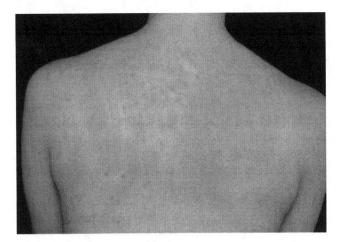

Figure 16 (*See color insert*) Wheals localized to areas on the back exposed to the sun, and sparing covered areas in a patient with solar urticaria.

eruption and 3% actinic reticuloid (242). These investigators found that the probability of resolution at 5, 10, and 15 years after diagnosis was 12%, 26%, and 46%, respectively; so the condition can last for many years. In a Belgian series the median persistence was 4 to 11 years (257), in an Italian series 50% were clear in five years (253), but none of 40 Japanese patients cleared (252).

Diagnosis can be confirmed by exposure to strong natural sunlight or to a solar simulator, and erythema and wheals occur in minutes, but it is important to exclude other forms of sunlight-induced urticaria such as heat urticaria. Testing is best on previously unexposed areas such as the back. The activating wavelengths may be categorized broadly by additional use of filters (257). The most sophisticated method is using a narrow band monochromator (263), to test the reactivity to individual wavelengths (Fig. 17). This also allows definition of the smallest irradiation dose at a waveband that will induce whealing– the minimal urticarial dose (MUD). This end point may be important in individual patients in assessing different forms of therapy. Lasers have been used to diagnose

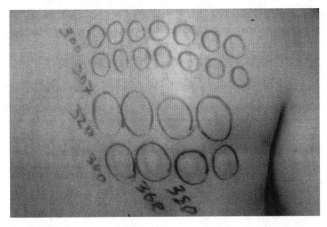

Figure 17 (*See color insert*) Wheals appearing at test sites with a monochromator at 320, 340, 360 nm, but not at 300 and 307 nm, in a patient with solar urticaria.

urticarial reactions to visible light (264). The activating wavelengths occur between 280 and 700 nm. The most common activating wavelenghts in the Scotland is the longer UVA and shorter visible light, though some also whealed with UVB (242), while it is visible light that is most common in a Japanese series (243). Sometimes there are changes in photosensitivity over time in an individual patient (265).

Various classifications relating to activating wavelengths have been proposed, the simplest by Ramsay (266). He suggested four categories: group 1 reacting to UVB, group 2 to UVA, group C to visible, and group 4 to a wide spectrum, but not all patients fit into these groups.

An unusual aspect of solar urticaria is the phenomenon of inhibition spectra. Here when the skin is exposed to wavelengths inducing solar urticaria and concurrently or immediately afterward exposed to the inhibition wavelengths, the urticarial response can be decreased. Inhibition spectra are found mainly in Japanese patients occurring in 69% (252). The inhibition spectra are usually of longer wavelengths than the action spectra, but rarely shorter wavelengths can inhibit longer-activating ones (267). Inhibitory wavelengths may inactivate photoallergens produced by the action spectrum and stabilize the mast cells (268).

The most common differential diagnosis is polymorphic light eruption where urticated papules, vesicles, or plaques can occur within 30 minutes from sun exposure, but these persist for days. It complicates the diagnosis when PLE and solar urticaria coexist, and phototesting may be particularly useful. Secondary causes such as medication, systemic lupus, or porphyria should be excluded.

Treatment can be difficult, but in the milder cases the newer broad-spectrum sunscreens providing some protection against UVA (but not against visible wavelengths) may be helpful. The treatment of choice is low sedation antihistamines (e.g., fexofenadine, cetirizine, desloratadine). In the Scottish study, 35% of patients showed improvement with sunscreens and a further 35% from antihistamines (242). For those who do not respond, other treatments include UVA therapy (269) and PUVA (270), but these must be administered carefully, with initial determination of the MUD dose and sometimes under oral steroid cover. In some patients tolerance can be induced, by graduated repeated exposures to the eliciting wavelengths (247,271,272). For the most severe unresponsive cases, plasmapheresis has been used with some success in a few patients (273–275), but not in others (276) by itself or in combination with PUVA (277). More recently, the successful use of intravenous immunoglobulin (278,279), cyclosporin (280), and photopheresis (281) has been reported in individual patients.

Variations of classical solar urticaria include solar erythema when itching erythema without whealing occurs (282). Solar urticaria localized to specific areas of the body (fixed solar urticaria) has been described (283,284). Solar urticaria may rarely have a delayed onset (285). Rarely solar urticaria has the histology of a vasculitis (286).

AQUAGENIC URTICARIA

In aqagenic urticaria contact with water at any temperature induces an eruption of small usually pruritic wheals, surrounded by a flare, resembling CU but sparser (287,288). It is rare, with less than 40 cases describe (289). It occurs in young adults (289), though it has been described in children (290,291). A few cases are familial (292), and in one family it was associated with lactose intolerance (293) and in another with Bernard-Soulier syndrome (294).

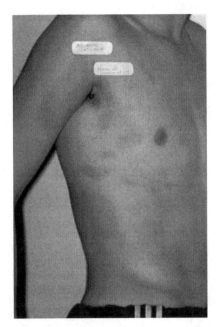

Figure 18 (*See color insert*) Aquagenic urticaria with small sparse wheals, resembling cholinergic urticaria, within minutes of bathing in water for 15 minutes at skin temperature.

It has been proposed that water carries an epidermal antigen to the sensitized mast cell (295). There is mast cell degranulation and histamine release (296,297). Some authors have implicated acectylcholine (296), but not others (289).

Usually all forms of water such as tap, swimming pool, distilled water (296), high humidity (298), tears (299), sweat (300), and saliva (297) can induce lesions within a few minutes. The upper trunk and neck are particularly affected, sparing the face (Fig. 18). Very occasionally it occurs on localized areas only such as the back of hands (300) and face (301) and neck, V of chest and shoulders in another (302). Systemic symptoms such as wheezing (289,297) and headache are rare (303). In two cases, induction of wheals was dependent on the salinity of the water (301,304). Organic solvents such as ethanol and acetone usually enhance the water-induced whealing (296), but occasionally they may induce wheals (297). Prior application of barrier applications such as petrolatum reduces whealing (296). Combinations with other physical urticarias occur such as with dermographisma, CU (305), and cold urticaria (306). Aquagenic urticaria has occurred it in association with HIV in one patient (307).

Diagnosis consists of excluding other urticarias that can also be induced by physical properties of water such as temperature water (cold urticaria, CU) and force of water (dermographism). Additionally, wheals should be induced within minutes under a wet swab kept at body temperature (at sites usually affected by aquagenic urticaria) for 20 to 30 minutes or after immersion in a body temperature bath for 15 minutes. It is a different entity from aquagenic pruritus where there is water-induced itching but no whealing (308,309). Aquagenic pruritus occurs predominantly on the legs and lower trunk. Very rarely the condition, can be associated with blood disorders such as polycythemia rubra vera.

Treatment is difficult. In some patients low sedation antihistamines may be helpful. Others respond to treatment with UVB (299) or photochemotherapy (PUVA) (310). Induction of tolerance by repeated bathing (311) was useful in one patient, though not in

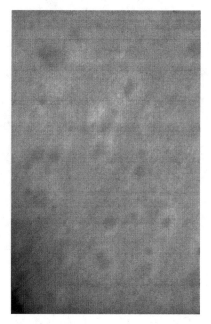

Figure 19 (*See color insert*) The appearance described for adrenergic urticaria. Small wheals 3 to 4 mm in diameter resembling cholinergic urticaria, surrounded by areas of blanching.

the author's experience. The patient with HIV responded to treatment with stanozolol (307). One patient's aquagenic urticaria responded to a combination of cyproheptadine and oral methscopolamine, but her associated headache was prevented only by a selective serotonin reuptake inhibitor (SSRI) (303).

ADRENERGIC URTICARIA

Adrenergic urticaria is characterized by development of multiple small wheals, induced by stress. It is said to be distinguished from CU by the presence of blanching and vasoconstriction surrounding the wheals (Fig. 19). Heat and exercise do not induce whealing, but they can be reproduced by intradermal injections of adrenaline and nonadrenaline but not by acetylcholine (312–314). β-Adrenergic blockers such as propanalol reduced the severity of adrenergic urticaria (312–314); they also improve CU.

REFERENCES

1. Kobza Black A. The physical urticarias. In: Champion RH, Greaves MW, Kobza Black A, Pye RJ, eds. The Urticarias. Edinburgh: Churchill Livingstone, 1985:168–190.
2. Dice JP. Physical urticaria. Immunol Allergy Clin North Am 2004; 24:225–246
3. Czarnetzki.The physical urticaris. In: Czarnetzki BM, ed. Urticaria. Berlin: Springer Verlag, 1986:55–88.
4. Zuberbier T, Bindslev-Jensen C, Canonica W, et al. EAACI/GA^{2}LEN/EDF guideline: definition, classification and diagnosis of urticaria. Allergy 2006; 61:316–320.
5. Kountou-Fili K, Borici Mazi R, Kapp A, et al. Physical urticaria:classification and diagnostic guidelines. An EAACI position paper. Allergy 1997;52:504–513.

6. Poon E, Seed PT, Greaves MW, et al. The extent and nature of disability in different urticarial conditions. Br J Dermatol 1999; 140:666–671.

7. Champion RH. Urticaria then and now. Br J Dermatol 1988; 119:427–436.

8. Humphreys F, Hunter JAA. The charactersistics of urticaria in 390 patients. Br J Dermatol 1998; 138:635–638.

9. Sibbald RG, Cheema AS, Lozinski A, et al. Chronic urticaria. Evaluation of the role of physical, immunologic and other contributory factors. Int J Dermatol 1991; 30:381–386.

10. Kozel MMA, Mekkes JR, Bossyut PMM, et al. The effectiveness of a history-based diagnostic approach in chronic urticaria and angioedema. Arch Dermatol 1998; 134:1675–1680.

11. Volonakis M, Katsarou-Katsari A, Stratigos J. Etiologic factors in childhood chronic urticaria. Retrospective evaluation and follow-up. Annals of Allergy 1992; 69:61–65.

12. Kauppinen K, Juntunen K, Lanki H. Urticaria in children. Allergy 1984; 39:469–472.

13. Breathnach SM, Allen R, Milford Ward A, et al. Symptomatic dermographism: natural history, clinical features, laboratory investigations and response to therapy. Clin Exp Dermatol 1983; 8:463–476.

14. Wong RC, Fairley JA, Ellis CN. Dermographism: a review. J Am Acad Dermatol 1984; 11: 643–652.

15. Lewis T. Vascular reactions of the skin to injury-1. Reaction to stroking: urticaria factitia. Heart 1924; 2:119–129.

16. Kirby JD, Matthews CNA, James J, et al. The incidence and other aspects of factitious wealing (dermographism). Br J Dermatol 1971; 85:331–335.

17. Jedele KB, Michels VV. Familial dermographism. Am J Med Genet 1991; 39:201–203.

18. Bart RS, Ackerman AB. Urticarial dermographism Arch Derm 1966; 94:716–719.

19. English JSC, Murphy GM, Winkelmann RK, et al. A sequential histological study of demographism. Clin Experimental Dermatol 1988; 13:314–317.

20. James MP, Eady RAJ, Kobza Black A, et al. Physical urticarias: a microscopical and pharmacological study of mast cell involvement. J Invest Dermatol 1980; 74:451A.

21. Lawlor F, Kobza Black A, Murdoch RD, et al. Symptomatic dermographism, wealing, mast cells and histamine are decreased in skin following long term application of a potent topical steroid. Br J Dermatol 1989; 121:629–634.

22. Newcomb RW, Nelson H. Dermographia mediated by immunoglobulin E. Am J Med 1973; 54: 174–180.

23. Horiko T, Aoki T. Dermographism (mechanical urticaria) mediated by IgM. Br J Dermatol 1984; 114:545–550.

24. Murphy GM, Zollman PE, Greaves MW, et al. Symptomatic dermographism (factitious urticaria) –passive transfer experiments from human to monkeys. Br J Dermatol 1987; 116:801–804.

25. Wallengren J, Moller H, Ekman R. Occurrence of substance P, vasoactive intestinal peptide, and cacitonin gene-related peptide in dermographism and cold urticaria. Arch Dermatol Res 1987; 279:512–515.

26. Lambiris A, Greaves MW. Dyspareunia and vulvodynia are probably common manifestations of factitious urticaria. Br J Dermatol 1997; 136:140–141.

27. Smith JA, Mansfield LE, Fokakis A, et al. Dermographia caused by IgE mediated penicillin allergy. Ann Allergy 1983; 51:30–33.

28. Warner DMcC, Ramos-Caro FA, Flowers FP. Famotidine (Pepcid)-induced symptomatic dermatographism. J Am Acad Dermatol 1994; 31:677–678.

29. Skrebova N, Nameda Y, Takiwaki H, et al. Severe dermographism after topical therapy with diphenylcyclopropenone for alopecia totalis. Contact Dermatitis 2000; 42:212–215.

30. Taskapan O, Harmanyeri Y. Evaluation of patients with symptomatic dermographism. JEADV 2006; 20:58–62.

31. Wu JJ, Huang DB, Murase JE, et al. Dermographism secondary to trauma from a coral reef. JEADV 2006; 20:1337–1338.

32. Watsky KL, McGovern T. Intolerance to topical products may be due to dermographism. Am J Contact Dermat 2003; 14:35–36.

33. James J, Warin RP. Factitious wealing at the site of previous cutaneous response. Br J Dermatol 1969; 81:882–824.

34. Termklinchan V, Kulthanan K, Bunyaratavej S. Assessment of dermographism at different anatomical regions by dermographometer. J Med Assoc Thai 2006; 89:992–996.

35. Grolnick M. An investigative and clinical evaluation of dermographism. Annals of Allergy 1970; 28:395–404.

36. Sharpe GR, Shuster S. In dermographic urticaria H_2 receptor antagonists have a small but therapeutically irrelevant additional effect compared with H_1 antagonists alone. Br J Dermatol 1993; 129:575–579.

37. Johnsson M, Falk ES, Volden G. UVB treatment of factitious urticaria. Photodermatology 1987; 4:302–304.

38. Logan RA, O'Brien TJ, Greaves MW. The effect of psoralen photochemotherapy (PUVA) on symptomatic dermographism. Br J Dermatol 1989; 14:25–28.

39. Pellicano R, Camassa F, Lomuto M. Localized dermographism at the site of a fixed drug eruption. Br J Dermatol 1995; 132:156–158.

40. Warin RP. Factitious urticaria: red dermographism. Br J Dermatol 1981; 104:285–288.

41. Mayou SC, Kobza Black A, Greaves MW. Cholinergic dermographism. Br J Dermatol 1986; 115:371–377.

42. Kalz F, Bower CM, Prichard H. Delayed and persistent dermographia. Arch Dermatol 1950; 61:772–779.

43. Baughman RD, Jillson OF. Seven specific types of urticaria with a special reference to delayed persistent dermographism. Ann Allergy 1963; 21:248–255.

44. Dover JS, Kobza Black A, Milford Ward A, et al. Delayed pressure urticaria. Clinical features, laboratory investigations, and response to therapy in 44 patients. J Am Acad Dermatol 1988; 18:1289–1298.

45. Grimm V, Mempel M, Ring J, et al. Congenital symptomatic dermographism as the first symptom of mastocytosis. Br J Dermatol 2000; 143:1109.

46. Lawlor F, Kobza Black A, Greaves MW. Immediate-pressure urticaria - a distinct disorder. Clin Exper Dermatol 1991; 16:155–157.

47. Parrillo JE, Lawley TJ, Frank MM, et al. Immunologic reactivity in the hypereosinophilic syndrome. J Allergy Clin Immunol 1979; 64:113–121.

48. Ryan TJ, Shim-Young N, Turk JL. Delayed pressure urticaria. Br J Dermatol 1968; 80: 485–490.

49. Sussman GL, Harvey RP, Schoket AL. Delayed pressure urticaria. J Allergy Clin Immunol 1982; 70:337–342.

50. Lawlor F, Black AK. Delayed pressure urticaria. Immunol Allergy Clinics North Am 2004; 24:247–258.

51. Barlow RJ, Warburton F, Watson K, et al. Diagnosis and incidence of delayed pressure urticaria in patients with chronic urticaria. J Am Acad Dermatol 1993; 29:954–958.

52. Barlow RJ, Ross EL, MacDonald DM, et al. Mast cells and T lymphocytes in chronic urticaria. Clin Exp Allergy 1995; 25:317–322.

53. Barlow RJ, Ross EL, Mac Donald DM, et al. Adhesion molecule expression and the inflammatory cell infiltrate in delayed pressure urticaria. Br J Dermatol 1994; 131:341–347.

54. Czarnetzki BM, Meentken J, Kolde G, et al. Morphology of the cellular infiltrate in delayed pressure urticaria. J Am Acad Dermatol 1985; 12:1253–1259.

55. Lawlor F, Bird C, Camp RDR, et al. Increased interleukin 6, but reduced interleukin 1, in delayed pressure. Br J Dermatol 1993; 128:500–503.

56. Hermes B, Prochazka A-K, Haas N, et al. Upregulation of TNF-α and IL-3 expression in lesional and uninvolved skin of different types of urticaria. J Allergy Clin Immunol 1999; 103:307–314.

57. Mijailovic BB, Karadaglic DM, Ninkovic MP, et al. Bullous delayed pressure urticaria; pressure testing may produce a systemic reaction. Br J Dermatol 1997; 136:434–436.

58. Kerstan A, Rose C, Simon D, et al. Bullous delayed pressure urticaria: a pathogenic role for eosinophilic granulocytes? Br J Derm 2005; 153:435–437.

59. Jauhar S, Staines K, McQueen M, et al. Dermographism and delayed pressure urticaria. Oral Surg Oral Med Oral Pathol Oral Radiol Endod 2007; 103:774–779.

60. Mc Fadden JP, Newton JA, Greaves MW. Dyspareunia as a complication of delayed pressure urticaria. Br J Sexual Med 1988; 15:61.

61. Poon E, Kobza Black A. Delayed pressure urticaria causing obstruction of urinary flow. Acta Derm Venereol 1998; 78:394.

62. Kobza Black A. Urticaria vasculitis. Clinics in Dermatology 1999; 17:565–569.

63. Warin RP. Clinical observations on delayed pressure urticaria. Br J Dermatol 1989; 121:225–228.

64. Illig L, Kunick J. Klinik und Diagnostik der physikalischen Urticaria I. Hautarzt 1969; 20: 167–178.

65. Lawlor F, Kobza Black A, Milford Ward A, et al. Delayed pressure urticaria, objective evaluation of a variable disease using a dermographometer and assessment of treatment using colchicine. Br J Dermatol 1989; 120:403–408.

66. Warin RP. A simple out-patient test for delayed pressure urticaria. Br J Dermatol 1987; 11: 742–743.

67. Pise GA, Thappa DM. Is it delayed pressure urticaria or demographism? Indian J Dermatol Venereol 2006; 72:155–156.

68. Estes SA, Yung CW. Delayed pressure urticaria: an investigation of some parameters of lesion induction. J Am Acad Dermatol 1981; 5:25–31.

69. Kontou-Fili K, Maniatakou G, Demaka P, et al. Therapeutic effects of cetirizine in delayed pressure urticaria: clinicopathologic findings. J Am Acad Dermatol 1991; 24:1090–1093.

70. Gould DJ, Campbell D, Dayani A. Delayed pressure urticaria. Successful treatment of 5 cases. Br J Dermatol 1991; 125(suppl. 38):25.

71. Engler RJM, Squire E, Benson P. Chronic sulfasalazine therapy in the treatment of delayed pressure urticaria and angioedema. Annals of Allergy, Asthma and Immunology 1995; 74: 155–159.

72. Kulthanan K, Thumpimukvatana N. Positive impact of chloroquine on delayed pressure urticaria. J Drugs Dermatol 2007; 6:445–446.

73. Berkun Y, Shalit M. Successful treatment of delayed pressure urticaria with montelukast. Allergy 2000; 55:203–204.

74. Shedden C, Highet AS. Delayed pressure urticaria controlled by tranexamic acid. Clin Exp Dermatol 2005; 31:295.

75. Nettis E, Colanardi MC, Soccio AL, et al. Desloratadine in combination with montelukast suppresses the dermographometer challenge test papule, and is effective in the treatment of delayed pressure urticaria: a randomized, double-blind, placebo-controlled study. Br J Dermatol 2006; 155:1279–1282.

76. Vena GA, D'Argento V, Cassano N, et al. Sequential therapy with nimesulide and ketotifen in delayed pressure urticaria. Acta Dermatovener 1998; 78:304–305.

77. Kalogeromitros D, Kempuraj D, Katsarou-Katsari A, et al. Theophylline as an "add-on" therapy in patients with delayed pressure urticaria: a prospective self-controlled study. Int J Immunopathol Pharmacol 2005; 18:595–602.

78. Barlow RJ, MacDonald DM., Kobza Black A, et al. The effects of topical corticosteroids on delayed pressure urticaria. Arch Derm Res 1995; 287:285–288.

79. Vena GA, Cassano N, D'Argento V, et al. Clobetasol proprionate 0.05% in a novel foam formulation is safe and effective in the short-term treatment of patients with delayed pressure urticaria: a randomized, double-blind, placebo-controlled trial. Br J Dermatol 2005; 154: 353–356.

80. Dawn G, Urcelay M, Ah-Weng A, et al. Effect of high-dose intravenous immunoglobulin in delayed pressure urticaria. Br J Dermatol 2003; 149:836–840.

81. Magerl M, Philipp S, Monasterski M, et al. Successful treatment of delayed pressure urticaria with anti-TNFα. J Allergy Clin Immunol 2007; 119:752–754.

82. Patterson R, Mellies CJ, Blankenship ML, et al. Vibratory angioedema: a hereditary type of hypersensitivity. J Allergy Clin Immunol 1972; 50:175–182.

83. Highet AS, Pye R, Felix RH. Vibratory urticaria. Br J Dermatol 1981; 105:40–41.

84. Metzger WJ, Kaplan AP, Beaven MA, et al. Hereditary vibratory angioedema: confirmation of histamine release in a type of physical hypersensitivity. J Allergy Clin Immunol 1976; 57: 605–608.

85. Kaplan AP, Beaven MA. In vivo studies of the pathogenesis of cold urticaria, cholinergic urticaria and vibration-induced angioedema. J Invest Dermatol 1976; 67:327–332.

86. Wener MH, Metzger WJ, Simon RA. Occupationally acquired vibratory angioedeama with secondary carpal tunnel syndrome. Annals Internal Medicine 1983; 48:44–46.

87. Ting S, Reiman BEF, Rauls DO, et al. Non-familial, vibration-induced angioedema. J Allergy Clin Immunol 1983; 71:547–551.

88. Lawlor F, Kobza Black A, Breathnach AS, et al. Vibratory angioedema: lesion induction, clinical features, laboratory and ultrastructural findings, and response to therapy. Br J Dermatol 1989; 120:93–99.

89. Mathelier-Fusade P, Vermeulen C, Leynadier F. Angio-oedeme vibraitoire. Ann Dermatol Venereol 2001; 128:750–753.

90. Keahey TM, Indrisano J, Lavker RM, et al. Delayed vibratory angioedema: insights into pathophysiologic mechanisms. J Allergy Clin Immunol 1987; 8:831–838.

91. Moore-Robinson M, Warin RP. Some clinical aspects of cholinergic urticaria. Br J Dermatol 1968; 80:794–799.

92. Hirschmann JV, Lawlor F, English JSC, et al. Cholinergic urticaria. A clinical and histologic study. Arch Dermatol 1987; 123:462–467.

93. Tupker RA, Doeglas HMG. Water vapour loss threshold and induction of cholinergic urticaria. Dermatologica 1990; 181:23–25.

94. Zuberbier T, Althaus C, Chantraine-Hess S, et al. Prevalence of cholinergic urticaria in young adults. J Am Acad Dermatol 1994; 31:978–981.

95. Onn A, Levo Y, Kivity S. Familial cholinergic urticaria. J Allergy Clin Immunol 1996; 98: 847–849.

96. Grant RT, Bruce Pearson RS, Comeau WJ. Observations on urticaria provoked by emotion, by exercise and by warming the body. Clin Sci 1936; 2:253–272.

97. Magnus IA, Thompson RS. Cholinesterase activity in human skin. Br J Dermatol 1954; 66: 163–173.

98. Shelley WB, Shelley E, Ho AS. Cholinergic urticaria: acetyl choline-receptor-dependent immediate–type hypersensitivity reaction to copper. Lancet i 1983; 843–846.

99. Murphy GM, Smith SE, Smith SA, et al. Autonomic function in cholinergic urticaria and atopic eczema. Br J Dermatol 1984; 110:581–586.

100. Illig L, Heinicke A. Zur Pathogenese der cholinergischen Urticaria. IV. Zur Frage einer echten Antigen-Antikörper Reaktion. Arch Klin Exp Dermatol 1967; 229:360–371.

101. Adachi J, Aoki T, Yamatodani A. Demonstration of sweat allergy in cholinergic urticaria. J Dermatol Sci 1994; 142:142–149.

102. Kobayashi H, Aiba S, Yamagishi T, et al. Cholinergic urticaria, a new pathogenic concept: hypohidrosis due to interference with the delivery of sweat to the skin surface. Dermatology 2002; 204:173–178.

103. Rho N-K. Cholinergic urticaria and hypohidrosis: a clinical reappraisal. Dermatology 2006; 213:357–358.

104. Fukunaga A, Toshinori B, Tsuru K, et al. Responsiveness to autologous sweat and serum in cholinergic urticaria classifies its clinical subtypes. J Allergy Clin Immunol 2005; 116: 397–402.

105. Sabroe RA, Grattan CEH, Francis DM, et al. The autologous serum skin test: a screening test for autoantibodies in chronic idiopathic urticaria. Br J Dermatol 1999; 140:446–452.

106. Wong E, Eftekhari N, Greaves MW, et al. Beneficial effects of danazol on symptoms and laboratory changes in cholinergic urticaria. Br J Dermatol 1987; 116:553–556.

107. Udassin R, Harari Z, Shoenfeld Y, et al. Cholinergic urticaria: a seasonal disease. Arch Intern Med 1981; 141:1029–1030.

108. Lawrence CM, Jorrizo JL, Kobza-Black A, et al. Cholinergic urticaria associated with angio-oedema. Br J Dermatol 1981; 105:543–550.

109. Kounis NG, McMahon RG. Cholinergic urticaria with systemic manifestations. Annals of Allergy 1975; 35:143–145.

110. Czarnetzki BM, Galinski C, Meister R. Cutaneous and pulmonary reactivity in cholinergic urticaria. Br J Dermatol 1984; 110:587–590.

111. Soter NA, Wasserman SI, Austen KF, et al. Release of mast-cell mediators and alterations in lung function in patients with cholinergic urticaria. N Engl J Med 1980; 302:604–608.

112. Kaplan AP, Natbony SF, Tawil AP, et al. Exercise-induced anaphylaxis as a manifestation of cholinergic urticaria. J Allergy Clin Immunol 1981; 68:319–324.

113. Sheffer AL, Soter NA, McFadden ER, et al. Exercise-induced anaphylaxis. A distinct form of physical allergy. J Allergy Clin Immunol 1983; 73:311–316.

114. Commens CA, Greaves MW. Tests to establish the diagnosis in cholinergic urticaria. Br J Dermatol 1978; 98:47–51.

115. Mc Clean SP, Arreaza EE, Lett-Brown MA, et al. Refractory cholinergic urticaria successfully treated with ketotifen. J Allergy Clin Immunol 1989; 83:738–41.

116. Tudoric N, Plavec D, Klepac T, et al. Adding montelukast leads to successful prevention of exercise-induced cholinergic urticaria. Allergy 2002; 57(suppl. 73):316 P.

117. Pachor ML, Lunardi C, Nicolis F, et al. Utilita del propranololo nel trattamento dell'orticaria colinergica. La Clinica Terapeutica 1987; 120:205–210.

118. Tsunemi Y, Ihn H, Saeki H, et al. Cholinergic urticaria successfully treated with scopolamine butylbromide. Int J Dermatol 2003; 42:850.

119. Nomland R. Cholinergic urticaria and cholinogenic itching. Arch Derm Syph 1944; 50: 247–250.

120. Berth-Jones J, Graham-Brown RAC. Cholinergic pruritus, erythema and urticaria: a disease spectrum responding to danazol. Br J Dermatol 1989; 121:235–237.

121. Duffull SB, Begg EJ. Terfenadine ineffective in the prophylaxis of exercise –induced pruritus. J Allergy Clin Immunol 1992; 89:916–917.

122. Murphy GM, Kobza Black A, Greaves MW. Persistent cholinergic erythema: a variant of cholinergic urticaria. Br J Dermatol 1983; 109:343–348.

123. Kaplan AP, Garofalo J. Identification of a new physically induced urticaria—cold induced cholinergic urticaria. J Allergy Clin Immunol 1981; 68:438–441.

124. Delorme P. Localized heat urticaria. J Allergy 1969; 43:284–291.

125. Greaves MW, Sneddon IB, Smith AK, et al. Heat urticaria. Br J Dermatol 1974; 90:289–292.

126. Chang A, Zic JA. Localized heat urticaria. J Am Acad Dermatol 1999; 41:354–356.

127. Martin-Munoz MF, Munoz-Robles ML, Gonzales P, et al. Immediate heat urticaria in a child. Br J Derm 2002; 147; 813–814.

128. Atkins PC, Zweiman B. Mediator release in local heat urticaria. J Allergy Clin Immunol 1981; 68:286–289.

129. Irwin RB, Lieberman P, Friedman MM, et al. Mediator release in local heat urticaria: Protection with combined H1 and H2 antagonists. J Allergy Clin Immunol 1985; 76:35–39.

130. Koro O, Dover JS, Francis DM, et al. Release of prostaglandin D2 and histamine in a case of localized heat urticaria, and effect of treatments. Br J Dermatol 1986; 115:721–728.

131. Koh YI. Choi IS, Lee S-H, et al. Localized heat urticaria associated with mast cell and eosinophil degranulation. J Allergy Clin Immunol 2002; 109:714–715.

132. Daman L, Lieberman P, Ganier M, et al. Localized heat urticaria. J Allergy Clin Immunol 1978; 61:273–278.

133. Johansson EA, Reunala T, Koskimies S, et al. Localized heat urticaria associated with a decrease in serum complement factor B (C3 proactivator). Br J Dermatol 1984; 110:227–231.

134. Grant JA, Findlay SR, Thueson DO, et al. Local heat urticaria/angioedema: evidence for histamine release without complement activation. J Allergy Clin Immunol 1981; 67:75–77.

135. Fukunaga A, Shimoura S, Fukunaga M, et al. Localized heat urticaria in a patient is associated with a wealing response to heated autologous serum. Br J Dermatol 2002; 147:994–997.

136. Willis I, Epstein JH. Solar-vs heat-induced urticaria. Arch Dermatol 1974; 110:389–392.

137. Baba T, Nomura K, Hanada K, et al. Immediate-type heat urticaria: report of a case and study of plasma histamine Br J Dermatol 1998; 138:326–328.

138. Neittaanmäki H, Fräki JE. Combination of localized heat urticaria and cold urticaria. Release of histamine in suction blisters and successful treatment of heat urticaria with doxepin. Clin Experimental Dermatol 1988; 13:87–91.

139. Darling M, Lambiase MC, Hodson DS. Localized heat induced urticaria: report of a case. J Drugs Dermatol 2004; 3:75–76.

140. Leigh IM, Ramsay CA. Localized heat urticaria treated by inducing tolerance to heat. Br J Dermatol 1975; 92:191–194.

141. Higgins EM, Friedmann PS. Clinical report and investigation of a patient with localized heat urticaria. Acta Derm Venereol (Stockh) 1991; 71:434–436.

142. Michäelsson G, Ros A-M. Familial localized heat urticaria of the delayed type. Acta Dermatovener (Stock) 1971; 51:279–283.

143. Black AK. Cold urticaria. Semin Dermatol 1987; 6:292–301.

144. Wanderer AA. Cold urticaria syndromes: historical background, diagnostic classification, clinical and laboratory characteristics, pathogenesis, and management. J Allergy Clin Immunol 1990; 85:965–981.

145. Neittaanmäki H. Cold urticaria. Clinical findings in 220 patients. J Am Acad Dermatol 1985; 13:636–644.

146. Claudy A. Cold urticaria. J Invest Dermatol Symposium Proceedings 2001; 6:141–142.

147. Siebenhaar F, Weller K, Mlynek A, et al. Acquired cold urticaria: clinical picture and update on diagnosis and treatment. Clin Exp Dermatol 2007; 32:241–245.

148. Alangari AA, Twarog FJ, Shih M-C, et al. Clinical features and anaphylaxis in children with cold urticaria. Pediatrics 2004; 113:313–317.

149. Bentley-Phillips CB, Kobza Black A, Greaves MW. Induced tolerance in cold urticaria caused by cold-evoked histamine release. Lancet 1976; ii:63–66.

150. Kaplan AP, Horakova Z, Katz SI. Assessment of tissue fluid histamine levels in patients with cold urticaria. J Allergy Clin Immunol 1978; 61:350–354.

151. Andersson T, Wardell K, Anderson C. Human in vivo cutaneous microdialysis: estimation of hiastamine release in cold urticaria. Acta Derm Venereol (Stock) 1995; 75:353–357.

152. Kobza Black A, Keahey TM, Eady RAJ, et al. Dissociation of histamine release and clinical improvement following treatment of acquired cold urticaria by prednisone. Br J Pharmac 1981; 12:327–331.

153. Lawlor F, Kobza Black A, Breathnach AS, et al. A timed study of the histopathology, direct immunofluorescence and ultrastructural findings in idiopathic cold- contact urticaria over a 24-h period. Clin Exp Dermatol 1989; 14:416–420.

154. Kaplan AP, Garofalo J, Sigler R, et al. Idiopathic cold urticaria: in vitro demonstration of histamine release upon challenge of skin biopsies. N Engl J Med 1981; 18:1074–1077.

155. Misch K, Kobza Black A, Greaves MW, et al. Passive transfer of idiopathic cold urticaria to monkeys. Acta Dermatovener (Stockh) 1983; 63:163–164.

156. Katayama I, Doi T, Nishioka K. Possibility of passive transfer of cold urticaria to guinea pigs. J Dermatol 1984; 11:259–262.

157. Wanderer AA, Maselli R, Ellis EF, et al. Immunological characterization of serum factors responsible for cold urticaria. J Allergy Clin Immunol 1971; 48:13–18.

158. Wanderer AA. A potential new therapy for cold urticaria. J Allergy Clin Immunol 2007; 119:517.

159. Marone G, Florio G, Petraroli A, et al. Dysregulation of the IgE/Fc epsilon network in HIV-1 infection. J Allergy Clin Immunol 2001; 107:22–30.

160. Doeglas HMG, Rijnten WJ, Schröder FP, et al. Cold urticaria and virus infections: a clinical and serological study. Br J Dermatol 1986; 114:311–318.

161. Wasserman SI, Soter NA, Center DM, et al. Cold urticaria. Recognition and characterization of a neutrophil chemoctactic factor which appears in the serum during experimental challenge. J Clin Invest 1977; 60:189–196.

162. Wasserman SI, Austen KF, Soter NA. The functional and physiochemical characterization of three eosinophilic activities released into the circulation by cold challenge of patients with cold urticaria. Clin Exp Immunol 1982; 47:570–578.

163. Ormerod AD, Heavey DJ, Kobza Black A, et al. Prostaglandin D2 and histamine release in cold urticaria unaccompanied by evidence of platelet activation. J Allergy Clin Immunol 1988; 82:586–589.

164. Maltby NH, Ind PW, Causon RC, et al. Leukotriene E4 release in cold urticaria. Clin Exp Allergy 1989; 19:33–36.

165. Nuutinen P, Harvima IT, Ackermann L. Histamine but not leukotriene C4, is an essential mediator of cold urticaria wheals. Acta Derm Venereol 2007; 87:9–13.

166. Grandel KE, Farr RS, Wanderer AA, et al. Association of platelet-activating factor with primary acquired cold urticaria. N Engl J Med 1985; 313:405–409.

167. Tillie-Leblond I, Gosset P, Janin A, et al. Tumor necrosis-α release during systemic reaction in cold urticaria. J Allergy Clin Immunol 1994; 93:501–509.

168. Doeglas H, Bleumink E. Protease inhibitors in plasma of patients with chronic urticaria. Arch Dermatol 1975; 111:979–985.

169. Buss Y-L, Sticherling M. Cold urticaria; disease course and outcome- an investigation of 85 patients before and after therapy. Br J Dermatol 2005; 153:440–441.

170. Mesko JW, Wu LYF. Infectious mononucleosus and cold urticaria. JAMA 1982; 248:828.

171. Morais-Almeida M, Marinho S, Gaspar A, et al. Cold urticaria and infectious mononucleosis in children. Allergologia et immunopathologia 2004; 32; 368–371.

172. Husz S, Toth-Kasa I, Kiss M, et al. Treatment of cold urticaria. Int J Dermatol 1994; 33:210–213.

173. Koeppel MC, Bertrand S, Abitan R, et al. Urticaire au Froid. 104 cas. Ann Dermatol Venereol 1996; 123:627–632.

174. Yu RC, Evans B, Cream JJ. Cold urticaria, raised IgE and HIV infection. J R Soc Med 1995; 88:294–295.

175. Hogendijk S, Hauser C. Wasp sting-associated cold urticaria. Allergy 1997; 52:1144–1145.

176. Kalogeromitros D, Gregoriou S, Papaioannou D, et al. Acquired primary cold contact urticaria after Hymenoptera sting. Clin Exp Dermatol 2004; 29:93–95.

177. Muller SA. Urticarial sensitivity to cold in the tropics. Arch Dermatol 1961; 83:930–933.

178. Visiuthorn N, Tuchida M, Vichyanond P. Cold urticaria in Thai children: comparison between cyproheptadine and ketotifen in the treatment. Asian Pacific J allergy Immunol 1995; 13: 29–33.

179. Van der Valk PGM, Moret G, Kiemeny LALM. The natural history of chronic urticaria and angioedema in patients visiting a tertiary referral centre. Br J Dermatol 2002; 146:110–113.

180. Sarkany I, Gaylarde PM. Negative reactions to ice in cold urticaria. Br J Dermatol 1971; 85:46–48.

181. Fitzgerald DA, Heagerty AHM, English JSC. Cold urticaria as an occupational dermatosis. Contact Dermatitis 1995; 32:238.

182. Mathelier-Fusade P, Aissaoui M, Bakhos D, et al. Clinical predictive factors of severity of cold urticaria. Arch Dermatol 1998; 134:106–107.

183. Burroughs JR, Patrinely JR, Nugent JS, et al. Cold urticaria: an under-recognized cause of postsurgical periorbital swelling. Ophthal Plast Reconstr Surg 2005; 21:327–30.

184. Johnston WE, Moss J, Philbin DM, et al. Management of cold urticaria during hypothermic cardiopulmonary bypass. New Engl J Medicine, 1882; 306:219–221.

185. Lancey RA, Schaefer OP, McCormick MJ. Coronary artery bypass grafting and aortic valve replacement with cold cardioplegia in a patient with cold-induced urticaria. Ann Allergy Asthma Immunol 2004; 92:273–275.

186. Möller A, Henning M, Zuberbier T, et al. Epidemiologie und Klinik der Kälteurtikaria. Hautarzt 1996; 47:510–514.

187. Henquet CJM, Martens BPM, Van Vloten WA. Cold urticaria: a clinico-therapeutic study in 30 patients; with special emphasis on cold desensitization. Eur J Dermatol 1992; 2:75–77.

188. Magerl M, Schmolke J, Siebenhaar F, et al. Acquired cold urticaria symptoms can be safely prevented by ebastine. Allergy 2007; 62:1465–1468.

189. Tosoni C, Lodi-Rizzini F, Bettoni L, et al. Cinnarazine is a useful and well-tolerated drug in the treatment of acquired cold urticaria (ACU). Europ J Dermatol 2003; 13:54–56.

190. Villas Martinez F, Contreras FJ, Lopez-Cazana JM, et al. A comparison of new nonsedating and classical antihistamines in the treatment of primary acquired cold urticaria. J Invest Allergol Clin Immunol 1992; 2:258–262.

191. Hani N, Hartmannn K, Casper C, et al. Improvement of cold urticaria by treatment with the leukotriene receptor antagonist montelukast. Arch Derm Vener 2000; 80:229.

192. Bonadonna P, Lombardi C, Gianenrico S, et al. Treatment of acquired cold urticaria with cetirizine and zafirkulast in combination. J Am Acad Dermatol 2003; 49:714–716.

193. Von Mackensen YA, Sticherling M. Cold urticaria: tolerance induction with cold baths. Br J Dermatol 2007; 157:835–836.

194. Kobza Black A, Sibbald RG, Greaves MW. Cold urticaria treated by induction of tolerance. Lancet II, 1979:964.

195. Keahey TM, Indrisano J, Kaliner MA. A case study on the induction of clinical tolerance in cold urticaria. J Allergy Clin Immunol 1988; 82:256–261.

196. Marsland AM, Beck MH. Cold urticaria responding to systemic ciclosporin. Br J Dermatol 2003; 149:214–215.

197. Boyce JA. Successful treatment of cold-induced urticaria/anaphylaxis with anti-IgE. J Allergy Clin Immunol 2006; 117:1415–1418.

198. Constanzi JJ, Coltman CA. Kappa chain cold precipitable immunoglobulin G (IgG) associated with cold urticaria. 1. Clinical observations. Clin Exp Immunol 1967; 2:167–178.

199. Smith SB, Arkin C. Cryofibrinogenemia: incidence, clinical correlations and a review of the literature. Am J Clin Pathol 1972; 58:524–530.

200. Houser DD, Arbesman CE, Ito K, et al. Cold urticaria: immunologic studies. Am J Med 1970; 49: 23–33.

201. Pruzanski W, Shumak KH. Biological activity of cold-reacting autoantibodies (Second of two parts). N Engl J Med 1977; 297:583–589.

202. Bäck O, Larsen A. Delayed cold urticaria. Acta Dermatovener 1978; 58:369–371.

203. Sarkany I, Turk JL. Delayed hypersensitivity to cold. Proc R Soc Med 1965; 58:622–623.

204. Juhlin L. Cold urticaria with persistent weals. Br J Dermatol 1981; 104:705–707.

205. Soter NA, Joshi NP, Twarog FJ, et al. Delayed cold-induced urticaria. J Allergy Clin Immunol 1977; 59:294–297.

206. Eady RAJ, Keahey TM, Sibbald RG, et al. Cold urticaria with vasculitis: report of a case with light and electron microscopic, immunofluorescence and pharmacological studies. Clin Exper Dermatol 1981; 6:355–366.

207. Solomon LM, Strauss H, Leznoff A. Localized secondary cold urticaria. Arch Dermatol 1966; 94:156.

208. Kurtz AS, Kaplan AP. Regional expression of cold urticaria. J Allergy Clin Immunol 1990; 86: 272–273.

209. Mathelier-Fusade P. Leynadier F. Localized cold urticaria. Br J Dermatol 1995; 132:666–667.

210. Garcia F, Blanco J, Perez R, et al. Localized cold urticaria associated with immunotherapy. Allergy 1998; 53:110–111.

211. Czarnetzki BM, Frosch PJ, Sprekeler R. Localized cold reflex urticaria. J Allergy Clin Immunol 1981; 104:83–87.

212. Matthews CNA, Warin RP. Cold urticaria and cold precipitated dermographism. Br J Dermatol 1970; 82:91.

213. Kaplan AP. Unusual cold-induced disorders: cold dependent dermographism and systemic cold urticaria. J Allergy Cilin Immunol 1984; 73:453–456.

214. Shelley WB, Caro WA. Cold erythema. A new hypersensitivity syndrome. JAMA 1962; 180: 639–642.

215. Hoffman HM, Wanderer AA, Broide DH. Familial cold autoinflammatory syndrome: phenotype and genotype of an autosomal dominant periodic fever. J Allergy Clin Immunol 2001; 108:615–620.

216. Aganna E, Martinin F, Hawkins PN, et al. Association of mutations in the NALP3/CIAS1/PYPAK1 gene with a broad phenotype including recurrent fever, cold sensitivity, sensineural deafness and AA amyloidosis. Arthritis Rheum 2002; 46:2445–2452.

217. Hoffman HM, Rosengren S, Boyle DL, et al. Prevention of cold –associated acute inflammation in familial cold autoinflammatory syndrome by interleukin-1 receptor antagonist. Lancet 2004; 364:1779–1785.

218. Shinkai K, McCalmont TH, Leslie KS. Cryopyrin-associated periodic syndromes and autoinflammation. Clin Exp Dermatol 2008; 33:1–9.

219. Ormerod AD, Smart L, Reid TMS, et al. Familial cold urticaria. Investigation of a family and response to stanozolol. Arch Dermatol 1993; 129:343–346.

220. Illig L, Paul E, Bruck K, Experimental investigations on the trigger mechanism of the generalized type of heat and cold urticaria by means of a climatic chamber. Acta Derm Venereol (Stockh) 1980; 60:373–380.

221. Kivity S, Schwartz Y, Wolf R, et al. Systemic cold-induced urticaria—Clinical and laboratory characterization. J Allergy Clin Immunol 1990; 85:52–54.

222. Geller M. Cold-induced cholinergic urticaria. Annals of Allergy; 63:29–30.

223. Horan RF, Sheffer AL. Exercise-induced anaphylaxis. Immunology and Allergy Clinics of North America 1992; 12:559–569.

224. Romano A, Di Fonso M, Giuffreda F. Exercise-induced anaphylaxis. International J Immunopathology & Parmacology 1997; 10:95–99.

225. Volcheck GW, Li JTC. Exercise-induced urticaria and anaphylaxis Mayo Clin Proc 1997; 72: 140–147.

226. Casale TB, Keahey TM, Kaliner M. Exercise-induced anaphylactic syndromes. Insights into diagnostic and pathophysiologic features. JAMA 1986; 255:2049–2053.

227. Chong SU, Worm M, Zuberbier T. Role of adverse reactions to food in urticaria and exercise-induced anaphylaxis. Int Arch Allergy Immunol 2002; 129:19–26.

228. Sheffer AL, Tong AKF, Murphy GF, et al. Exercise-induced anaphylaxis: a serious form of physical allergy associated with mast cell degranulation. J Allergy Clin Immunol 1985; 75:479–484.

229. Wade S, Liang MH, Sheffer AL. Exercise-induced anaphylaxis: epidemiologic observations. Prog Clin Biol Res 1989; 297:175–182.

230. Longley S, Panush RS. Familial exercise-induced anaphylaxis. Ann Allergy 1987; 68: 257–259.

231. Dohi M, Suko M, Sugiyama H, Food-dependent, exercise-induced anaphylaxis: a study of 11 Japanese cases. J Allergy Clin Immunol 1991; 87:34–40.

232. Kivity S, Sneh E, Greif J, et al. The effect of food and exercise on the skin response to compound 48/80 in patients with food-associated exercise-induced urticaria-angioedema. J Allergy Clin Immunol 1988; 81:1155–1158.

233. Hanakawa Y, Tohyama M, Shirakata Y, et al. Food-dependent exercise-induced anaphylaxis: a case related to the amount of food allergen ingested. Br J Dermatol 1998; 138:898–900.

234. Harada S, Horikawa T, Ashida M, et al. Aspirin enhances the induction of type 1 allergic symptoms when combined with food and exercise in patient with food-dependent exercise-induced anaphylaxis. Br J Dermatol 2001; 145:336–339.

235. Briner WW Jr. Physical allergies and excercise. Clinical implications for those engaged in sports activities. Sports Medicine 1993; 15:365–373.

236. Caffarelli C, Cavagni G, Giordano S, et al. Reduced pulmonary function in multiple food-induced, exercise-related episodes of anaphylaxis. J Allergy Clin Immunol 1986; 98:762–765.

237. Juji F, Suko M. Effectiveness of disodium cromoglycate in food-dependent, exercise-induced anaphylaxis: a case report. Annals of Allergy 1994; 72:452–454.

238. Kidd III JM, Cohen SH, Sosman AJ, et al. Food-dependent exercise-induced anaphylaxis. J Allergy Clin Immunol 1983; 71:407–411.

239. Ii M, Sayama K, Tohyama M, et al. A case of cold-dependent exercise-induced anaphylaxis. Br J Dermatol 2002; 147:368–370.

240. Leenutaphong V, Hölzle E, Plewig G. Pathogenesis and classification of solar urticaria: a new concept. J Am Acad Dermatol 1989; 21:237–40.

241. Roelandts R. Diagnosis and treatment of solar urticaria. Dermatologic Therapy 2003; 16:52–56.

242. Beattie PE, Dawe RS, Ibbotson SH, et al. Characteristics and prognosis of idiopathic solar urticaria. Arch Dermatol 2003; 139:1149–1154.
243. Horio T. Solar urticaria-idiopathic? Photodermatol Photoimmunol Photomed 2003; 19:147–154.
244. Mekkes JR, de Vries HJC, Kammeyer A. Solar urticaria inducd by infrared radiation. Clin Exp Dermatol 2003; 28:222–223.
245. Kojima M, Horiko T, Nakamura Y, et al. Solar urticaria. The relationship of photoallergen and action spectrum. Arch Dermatol 1986; 122:550–555.
246. Hawk JLM, Eady RAJ, Challoner AVJ, et al. Elevated blood histamine levels and mast cell degranulation in solar urticaria. Br J Clin Pharmac. 1980; 9:183–186.
247. Keahey TM, Lavker RM, Kaidbey KH, et al. Studies on the mechanism of clinical tolerance in solar urticaria. Br J Dermatol 1984; 110:327–338.
248. Norris PG, Murphy GM, Hawk JLM, et al. A histological study of the evolution of solar urticaria. Arch Dermatol 1988; 124:80–83.
249. Neittaanmäki H, Jääskeläinen T, Harvima RJ, et al. Solar urticaria: demonstration of histamine relase and effective treatment with doxepin. Photodermatology 1989; 6:52–55.
250. Soter NA, Wasserman SI, Pathak MA, et al. Solar urticaria: release of mast cell mediators into the circulation on experimental challenge. J Invest Dermatol 1979; 72:282A.
251. Kerr HA, Lim HW. Photodermatoses in African Americans: a retrospective analysis of 135 patients over a 7-year period. Am J Acad Dermatol 2007; 57:638–643.
252. Uetsu N, Miyauchi-Hashimoto H, Okamoto H, et al. The clinical and photobiological characteristics of solar urticaria in 40 patients. Br J Dermatol 2000; 142:32–38.
253. Monfrecola G, Masturzo E, Riccardo AM, et al. Solar urticaria: a report of 57 cases. Am J Contact Dermatitis 2000; 11:89–94.
254. Harris A, Burge SM, George SA. Solar urticaria in an infant. Br J Dermatol 1997; 136:105–107.
255. Williams-Arya P, Hogan MB, Wilson NW. Solar urticaria in a 6-year old child. Ann Allergy Asthma Immunol 1996; 76:141–143.
256. Farr PM. Solar urticaria. Br J Dermatol 2000; 142:4–5.
257. Ryckaert S, Roelandts R. Solar urticaria: a report of 25 cases and difficulties in phototesting. Arch Dermatol 1998; 134:71–74.
258. Rose RF, Bhusan M, King CM, Rhodes. Solar angioedema: an uncommonly recognized condition? Photodermatol Photoimmunol Photomed 2005; 21:226–228.
259. Dawe RS, Clark C, Ferguson J. Porphyria cutanea tarda presenting as solar urticaria. Br J Dermatol 1999; 141:590–591.
260. Yap LM, Foley PA, Crouch RB, et al. Drug-induced solar urticaria due to tetracycline. Australas J Dermatol 2000; 41:181–184.
261. Kurumaji Y, Shono M. Drug-induced solar urticaria due to repirinast. Dermatology 1994; 188: 17–21.
262. Morison WL. Solar urticaria due to progesterone compounds in oral contraceptives. Photodermatol Photoimmunol Photomed 2003; 19:155–156.
263. Ive H, Lloyd J, Magnus IA. Action spectra in idiopathic solar urticaria. A study of 17 cases with a monochromator. Br J Dermatol 1965; 77:229–243.
264. Alora MB, Taylor CR. Solar urticaria: a case report and phototesting with lasers. J Am Acad Dermatol 1998; 38:341–343.
265. Ng JCH, Foley PA, Crouch RB, et al. Changes of photosensitivity and action spectrum with time in solar urticaria. Photodermatol Photoimmunol Photomed 2002; 18:191–195.
266. Ramsay CA. Solar urticaria. Int J Dermatol 1980; 19:233–236.
267. Leenutaphgong V, Von Kries R, Hölzle E, et al. Solar urticaria induced by visile light and inhibited by UVA. Photodermatol 1988; 5:170–174.
268. Watanabe M, Matsunaga Y, Katayama I. Solar urticaria: A consideration of the mechanism of inhibition spectra. Dermatology 1999; 198:252–255.
269. Beissert S, Ständer H, Schwartz. UVA rush hardening for the treatment of solar urticaria. J Am Acad Dermatol 2000; 42:1030–1032.
270. Parrish JA, Jaenicke KF, Morison WL, et al. Solar urticaria: treatment with PUVA and mediator inhibitors. Br J Dermatol 1982; 106:575–580.

271. Ramsay CA. Solar urticaria. Treatment by inducing tolerance to artificial radiation and natural sunlight. Arch Dermatol 1977; 113:1222–1225.

272. Leenatuphong V, Hölzle E, Plewig G. Solar urticaria: studies on the mechanism of tolerance. Br J Dermatol 1990; 122:601–606.

273. Duschet P, Leyen P, Schwarz T, et al. Solar urticaria- effective treatment by plasmapheresis. Clin Experimental Dermatol 1987; 12:185–158.

274. Leenutaphong V, Hölzle E, Plewig G, et al. Plamapheresis in solar urticaria. Photo-dermatology 1987; 4:308–309.

275. Bissonnette R, Buskard N, McLean DI, et al. Treatment of refractory solar urticaria with plasma exchange. J Cutan Med Surg 1999; 3:236–238.

276. Collins P, Ahamat R, Green C, et al. Plasma exchange therapy for solar urticaria. Br J Dermatol 1996; 134:1093–1097.

277. Hudson-Peacock MJ, Farr PM, Diffey BL, et al. Combined treatment of solar urticaria with plasmapheresis and PUVA. Br J Dermatol 1993; 128:440–442.

278. Puech-Plottova I, Michel JL, Rouchouse B, et al. Urticaire solaire: un cas traite par immunoglobulines polyvalentes. Ann Dermatol Venereol 2000; 127:831–835.

279. Darras S, Ségard M, Mortier L, et al. Treatment of solar urticaria by intravenous immunoglobulins and PUVA therapy. (article in Fr) Ann Dermatol Venereol 2004; 131:65–69.

280. Edstrom DW, Ros AM. Cyclosporin therapy of severe solar urticaria. Photodermatol Photoimmunol Photomed. 1997; 13:61–63.

281. Mang R, Stege H, Budde MA, et al. Successful treatment of solar urticaria by extracorporeal photochemotherapy (photopheresis)- case report. Photodermatol Photoimmunol Photomed 2002; 18:196–198.

282. Torinuki W. Two patients with solar urticaria manifesting pruritic erythema. The J of Dermatol 1992; 19:635–637.

283. Reinauer S, Leenutaphong V, Hölzle E. Fixed solar urticaria. J Am Acad Dermatol 1993; 29: 161–165.

284. Schwarze HP, Marguery MC, Journe F, et al. Fixed solar urticaria to visible light sucessfully treated with fexofenadine. Photodermatology and Immunology and Photomedicine 2001; 17: 39–41.

285. Monfrecola G, Nappa P, Pini D. Solar urticariawith a delayed onset: a case report. Photodermatology 1988; 5:103–104.

286. Armstrong RB, Horan DB, Silvers DN. Leukocytoclastic vasculitis in urticaria induced by ultraviolet irradiation. Arch Dermatol 1985; 121:1145–1148.

287. Shelley WB, Rawnsley HM. Aquagenic urticaria. JAMA 1964; 189:895–898.

288. Panconesi E, Lotti T. Aquagenic urticaria. Clin Dermatol 1987; 5:49–51.

289. Luong KV, Nguyen LT. Aquagenic urticaria: a case report and review of the literature. Ann Allergy Asthma Immunol 1998; 80:483–485.

290. Wasserman D, Preminger A, Zlotogorski A. Aquagenic urticaria in a child. Pediatr Dermatol 1994; 11:29–30.

291. Frances AM, Fiorenza G, Frances RJ. Aquagenic urticaria: report of a case. Allergy Asthma Proc. 2004; 25:195–197.

292. Bonnetblanc JM, Andrieu-Pfahl F, Meraud JP, et al. Familial aquagenic urticaria. Dermatologica 1979; 158:468–470.

293. Treudler R, Tebbe B, Steinhoff M, et al. Familial aquagenic urticaria associated with familial lactose intolerance. J Am Acad Dermatol 2002; 47:611–613.

294. Pitarch G, Torrijos A, Martinez-Menchón T, et al. Familial aquagenic urticaria and Bernard-Soulier Syndrome. Dermatology 2006; 212:96–97.

295. Czarnetzki BM, Breetholt K-H, Traupe H. Evidence that water acts as a carrier for an epidermal antigen in aquagenic urticaria. J Am Acad Dermatol 1986; 15:623–627.

296. Sibbald RG, Kobza Black A, Eady RAJ, et al. Aquagenic urticaria: evidence of cholinergic and histaminergic basis. Br J Dermatol 1981; 105:297–302.

297. Giminez - Arnau A, Serra-Baldrich E, Camarasa JG. Chronic aquagenic urticaria. Acta Derm Venereol 1992; 72:389.

298. Harwood CA, Kobza Black A. Aquagenic urticaria masquerading as occupational penicillin allergy. Br J Dermatol 1992; 127:547–548.

299. Martinez-Escribano JA, Quecedo E, De la Cuedra J, Treatment of aquagenic urticaria with PUVA and astemizole. J Am Acad Dermatol 1997; 36:118–119.

300. Blanco J, Ramirez M, Garcia F, et al. Localized aquagenic urticaria. Contact Dermatitis 2000; 42:303–304.

301. Gallo R, Cacciapuoti M, Cozzani E, et al. Localized aquagenic urticaria dependent on saline concentration. Contact Dermatitis 2001; 44:110–111.

302. Bayle P, Gadroy A, Messer L, et al. Localized aquagenic urticaria: efficacy of a barrier cream. Contact Dermatitis 2003; 49:160–161.

303. Baptist AP, Baldwin JL. Aquagenic urticaria with extracutaneous manifestations. Allergy and Asthma Proc. 2005; 217:217–220.

304. Hide M, Yamamura Y, Sanada S, et al. Aquagenic urticaria: a case report. Acta Derm Venereol 2000; 80:148–149.

305. Davis RS, Remigio LK, Schocket AL, et al. Evaluation of a patient with both aquagenic and cholinergic urticaria. J Allergy Clin Immunol 1981; 68:469–483.

306. Mathelier-Fusade P, Aissaoui M, Chabane MH, et al. Association of cold and aquagenic urticaria. Allergy 1997; 52:678–679.

307. Fearfield LA, Gazzard B, Bunker CB. Aquagenic urticaria and human deficiency virus infection: treatment with stanozolol. Br J Dermatol 1997; 137:620–622.

308. Greaves MW, Black AK, Eady RAJ, et al. Aquagenic pruritus. Br Med J 1981; 282:2007–2010.

309. Steinman H, Greaves MW. Aquagenic pruritus. J Am Acad Dermatol 1985; 13:91–96.

310. Juhlin L, Malmros-Enander I. Familial polymorphous light eruption associated with aquagenic urticaria: successful treatment with PUVA. Photodermatol 1986; 3:346–349.

311. Chalamidas SL, Charles CR. Aquagenic urticaria. Arch Dermatol 1971; 104; 541–546.

312. Shelley WB, Shelley ED. Adrenergic urticaria: a new form of stress-induced hives. Lancet 2 1985; 1031–1033.

313. Haustein U-F. Adrenergic urticaria and adrenergic pruritus. Acta Derm Venereol (Stock) 1990; 70:82–84.

314. Maerens-Tchokokam B, Vigan M, Breuillard F, et al. Guess what! Adrenergic urticaria. Eur J Dermatol 1999; 9:137–138.

12

Urticaria and Angioedema in Infancy and Early Childhood

Michael C. Zacharisen
Department of Pediatrics, Medical College of Wisconsin,
Milwaukee, Wisconsin, U.S.A.

INTRODUCTION

When urticaria and angioedema occur in young children, parents can become distressed and frustrated, resulting in multiple calls or visits searching for the cause, hoping to eliminate the culprit, and thus curing the hives. Similarly, urticaria can be frustrating to physicians who weigh the utility of obtaining costly laboratory tests or implementing an elimination diet realizing that both frequently lead to disappointing results. While it is common to treat urticaria and angioedema symptomatically, parental concerns are generally aimed at determining the underlying cause. In young children, there are diverse triggers and disease states that must be borne in mind. While most urticaria is acute, limited and benign in nature, it can be chronic, a sign of a systemic disease, or part of a multisystem allergic reaction.

HISTOLOGY AND PATHOPHYSIOLOGY

The histology in both acute and chronic urticaria is similar despite the various pathogenic mechanisms involved and is the same as urticaria occurring at other ages. Acute urticarial lesions exhibit (*i*) vasodilation, engorgement of capillaries, and small venules; (*ii*) superficial dermal lymphatic vasodilation; (*iii*) widening of dermal papillae; (*iv*) flattening of rete pegs secondary to fluid extravasation and swelling of collagen fibers; and (*v*) minimal perivascular cell infiltrate with or without eosinophils. In contrast to urticarial vasculitis, there is no vascular damage, red cell extravasation, or nuclear debris (1).

Urticaria results from mast cell degranulation releasing preformed mediators such as histamine and newly generated mediators such as eicosanoids, leukotrienes, and prostaglandins. Other mediators include kinins, neuropeptides (substance P, vasoactive intestinal polypeptide, calcitonin gene-related peptide, neuropeptide Y), adenosine triphosphate, neutral proteases, cytokines, and platelet-activating factor.

In chronic urticaria a late-phase-like reaction can occur with the early influx of neutrophils followed within 24 hours by CD4+ lymphocytes. The role of lymphocytes in urticaria is not well defined. In 14 children aged 2 to 11 years with milk-induced urticaria, memory T lymphocytes expressing cutaneous lymphocyte antigen (CLA), a unique skin-homing receptor, were selectively activated compared with children with milk-induced GI symptoms, and control subjects (2). The results are similar to children with milk-induced atopic dermatitis, suggesting a role for CLA antigen in allergic skin conditions.

Pathophysiologic mechanisms to explain urticaria include immune-mediated, complement-mediated, and nonimmune-mediated. Immune-mediated refers to specific IgE bound on mast cells and circulating basophils that release mediators after interaction with a protein. The protein cross-links the bound IgE, resulting in a cascade of events leading to the release of multiple mediators. Complement-mediated urticaria occurs when C3a, C4a, or C5a trigger mast cell degranulation in such disorders as collagen vascular diseases, serum sickness, and blood product reactions. Nonimmune mechanisms include direct degranulation of mast cells without requiring IgE or complement. Urticaria and angioedema can occur after antigen exposure by many routes including, direct local contact, ingestion, inhalation, and injection or through mechanisms occurring internally due to disease states.

EPIDEMIOLOGY

Approximately 15% to 20% of children experience at least one episode of acute, transient urticaria by adolescence (3). A prospective study of 57 children ages 1 to 36 months hospitalized with acute urticaria were evaluated, and 40 of them followed for one to two years. In 92% of cases, a cause was identified or suspected. Infection either associated with or not with drug intake was suspected in 81% of cases. Viral infections predominated. Amoxicillin and cephalosporins were used most commonly and the timing of the urticaria suggested serum sickness. Hemorrhagic lesions were seen in nearly half of these children and in addition to articular symptoms were more frequent in those with infections. Urticaria caused by foods (11%) was accompanied by lip angioedema and frequently associated with atopic dermatitis. Angioedema occurred in 60% of cases. Half of the patients were atopic. This cohort likely represents the more severe spectrum of urticaria since they required hospitalization (4). Compared with adults, the etiologic factors are more readily identified in infants (65%). Acute urticaria is the most common presentation occurring in 85% of children (3); however, a study of 44 children younger than 14 years old, evaluated at a referral center, reported 80% had chronic urticaria (5). Of interest and contrary to the adult population, an etiology was identified in 74% of these children (5).

The trigger of urticaria is influenced by age. Cow's milk allergy is the most common trigger before six months of age, while drug allergy and infections are more frequent triggers between 6 months and 2 years (6).

The natural history of urticaria in children is distinct from adults. A review of 94 children with chronic urticaria revealed that 58% became symptom-free for six months or more, whereas 42% continued to have episodic urticaria (7). A cause in this study was determined in only 16%. In another report of 226 children ages 1 to 14 years with chronic urticaria, only 21% were determined to have a cause. In descending order of frequency, these were 6.2% physical, 4.4% infection, 4% food allergy, 2.6% food additive, 2.2% aeroallergens, and 1.8% drugs (8). The age distribution was not provided, but the mean age was eight years. This contrasts to study of chronic pediatric urticaria, where physical factors were the most common, occurring in 25%, followed by infections (7.3%), food allergy (9%), food additive (1.8%), and drugs (1.7%) (9).

CLINICAL MANIFESTATIONS

Urticaria and angioedema are divided into acute and chronic on the basis of the duration. Symptoms persisting beyond six weeks are classified as chronic.

Urticaria can affect any area of the body, although it usually is absent on the mucus membranes, with the exception of cold urticaria on the tongue or palate. The skin findings can be impressive and occur rapidly with a fluctuating course. The lesions are characteristically pruritic and occur in various patterns ranging from several millimeter-sized wheals with a large, blanching, erythematous flare to round to oval, erythematous raised individual lesions (wheals) with a pale center and pseudopodia with surrounding erythema (Figs. 1, 2). They can appear as diffuse confluent plaques with erythema. The eruption

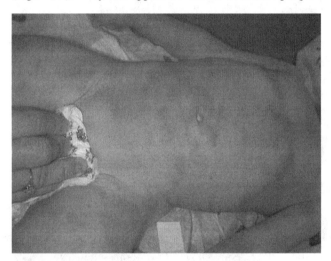

Figure 1 (*See color insert*) Young child with acute urticaria following a viral infection.

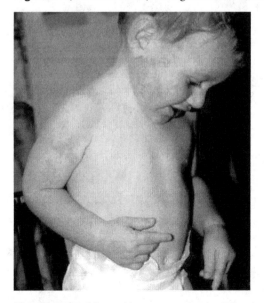

Figure 2 Toddler with acute urticaria following generalized cold air exposure. Note the distribution on the face and extremities.

may last from days to months, but an individual lesion typically lasts less than 24 hours. In urticarial vasculitis, individual lesions persist beyond 48 hours. There is no associated scaling of the skin. Infants may demonstrate extreme fussiness or crying as the intense pruritus may be interpreted as painful stimuli.

Angioedema is similar to urticaria, but affects the deep dermal and subcutaneous or submucosal tissues resulting in non-pitting, nondependent swelling with or without the erythema of urticaria and oftentimes without pruritus. Angioedema can occur on any area of the body, but occurs more frequently in the periorbital region, tongue, lips, and genitals. The frequency that angioedema occurs with urticaria in children ranges from 6% to 60% (4,5,7,10).

CAUSES OF URTICARIA AND ANGIOEDEMA

The various causes of urticaria are outlined in Table 1.

Allergic

Inhalant-Induced Urticaria

Airborne allergens are usually associated with rhinitis or asthma, but the target tissue can be the skin. Of 226 children with chronic urticaria, 3 had symptoms during the grass and tree pollen season only. Two children had cat dander–induced urticaria (8). All of these children also had asthma and/or rhinoconjunctivitis. As most seasonal allergies require two pollen seasons of exposure to sensitize, seasonal airborne allergen triggers would be unlikely in infants.

Food-Induced Urticaria

Urticaria is second only to exacerbations of atopic dermatitis in the manifestation of food allergies. Food allergy accounts for nearly 20% of acute urticaria (11). It can occur via direct contact termed "contact urticaria" (12) or after ingestion leading to perioral or generalized urticaria with or without angioedema. Onset of symptoms after ingestion or contact is minutes to several hours, but less than 24 hours. Two hypotheses account for local and systemic manifestations of food allergy: (*i*) absorption-deposition hypothesis and (*ii*) immune-response hypothesis. The skin as the hyperreactive target organ develops overt hives after exposure within the GI tract (11).

Urticaria induced by foods varies by age; 22% of children zero to three years who have food allergy present with urticaria, while over 40% of children with food allergy 3 to 15 years present in this manner (11). While virtually any food can elicit an allergic reaction, a short list (egg, cow's milk, soybean, wheat, seafood, peanut, and tree nuts) accounts for the vast majority of reactions (11). The most common food allergen to elicit acute urticaria in infants less than six months is cow's milk (6). Occasionally an infant will present with urticaria on the first known exposure to that food. Milk, egg, and peanut proteins may cross into human milk and potentially sensitize the infant during breastfeeding. When the child ingests that food for the "first time," acute urticaria occurs. While in utero sensitization to food proteins has been postulated, other disorders with onset in the neonatal period need to be considered. Food allergy was reported in 2% to 9% of children with chronic urticaria with milk being the most common (7–9).

Other implicated foods include grapes, causing lip angioedema in a five-year-old (13) and urticaria to white potato in two infants less than six months (14). Although tomato is commonly believed responsible for hives, IgE-mediated tomato allergy is very

Table 1 Triggers of Urticaria and Angioedema in Infants and Young Children

Ingestants	Injectants	Contactants	Inhalants	Infectious agents	Physical	Systemic disease/other
Foods	Drugs	Plant substances	Foods	Viral	Dermographism	Vasculitis
Milk	Antibiotics	Latex	Fish/seafood	Hepatitis B	Cold	Henoch-Schonlein purpura
Egg	Blood products	Stinging Nettle		Influenza	Primary acquired	Urticarial vasculitis
Wheat	Antisera		Pollen	Adenovirus	Secondary acquired	SLE, JRA
Soy	Vaccines	Foods	Grass and tree	Enterovirus		
Peanut	IV contrast media	Milk		RSV	Heat	Mast cell infiltration
Fruits/berries	Insulin	Peanut butter		VZV	Cholinergic	Urticaria pigmentosa
Tree nuts	Prostaglandin E1			EBV	Localized heat	Mastocytoma
Seafood		Animal saliva		Rotavirus		
	Stings/bites	Cat and dog			Other	Autoinflammatory syndromes
Additives	Papular urticaria			Bacterial	Solar	NOMID/CINCA
Tartrazine	Mosquito	Insects		Group A strep	Aquagenic	FCAS (cold trigger)
Azo dyes	Flea	Moths		E. coli	Vibratory	Muckle-Wells syndrome
Salicylates	Bedbug	Butterflies				TRAPS
		Caterpillars		Protozoan		
Medications	Hymenoptera			H. pylori		Serum sickness
Antibiotics	vespids	Sealife		Giardia		ALL with eosinophilia
Aspirin	Bees	Portuguese				Langerhans sell
NSAID	Fire ants	Man-o-War				Histiocytosis
Opiates	Spiders					

Abbreviations: NOMID: Neonatal onset multisystem inflammatory disorder; CINCA: Chronic infantile neurologic cutaneous and articular syndrome; TRAPS: TNF-receptor-associated periodic syndrome; FCAS: Familial cold autoinflammatory disorder; SLE: Systemic lupus erythematosus; JRA: Juvenile Rheumatoid arthritis; ALL: Acute lymphoblastic leukemia.

uncommon or not reported. Fresh fruits and berries are also frequently implicated in urticaria, although published data are scarce. Direct histamine-releasing factors may be present in egg white, strawberry, and shellfish. Alternatively, the currently available commercial food extracts for skin testing may lack factors that are present in fresh foods, thus resulting in false-negative skin tests. Prick-on-prick skin testing with fresh fruit has been advocated. Histamine may be present in some foods or as the result of spoilage of various fish species, whereby histadine is converted to histamine, resulting in urticaria upon ingestion.

Food Additive-Induced Urticaria

Preservatives and dyes may be responsible for chronic urticaria through nonimmunologic mechanisms. The difficulty in diagnosis is the lack of a confirmatory skin or in vitro test, thus relying on challenge tests. The wide variation in positive challenge tests may be attributed to predisposing factors, the difference in the quantity of the additive, and the inclusion of uncertain reactions (15). In pediatric studies, the incidence ranges from 2.6% to 18% (8,9). Tartrazine (yellow dye) and salicylates appear to be the most commonly implicated foods (8), yet controlled studies are lacking. Data on natural salicylates in food are contradictory and scarce (16). Commonly reported foods include fruits and vegetables (apple, apricot, orange, cucumber), herbs/spices (cinnamon, curry, thyme), and honey. Other reported sources are birch bark, wintergreen and willow bark. Mint flavored candy, pills, foods, and beverages contain higher levels of salicylates. Aspartame used as a sweetener has been reported to cause urticaria in adults, but has not been reported in children.

Contact Urticaria

Direct antigen exposure and penetration of intact skin resulting in urticaria within minutes to an hour was first described in 1975. Examples of contact urticaria include transfer of the affected allergen by kissing, licking, or spilling upon oneself. This commonly occurs with foods (milk, peanut, egg) and animal saliva or hair (12). Contact with animal saliva or dander can produce acute urticaria either by inhalation or direct skin absorption. Red food colorings E124 and E129 in play dough were responsible for acute contact urticaria on the hands and forearms in a three-year-old child (17).

Latex Allergy–Induced Urticaria

Latex allergy is uncommon in healthy children, but in high-risk groups such as those with neural tube defects, the incidence can reach up to 60%. An atopic two-month-old infant suckling a latex nipple had repeated stridor, suggesting laryngeal angioedema (18). Children with contact urticaria to latex frequently have other IgE-mediated symptoms such as rhinitis and asthma.

Physical Urticaria

This is a common cause of chronic urticaria in children, occurring in 24% (5).

Dermographism

This common urticaria occurs after firm stroking of the skin. This can be performed using a dermographometer or simply stroking the skin with a tongue blade or other rigid object.

Stroking of normal-appearing skin will result in linear wheals along the line of stroking. This commonly occurs after rubbing with a towel or along areas of skin prone to friction.

Cholinergic/Heat-Induced Urticaria

Increases in core body temperature achieved through exercise or external sources such as hot baths or over-bundling result in classic two to four mm punctate wheals with surrounding erythema. The lesions are transient, resolving within two hours. Fever is not a trigger. This frequently coincides with symptomatic dermographism and is most common among teenagers (1). Studies in young children are lacking.

Localized Heat Urticaria

Less than 50 cases of localized heat urticaria have been described and none were in infants, although a familial pattern was reported where older children were affected. Most cases occur in adult females. Treatment options are limited and have been variably effective (19).

Cold Urticaria

In children with primary acquired cold urticaria, wheals and pruritus occur within a few minutes of applying a cold stimulus to the skin. The wheal fades after 30 minutes. Urticaria may occur in the mouth after drinking a cold beverage, while systemic symptoms may occur after immersion in cold water. This type of urticaria is more common in older children and may follow an infection producing cold agglutinins. Histamine is released after cold challenge and can be measured in the plasma (20). Leukotriene E4 is released into the blood draining the site of cold-induced urticaria (21). Secondary acquired cold urticaria is associated with an underlying disorder that results in the production of cryoglobulin, cryofibrinogens, or cold agglutinins. Familial cold urticaria is an autoinflammatory syndrome and addressed in that section.

Vibratory Angioedema

A rare familial form with autosomal dominance has been described in infants (22). It is characterized by swelling without urticaria occurring within minutes of a vibratory stimulus. Symptoms are proportional to the duration and intensity, lasting up to 24 hours.

Solar Urticaria

Six categories of solar urticaria have been described on the basis of the wavelength of light that induces the lesion. While photosensitivity reactions are not uncommon in children, pediatric idiopathic solar urticaria is exquisitely rare. Therefore, in children with recurrent photosensitivity reactions, evaluation for erythropoietic protoporphyria, drug reactions, systemic lupus erythematosus (SLE), xeroderma pigmentosum, polymorphous light eruption, hydroa vacciniforme, and Hartnup's disease should be considered (23). Drugs causing photosensitivity reactions are sulfonamides, chlorpromazine, grizeofulvin, tetracycline, and phenothiazines. Xeroderma pigmentosum is an autosomal-recessive disorder where UV light–induced thymidine dimers cannot be repaired, resulting in severe sunburns in early childhood.

Aquagenic Urticaria

Aquagenic urticaria is extremely rare. Contact with water, regardless of temperature or salinity, induces urticaria through mast cell degranulation. This is distinct from aquagenic pruritus without urticaria. The youngest reported case is a three-year-old. A familial pattern has been described (24,25). Diagnosis is with a room temperature water compress. Small wheals with erythema develop within 30 minutes. Treatment includes rapid drying after bathing, water-occlusive agents, and antihistamines. Other modalities with limited success include PUVA or UVB with hydroxyzine.

Delayed Pressure Urticaria

Delayed pressure urticaria frequently occurs concurrently with chronic idiopathic urticaria (CIU) in adults, but is rare in children. Delayed pressure urticaria was described in a five-year-old child. A majority of patients will have generalized flu-like symptoms and disabling, unremitting symptoms. Over 25% of affected patients will have angioedema. Oral steroids remain the only effective treatment.

Medication-Induced Urticaria

While any medication can cause urticaria, the most commonly implicated agents in pediatrics are antibiotics in the classes of penicillin, cephalosporin, and sulfa. Drugs received orally or parenterally can cause acute urticaria. Drug-induced urticaria may occur through IgE-mediated, complement-mediated, or serum-sickness type reactions.

Antibiotics

Multiple courses of an antibiotic can sensitize and eventually trigger a reaction in a predisposed individual. Penicillin is the most common antibiotic implicated in causing urticaria in infants, likely because this is the most commonly prescribed antibiotic class. Cephalosporins are structurally related to penicillin and by virtue of cross-reactivity can trigger urticaria. Serum sickness is a type III reaction mediated by antigen-antibody complexes deposited in small blood vessels leading to urticaria, fever, and arthralgia within 20 days (typically 7–11 days) of drug exposure. While there is an excess risk of serum sickness–like reaction with Cefaclor, direct evidence of immune-complex formation has not been sought (26).

Aspirin

Salicylates are rarely used in young children because of the risk of Reye's syndrome, yet nonsteroidal anti-inflammatory drugs (NSAIDs) are commonly used. Ibuprofen-induced urticaria in pediatrics has only been reported in two children (7 and 14 years old) (27). The pathophysiologic mechanism for aspirin is likely through blockade of cyclo-oxygenase resulting in increased leukotrienes via the lipoxygenase pathway. Aspirin and NSAIDs can produce phototoxic reactions, pruritus, urticaria, and erythema multiforme. No available skin or in vitro test is available. Escalating doses in a challenge test or oral desensitization protocols can be employed if acceptable substitutes are not available.

Vaccines

Immunizations are routinely administered at birth and thereafter at two months of age. All vaccines have been associated with acute urticaria. There are several vaccine components that may be responsible, such as egg protein in the influenza vaccine and gelatin in the measles-mumps-rubella (MMR) and varicella vaccines. Initially allergic reactions to MMR were believed to be due to egg protein, but it is likely that gelatin is causative as most reactions occurred in children who could tolerate egg (28). Gelatin was the trigger in four children ages one to four years who developed urticaria with or without systemic symptoms after varicella vaccine (29).

Opiates

Opiate analgesics are commonly associated with pruritus and urticaria. The mechanism of action is direct mast cell degranulation. Implicated drugs include demerol, morphine, oxycodone, hydrocodone, and codeine. Fentanyl appears to have less such activity and may be an alternative. Skin testing to codeine is not valuable, as it would be expected to induce a wheal and flare.

Steroid-Induced Urticaria

Corticosteroid allergy is suspected when dermatitis worsens with topical steroid therapy. A two-year-old with asthma and atopic dermatitis developed contact urticaria with clobetasone. He had positive immediate skin and patch tests to several topical steroids, including clobetasone. He tolerated oral, nasal, and inhaled steroids. Similarly, a five-year-old developed immediate urticaria and angioedema after ingestion of cortisone, prednisolone, and dexamethasone. Skin puncture but not patch tests were positive (30).

Other Medication-Induced Urticaria

A two-day-old infant with heart disease developed recurrent acute urticaria with infusions of Prostaglandin E1. The severity of urticaria was proportional to the dose of PGE1 (31). Experimental evidence suggests the mechanism is direct mast cell degranulation. This report is in contrast to facial flushing which is very common. An eight-week-old infant had hand puffiness and generalized urticaria two hours after the third dose of oral vitamin K (32).

Urticaria Associated with Infections

It is challenging to confirm infections as the etiologic agent, and most often the diagnosis is presumptuous, being based on circumstantial evidence at best.

Viral

Viruses suspected of triggering urticaria include hepatitis B, Epstein–Barr, influenza, adenovirus, enterovirus, respiratory syncytial virus, rotavirus, and varicella-zoster (4,33,34). Although it is commonplace to observe transient urticarial lesions in children with the "common cold," data on rhinovirus-associated urticaria is lacking. Chronic urticaria with HIV (35) and hepatitis C infection has been reported in adults only (36).

Bacterial

Bacterial infections are controversial causes of urticaria. Group A β-hemolytic streptococcal infection was diagnosed in 16% of cases of acute urticaria. Thirteen of the thirty-three children who were assessed for streptococcal infection were positive by either serology or throat culture (37). The youngest child was four years. Since 1947, anecdotal reports have associated urticaria in adults with dental abscess (9 cases), sinusitis (3 cases), cholecystitis (3 cases), prostatitis, rectal abscess (1 case), and urinary tract infection (2 cases). In many of these cases, the infection was asymptomatic. The association between local bacterial infections and urticaria is probably coincidental rather than causal. Histamine-releasing factors other than IgE have been postulated to be the underlying mechanism for infection-induced urticaria (38), but this remains controversial. *Escherichia coli* infection was a presumptive cause of urticaria in a young child with gastroenteritis (38), but again the occurrence could have been fortuitous.

Protozoa

Urticaria in association with protozoal infections is rare, with only 10 cases (2 pediatric) reported. In 1949, a 16-year-old and over 20 years ago a 4-year-old girl was believed to have Giardia as a trigger of acute urticaria. She had normal-appearing stools, but Giardia lamblia cysts were identified. Within one hour of the second dose of metronidazole, she experienced worsening of urticaria, postulated to be due to the release of large amounts of parasite antigen entering the blood. After drug completion, she had resolution of urticaria and negative stool samples (39). A review of 44 children from India with urticaria revealed that 25% had evidence of Giardia or helminthes; however, eradication of the infestation did not improve the urticaria (6). A direct role of *Helicobacter pylori* infection in adult CIU is controversial due to the lack of controlled trials (40,41).

Fungal

No cases of fungal infection could be found that were associated with urticaria in children. However, Trichophyton-specific IgE was elevated in adults with recurrent urticaria (42). Whether the absorption of dermatophyte allergen is contributing to symptoms is uncertain.

Stings and Bites

Hymenoptera

The venom from the stings of honeybees, yellow jackets, wasps, and hornets can induce urticaria with or without angioedema through an IgE-mediated mechanism. A local reaction with pain and swelling is normal. Large local reactions can be delayed and be confused with cellulitis. In contrast to adults, generalized cutaneous reactions in children do not significantly increase the risk of anaphylactic reactions. For children experiencing a systemic reaction, skin testing with venom can identify the culprit insect, and venom immunotherapy can significantly reduce the risk of an anaphylactic reaction in the event of a subsequent sting.

Fire Ants

In the southern United States, imported fire ants live in tall mounds. Their venom can induce IgE-mediated reactions ranging from urticaria to anaphylaxis. At the site of the sting are sterile pustules in a ring formation caused by the stinger as the ant pivots. Skin testing with whole body extract is available and desensitization recommended for those experiencing systemic reactions.

Mosquitoes/Fleas/Bedbugs

Some infants will experience large local reactions to insect bites. Papular urticaria refers to pruritic 3 to 10 mm firm urticated papules often with a central punctum that occur in crops or clusters in response to the bite of mosquitoes, fleas, bedbugs, or other insects

(43). Also known as lichen urticatus, papular urticaria has been described in infants as young as two weeks, although primarily affects children ages two to seven years. Lesions persist for 2 to 10 days, resulting in temporary post-inflammatory erythema. If exposure continues, attacks may persist for years. Histopathologically, papular urticaria is identical to insect bites, although the reaction may be IgE-mediated. Treatment consists of disinfecting pets, home fumigation, topical steroids, and oral antihistamines. Some reports identify specific IgE against mosquito. Mosquito skin testing extract is available, but not generally warranted.

Spiders

Acute generalized urticaria can be the result of spider bites. In a young child, history revealed that urticaria began on the back. Close examination revealed two fang marks, presumably from a spider. These reactions are likely non-IgE-mediated, although specific studies are lacking.

Vasculitis

Urticarial vasculitis can be differentiated from other forms of urticaria by the presence of persistent, tender, or burning erythematous wheals with central clearing. Typically, there is petechia or purpura with individual lesions persisting for 48 to 72 hours, resulting in skin hyperpigmentation. Associated symptoms include fever, arthralgia or arthritis, proteinuria or hematuria, vomiting and abdominal pain, and cough, dyspnea, or rarely hemoptysis (44). Urticarial vasculitis has been associated with SLE, rheumatic fever, juvenile rheumatoid arthritis (JRA) (Still's disease), and other collagen vascular diseases.

Henoch-Schonlein purpura (HSP) or anaphylactoid purpura is a common cause of small vessel vasculitis in children ages 2 to 12 years, affecting boys twice as often as girls. The cause is unknown, although cases associated with acute rheumatic fever and rheumatic carditis have been reported, suggesting group A streptococcus as an inciting antigen. The clinical cutaneous feature is the sudden onset of palpable purpura distributed symmetrically and predominately on the lower extremities and buttocks. The rash may initially appear urticarial or petechial, but evolves within hours to the classic rash. The purpura slowly darken, fade, and become flat over two to three weeks, leaving a transient pigmentation. Occasionally there is soft tissue swelling over the head or extremities. Commonly there are gastrointestinal (abdominal pain, vomiting, guaiac-positive stools, or melena) and joint (arthralgia and peri-articular swelling) manifestations that typically follow, but may precede the rash. Transient microscopic hematuria/proteinuria is present in nearly 30% of cases; renal failure is responsible for most of the 1% to 3% mortality. Tissue deposition of IgA-containing immune complexes is the pathologic hallmark. Skin and blood vessel biopsies reveal IgA deposits, C3, and occasionally IgG and IgM. Direct immunofluorescence staining of the involved skin confirms the diagnosis. While no specific treatment affects the rash or renal involvement, systemic steroids may improve joint and GI symptoms. Aspirin should be avoided as it may increase the risk of GI hemorrhage.

Infantile HSP, also known as acute hemorrhagic edema of infancy or acute benign cutaneous leukocytoclastic vasculitis of infancy, affects children ages four months to two years. In a series of 12, all had angioedema affecting primarily the feet, hands, scalp, lips, or scrotum. The purpuric rash was more likely to be distributed over the face, although all had lower extremity involvement. Inflammatory subcutaneous edema is common. Involvement of the GI tract, joints, and kidneys was significantly less common. All patients recovered completely (45). No specific therapy is necessary.

JRA of the systemic form in infants or young children is associated with a rash in 95% of cases. The rash is characterized by recurrent, evanescent, small, pale, pink-red macules with central pallor on the trunk and proximal extremities. It appears with fever, emotional stress, heat, and skin trauma.

Underlying Systemic Disorders

Urticaria may be a presenting sign of an autoinflammatory syndrome where there are recurrent inflammatory symptoms without autoantibodies or antigen-specific T cells. Subgroups of autoinflammatory diseases include periodic fever syndromes and cryopyrin-associated periodic syndromes (CAPS). Lack of improvement of hives or blanching rashes with antihistamines is common, and one should alert the clinician.

The CAPS include familial cold autoinflammatory syndrome (FCAS), Muckle-Wells syndrome (MWS), and Neonatal onset multisystem inflammatory disorder (NOMID). These disorders are autosomal-dominant with variable penetrance and result from mutations in the gene CIAS1 on chromosome 1, encoding the cryopyrin protein known as NALP3 and PYPAF1. This gene mutation promotes aberrant formation of the inflammasone, leading to inappropriate production of the active proinflammatory cytokine IL-1-β.

FCAS, formerly called familial cold urticaria, is a rare autosomal-dominant disorder with episodic macular papular erythematous pruritic patches or confluent plaques on the extremities after exposure to cold. Petechia may be present. The onset is within six months, but can appear in the first days of life in 60% of those affected. After one hour of generalized cold exposure, skin lesions appear and last less than 24 hours. Fever and polyarthralgia occur in nearly all patients; conjunctivitis without periorbital edema, profuse sweating, drowsiness, headache, extreme thirst, and nausea occur with variable frequency. The ice cube test is negative, but WBC count and markers of inflammation are elevated. This syndrome is linked to chromosome 1q44, and the gene mutation (T1058C) has been sequenced and designated CIAS1. It is one of the hereditary periodic fever syndromes, but the only one associated with cold exposure (46,47). Treatment includes rest, warming, and analgesics for joint pain. Antihistamines, steroids, and colchicine have minimal effect. The IL-1 receptor antagonist anakinra, may prevent cold-induced attacks and reduce daily symptoms. If left untreated, chronic FCAS can lead to secondary AA amyloidosis.

MWS is a rare condition characterized by episodic episodes of fever, urticarial rash and joint pain, progressive sensorineural deafness, and amyloidosis with nephropathy. Episodes of fever last 12 to 36 hours, occurring at intervals of three weeks and resolve spontaneously. The age of onset is variable and triggers may include both heat and cold.

NOMID also known as "chronic infantile neurologic cutaneous and articular syndrome" (CINCA), presents with an urticarial rash within the first days of life and is chronic, may or may not be pruritic, fluctuates, and is unresponsive to antihistamines. Arthropathies ranging from transient arthritis to deforming polyarthritis may follow the rash by 18 months. This is associated with limb and joint pain, fever, impaired growth, and abnormal facies with saddle-shaped nose, frontal bossing, and protruding eyes. Developmental delay is nearly universal. Other CNS findings include CSF pleocytosis, papilledema, uveitis, deafness, seizures, and macrocephaly with brain atrophy. Hematologic abnormalities are common and include anemia, thrombocytosis, and elevated peripheral WBC. Autoantibodies are negative. The etiology is unknown (48). Effective treatment for some includes anakinra (49), thalidomide, and humanized anti-IL-6 receptor monoclonal antibody.

TNF-receptor-associated periodic syndrome (TRAPS) is a periodic fever syndrome. Twenty missense mutations in the TNF-receptor have been described that result in this rare auto-dominant syndrome. The median age of onset is three years, but can present as early as two weeks. Symptoms include recurrent episodes of fever, severe myalgia, severe abdominal pain, ocular symptoms (conjunctivitis, periorbital edema, and uveitis), and rash often lasting longer than five days. Distinguishing features are the migratory nature of the myalgia and rash with symptoms lasting on average 21 days per month and occurring at irregular intervals every five to six weeks. The rash most commonly is a centrifugal migratory, erythematous patch overlying a local area of myalgia on the limbs and torso. Lesions ranging in size from 1 to 28 cm are tender, warm, and blanchable. Skin biopsy reveals superficial and deep lymphocytic and monocytic perivascular and interstitial infiltrate without granuloma, vasculitis, or eosinophilic infiltration. Laboratory studies display elevated acute phase reactants. Treatment options include NSAIDs, steroids, anakinra, and etanercept (50). The response to colchicine is poor.

Hashimoto-Pritzker Langerhans cell histiocytosis (LCH) is a benign condition without systemic involvement compared with the more aggressive systemic forms of LCH. In these conditions, there is an abnormal proliferation of bone marrow–derived cells, which can manifest clinically as red-brown papules. A two-month-old infant had urticaria and a positive Darier's sign due to the increased number of mast cells in LCH (51).

Acute lymphoblastic leukemia with eosinophilia is a rare malignancy that can present as young as two years with eosinophilia greater than $5000/mm^3$ and chronic urticaria preceding systemic symptoms (52). This can be mistaken for idiopathic hypereosinophilia syndrome.

Angioedema

Angioedema can occur with or without urticaria. Angioedema without associated urticaria is a presenting symptom of C1 esterase inhibitor deficiency.

Hereditary angioedema (HAE) is an autosomal-dominant disease that affects 1:1,000 to 1:150,000 persons and has been described in all races and without gender predominance. It is caused by a 30% reduction of serum C1 inhibitor in 85% of patients (HAE type I) or by a nonfunctional C1 inhibitor in 15% of patients (HAE type II). Type III HAE only affects females (53). The clinical presentation is the same regardless of the type. A deficiency of the activity or function of C1 inhibitor leads to C1 activation and uncontrolled C1s activity and a cascade of events in the complement and kallikrein/bradykinin system resulting in recurrent, non-pitting edema. Acquired C1 esterase inhibitor deficiency is a rare condition associated with autoimmune or B-cell lymphoproliferative disorders occurring primarily in middle-aged adults and elderly (54). This type of angioedema has not been described in children.

The hereditary form can present within the first two years of life with rapid painless swelling affecting any part of the body without urticaria, itching, discoloration, or redness. Abdominal pain can be mistaken for infantile colic or an "acute abdomen." Other symptoms include watery, non-bloody diarrhea and laryngeal edema that can progress to complete airway obstruction and is potentially fatal. Severe attacks typically do not occur until late childhood. Attacks last two to three days and resolve spontaneously. Triggers include minor trauma, menstruation, increased estrogen (oral contraceptive), exercise, and emotional stress.

Diagnostic studies include a marked reduction of serum C4 in 80% to 85% of cases and serum C2 levels during an attack. Between attacks serum C4 is characteristically low;

C3 and C2 are normal. Quantitative and functional measurements of C1 esterase inhibitor confirm HAE. In children younger than one year, tests may be unreliable and requires genetic typing followed by repeat testing for children older than one year. In type III, all the above studies are normal both during and between attacks and require genetic testing to confirm (55).

Acute treatment of HAE in the United States is fresh frozen plasma (FFP), as it contains adequate amounts of C1 inhibitor; however, FFP administration is controversial as it also contains the complement components that could fuel ongoing symptoms. Other risks include the transmission of infections, alloimmunization, and anaphylaxis. In Europe, IV administration of C1 inhibitor concentrate 500 to 1000 units will begin to resolve the edema in 30 to 120 minutes with complete remission by 24 hours. There is little if any effect of epinephrine, antihistamines, or corticosteroids, although a trial is warranted. With laryngeal involvement, endotracheal intubation or tracheostomy may be necessary. ACE inhibitors and estrogen contraceptives should be avoided as they may trigger or worsen angioedema in HAE patients.

For children requiring long-term therapy, prophylactic treatment includes avoidance of precipitating factors, attenuated androgens, or antifibrinolytic agents such as tranexamic acid and epsilon aminocaproic acid (EACA) (55). EACA, a plasmin inhibitor, is given as a loading dose, followed by 7 to 10 g daily. Side effects may include myalgia, muscle weakness, hypotension, and fatigue. Attenuated androgens such as danazol are generally more effective than EACA and have relatively mild adverse effects but are contraindicated in young children. They should be used with caution as they can impact growth and promote virilization in females. The lowest effective dose and alternate-day therapy may decrease the potential for adverse effects. Liver function and lipid profiles should be monitored while on androgen therapy, as atherogenesis and liver disorders are associated with androgens. Emerging therapies with favorable safety profiles include kinin pathway modulators such as DX-88 (Ecallantide) and Icatibant. Bradykinin levels are elevated during HAE attacks, and the edema formation is likely due to microvascular leakage due to bradykinin. Subcutaneous injections of DX-88 inhibits plasma kallikrein and in clinical trials in subjects 10 years and older, efficacy was achieved in four hours for HAE attacks (56). Icatibant, a potent antagonist of bradykinin B2 receptor, demonstrated relief in two and a half hours for acute attacks.

Other

Acute annular urticaria (AAU), a type of giant urticaria, occurs from four-months-old to four-years-old. There is sudden onset of numerous small, round, erythematous wheals that rapidly spread across the body enlarging into polycyclic, blanching wheals with a bright violaceous center. The lesions fade within one to two hours, but new lesions wax and wane over 10 days, then resolve completely. There may be transient periorbital, hand or foot edema, fever to 39°C, and pruritus in half the patients. While the etiology is uncertain, nearly two-thirds of children had diarrhea treated with furazolidone. Laboratory tests were normal. Treatment was symptomatic. Since furazolidone has been replaced with newer drugs, AAU is rarely seen (57).

Idiopathic

CIU is reserved for cases where an etiology has not been established. CIU and chronic idiopathic angioedema are less common in childhood compared with adults (5). Recurrent intermittent hives are not well characterized in either children or adults. The findings of functional autoantibodies directed against the α-chain of the high-affinity IgE receptor or less commonly IgG is approximately 40% in adults. This is termed autoimmune urticaria. In 93 children, 9-months- to 16-years-old with chronic urticaria, 31% were found to have autoimmune urticaria as diagnosed by autologous serum skin test or serum-induced basophil histamine release (58). The autoantibodies were found in children with known eliciting agents (physical, allergic, infectious), but none had concomitant autoimmune disease, signs of thyroid autoimmunity, celiac disease, or *H. pylori* infection.

Differential Diagnosis

Urticaria

While recognizing urticaria does not usually pose a significant clinical dilemma, there are a several skin eruptions that can masquerade as urticaria and in turn may be treatable. Tissue swelling that resembles angioedema can be due to unrelated disorders (59). The differential diagnosis is extensive and outlined in Table 2. Benign facial flushing associated with bottle- or breast-feeding is frequently reported by parents. This is not associated with other symptoms and resolves spontaneously. The underlying mechanism has yet to be established.

Urticaria Pigmentosa

This disorder refers to collections of mast cells in the skin appearing as well-demarcated tan macules and papules beginning in the first six months of life. The lesions enlarge to become plaques several centimeters in diameter. These are mastocytomas and can be either solitary or multiple. They urticate with gentle trauma such as stroking the skin (Darier's sign). The formation of bullae or vesicles is more common in children younger than two years. Mastocytomas and urticaria pigmentosa are the most common forms of mast cell disease in children. When mast cells infiltrate the bone marrow, spleen, lymph

Table 2 Masqueraders of Urticaria/Angioedema in Infants and Young Children

Urticaria		Angioedema	
Well-circumscribed rashes		**Skin swelling**	
Diffuse mastocytosis	Urticaria pigmentosa	Dermatomyositis	Scleroderma
Erythema marginatum	Erythema multiforme	**Periorbital/infraorbital swelling**	
Erythema annular centrifugum	Familial annular erythema	Blunt trauma	Sinusitis
Neonatal lupus		Parasitic disease	Melkersson-Rosenthal syndrome
			Superior vena cava syndrome
Food-associated erythematous rashes			
Gustatory flushing	Frey syndrome	**Scalp swelling**	
Irritant dermatitis	Benign facial flushing	Blunt trauma	Cellulitis/abscess
Food additive intolerance		Bleeding diathesis	Tumor (neuroblastoma, leukemia)
Infections/infestations		**Periorbital, face, extremity swelling**	
Parasite (Strongyloides)	Scabies	Nephrotic syndrome	Lymphedema
Lyme disease		Myxedema	

nodes, or liver, the disorder is termed "systemic mastocytosis." Triggers of mast cell degranulation include exercise, change in body temperature, infections, and certain drugs. The result is pruritus, flushing, and hypotension (59). When the lesions appear nodular, they should be differentiated from nodular scabies, (LCH), insect bite reactions, and localized pseudolymphoma. Diffuse cutaneous mastocytosis often presents by age three years with either normal-appearing skin or reddish-tan, thickened skin with an orange peel texture. On microscopy, there is infiltration of the entire skin by mast cells. Bullae are common and systemic mastocytosis is more likely to develop.

Erythema Multiforme

This is rare in young children. The lesions are typically target-shaped macules, papules, or bullae and extend across the extremities, lips, and face. Unlike typical urticaria, these lesions remain fixed and persist for several days. Associated symptoms include malaise, fever, and arthralgia. The rash is resistant to treatment with epinephrine.

Infections

Scabies. Scabies is caused by burrowing into the skin and release of toxic substances by the female mite *Sarcoptes scabiei*. Symptoms are intense pruritus and a 1 to 2 mm erythematous papular rash that becomes scaly, excoriated, and crusted. The classic lesion of threadlike burrows may not be seen in infants, although bullae and pustules are common. Wheals and papules can be mistaken for urticaria and papular urticaria, respectively. In infants, the palms, soles, face, and scalp are frequently affected. Diagnosis is by microscopic identification of the mite, ova, or scybala in skin scrapings from burrows, eczematous lesions, or fresh papules.

Spirochete disease. Lyme borreliosis is associated with a single annular erythematous rash termed "erythema chronicum migrans," occurring after an arthropod bite and infection. There may be multiple lesions that slowly enlarge over weeks or months, followed by arthritis. The skin lesion may not feel hot to the touch, but the child may complain of itching or burning. In nearly half of patients, multiple, smaller, annular secondary lesions will occur that are recurrent and evanescent.

Parasitic disease. Strongyloides stercoralis is a nematode of worldwide distribution including Southern Appalachia that can infect humans through direct skin invasion and eventually reside in the upper GI system. With repeated skin invasion, a papular rash may occur. Larva currens describes a large erythematous urticarial–like lesion with rapidly spreading edges usually localized within 30 cm of the anus. Peripheral eosinophilia is common and associated symptoms include colicky abdominal pain, vomiting, mucus diarrhea, and failure to thrive (60).

Other. Erythema annulare centrifugum is characterized by red plaques with a scaly leading edge that can persist for years. Annular erythema of infancy presents as erythematous papules that develop into arcs and polycyclic lesions. While individual lesions resolve in two days, eruptions can occur for months to years (61). Familial annular erythema was described in one family and inherited as autosomal-dominant. Infiltrated papules gradually enlarge to form erythematous rings with areas of central fading and transient residual hyperpigmentation (62).

Frey syndrome, also known as auriculotemporal nerve syndrome, can be mistaken for urticaria related to food allergy. After unilateral injury to the nerve by birth trauma, aberrant reinnervation of the nerve to the skin as opposed to the salivary gland can result in a unilateral flushing erythematous rash occurring within minutes of eating, especially tart foods. The absence of pruritus and angioedema and the unilateral distribution differentiates this from urticaria.

Acute nonlymphocytic leukemia presented as asymptomatic erythematous wheal-like papules, macules, and nodules in a 15-month-old male who had been treated for urticaria for six months (63). Leukemic infiltration of the skin is termed "leukemia cutis."

The rash of neonatal lupus erythematosus (NLE) is usually annular, erythematous with central clearing, and has a raised border affecting predominantly the face and scalp, but also the trunk, extremities, and diaper area. The rash begins within days to weeks of birth and heals with minimal scarring, but potentially permanent telangiectasia (64). NLE is associated with congenital heart block in infants with a structurally normal heart. Over 85% of infants and their mothers will have La (SSB) and/or Ro (SSA) serum antibodies.

Angioedema

Child Abuse

Recurrent scalp edema was misdiagnosed as child abuse in an 18-month-old child (65).

Nephrotic Syndrome

This is characterized by edema, proteinuria, hypoproteinemia, and hyperlipidemia. Over 90% of children with nephrotic syndrome have minimal change disease. It occurs in children ages two to six years, affecting boys twice as often as girls. Children presenting with morning, bilateral, periorbital edema that is unresponsive to antihistamines, but gradually resolves over the day should be assessed for nephrotic syndrome. The lower extremity pitting edema may progress to generalized edema, weight gain, ascites, and pleural effusion. Urinalysis reveals protein and occasionally microscopic hematuria.

Superior Vena Cava Syndrome

In children, this presents as head and neck edema with distended neck veins, plethora, cyanosis, and proptosis. Superior mediastinal masses such as lymphoma could precipitate this.

Myxedema

Congenital hypothyroidism can present with non-pitting edema of the extremities and genitals and facial puffiness. In the first month of life, associated symptoms include enlarged head size, prolonged physiologic icterus, and feeding difficulties. Thereafter, somnolence, sluggishness, poor appetite, constipation, low temperature, pericardial effusion, heart murmur, bradycardia, and large abdomen with umbilical hernia can be seen. Despite the routine newborn screen, laboratory errors can occur. Thyroid function studies confirm the diagnosis.

Dermatomyositis

This multisystem disease of unknown etiology is characterized by inflammation of striated muscle and cutaneous lesions. Presentation is insidious onset and gradual progression of proximal muscle weakness. Non-pitting edema and skin thickening can occur. It rarely presents before age tow with average age of onset at eight to nine years. Elevated levels of serum muscle enzymes and abnormal electromyogram support the diagnosis. Early treatment has a favorable prognosis.

Scleroderma

Morphea and linear scleroderma are cutaneous manifestations of a chronic fibrotic disturbance of connective tissue. This rare disease of unknown etiology can occur at any time in childhood. Early skin findings include slightly erythematous and edematous patches often in a linear pattern and commonly unilateral. The child may complain of a prickly sensation or pain. With disease progression, the involved skin becomes indurated and enlarges peripherally, exhibiting a violaceous center. It may progress to involve an entire extremity resulting in atrophic and shiny skin with scarring, limb shortening, and flexion contractures. Laboratory findings are nonspecific, and no specific therapy is available (66).

Parasitic Disease

Trichinosis is caused by Trichinella spiralis through ingestion of undercooked pork, walrus, bear, or horse meat. Periorbital and facial edema occur in up to 80% of cases and follows gastroenteritis by one week and lasts another two to three weeks. The edema phase is due to larval invasion and is associated with myalgia, fever, and peripheral eosinophilia. Affected muscles include the masseters, intercostals, and diaphragm. Diagnosis is by serology and muscle biopsy.

DIAGNOSTIC STRATEGIES

The evaluation of urticaria in childhood may require the combined skills of the pediatrician, allergist, and dermatologist. Table 3 outlines a suggested approach to evaluation.

Acute Urticaria and Angioedema

The most important factor in determining the trigger in urticaria is a detailed history (Table 3). A thorough physical examination can identify findings beside cutaneous features and help confirm that the eruption is indeed urticaria or the edema is angioedema. A laboratory evaluation of acute urticaria or angioedema is not required. As part of the examination, assess for dermographism by briskly stroking the skin. Within two to five minutes, linear pruritic wheals with a flare develop at the site. Dermographism may follow a viral infection or drug reaction, and its presence can invalidate allergy skin testing that relies on a wheal-and-flare reaction.

When urticaria occurs during the course of a febrile illness and antibiotics are administered concomitantly, it may be necessary to determine whether the causative trigger was the antibiotic or a cutaneous manifestation related to the infection itself. While there is no commercially available skin test preparation for antibiotics or other medications in the United States, Diater S.A. in Madrid, Spain has benzylpenicilloyl polylysine (PPL) and minor determinant mixture (sodium benzylpenicillin, disodium benzylpenicilloate, and benzylpenicilloic acid) for purchase. A minor determinant mixture can also be made by alkaline hydrolysis of penicillin. Furthermore, as a partial source of minor determinants, penicillin G 10,000 U/mL can be used for skin testing. With this approach, 85% of patients with a history of allergy to penicillin who have

Table 3 Evaluation of Young Children with Urticaria and/or Angioedema

History (acute/chronic)

Onset, duration (individual lesions vs. all lesions), distribution, and pattern
Relation to meals or specific food, medication, infectious illness, exertion, sting, or bite
Pruritus: presence or absence of
Physical stimulus: cold, heat, vibratory, sunlight, and water (see below)
Associated symptoms: rhinitis, fever, arthritis, cough, vomiting, diarrhea, weight loss
Medical History: atopy: eczema, allergic rhinitis, asthma
Diet: formula, foods
Medications: Specifically ASA, NSAIDs, antibiotics, narcotics, OTC, herbal remedy
Immunizations: gelatin or egg-based vaccines
Environment: pets (fleas), roaches, insect infestation, daycare; travel: tropical, drinking water
Family history: angioedema, atopy
Growth and development: developmental delay

Laboratory (acute)

Specific IgE
Skin testing or in vitro (RAST or ELISA)
Foods, inhalants, latex
Penicillin skin testing (if indicated by history)
Throat culture (for strep) if >4 yr

Laboratory (chronic)

Total serum IgE
Specific IgE: Skin testing or in vitro assay: foods, latex, inhalants
Basophil histamine release assay (research applications)
CBC with differential (evaluate for eosinophilia)
ESR, CR-P, ANA, Serum complement levels: C2, C4
C1 esterase inhibitor level and functional assay (if angioedema only)
Viral titers: Hepatitis B and C panel, HIV, EBV, HSV
Cryoglobulins
Urinalysis for WBC, bacteria, protein
Anti-IgE or IgE receptor antibodies
Free red blood cell protoporphyrin and fecal protoporphyrins (if solar induced)

Procedures

Tests for physical urticaria
Dermographism: stroking skin for Darier's sign
Cold: Ice cube test
Vibratory: laboratory vortex
Cholinergic: partial submersion in 40°C water
Tests for urticarial vasculitis
Skin biopsy: lesional skin
Tests for food allergy: elimination diet and reintroduction
Open food challenge vs. DBPCFC

Physical examination

Vital signs, temperature, weight, height, OFC
Skin, chest, abdomen, musculoskeletal

Abbreviations: OFC: Occipital frontal circumference; CBC: complete blood count; ESR: erythrocyte sedimentation rate; CR-P: C-reactive protein; ANA: antineutrophil antibody; RAST: Radioallergosorbent test; ELISA: enzyme-linked immunosorbent assay; DBPCFC: double blind placebo-controlled food challenge.

negative reactions to skin tests will tolerate penicillin. For penicillin, the major determinant penicilloyl appears to be responsible for most cases of urticaria, while the minor determinants are involved in anaphylaxis. Skin testing with drugs of low molecular weight is problematic and not predictive as these drugs combine with serum proteins to form haptens to which the antibody is then directed. A negative skin test to a low molecular weight medication is not satisfactory to confirm safe use of that drug. A positive skin test may indicate an irritant reaction but nevertheless be avoided. High molecular weight drugs that can act as complete antigens may be used for skin testing. IgE RAST test for penicillin is not sensitive enough to exclude penicillin as the culprit.

Food allergy evaluation includes a detailed history where symptoms improve after elimination of the suspect food. An extreme or prolonged elimination diet should be avoided to prevent nutritional deprivation. Identification of specific IgE using percutaneous skin testing or an in vitro method such as Radioallergosorbent test (RAST) or enzyme-linked immunosorbent assay (ELISA) can be used. Currently available CAP RAST are of sufficient sensitivity and specificity to provide 95% confidence intervals for peanut, milk, and egg, allowing a decision to pursue open challenge if the result is low or conversely to continue avoidance if the level is elevated (67). Skin tests are helpful if negative in ruling out a food allergy as there is a good predictive value. False-positive skin tests with foods approach 50%, thus highlighting the importance of clinical correlation. Intradermal skin testing with food allergens frequently causes irritant reactions and is not recommended. An elimination diet of two weeks, followed by reintroduction of the food may reveal the culprit. Open, single blind and double blind food challenges can be performed in the office where immediate treatment can be provided if a reaction occurs. While the double blind placebo-controlled food challenge is the gold standard and utilized in research protocols, it is time consuming in both preparation and administration. In young children, blinding is not necessary as a psychological component is unlikely.

Chronic Urticaria and Angioedema

The history and examination are of key importance. Special attention to non-dermal organ systems may uncover a systemic disease. Tests for physical urticaria should be performed. Laboratory tests may indicate an underlying disorder (Table 3). However, an extensive laboratory evaluation in the absence of other organ system involvement either identified by history or examination is not warranted except for the evaluation for chronic autoimmune urticaria. Several methods are available in a research setting, including basophil histamine release assay, basophil expression of CD203c, and anti-IgE assay. To the clinician, autologous serum skin testing has been all but replaced with assays for IgG anti-Fc_ε RI_α available at reference laboratories. An elimination diet, if undertaken, should not be extended. A skin biopsy may prove helpful in atypical lesions or where urticarial vasculitis is suspected.

MANAGEMENT

Treatment is directed at identifying the underlying trigger and if possible, avoiding it. Additional treatment is aimed at relieving the pruritus and decreasing the size and number of urticaria (Table 4). A variety of therapeutic options have been used to treat urticaria and angioedema in adults. Less published experience is available in the pediatric age groups. Likely the most important aspect of management is reassurance to the parents and child.

Table 4 Treatment of Infants and Young Children with Urticaria and/or Angioedema

Avoidance
Avoid Aspirin

If a drug is suspected, discontinue and monitor for symptom resolution
If a food/food additive is suspected, discontinue for 2 wk and monitor for symptom resolution, consider reintroduction

Pharmacotherapy

First line	H1-antagonist antihistamines
	Combine H1 with H2-antagonist antihistamine
If severe	oral corticosteroids and epinephrine intramuscularly if airway angioedema
Other	Leukotriene modifiers: LTC4, LTD4, LTE4 receptor antagonists
	Oral β-2-agonists	Calcium channel antagonists
	Tricyclic antidepressants	Mast cell stabilizer (not available in U.S.A.)

	Generic	Trade	Formulation	Dosing	Age
H1-antagonist	Cetirizine	Zyrtec	1 mg/mL	2.5 mg qd	6–12 mo
				2.5 mg qd–bid	1–5 yr
	Levocetirizine	Xyzal	0.5 mg/mL	1.25 mg bid	2–6 yr
	Loratadine	Claritin	1 mg/mL	5 mL qd	2–5 yr
	Desloratadine	Clarinex	0.5 mg/mL	1 mg qd	6–11 mo
				1.25 mg qd	1–5 yr
	Fexofenadine	Allegra	6 mg/mL	15 mg bid	6–23 mo
				30 mg bid	2–11 yr
H2-antagonist	Ranitidine	Zantac	50 mg/mL	1–2 mg/kg bid	1 mo–16 yr
Leukotriene modifier	Montelukast	Singulair	4 mg chewable or oral granule	4 mg qd	6 mo–5 yr[a]
	Zafirlukast	Accolate	10 mg	bid	5–11 yr[b]

[a]Age indication for perennial allergic rhinitis.
[b]Age indication for asthma.

Antihistamines

Systemic H1-Antagonists

While oral H1-antagonists are effective in the treatment of pediatric allergic rhinitis, the evidence base for their use in children with urticaria contains large gaps. The first-generation antihistamines are presumed safe for young children and have undoubtedly been administered without apparent harm in this age group for over 50 years. However, CNS impairment beyond the typical drowsiness may be more common than realized, but has not been studied in children with chronic urticaria. Use of these antihistamines should probably be restricted to children with either urticaria or atopic dermatitis whose pruritus is so severe that the sedative effect is a benefit rather than a risk (68).

The second-generation antihistamines are virtually free of CNS effects and becoming the preferred medication particularly since pediatric formulations are available. Cetirizine, the metabolite of hydroxyzine, is available as a 1 mg/mL syrup approved for children ages six months and older for the treatment of urticaria. Loratadine is available in a 1 mg/mL syrup. Fexofenadine is available in a 6 mg/mL syrup for tid use. The 30 mg tab is approved for CIU in children over 12 years (69,70). The pharmacokinetics of 30 mg bid to 60 mg daily of fexofenadine in children ages 8 to 12 years is similar to adults with 80% of a dose eliminated unchanged in the feces. Onset of action based on suppression of histamine-induced wheal-and-flare reactions was one to two hours and duration was 24 hours (71).

Topical H1 Antagonists

While diphenhydramine is available for topical use and parents frequently report using this method, the efficacy is unclear and not studied. The nature of urticaria limits its potential for efficacy and the risk of contact dermatitis is increased with topical administration.

H2 Antagonists

While data is lacking in pediatric patients, adding H2 antagonists to H1 antagonists has reduced wheal formation and pruritus in adults, although this remains an area of controversy. In most adult studies, cimetidine was used. Few studies using ranitidine have been reported. Monotherapy does not appear to be beneficial.

β-Agonists

Epinephrine is beneficial in acute, severe urticaria, and angioedema. The effect, however, is short-lived. Intermediate-acting epinephrine is no longer available. Orally administered drugs have mixed results and data is absent in young children.

Tricyclic Antidepressants

Many compounds in this category have H1-antihistaminic properties. Doxepin, a highly potent H1-antagonist with weak H2-antagonist properties, is effective in adults with chronic urticaria at doses as low as 10 mg daily. Pediatric results are not available.

Calcium-Channel Antagonists

Since calcium influx is required for allergen-induced mast cell activation and release of histamine and leukotrienes, it stands to reason that calcium channel blockers could inhibit release of these mediators. Nifedipine demonstrated a beneficial effect in adults with CIU (72). Two small studies in adults with CIU exhibited mild improvement. Pediatric studies are lacking.

Mast Cell Stabilizers

Ketotifen possesses H1-antagonistic activities and mast cell–stabilizing properties. In adults, it has shown partial effectiveness in cold urticaria, dermographism, and exercise-induced urticaria. Studies in young children are not available. Cromolyn and nedocromil, although effective at stabilizing mast cells in the nose, conjunctiva, and lungs, do not effectively stabilize skin mast cells.

Anabolic Steroids

Attenuated androgens such as danazol are useful as prophylactic therapy in HAE as well as cholinergic urticaria and steroid-dependent urticaria. Androgens may act through their ability to augment protease inhibitor levels that could thereby inhibit pro-inflammatory mediators. Side effects limit their widespread use, particularly in young children. The adverse effects are relatively mild and efficacy greater than the fibrinolytic agents.

Corticosteroids

Systemic

Oral or injectable corticosteroids, while highly effective in treating urticaria and angioedema, in general, should be reserved for severe symptoms. This form of therapy is ineffective in HAE.

Topical

Data is unavailable on the efficacy of topical steroids in urticaria. It is common to hear that patients have attempted steroid creams without symptom relief. Because of the potential for widespread involvement, it is unlikely that a topical approach would be beneficial.

Leukotriene Modifiers

Leukotriene receptor antagonists, including zafirlukast and montelukast have demonstrated improvement in CIU in small open-label and one single blind trial in adults when used alone or in combination with antihistamines (73–75). In addition to symptom reduction, antihistamine rescue was reduced. Although pediatric studies in urticaria are not available, safety in this age group has been established down to one year of age. Zilueton, a 5-LO inhibitor, has similarly shown improvement in urticaria in adults. Its use in pediatrics is limited by the lack of appropriate formulation, four times daily dosing and need for liver function testing. In some cases, the use of leukotriene modifiers has allowed the discontinuation of steroids. Leukotrienes play a role in urticaria (1). When injected into the skin, they induce a dose-dependent wheal-and-flare response similar to histamine (76).

Immunosuppressive Therapy

Cyclosporin inhibits the release of mediators from mast cells as well as inhibiting the effect of interleukins. Cyclosporin 2 mg/kg/day eliminated the need for oral steroids in four of six adults whose urticaria was refractory to combination therapy with a leukotriene modifier and H1 and H2 antagonists (77). Serious side effects limit widespread use. Pediatric experience in the treatment of urticaria with cyclosporin is preliminary, but promising.

Other Therapies

Because of the recurrent nature of chronic urticaria, or unresponsiveness of severe urticaria to standard therapy, many unconventional treatments have been attempted. Sulfasalazine induced remission of steroid-dependent CIU in three adults (78). Methotrexate, antimalarial drugs, dapsone, gold, colchicine, and plasmapheresis have been utilized in either small, uncontrolled series or individual adult patients with limited benefit. Pediatric data is not available. Data is lacking to support empiric antibiotics for treatment of presumed bacterial infection.

CONCLUSIONS

Urticaria and angioedema in infants and young children is clinically and etiologically different from older children and adults. Angioedema is more common and pruritus is less consistent or more difficult to recognize. Generally the acute form is more common, uncomplicated, short-lived, and easily managed with H1 antagonists. Depending on the age of the child, food allergy, and medication reactions are the most common triggers for acute urticaria in children, while physical urticaria is common for chronic urticaria. Parental reassurance is necessary in addition to measures to decrease symptoms. An extensive search utilizing laboratory studies is typically not necessary.

REFERENCES

1. Greaves M. Chronic urticaria. J Allergy Clin Immunol 2000; 105:664–672.
2. Beyer K, Castro R, Feidel C, et al. Milk-induced urticaria is associated with the expansion of T cells expressing cutaneous lymphocyte antigen. J Allergy Clin Immunol 2002; 109:688–693.
3. Legrain V, Taieb A, Sagi T, et al. Urticaria in infants: a study of forty patients. Pediatr Dermatol 1990; 7:101–107.
4. Mortureux P, Leaute-Labreze C, Legrain-Lifermann V, et al. Acute urticaria in infancy and early childhood. Arch Dermatol 1998; 134:319–323.
5. Ghosh S, Kanwar AJ, Kaur S. Urticaria in children. Ped Derm 1993; 10:107–110.
6. Legrain V, Taieb A, Maleville J. Epidemiology of urticaria in infants. Allergie et Immunologie 1993; 25(8):324–326.
7. Harris A, Twarog FJ, Geha RS. Chronic urticaria in childhood: natural course and etiology. Ann Allergy 1983; 51:161–165.
8. Volonakis M, Katsarou-Katsari A, Stratigos J. Etiologic factors in childhood chronic urticaria. Ann Allergy 1992; 69:61–65.
9. Kauppinen K, Juntunen K, Lanki H. Urticaria in children. Retrospective evaluation and follow-up. Allergy 1984; 39:469–472.
10. Tuchinda M, Srimurta N, Habananda S, et al. Urticaria in Thai children. Asian Pac J Allergy Immunol 1986; 4:41–45.
11. Sicherer SH. Determinants of systemic manifestations of food allergy. J Allergy Clin Immunol 2000; 106:S251–S257.
12. Oranje AP, Van Gysel D, Mulder PGH, et al. Food-induced contact urticaria syndrome (CUS) in atopic dermatitis: reproducibility of repeated and duplicate testing with a skin provocation test, the skin application food test (SAFT). Contact Derm 1994; 31:314–318.
13. Rodriguez A, Trujillo MJ, Matheu V, et al. Allergy to grape: a case report. Pediatr Allergy Immunol 2001; 12:289–290.
14. De Swert L, Cadot P, Ceuppens JL. Allergy to cooked white potatoes in infants and young children: a cause of severe, chronic allergic disease. J Allergy Clin Immunol 2002; 110:524–529.
15. Simon RA. Adverse reactions to food additives. Curr Allergy Asthma Rep 2003; 3:62–66.
16. Perry CA, Dwyer J, Gelfand JA, et al. Health effects of salicylates in foods and drugs. Nutr Rev 1996; 54:225–240.
17. Baron SE, Moss C. Contact urticaria to play dough: a possible sign of dietary allergy. Br J Dermatol 2004; 151:927–952.
18. Freishtat RJ, Goepp JG. Episodic stridor with latex nipple use in a 2 month-old infant. Ann Emerg Med 2002; 39:441–443.
19. Chang A, Zic JA. Localized heat urticaria. J Amer Academy Dermatol 1999; 41:354–6.
20. Capulong MC, Tomikawa M, Tahara K, et al. Cold stimulation test and histamine release in primary acquired cold urticaria. Intern Arch Allergy Immunol 1997; 114:400–403.
21. Maltby NH, Ind PW, Causon RC, et al. Leukotriene E4 release in cold urticaria. Clin Exp Allergy 1989; 19:33–36.
22. Patterson R, Mellies CJ, Blankenship ML, et al. Vibratory angioedema: a hereditary type of physical urticaria. J Allergy Clin Immunol 1972; 50:174–182.
23. Williams-Arya P, Hogan MB, Wilson NW. Solar urticaria in a 6-year-old child. Ann Allergy Asthma Immunol 1996; 75:141–143.
24. Wasserman D, Preminger A, Zlotogorski A. Aquagenic urticaria in a child. Pediatr Dermatol 1994; 11:29–30.

25. Luong KVQ, Nguyen LTH. Aquagenic urticaria: report of a case and review of the literature. Ann Allergy Asthma Immunol 1998; 80:483–485.

26. Heckbert SR, Stryker WS, Coltin KL, et al. Serum sickness in children after antibiotic exposure: estimates of occurrence and morbidity in a health maintenance organization population. Amer J Epidemiol 1990; 132:336–342.

27. Diaz JM, Perez Montero A, Gracia Bara MT, et al. Allergic reactions due to ibuprofen in children. Pediatr Dermatol 2001; 18:66–67.

28. Kelso JM, Jones RT, Yunginger JW. Anaphylaxis to measles, mumps, and rubella vaccine mediated by IgE to gelatin. J Allergy Clin Immunol 1993; 91:867–872.

29. Sakaguchi M, Yamanaka T, Ikeda K, et al. IgE-mediated systemic reactions to gelatin included in the varicella vaccine. J Allergy Clin Immunol 1997; 99:263–264.

30. Peng YS, Shyur SD, Lin HY, et al. Steroid allergy: report of two cases. J Microbio Immunol Infect 2001; 34(2):150–154.

31. Carter EL, Garzon MC. Neonatal urticaria due to prostaglandin E1. Pediatr Dermatol 2000; 17:58–61.

32. Ford G. Possible skin allergy reaction to oral vitamin K. J Paediatr Child Health 1993; 29:241.

33. Forman M, Cherry JD. Enanthems associated with uncommon viral syndrome. Pediatr 1968; 41:873.

34. Cherry JD, John CL. Virologic studies of enanthems. J Pediatr 1966; 68:204.

35. Aftergut K, Cockerell CJ. Update on the cutaneous manifestations of HIV infection. Clinical and pathologic features. Dermatol Clin 1999; 17:445–471.

36. Reichel M, Mauro TM. Urticaria and hepatitis C. Lancet 1990; 336:822–823.

37. Schuller DE, Elvey SM. Acute urticaria associated with Streptococcal infection. Pediatr 1980; 65:592–596.

38. Ostrov MR. Dramatic resolution of chronic urticaria. Ann Allergy Asthma, Immunol 1995; 75:227–231.

39. Hamrick HJ, Moore GW. Giardiasis causing urticaria in a child. Am J Dis Child 1983; 137: 761–763.

40. Gaig P, Garcia-Ortega P, Enrique E, et al. Efficacy of the eradication of Helicobacter pylori infection in patients with chronic urticaria. A placebo-controlled double blind study. Allergolo et Immunopathol 2002; 30:255–258.

41. Wedi B, Kapp A. Helicobacter pylori infection in skin diseases: a critical appraisal. Amer J Clin Dermatol 2002; 3:273–282.

42. Platts-Mills T, Fiocco G, Hayden M, et al. Serum IgE antibodies to Trichophyton in patients with urticaria, angioedema, asthma, and rhinitis: development of Radioallergosorbent test. J Allergy Clin Immunol 1987; 79:40–45.

43. Stibich AS, Schwartz RA. Papular urticaria. Cutis 2001; 68:89–91.

44. Kaplan AP. Chronic urticaria and angioedema. N Engl J Med 2002; 346(3):175–179.

45. Al-Sheyyab M, El-Shanti H, Ajlouni S, et al. The clinical spectrum of Henoch-Schonlein purpura in infants and young children. Eur J Pediatr 1995; 154:969–972.

46. Hoffman HM, Wanderer AA, Broide DH. Familial cold autoinflammatory syndrome: phenotype and genotype of an autosomal dominant periodic fever. J Allergy Clin Immunol 2001; 108:615–620.

47. Johnstone RF, Dolen WK, Hoffman HM. A large kindred with familial cold autoinflammatory syndrome. Ann Allergy Asthma Immunol 2003; 90:233–237.

48. Ferdman RM, Shaham B, Church JA. Neonatal urticaria as a symptom of a multisystem inflammatory disease. J Allergy Clin Immunol 2000; 106:986–987.

49. Hawkins PN, Lachmann HJ, Aganna E, et al. Spectrum of clinical features in Muckle-Wells syndrome and response to anakinra. Arthritis Rheum 2004; 50:607–611.

50. Hull K, Drewe E, Aksentijevich I, et al. The TNF receptor-associated periodic syndrome (TRAPS). Medicine 2002; 81:349–368.

51. Butler DF, Ranatunge BD, Rapini RP. Urticating Hashimoto-Pritzker Langerhans cell histiocytosis. Pediatr Dermatol 2001; 18:41–44.

52. Hill A, Metry D. Urticarial lesions in a child with acute lymphoblastic leukemia and eosinophilia. Ped Dermatol 2003; 20:502–505.
53. Bork K, Barnstedt S, Koch P, et al. Hereditary angioedema with normal C1-inhibitor activity in women. Lancet 2000; 356:213–217.
54. Orfan N, Kolski GB. Angioedema and C1 inhibitor deficiency. Ann Allergy 1992; 69:167–172.
55. Bowen T, Cicardi M, Bork K, et al. Hereditary angioedema: a current state-of-the-art review. Ann Allergy Asthma Immunol 2008; 100:S30–S40.
56. Bernstein JA. Hereditary angioedema: a current state-of-the-art review, VIII: current status of emerging therapies. Ann Allergy Asthma Immunol 2008; 100:S41–S46.
57. Tamayo-Sanchez L, Ruiz-Maldonado R, Laterza A. Acute Annular urticaria in infants and children. Pediatr Dermatol 1997; 14:231–234.
58. Brunetti L, Francavilla R, Mineillo V, et al. High prevalence of autoimmune urticaria in children with chronic urticaria. J Allergy Clin Immunol 2004; 114.
59. Hartmann K, Metcalfe DD. Mast cell Disorders, Pediatric mastocytosis. Hematol/Oncol Clin North Amer 2000; 14:625–640.
60. Van Dellen RG, Maddox DE, Dutta EJ. Masqueraders of angioedema and urticaria. Ann Allergy Asthma Immunol 2002; 88:10–15.
61. Hebert A, Esterly N. Annular erythema of infancy. J Am Acad Dermatol 1986; 14:339–343.
62. Beare J, Froggatt P, Jones J, et al. Familial annulare erythema. Br J Dermatol 1966; 78:59–68.
63. Chen MJ, Huang ML, Hung IJ, et al. Leukemia cutis as the initial manifestation of acute nonlymphocytic leukemia in a young child. Cutis 1997; 60:263–264.
64. Carder KR. Hypersensitivity reactions in neonates and infants. Dermatol Ther 2005; 18: 160–175.
65. Thakur BK, Kaplan AP. Recurrent "unexplained" scalp swelling in an eighteen-month old child: atypical presentation of angioedema causing confusion with child abuse. J Pediatr 1996; 129:163–165.
66. Ansell BM, Falcini F, Woo P. Scleroderma in childhood. Clin Dermatol 1994; 12:299.
67. Sampson HA, Ho DG. Relationship between food-specific IgE concentrations and the risk of positive food challenges in children and adolescents. J Allergy Clin Immunol 1997; 100: 444–451.
68. Simons FE. H1-antihistamines in children. Clin Allergy Immunol 2002; 17:437–464.
69. Nelson HS, Reynolds R, Mason J. Fexofenadine HCL is safe and effective for treatment of chronic idiopathic urticaria. Ann Allergy Asthma Immunol 2000; 84:517–522.
70. Finn AF, Kaplan AP, Fretwell R, et al. Double blind, placebo controlled trial of fexofenadine in the treatment of chronic idiopathic urticaria. J Allergy Clin Immunol 1999; 103:1071–1078.
71. Simons FE, Bergman JN, Watson WTA, et al. The clinical pharmacology of fexofenadine in children. J Allergy Clin Immunol. 1996; 98:1062–1064.
72. Bressler RB, Sowell K, Huston DP. Therapy of chronic idiopathic urticaria with nifedipine: demonstation of beneficial effect in a double-blinded, placebo-controlled, crossover trial. J Allergy Clin Immunol 1989; 83:756–763.
73. Bensch G, Borish L. Leukotriene modifiers in chronic urticaria. Ann Allergy Asthma Immunol 1999; 83:348.
74. Nettis E, Dambra P, Loria M, et al. Comparison of montelukast and fexofenadine for chronic idiopathic urticaria. Arch Dermatol 2001; 137:99–100.
75. Erbagci Z. The leukotriene receptor antagonist montelukast in the treatment of chronic idiopathic urticaria: single blind, placebo-controlled, crossover clinical study. J Allergy Clin Immunol 2002; 110:484–488.
76. Maxwell DL, Atkinson BA, Spur BW, et al. Skin responses to intradermal histamine and leukotrienes C4, D4, and E4 in patients with chronic idiopathic urticaria and in normal subjects. J Allergy Clin Immunol 1990; 86:759–765.
77. Norris JG, Sullivan TJ. Leukotrienes and cytokines in steroid-dependent chronic urticaria. J Allergy Clin Immunol 1998; 101:S128.
78. Jaffer AM. Sulfasalazine in the treatment of corticosteroid-dependent chronic idiopathic urticaria. J Allergy Clin Immunol 1991; 67:964–965.

13
Papular Urticaria

Timo Reunala
Tampere University and University Hospital, Tampere, Finland

PAPULAR URTICARIA

Definition

"Papular urticaria" (PU) is a term, used over 100 years, for an eruption suspected as being caused by insect bites (1). Other terms used earlier for this condition are strophulus and lichen urticatus. At present, PU can be defined as a chronic or recurrent eruption of pruritic papules, vesicles, and wheals resulting from a hypersensitivity reaction to biting insects or mites (2). Dog and cat fleas and bedbugs had been considered to be the principal insects causing PU (1). Recent studies have shown that hypersensitivity to mosquito bites is common around the world, and children in particular, experience papular bite reactions similar to PU (34). Theoretically recurrent bites over a period of time from any arthropod species may cause PU (Table 1).

Young children are mainly affected by PU and typical eruption consists of grouped, often long-lasting papules. Preceding or accompanying wheals are rarely noticed by the parent or seen by the physician, and therefore the term urticaria in the name of this entity is not the best one. A suggestion that a more appropriate term for PU would be insect bite–induced hypersensitivity was recently made by Hernandez and Cohen (2).

Epidemiology

There is agreement that PU affects mostly children from 2 to 10 years of age (1). A recent study in the United States showed that 5% of the visits to a pediatric dermatology clinic during a four-week period were attributed to PU or insect bite reactions (2). It has been speculated that the prevalence of PU would increase in the spring and summer months when insect populations peak (5). In contrast, Howard and Frieden (6) reported that in San Francisco, children with PU due to flea bites present to a dermatologic practice year round. In Baltimore, Hernandez and Cohen (2) observed that PU invariably recurred during the fall and winter months. Adults are also vulnerable to PU, and especially newcomers to flea or other insect-infested areas are known to suffer from bite reactions in

Table 1 Insects and Mites Causing PU

	Occurrence	Cause of PU	Typical findings
Insects			
Cat and dog fleas (Ctenocephalides) Bird fleas (Ceratophyllus)	Cosmopolitan Indoors and outdoors	++	Small papules or vesicles in linear fashion or in crops. Clusters around ankles and waistline, also under clothing.
Bedbug (Cimex)	Increasing in all developed countries	++	Nocturnal bites indoors. Large papules or vesicles in
Kissing bug (Triatoma)	In the United States and Central and South Americas	+	crops or linear fashion on uncovered skin.
Mosquitoes (Aedes, Culex, Anopheles)	Cosmopolitan Outdoors and indoors	++	Daytime and nocturnal bites on uncovered skin. Immediate wheals and delayed bite papules very common, blisters rare.
Black flies and biting midges (Simulidium, Ceratopogonidae)	Cosmopolitan Outdoors	+	Small hemorrhagic macules or papules mainly on lower legs.
Sandflies (Plebotomus)	Old World Indoors and outdoors	+	Firm red papules on hands, forearms, and lower legs.
Horse and deer flies (Tabanus, Chrysops)	Cosmopolitan. Outdoors.	+	Painful bites on uncovered skin. Wheals, papules rare.
Deer ked (Lipoptena)	Northern Europe Outdoors	++	Large firm papules on scalp and back under clothing.
Mites			
Bird mites (Dermanyssus)	Domestic and wild birds Poultry handling	++	Bites mainly nocturnal. Clusters of small itchy papules.
Dog mites (Cheyletiella)	Cosmopolitan Dog handling.	++	Small itchy papules on dog contact areas.
Grain mites (Pyemotes)	Cosmopolitan Farmers and grain handlers.	++	Very small papules on grain contact areas. Severe itch.
Chiggers (Trombiculid mite larvae)	Common in tropical and subtropical areas	++	Ankles and lower legs. Small itchy macules and papules.

Abbreviation: PU, papular urticaria.

contrast to indigenous population (1). In agreement with this, a recent study after the hurricane disaster in New Orleans showed that PU was the most common diagnosis in construction workers suffering from skin problems (7).

Several reports suggest that PU is a common disorder in Central and South America, Africa, and Asia, where children seem to be frequently sensitized to mosquito and flea bites (3,8–10). In the rainy season mosquito-bite exposure increases in Senegalese children, but whether the occurrence of PU peaks when mosquitoes are prominent is not known (11). In Africa, poverty seems to play an important role in the prevalence of insect bites and results in PU (10).

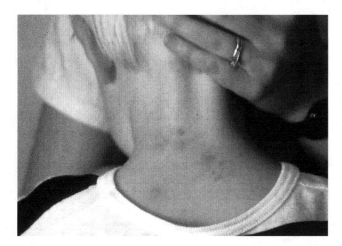

Figure 1 Papular Aedes-mosquito bites on the neck of a boy who presented also with immediate wheals.

In northern countries such as Canada and Finland, the mosquito season is short, but almost all exposed children and many adults suffer from the pruritic-bite papules (Fig. 1) usually preceded by wheals (3,4). Because this condition affects almost every child and is easily linked by the parents and physicians to mosquito bites, the term used has always been "mosquito bites" or "mosquito-bite allergy," and not PU. In Finland, a second season of insect bite reactivity could also be termed "PU," since it is because of bird flea hypersensitivity. It peaks in the spring before the mosquito season and is caused by fleas originating from bird nests in the human houses or nearby trees. (12). The third common seasonal increase in PU occurs mainly in adults in the fall and is caused by deer keds (13).

Clinical Features and Differential Diagnosis

The PU lesions caused by flea or bedbug bites are most commonly grouped in crops or linear clusters on exposed areas (Table 1). Flea bites have a tendency to cluster around the waistline and areas where tight clothing forms a barrier to the flea's progress whereas mosquito- and bedbug-bite lesions appear in uncovered sites. The deer ked seeks hairy areas, and the bite papules are typically in the scalp. When the bite lesions recur, all stages can be seen simultaneously, and the patients may present with a fresh wheal or red macula with central puncta, accompanied by more persistent papules, vesicles, or even bullae. The size of the papules varies; flea and mosquito bites usually cause rather small papules whereas bedbug-bite lesions are often 5 to 10 millimeters or even larger (Fig. 2). Intense pruritus accompanies the eruption in PU resulting in excoriations, secondary infection, scarring, and long-lasting hyper- or hypopigmentation particularly in darkly pigmented individuals (1,2). When new bites occur, a clinical feature rather typical for PU is the flare-up of older bite lesions. The lesions caused by biting flies such as black flies and biting midges consist of small hemorrhagic macules and papules that seem to appear in every bitten subject (Table 1). Therefore, a toxic substance in the saliva or tissue damage from the bite seems to cause these lesions. PU-like hypersensitivity reactions can occur from the biting flies, and the same is true for the various mite species also biting man (Table 1).

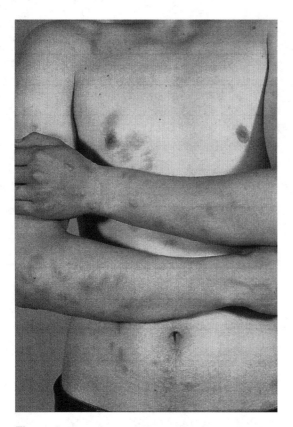

Figure 2   Numerous macular and papular bedbug bites received in an infested apartment.

The history and clinical appearance of the papular lesions that occur mainly in young children and have a tendency to recur in the same time of the year are almost diagnostic for PU. Bee, wasp, and especially fire ant stings can be difficult to differentiate from PU (14). Several dermatological conditions should also be considered in the differential diagnosis of PU (Table 2). Scabies and atopic dermatitis are common in children, and both can present with papular itchy lesions resembling PU. In scabies, multiple family members are generally affected and typical furrows can be seen (15). In children with atopic dermatitis, the eczematous lesions have a predilection for the face and flexural surfaces, and there is generally a positive family history of atopy. When PU is accompanied with secondary infected lesions, the differential diagnosis includes pyogenic infections such as impetigo and ecthyma.

Histopathology

Histopathologic findings in PU have shown to vary with the age of the lesion. Jordaan and Schneider (16) studied 30 South African children with PU. Features that presented in more than 50% of cases included mild acanthosis, spongiosis, and subepidermal edema. A superficial and deep mixed inflammatory cell infiltrate was also common, and eosinophils were present in 86% of the samples. Immunohistochemistry revealed abundant T-lymphocytes and macrophages in all cases. The authors concluded that PU with marked spongiosis and a dense inflammatory cell infiltrate cannot be reliably distinguished from arthropod bites on histopathologic grounds.

Table 2 Differential Diagnosis of Papular Urticaria

Disorder	Differential findings
Mites and insect stings	
Scabies	Furrows with mites. Multiple family members generally affected.
Fire ant stings	Mostly in lower legs. Severe pain at onset. Pustules with surrounding erythema, later papules.
Bee and wasp stings	Sting painful. Small to large local swelling. Systemic symptoms when severe venom allergy.
Miscellaneous skin disorders presenting with papules	
Papular eczema	Common in atopic children. Accompanied generally by typical eczematous lesions on face and/or flexures.
Polymorphous light eruption	A history of relapses after sun exposure. Predilection sites on face, ears, and hands; vesicles often present.
Papular drug reaction	A history of drug intake. Generally symmetric distribution on the trunk and extensor surfaces.
Papular acrodermatitis of childhood (Gianotti-Crosti syndrome)	A self-limited papular rash with symmetric acral distribution. Buttocks and face may also be affected. Associated with viral infections.
Urticaria	
Cholinergic urticaria	A history of relapses after exercise and sweating. Small papules of short duration.
Urticaria pigmentosa (mastocytosis)	Solitary mastocytoma or several darkly pigmented macules and papules scattered around the trunk. Scratching produces typical wheal-and-flare reaction.
Autoimmune skin diseases	
Linear IgA bullous dermatosis	Vesicular lesions grouped in annular fashion. IFL biopsy diagnostic.
Dermatitis herpetiformis	Polymorphic vesicular, papular, and crusted lesions. Predilections sites on elbows, knees, and buttocks. IFL biopsy shows granular IgA deposits

Table 3 Developmental Stages of Skin Reactions to Repeated Insect Bites

Stage 1	No reactivity/induction of hypersensitivity
Stage 2	Delayed reaction (papule)
Stage 3	Delayed reaction and immediate reaction (wheal)
Stage 4	Immediate reaction
Stage 5	No reactivity/acquired tolerance

Source: Adapted from Refs. 17,18.

Immune Pathophysiology

Infants never bitten by mosquitoes or fleas showed no reaction to the first bites (1).

Subsequent bites sensitize children, which happens in the second year of age or thereafter.

Animal experiments and observations in man show that skin reactivity to recurrent exposure to flea or mosquito bites can be characterized by five different stages (Table 3). Stage 1 is a period of induction of hypersensitivity with no observable bite reactions.

Stage 2 shows a delayed (papule) skin reaction, stage 3 an immediate reaction (wheal) followed by delayed reaction, and stage 4 an immediate reaction only. Finally, in stage 5 the reactivity to the bites has disappeared, i.e., a stage of tolerance has been achieved. Recently, Peng and Simons (17) exposed a nonreactive male subject every second week to 100 *Culex* mosquito bites for 10 months. Delayed and immediate cutaneous bite reactions appeared at week 3, peaked at weeks 5 to 19, and returned to nonreactive baseline by week 26. This experiment confirms that an intense mosquito bite exposure can produce a sequence of delayed and immediate bite reactions in a person, and then after several weeks desensitize the subject.

Several mosquito and a few flea and bedbug saliva allergens have been characterized at the molecular level (19–21). Children reacting to *Aedes* mosquito bites in various parts of the world frequently show antisaliva-IgE and IgG4 antibodies, and antisaliva IgE concentration correlates with the size of the wheal bite (3,22). Declining frequencies of antisaliva IgE and IgG antibodies throughout childhood and adolescence has been observed in Canada suggesting that natural desensitization can also be achieved in areas where the annual mosquito season is short (4). The reactivity to mosquito bites can be species-specific but often the sensitized subject reacts to the bites of several species cross-reactive epitopes of the saliva allergens (3,21). It seems that IgG antibodies in patients with PU could also be cross-reactive to bedbug, mosquito, and flea saliva antigens (23).

Karppinen et al. (24) took serial biopsies from experimental mosquito bites in 26 adult subjects. Most of them reacted with immediate wheals followed by delayed bite papules. Biopsy specimens taken at 2 hours showed a marked influx of eosinophils and fewer neutrophils. Biopsies from 24 hour bite papules showed an intense influx of CD4+ T cells. Garcia et al. (8) took biopsies from 45 patients with PU caused by flea bites, and also found a predominance of eosinophils and CD4+ T cells. Consistent with an influx of CD4+ T cells into the skin, the subjects with delayed mosquito-bite reactions show high lymphocyte proliferation indices to mosquito antigens (25). Similarly, flea antigen extracted together with lipopolysaccharide activates dendritic cells in children with PU (26). Bone marrow transplantation transferred PU to a nonreactive recipient also highlighting the importance of allergen-specific T cells (27). It is also of great interest that patients with HIV infection and chronic lymphocytic leukemia can present with variable long-lasting bite reactions from mosquitoes and other insects (28,29). Whether the reason for exaggerated bite reactivity in these disorders is breakage of acquired natural tolerance is possible but not confirmed.

In conclusion, the present evidence indicates that PU caused by mosquito or flea bites, and obviously also from other arthropod bites, can be mediated by antisaliva IgE antibodies leading to subsequent activation of eosinophils and T-lymphocytes, i.e., this reaction pattern is a type I allergic late-phase reaction. The delayed papular skin lesions appearing without preceding wheals in PU patients seem to be caused by a cell-mediated type IV immune response to arthropod saliva antigens. It is, however, obvious that depending on the stage of bite exposure (Table 3) a particular subject can, in the course of time, be affected by skin lesions caused by either of the two immunological mechanisms or by the combined effect of the two.

Treatment

Moderate topical steroids may help children with milder PU lesions (2). Chronic papular lesions especially in adults need high-potency topical steroids or even a short course of oral prednisolone. Control of itch in PU is important because erosions caused by scratching are prone to secondary bacterial infections. Placebo-controlled studies have shown that prophylactically taken antihistamine (cetirizine, ebastine) decreases the size of mosquito-bite wheals about 50% and accompanying pruritus by 70% (30). Levocetirizine 5 mg has also been shown to have a significant effect on the delayed mosquito bite papules (31). These results suggest that the new-generation antihistamines would also be effective when PU is caused by flea or bedbug bites.

Prophylactic measures can be best targeted when the insect or mite species causing PU has been identified. Repellents containing deet (N,N-diethyl-3-methylbenzamide) and permethrin-impregnated nets used over the beds are most effective against mosquito bites (32). When fleas or mites derive from a pet animal, a visit to a veterinarian is of help. Eradication of bedbugs from human dwellings needs spraying with special chemicals.

REFERENCES

1. Alexander JO'D. Arthropods and human skin. Berlin, Germany: Spinger-Verlag, 1984:166–171.
2. Hernandez RG, Cohen BA. Insect bite-induced hypersensitivity and the SCRATCH principles: a new approach to papular urticaria. Pediatrics 2006; 118:e189–e196.
3. Reunala T, Brummer-Korvenkontio H, Palosuo K, et al. Frequent occurrence of IgE and IgG4 antibodies against saliva of Aedes communis and Aedes aegypti mosquitoes in children. Int Arch Allergy Immunol 1994; 104:366–371.
4. Peng Z, Ho MK, Li C, et al. Evidence for natural desensitization to mosquito salivary allergens: mosquito saliva specific IgE and IgG levels in children. Ann Allergy Asthma Immunol 2004; 93:553–556.
5. Steen CJ, Carbonaro PA, Schwartz RA. Arthropods in dermatology. J Am Acad Dermatol 2004; 50: 819–862.
6. Howard R, Frieden IJ. Papular urticaria in children. Pediatr Dermatol 1996; 13:246–249.
7. Noe R, Cohen AL, Lederman E, et al. Skin disorders among construction workers following Hurricane Katrina and Hurricane Rita: an outbreak investigation in New Orleans, Louisiana. Arch Dermatol 2007; 143:1393–1398.
8. Garcia E, Halpert E, Rodriguez A, et al. Immune and histopathologic examination of flea-bite induced papular urticaria. Ann Allergy Asthma Immunol 2004; 92:446–452.
9. Karthikeyan K, Thappa DM, Jeevankumar B. Pattern of pediatric dermatoses in a referral center in South India. Indian Pediatr 2004; 41:373–377.
10. Naafs B. Allergic skin reactions in the tropics. Clin Dermatol 2006; 24:158–167.
11. Remoue F, Alix E, Cornelie S, et al. IgE and IgG4 antibody responses to Aedes saliva in African children. Acta Trop 2007; 104:108–115.
12. Reunala T, Ulmanen I, Siltanen I. Animal fleas attacking man (in Finnish). Duodecim 1979; 95: 119–123.
13. Rantanen T, Reunala T, Vuojolahti P, et al. Persistent pruritic papules from deer ked bites. Acta Derm Venereol 1982; 62:307–311.
14. Kemp SF, de Shazo RD, Moffitt JE, et al. Expanding habitat of the imported fire ant (Solenopsis invicta): a public health concern. J Allergy Clin Immunol 2000; 105683–105691.
15. Chosidow O. Clinical practices. Scabies. N Engl J Med 2006; 354:1718–1727.
16. Jordaan HF, Schneider JW. Papular urticaria: a histopathologic study of 30 patients. Am J Dermatopathol 1997; 19:119–126.
17. Peng Z, Simons FE. A prospective study of naturally acquired sensitization and subsequent desensitization to mosquito bites and concurrent antibody responses. J Allergy Clin Immunol 1998; 101:284–286.
18. Mellanby K. Man's reactions to mosquito bites. Nature 1946; 158:554.
19. McDermott MJ, Weber E, Hunter S, et al. Identification, cloning, and characterization of a major cat flea salivary allergen (Cte f 1). Mol Immunol 2000; 37:361–375.

20. Leverkus M, Jochim RC, Schäd S, et al. Bullous allergic hypersensitivity to bed bug bites mediated by IgE against nitrophorin. J Invest Dermatol 2006; 126:91–96.

21. Peng Z, Simons FE. Advances in mosquito allergy. Curr Opin Allergy Clin Immunol 2007; 7: 350–354.

22. Brummer-Korvenkontio H, Palosuo K, Palosuo T, et al. Detection of mosquito saliva-specific IgE antibodies by capture ELISA. Allergy 1997; 52:342–345.

23. Abdel-Naser MB, Lotfy RA, Al-Sherbiny MM, et al. Patients with papular urticaria have IgG antibodies to bedbug (Cimex lectularius) antigens. Parasitol Res 2006; 98:550–556.

24. Karppinen A, Rantala I, Vaalasti A, et al. Effect of cetirizine on the inflammatory cells in mosquito bites. Clin Exp Allergy 1996; 26:703–709.

25. Peng Z, Yang M, Simons FE. Immunologic mechanisms in mosquito allergy: correlation of skin reactions with specific IgE and IgG antibodies and lymphocyte proliferation response to mosquito antigens. Ann Allergy Asthma Immunol 1996; 77:238–244.

26. Cuéllar A, García E, Rodríguez A, et al. Functional dysregulation of dendritic cells in patients with papular urticaria caused by fleabite. Arch Dermatol 2007; 143:1415–1419.

27. Smith SR, Macfarlane AW, Lewis-Jones MS. Papular urticaria and transfer of allergy following bone marrow transplantation. Clin Exp Dermatol 1988; 13:260–262.

28. Pedersen J, Carganello J, van der Weyden MB. Exaggerated reaction to insect bites in patients with chronic lymphocytic leukemia. Clinical and histological findings. Pathology 1990; 22: 141–143.

29. Smith KJ, Skelton HG III, Vogel P, et al. Exaggerated insect bite reactions in patients positive for HIV. J Am Acad Dermatol 1993; 29:269–272.

30. Karppinen A, Kautiainen H, Petman L, et al. Comparison of cetirizine, ebastine and loratadine in the treatment of immediate mosquito-bite allergy. Allergy 2002; 57:534–537.

31. Karppinen A, Brummer-Korvenkontio H, Petman L, et al. Levocetirizine for treatment of immediate and delayed mosquito bite reactions. Acta Derm Venereol 2006; 86:329–331.

32. Fradin MS. Mosquitoes and mosquito repellents: a clinician's guide. Ann Intern Med 1998; 128: 931–940.

14

Diagnosis of Difficult Urticaria and Angioedema

Allen P. Kaplan
Department of Medicine, Medical University of South Carolina, Charleston, South Carolina, U.S.A.

Malcolm W. Greaves
St. John's Institute of Dermatology, St. Thomas's Hospital, London, U.K.

INTRODUCTION

Most types of urticaria can be readily diagnosed on the basis of history and tests (provocation or laboratory) that are relatively simple. However there are clearly patients who present with a confusing array of symptoms, and the hives may or may not be present at the time of the initial presentation. A wide variety of possibilities need to be considered until a definitive diagnosis is made, including the possibility that more than one type of urticaria may be present. Before considering the specific possibilities one may encounter, some general guidelines may be helpful in an initial consideration of any patient.

SKIN CONDITIONS THAT CLINICALLY MIMIC URTICARIA AND ANGIOEDEMA

Even experienced specialists in allergy or dermatology can be taken in by urticaria-like skin manifestations of nonurticarial disease. The following are actual examples; a more detailed (but not fully comprehensive) list is included in Table 1.

Contact Allergic Dermatitis

A 50-year-old Afro-Caribbean woman with a long history of admissions for psoriasis vulgaris was admitted for in-patient treatment by the Ingram regimen (tar bath, ultraviolet phototherapy, and dithranol [anthralin]). Soon after admission she developed swelling, redness, and itching of the eyelids and scattered irritant red lesions on the trunk and limbs. Initially diagnosed as urticaria and angioedema, the lesions proved to be persistent and eventually peeled, leading to a revised diagnosis of contact dermatitis to synthetic rubber,

Table 1 Some Skin Conditions Clinically Mimicking Urticaria and Angioedema

Contact allergic dermatitis (especially of the face)
Dermatomyositis (especially of the face)
Acute photosensitivity (especially polymorphous light eruption)
Recurrent cellulitis, erysipelas
Fixed drug eruption
Erythropoietic protoporphyria (early childhood)
Hypoalbuminaemia (especially the nephrotic syndrome)
Crohn's disease (granulomatous cheilitis with lymphoedema)
Melkersson–Rosenthal syndrome (lymphoedema, fissured tongue, facial nerve palsy)
Myxedema

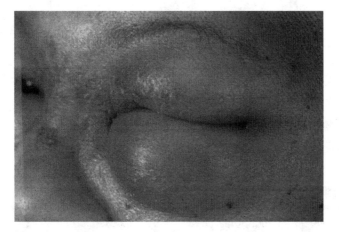

Figure 1 (*See color insert*) Allergic contact dermatitis—LATEX.

finally confirmed by patch testing. She had been in the habit of self-applying her dithranol using rubber gloves she had obtained at home (Fig. 1).

Crohn's Disease

A 35-year-old man presented with recurrent swelling of the lower lip for three months. The lips, especially the lower lip would swell for two to three days and then partially subside. There was no itching and no other cutaneous signs or symptoms. Examination showed non-ender swelling of the lower lip with some induration. An initial diagnosis of recurrent angioedema was made, and the patient underwent a panel of allergy skin tests. A subsequent, more thorough examination of the mouth revealed cobblestone thickening of the oral mucosa and the liver was found to be enlarged. A revised diagnosis of Crohn's disease with secondary lymphoedema was made. Further questioning revealed a history of intermittent bowel disturbance, previously labeled as irritable bowel syndrome, and endoscopic bowel investigations, a liver biopsy and oral mucosal biopsy confirmed Crohn's disease. It should be noted that Melkersson–Rosenthal syndrome (facial lymphoedema, facial nerve palsy, and scrotal tongue) can produce a similar clinical and granulomatous histological picture (Fig. 2). The swelling may be present for weeks (or longer).

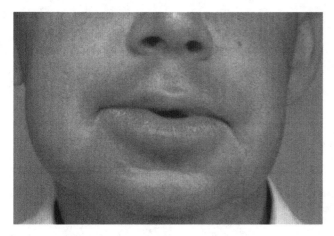

Figure 2 (*See color insert*) Granulomatous cheilitis: Crohn's disease.

Recurrent Erythema Multiforme

A 42-year-old man presented with a two-year history of red tender and itchy lesions mainly on the hands, feet, and limbs, and there was an accompanying variable crusted cheilitis with labial edema. The eyes, genitalia, and interior of the mouth were unaffected. Individual skin lesions lasted one to two weeks and desquamated. Initially the patient was referred with a presumptive diagnosis of intermittent urticaria and angioedema. However this was ruled out on the basis of prolonged duration of individual skin lesions and the presence of desquamation (urticaria and angioedema do not peel). Urticarial vasculitis was considered, but a skin biopsy showed upper dermal lymphocytic infiltration, exocytosis of CD8+ cells into the epidermis and satellite cell necrosis, indicative of erythema multiforme. Polymerase chain reaction (PCR) examination of the skin biopsy material revealed Herpes simplex DNA and the patient's attacks were greatly reduced following long-term acyclovir treatment. The final diagnosis was recurrent erythema multiforme secondary to chronic Herpes simplex infection (Fig. 3).

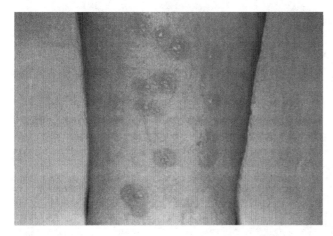

Figure 3 (*See color insert*) Erythema multiforme.

Recurrent Erysipelas of the Forearms

An obese 45-year-old woman presented with a two-year history of six episodes of acute swelling of the right forearm and three similar episodes of swelling of the left forearm. Each attack was painless, accompanied by fever, lasted a month, and resolved with scaling. The patient was referred for investigation of angioedema, but examination of the hands revealed bilateral cheiropompholyx (vesicular eczema of the palms) and careful observation showed that episodes of swelling were accompanied by signs of forearm lymphangitis. The overall picture was that of recurrent erysipelas, the portal of entry for infection being the palmar eczema. The patient experienced a reduction in attacks after commencing long-term penicillin treatment and topical corticosteroids for the eczema.

URTICARIA AND ANGIOEDEMA: ACUTE VS. CHRONIC

It is useful to differentiate acute from chronic disease because an acute, brief ($<$6 weeks) episode of urticaria/angioedema is likely due to some identifiable allergen (drug, food, infection) (1). Urticaria/angioedema that is persistent and exceeds six weeks is more likely to be endogenous and many in fact represent either autoimmune chronic urticaria/ angioedema or idiopathic urticaria/angioedema (2). This distinction, however, breaks down in a variety of circumstances. The various types of physical urticaria typically persist for many months or even years, and in that sense are "chronic," yet these need to be distinguished from the aforementioned types of chronic urticaria/angioedema. Statistics regarding the incidence of finding a "cause" for chronic hives vary tremendously in the literature, not only because of the erroneous attribution of some ingested substance as a cause of chronic urticaria, but also by the inclusion of the physical urticarias within the groups where a definite diagnosis has been made and in that sense, the cause already found. It is also possible that any patient presenting with urticaria/ angioedema of only a few weeks' duration may have disease that represents the beginning of a more chronic process. The diagnosis will not become evident until a much longer period has passed, with persistence of symptoms.

PHYSICAL URTICARIA VS. OTHER CAUSES

One of the important distinctions to be made between different causes of hives is the duration of individual lesions. Most types of hives that are physically induced have lesions that last less than two hours. This is generally true of cold urticaria, cholinergic urticaria, dermatographism, and solar urticaria. The major exception is pressure-induced urticaria (often designated delayed-pressure urticaria) in which not only is there a delay of 4 to 8 hours before urticaria appears after a pressure stimulus, but the duration of the hives certainly exceeds 2 hours and may remain 12 to 36 hours (3). Other causes of hives e.g., allergic reactions to foods or drugs or chronic urticaria (whether idiopathic or autoimmune) may result in individual lesions that last longer than 2 hours and typically last between 4 hours and 24 hours. Thus it is extremely helpful to inquire about the duration of individual lesions besides asking about the stimulus, shape, and location of lesions particularly when a physically induced hive is suspect. If angioedema occurs concurrently with the urticarial process (e.g., a cold urticaria patient who places one hand in ice water rather than doing an ice cube test), the swelling will remain for most of the day because it takes much longer to resorb the interstitial fluid, although the swelling will stop increasing in less than two hours if it is part of the aforementioned physical processes.

Next we will consider some of the more difficult presentations of patients with urticaria and angioedema.

COLD URTICARIA, CHOLINERGIC URTICARIA, AND DERMATOGRAPHISM

Although most patients with one of these disorders are readily identified, (i.e., hives due to touching cold objects vs. exercising, sweating, and hot showers vs. hives caused by scratching), historical clues can sometimes be misleading. There are patients with cholinergic urticaria who will describe hives occurring while swimming (a typical complaint of patients with cold urticaria), who do not have cold urticaria but induce hives as a results of the exercise of swimming. Many patients with severe dermatographism have hives when they shower, and the urticaria is caused by the fine spray hitting their skin regardless of the temperature. However, because it is more common to take a hot rather than cold shower, one might thus think that cholinergic urticaria is present. An exercise challenge (running on the spot in a heated room for 10 minutes or exercising on a stationary bicycle in a warmed room for 10–15 minutes) should be negative, but clothing rubbing against the skin while exercising can cause hives in patients with severe dermatographic disease. Once the diagnosis of severe dermatographism is made by scratching the person's skin, the diagnosis of concomitant cholinergic urticaria can only be made on the basis of distribution and appearance of the hives. For example, do hives appear on the face, or will exercise without clothing still cause hives?

Combinations of these physically induced hives can occur. For example, cold urticaria and cholinergic urticaria (4,5) may both be present; thus patients will have both a positive ice cube test and a positive exercise challenge, fulfilling criteria for each disorder. Dermatographism can also occur in combination with cold urticaria or cholinergic urticaria although this is infrequent. With severe dermatographism, the diagnosis of concomitant cholinergic urticaria (as described above) or cold urticaria can be difficult to affirm. We have seen an occasional dermatographic patient whose ice cube test was positive only because the ice cube was moved somewhat when the test was done, whereas other types of cold challenges, for example, placing one hand in the water or holding an ice-filled glass, were negative. Disorders that can be missed are those in which combinations of physical stimuli are needed to produce urticaria, but a single challenge is negative. Examples are cold-induced cholinergic urticaria and cold-dependent dermatographisms (6,7). In cold-induced cholinergic urticaria, exercise produces symptoms only when it occurs in a cold environment. The ice cube test is negative, and exercise in a heated room is negative as well. The term "cholinergic urticaria" was used here because the lesions had the appearance of cholinergic hives and were exercise related, but there is no evidence that released acetylcholine into the skin causes the urticaria, as is true of classical cholinergic urticaria. Cold-dependent dermatographism is seen in patients in whom scratching the skin causes linear hives only when the skin has been cooled, e.g., scratching while outside during the winter.

SOLAR URTICARIA

Difficulties regarding the diagnosis of solar urticaria arise because of confusion with other light sensitive rashes, most of which are not urticarial. The fact that patients may present without a rash and most offices lack the equipment to challenge patients with the appropriate wavelength contributes to this. Type I solar urticaria (8) is due to medium-wavelength UV light which does not pass through ordinary window glass and does not typically occur indoors. It should be distinguished from rare causes of solar urticaria occurring within the visible spectrum that can be induced by standing near a closed window on sunny days. These patients may also react to local heat, since infrared is adjacent to visible light in the solar emission spectrum. Exposure to either natural sunlight or a solar simulator can evoke an immediate wheal and flare response and thereby affirm the diagnosis and the wavelength specificity. Most patients who have solar urticaria will have lesions that last less than two hours if they are removed from the stimulus, whereas most other photosensitive rashes, whether urticarial or not, last for many hours and often days to weeks. Alternative considerations are photoallergic or phototoxic contact dermatitis, photosensitivity due to an ingested medication, or polymorphous light eruption, a particular delayed hypersensitivity-type rash, or cutaneous manifestations or one of the porphyrias.

CHRONIC INTERMITTENT URTICARIA/ANGIOEDEMA AND IDIOPATHIC ANAPHYLAXIS

When urticaria occurs intermittently, the diagnostic possibilities actually increase, although persistent urticaria can be far more troublesome for the patient. For example, a patient may have hives for one to two weeks, a respite of two to three weeks, and then recurrence that follows such a pattern for six months. The patient does not fulfill criteria for chronic urticaria and the intermittent nature makes one consider that some allergen may be responsible. Skin testing for IgE-mediated hypersensitivity to foods, spices, or condiments should be done even if the history provides no clues regarding foods that might be ingested in such an intermittent fashion. A thorough consideration of any medication used intermittently must also be made, including nonsteroidal anti-inflammatory drugs, (NSAIDS), hormone preparations, vitamins, and others. Such patients may have chronic urticaria with a presentation that is intermittent and perhaps less severe. The idiopathic version becomes a diagnosis of exclusion, whereas a positive test for IgG antibody to the IgE receptor or IgE itself suggests autoimmune chronic urticaria. Thyroid function tests and thyroid antibodies (antithyroglobulin and antimicrosomal) should be done since the incidence is 24% in patients with chronic urticaria (9) and provides a clue to this diagnosis. These antithyroid antibodies segregate with the autoimmune subtype of chronic urticaria rather than those that remain idiopathic (10), suggesting a more general immune abnormality in patients within the autoimmune subgroup of chronic urticaria patients. The incidence of these antibodies in the population at large is 7% to 8%, which is about the same percentage of antithyroid antibodies in patients lacking antibody to the IgE receptor or to IgE (10%) (11).

Angioedema occurs in approximately 40% of patients with chronic urticaria and can also be present intermittently in association with urticaria. If severe, the symptoms can be confused with idiopathic anaphylaxis, which is always intermittent and has an unpredictable frequency. One major difference, however, is that episodes of idiopathic anaphylaxis typically last one to two days, while episodes of intermittent chronic urticaria/angioedema usually (but not always) last much longer. The identifying features depend on the presence or absence of other hallmarks of anaphylaxis or, in the absence of such symptoms, the severity of the angioedema.

Idiopathic anaphylaxis presents with symptoms that can include facial flushing, urticaria, angioedema, asthma, nausea, vomiting, cramps, diarrhea, and hypotension. Chronic urticaria and angioedema is not associated hypotension and rarely if ever with gastrointestinal complaints or wheezing. On the other hand, a patient with flushing, urticaria, and angioedema in the absence of other symptoms most likely has chronic urticaria and angioedema, but there may be exceptions. Chronic urticaria can be associated with angioedema of the tongue or pharynx, but not laryngeal edema, and the swelling of the tongue and throat should not be of such severity as to cause respiratory embarrassment (e.g., inability to handle secretions, or pharyngeal or glottal swelling of such magnitude that intubation is a serious consideration). The latter patients have been considered to have idiopathic anaphylaxis (12). The distinction in the absence of other anaphylactic manifestations is, in part, semantic since there is no laboratory test for idiopathic anaphylaxis (anti FcεR1 autoantibody test is negative) (Lieberman P, Kaplan AP; unpublished observations.), but therapy will be influenced by the distinction. Although alternate day steroids have been advocated for each disorder, when severe (12,13), the dosage of prednisone in idiopathic anaphylaxis often begins at 40 to 60 mg every other day for months at a time. Chronic urticaria and angioedema can typically be treated with 20 to 25 mg prednisone q.o.d. (1), with decrements of 2.5 to 5.0 mg every two to three weeks (14). An alternative approach for chronic urticaria is prednisone at 10 mg daily, with decrements of 1 mg every 7 to 10 days (15).

ANAPHYLAXIS: WHAT MAKES IT IDIOPATHIC

In cases when anaphylaxis is recurrent and the diagnosis is not obviously due to latex hypersensitivity, fire ant stings, drugs, foods, or other identifiable stimuli it is deemed idiopathic: a cause cannot be found. Extensive skin testing is typically done in an attempt to identify an exogenous allergen. Some unusual causes of anaphylaxis are listed in Table 2 that should be kept in mind. Patients in whom a diagnosis of idiopathic anaphylaxis has been made should be reassessed if alternative possibilities become evident that had not previously been considered.

It is not uncommon that patients initially presenting with symptoms consistent with idiopathic anaphylaxis are also considered to possibly have systemic mastocytosis or

Table 2   Unusual Ingestants Reported to Cause Anaphylaxis (with Urticaria)

Coriander in teriyaki sauce
Carrageenan
Thiamine
Anisakis Simplex, a parasite of fish
Wheat flour contaminated with dust mite in dust mite allergic subject
Cumin
Oregano
Thyme
Caraway seeds
Carmine (naturally derived red dye)
Sesame seeds
Saffron
Condurango bark in herbal tea
Prednisone
Methylprednisolone succinate
Diphenhydramine
Omeprazole
Celecoxib

Source: From Refs. 16–22.

carcinoid syndrome. Patients with systemic mastocytosis may have flushing, cramps or diarrhea, and hypotension, in common with idiopathic anaphylaxis. They rarely have hives and swelling of the type seen in chronic urticaria and angioedema. The skin lesions vary from urticaria pigmentosa (i.e., pigmented lesions that urticate with scratching), or frank dermatographism, where the cutaneous mast cell infiltration is more generalized. These can be differentiated biochemically by the increased tryptase (and total α tryptase) seen in patients with systemic mastocytosis. Patients with idiopathic anaphylaxis have a normal tryptase level between episodes and elevated tryptase (particularly β tryptase) levels when anaphylaxis occurs. Skin biopsy or bone marrow examination, may reveal evidence of mast cell proliferation in systemic mastocytosis, whereas mast cell numbers are normal in idiopathic anaphylaxis. This is considered in greater detail in chapters 22 and 24.

ANGIOEDEMA: OTHER CONSIDERATIONS

Angioedema occurring in the absence of any urticaria requires evaluation for hereditary or acquired C1 INH deficiency (see chapter 16), allergic reaction to foods or drugs, and use of angiotensin-converting enzyme (ACE) inhibitors, before it is assumed to be idiopathic. The swelling typically affects the face, lips, tongue, pharynx, genitalia (in men), hands and feet, and to a lesser degree on the trunk or more proximal extremities. Gastrointestinal symptoms due to edema of the bowel wall may be seen. If true laryngeal edema occurs, the C1 INH deficiency, use of an ACE inhibitor, or idiopathic anaphylaxis is much more likely than idiopathic angioedema in which laryngeal edema virtually never occurs. Pharyngeal edema, is however, relatively common. The newly described hereditary angioedema with normal C1 INH (23,24) occurs predominantly (but not exclusively) in women and is associated with estrogen use. A mutant Factor XII with abnormally elevated activity when activated is present in many such cases. In the absence of a family history, a sporadic case may be assumed to be idiopathic angioedema. Gastrointestinal symptoms or true laryngeal edema may provide a clue as well as being refractory to most therapeutic modalities, particularly antihistamines.

Angioedema is episodic: after a period of many hours to a maximum of two to three days, it completely resolves and may later occur at the same site or other sites. Swelling that persists, particularly involving the face, is more likely Melkersson–Rosenthal syndrome. This is a persistent granulatomous inflammation, most commonly involving the lips and lower face, which may be associated with a fissured tongue, chronic facial lymphoedema, and Bells palsy (25–27) (Table 1). More general persistent and symmetrical facial swelling (or swelling elsewhere) can be a manifestation of nephrotic syndrome, cardiac or liver failure, myxedema, trichinosis, or lymphatic obstruction. Granulomatous cheilitis, virtually indistinguishable from the lip swelling of Melkersson–Rosenthal syndrome can be seen with Crohn's disease (28).

CONCLUDING COMMENTS

A specific diagnosis can be readily made in most patients presenting with urticaria and angioedema on the basis of history, appearance of lesions, and simple challenge tests or laboratory studies. However occasionally patients present with confounding symptoms that do not correspond to any particular entity. In those circumstances, one should consider the possibility that multiple types of urticaria/angioedema are present simultaneously, or that the diagnosis is an unusual type of hives or swelling, or that the presumption of urticaria and angioedema is not correct, and that some other cutaneous disorder or manifestation is present. It is important to see the lesions rather than rely on a description of the rash; obtain photographs of lesions if the lesions cannot be visualized; and, where appropriate, try to induce hives or swelling. Some dermatitides can have an appearance that resembles urticaria and a skin biopsy demonstrating spongiosis or other nonurticarial skin pathologic findings can help to resolve the issue. Even more difficult can be the occasional simultaneous occurrence of hives and some other skin rash, such as a dermatitis or rash associated with systemic lupus erythematosus.

REFERENCES

1. Kaplan AP. Urticaria and angioedema. In: Middleton E Jr., Reed CE, Ellis EF, et al. eds. Allergy – Principles of Practice. 5th ed. Vol. 2. St. Louis, MO: Mosby, 1998:1104–1122.
2. Greaves MW. Chronic urticaria. N Engl J Med 1995; 332:1767–1772.
3. Estes SA, Yang CW. Delayed pressure urticaria: an investigation of some parameters of lesion induction. J Am Acad Dermatol 1981; 5:25–31.
4. Ormerod AD, Lobza-Black A, Milford-Ward A, et al. Combined cold urticaria and cholinergic urticaria – clinical characteristics and laboratory findings. Br J Dermatol 1988; 118:621–627.
5. Sigler RW, Levinson AI, Evans R III, et al. Evaluation of a patient with cold and cholinergic urticaria. J Allergy Clin Immunol 1979; 60:35–38.
6. Kaplan AP. Unusual cold-induced disorders: cold dependent dermatographism and systemic cold urticaria. J Allergy Clin Immunol 1984; 73: 453–456.
7. Kaplan AP, Garolalo J. Identification of a new physically induced urticaria: cold induced cholinergic urticaria. J Allergy Clin Immunol 1981; 63:438–441.
8. Sams WM Jr., Epstein JH, Winkelmann RK. Solar urticaria: investigation of pathogenic mechanisms. Arch Dermatol 1969; 99:390–397.
9. Kaplan AP, Finn A. Autoimmunity and the etiology of chronic urticaria. Can J Allergy Clin Immunol 1999; 4:286–292.
10. Kikuchi Y, Fann T, Kaplan AP. Antithyroid antibodies in chronic urticaria and angioedema. J Allergy Clin Immunol 2003; 112(1):218.
11. Ajjan RA, Weetman AP. Autoimmune thyroid disease, Addison's Disease, and Autoimmune polyglandular syndromes. In: Austen KF, Frank MM, Atkinson JP, et al. eds. Samter's Immunologic Diseases. Vol. 2. Philadelphia: Lippincott, Williams, and Wilkins, 2001:605–626.
12. Patterson R, Stoloff RS, Greenberger PA, et al. Algorithms for the diagnosis and management of idiopathic anaphylaxis. Ann Allergy 1993; 7:40–44.
13. Patterson R, Wong S, Dykewicz MS, et al. Malignant idiopathic anaphylaxis. J Allergy Clin Immunol 1990; 85:86–66.
14. Kaplan AP. Chronic urticaria and angioedema. N Engl J Med 2002; 346:175–179.
15. Kaplan AP. Urticaria and Angioedema. In: Wolff K, Goldsmith LA, Katz SI, et al. eds. Fitzpatrick's Dermatology in General Medicine. 7th ed. New York: Magraw Hill Publishing, 2007:330–343.
16. Proebstle TM, Gall H, Jugert FK, et al. Specific IgE and IgG serum antibodies to thiamine associated with anaphylactic reaction. J Allergy Clin Immunol 1995; 95:1059–1060.
17. Audieana MT, de Corres LF, Munoz D, et al. Recurrent anaphylaxis caused by anisakis simplex parasitizing fish. J Allergy Clin Immunol 1995; 96:558–560.
18. Bianco C, Quiralte J, Castillo R, et al. Anaphylaxis after ingestion of wheat flour contaminated with mites. J Allergy Clin Immunol 1997; 99:308–313.
19. Boxer M, Roberts M, Grammer L. Cumin anaphylaxis: a case report. J Allergy Clin Immunol 1999; 99:722–723.
20. Wuthrich B, Kagi MK, Stucker W. Anaphylactic reactions to ingested carmine. Allergy 1997; 52: 1133–1137.
21. Wuthrich B, Schmid-Grendelmeyer P, Lundberg M. Anaphylaxis to saffron. Allergy 1997; 52: 474–475.

22. Burgdorff T, Venemalm L, Vogt T, et al. IgE medicated anaphylactic reaction induced by succinate ester of methylprednisolone. Ann Allergy 2002; 89:425–428.
23. Bork K, Gul D, Dewald G. Hereditary angioedema with normal C1 inhibitor in a family with affected women and men. Br J Dermatol 2006; 154:542–545.
24. Dewald G, Bork K. Missense mutations in the coagulation factor XII (Hageman factor) gene in hereditary angioedema with normal C1 inhibitor. Biochem Biophys Res Commun 2006; 343(4): 1286–1289.
25. Greene RM, Rogers RS III. Melkersson-Rosenthal syndrome: a review of 36 patients. J Am Acad Dermatol 1989; 21:1263–1270.
26. Sussman GL, Yang WH, Steinberg S. Melkersson-Rosenthal syndrome: clinical, pathologic, and therapeutic considerations. Ann Allergy 1992; 69:187–1994.
27. Zimmer WM, Rogers RS III, Reeve CM, et al. Orofacial manifestation of Melkersson-Rosenthal syndrome. A study of 42 patients and review of 220 cases from the literature. Oral Surg Oral Med Oral Pathol 1992; 74:610–619.
28. Kano Y, Shiohara T, Yagita A, et al. Granulomatous cheilitis and Crohn's disease. Br J Dermatol 1990; 123:409–412.

15

Hereditary Disorders with Urticaria or Angioedema

Hal M. Hoffman
Division of Rheumatology, Allergy, and Immunology, University of California, San Diego, La Jolla, California, U.S.A.

Alan A. Wanderer
Department of Pediatrics–Allergy, University of Colorado Health Sciences Center, Allergy and Asthma Consultants of Montana, Bozeman, Montana, U.S.A.

INTRODUCTION

In a typical clinical practice it is not uncommon to see urticaria/angioedema patients that report relatives with urticaria/angioedema, suggesting that there is a genetic influence on these disorders. However, the diagnosis of true hereditary urticaria/angioedema is rare, because most diseases do not follow a classic hereditary pattern. In the first section of this chapter we will discuss the initial diagnostic evaluation and counseling of patients with a family history of these disorders. We will also discuss models of heredity and the methods used by investigators to identify the genetic bases of diseases. In the second section, we describe a group of rare inherited systemic inflammatory diseases that present with atypical urticaria as a prominent feature. Finally, we discuss several disorders with urticaria and/or angioedema that appear to be inherited.

Hereditary Disease

Evaluation and Counseling of Patients with Inherited Diseases
It can be difficult to confirm the presence of an inherited disease, since most illnesses seen in clinical practice have complex etiologies, and accurate information about family members is often limited. As there are only a few known genes that cause disorders with urticaria or angioedema, one must rely on history and physical examination. A detailed family history of urticaria or angioedema as well as immunologic diseases, neonatal deaths and miscarriages, and unexplained deaths or illnesses is important. The creation of a complete and accurate pedigree, while difficult, can help identify patterns of inheritance. Ideally this is done by direct evaluation of family members; however, when necessary some information can be obtained from others.

It is also important to identify environmental exposures (e.g., toxic or infectious), as the significance of genetics can be overestimated because close family members have had similar environmental exposures. An example might be a brother and sister who develop cold urticaria, with a history of a father who developed cold urticaria as a child. At first glance, this might suggest a hereditary disease. However, further questioning reveals that the hives of both siblings developed weeks after confirmed mononucleosis, suggesting a nongenetic cause for the hives. However, it is possible that these two siblings and their father are genetically predisposed to the development of cold urticaria, and this was triggered by viral infection. The difficulty of definitive diagnosis, such as in this case, illustrates the complexity of accurately counseling parents about the risk of transmission for most diseases.

Physical examination of the patient as well as presumed affected family members during symptoms is crucial, because patients often assume that what they are experiencing is the same as that of their relative. Photographs of rashes may be used in place of a direct physical examination. Skin biopsies may also be helpful to confirm a diagnosis. Genetic testing may be performed in patients whose symptoms and family history are consistent with one of the illnesses for which a genetic basis has been identified.

In all but the most extensively studied inherited conditions, it is difficult to be confident of inheritance patterns. In suspected cases of inherited diseases, consider referral to a genetic counselor. Multiple complicating factors make risk determination an intricate task, even for experienced counselors. Fortunately, this may become easier as the underlying genetic defects in diseases are elucidated.

Mendelian Disease Inheritance Patterns

There are four basic Mendelian inheritance patterns seen in human disease: autosomal recessive, autosomal dominant, X-linked recessive, and X-linked dominant. These patterns are based on the assumption that mutations in a single gene are responsible for a disease and that no other complicating factors are involved. Often one can only infer a disease's mode of inheritance because of the limited size of families, but there are several distinguishing features that aid in this determination. Diseases with autosomal inheritance (genes on chromosome 1–22) affect either sex equally, and recessive diseases generally skip generations. X-linked diseases (genes on the X chromosome) are never passed from father to son (1).

Figure 1 A demonstrates a classic autosomal recessive mode of inheritance in which affected individuals possess two copies of a mutated gene (one from each parent) and carriers possess only one mutated gene. Affected individuals or carriers can be either male or female, and affected individuals are usually born to unaffected parents who are carriers. Diseases with this inheritance are often seen in physically or culturally isolated populations, and are particularly frequent in cases of parental consanguinity. If both parents are carriers, each child has a 25% chance of being affected. Adenosine deaminase deficiency, a type of severe combined immune deficiency, is an example of an autosomal recessive inherited disease.

The pedigree in Figure 1 B shows a classic autosomal dominant mode of inheritance in which possession of one mutated gene inherited from either parent results in disease. In this example affected individuals can be either male or female and have one affected parent. An affected parent has a 50% chance of having an affected child. Hereditary angioedema (HAE) discussed elsewhere in this book is an example of an autosomal dominant disease.

Figure 1 C demonstrates an X-linked recessive inheritance pattern in which males are exclusively affected because the Y chromosome does not possess a normal copy of the

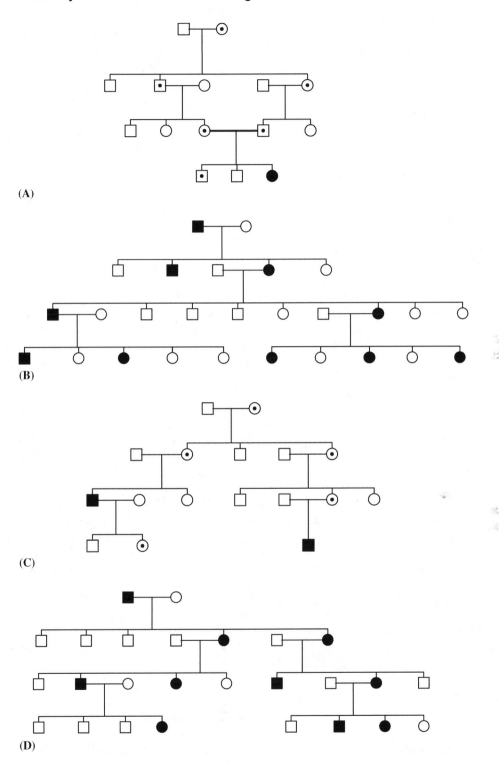

Figure 1 Mendelian inheritance patterns. (**A**) Pedigree of autosomal recessive disorder. (**B**) Pedigree of autosomal dominant disorder (FCAS family). (**C**) Pedigree of X-linked recessive disorder. (**D**) Pedigree of X-linked dominant disorder. *Filled squares* (males) and *circles* (females) indicate affected individuals and *open squares* and *circles* indicate unaffected individuals; *dotted squares* and *circles* indicte carrier individuals.

mutated gene located on the X chromosome. Females can be asymptomatic carriers and often have affected male relatives. One half of the male offspring of female carriers will be affected. Bruton's agammaglobulinemia, a humoral immunodeficiency, is an example of X-linked recessive disease.

X-linked dominant disorders (Fig. 1 D) are extremely rare. Pedigrees are similar to autosomal dominant transmission, except that affected fathers never have affected sons. In general, more females are affected than males, but females are often more mildly affected than males (sometimes lethal). The child of an affected female has a 50% chance of being affected. Hypophosphatemia, a form of vitamin D–resistant rickets, is an example of a disease with this mode of inheritance.

Complex Inheritance

There are a number of factors that complicate Mendelian inheritance of human diseases. Many individuals display no symptoms despite having an alteration in a dominantly inherited disease gene, but they still transmit the disease gene and disease to their offspring. This phenomenon is called nonpenetrance. While the hallmark of many inherited diseases is an early age of onset, some genetic diseases do not present until later in life, such as Huntington disease. This is referred to as age-dependent penetrance. Another complicating factor is variable expression in which individuals with mutations in the same gene display different signs and symptoms or different levels of severity, to the point where relatives with mutations can be indistinguishable from members without mutations. Sporadic cases with no family history of affected parents or offspring may not appear to have a genetic basis, but many autosomal dominant diseases arise from spontaneous mutations in the absence of affected parents, and some inherited diseases affect lifespan or reproductive capacity, so no affected offspring are generated. Finally, it is common for abnormalities in different genes to cause the same or similar clinical picture. This is referred to as genetic heterogeneity and is seen in common conditions such as anemia and cancer (1).

Few diseases are inherited in a purely Mendelian fashion. Most diseases or clinical syndromes are inherited in a complex fashion because of the contribution of one or multiple genes and/or environmental influences. The number of genes and the relative impact of genetic and environmental factors vary among conditions. In some diseases, such as X-linked lymphoproliferative disease, patients possess a single susceptibility gene and develop symptoms only after they are exposed to Epstein–Barr virus. It is predicted that several diseases possess a few major susceptibility genes, with contributions from many minor modifying genes. Asthma is an example of a complex disease that probably has multiple major and minor susceptibility genes as well as several factors in the environment that modify the disease presentation. Although significant advances have been made in our knowledge of the role of genetics in illness, the complex interactions between "nature and nurture" make it difficult to definitively describe the etiology in most diseases.

Identifying Genes and Diagnosing Genetic Diseases

The development of molecular genetic methods over the last decade has made it more feasible to identify the genetic basis of diseases. The physical mapping and sequencing performed by the Human Genome Project and the creation of databases of genes, genetic markers, and single nucleotide polymorphisms (SNPs) over the last 5 to 10 years have provided very powerful tools for human geneticists. Initially, disease genes were identified using clues on the basis of the known pathophysiology of the disease, but with modern mapping techniques it is possible to identify these genes with little or no understanding of the underlying mechanisms involved. Genetic mapping utilizes numerous identifiable markers (or SNPs) with known locations throughout the genome. When a marker is identified that consistently segregates with illnesses in affected families, it is said to be genetically linked to the disorder and points to the approximate chromosomal location of a disease gene. By systematically surveying the chromosomes with enough markers, one can identify the specific location of a disease gene. Candidate genes in the region can then be screened using a number of techniques that identify specific alterations in the DNA sequence. The application of these methods to a wide range of genetic illnesses has had spectacular success in the last few years, resulting in the identification of genes responsible for disorders such as cystic fibrosis and Duchenne's muscular dystrophy (1). The process of identifying the gene responsible for familial cold autoinflammatory syndrome (FCAS) is discussed later in the chapter.

The identification of genes often improves our understanding of the underlying pathophysiology, which may lead to new targeted therapies in the future. It has also become a diagnostic tool and will have a significant impact on clinical practice in the future. Increasingly, genetic information will be used with clinical findings to delineate specific groups that may have certain prognostic features or therapeutic responses. However, several limitations, including genetic heterogeneity and environmental influences, will ensure that careful clinical evaluations will always be necessary.

Hereditary Disorders with Atypical Urticaria or Angioedema: Cryopyrinopathies

There are now several diseases associated with urticaria or angioedema for which genes have been identified. HAE (discussed elsewhere in this book) has been associated with mutations in the C1 inhibitor gene in several families. Sporadic or familial cases of mastocytosis/urticaria pigmentosa have been associated with mutations in the c-kit gene (discussed elsewhere in this book). In this section, we will discuss three inherited inflammatory syndromes whose symptoms include an atypical urticarial rash.

The category of autoinflammatory disorders is a relatively new classification used to describe a group of diseases characterized by recurrent episodes of inflammation without the high-titer autoantibodies or antigen-specific T cells that are commonly seen in traditional autoimmune disease (2). These disorders are characterized by dysregulation of the innate immune system and involve abnormal cytokine responses and neutrophilic inflammation. The inherited recurrent fever disorders such as familial Mediterranean fever (FMF), hyper IgD with periodic fever (HIDS), and tumor necrosis factor (TNF)-associated periodic syndrome (TRAPS) are the classic illnesses in this group. There have been significant advances in understanding the pathophysiology of these disorders in the last decade, since the molecular basis of each of these inherited diseases has been elucidated. Pyrin, a protein involved in interleukin-1 (IL-1) signaling is altered in FMF. Mevalonate Kinase, a protein involved in cholesterol biosynthesis, is altered in HIDS, and the TNF receptor, a receptor involved in inflammatory cytokine responses, is altered in TRAPS. These diseases are all characterized by intermittent, but not necessarily periodic, episodes of systemic inflammation that can last from two to three days with FMF to more than a week with TRAPS. Fever is the most common symptom, but is not always the chief complaint. Other symptoms that can occur during episodes include arthritis, myalgia, abdominal pain, chest pain (FMF), lymphadenopathy and splenomegaly (HIDS), and periorbital swelling (TRAPS) (2,3). Rash is a prominent feature in these disorders, but urticaria is unusual. Recently, three additional diseases with an atypical urticaria as a prominent feature have been added to the group of autoinflammatory syndromes. These disorders known collectively as the cryopyrinopathies are caused by mutations in the same gene, and they represent a clinical continuum of varying severity.

Clinical Features and Heredity

Familial cold autoinflammatory syndrome. In 1940, Kile and Rusk described a large North American family with members who developed urticaria-like eruptions after cold exposure (4). These physicians clearly demonstrated that this syndrome was distinct from classic cold urticaria (discussed elsewhere in this book) in that patients did not develop localized urticaria immediately after direct contact with cold water, but instead developed rash hours after a generalized cold exposure. Additionally, the family in that report described symptoms of fever, chills, and arthralgias associated with the rash. Since that time there have been approximately 25 families reported with this same clinical picture primarily in North America and Europe. This syndrome has been referred to as cold hypersensitivity, familial cold polymorphous eruption, cold pathergy, and cold-specific vasomotor neuropathy. It is most commonly known as familial cold urticaria, but recently was renamed familial cold autoinflammatory syndrome (FCAS) to accurately reflect the systemic nature of this disease and to prevent confusion with the more common acquired cold urticaria (ACU) (5).

In our cohort, up to 60% of FCAS patients developed rash at birth and 95% developed rash in the first six months of life. Other symptoms developed later in childhood and persisted throughout a patient's life. Longevity was usually normal in FCAS patients. Most patients experienced some baseline daily symptoms in the absence of cold exposure; however, exposure to mild temperatures, such as air-conditioned rooms, was sufficient to elicit attacks. Most attacks lasted less than one day and several patients described a diurnal pattern of attacks in the afternoon or evening that resolve by morning. The rash occasionally has urticarial features, but is more commonly characterized by erythematous and edematous papules and plaques. (Fig. 2) The rash can be pruritic, but is often described as tender. Additional symptoms experienced by patients were conjunctivitis, sweating, headache, drowsiness, thirst, and nausea (5). Rarely, FCAS patients develop AA (Amyloid type A) amyloidosis because of chronic inflammation. While

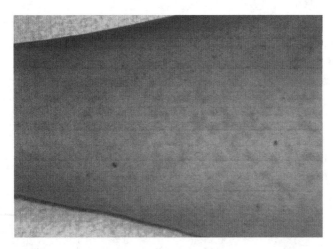

Figure 2 (*See color insert*) Photograph of the lower leg of a patient with FCAS. The leg was not directly exposed to cold prior to onset of rash.

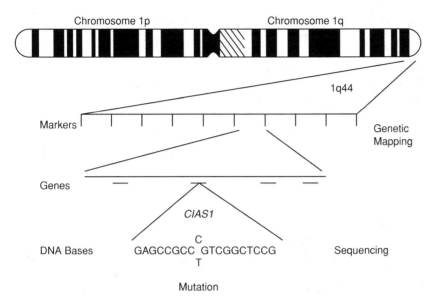

Figure 3 Mapping of the CIAS1 gene. Chromosomal location is identified by genetic mapping and further limited by fine genetic mapping. Potential genes in the region of interest are screened by DNA sequencing to identify DNA base changes (mutations).

FCAS has limited morbidity and mortality, the disease has significant impact on quality of life affecting school, work, and relationships (6).

FCAS is transmitted in a classic autosomal dominant fashion, with complete or near complete penetrance (Fig. 1 B). Sporadic cases have been documented, as is common for autosomal dominant diseases. There is variable expression in the clinical picture of FCAS in that some family members have more severe symptoms, and a few families have members that have developed amyloidosis. Two groups used genetic mapping of large families to identify a single locus on chromosome 1q44 for FCAS (7,8). Our group narrowed the chromosomal region of interest to approximately 1 million nucleotides (~0.4% of chromosome 1), a region that allowed for a gene-by-gene search. After screening approximately 80 potential genes (expressed sequence tags), we identified mutations in patients from families with FCAS in a single novel gene we termed "*CIAS1*" (cold induced autoinflammatory syndrome-1) that is now referred to as "*NLRP3*" (9) (Fig. 3). Since that time, we and several other investigators have identified a total of 14 mutations in exon 3 of *NLPR3* in patients with FCAS (10). Recently, two patients with a similar clinical presentation were found to have a mutation in a structurally related gene know as *NLRP12* (11). There are patients with classic FCAS features that do not possess *NLRP3* mutations, suggesting additional genetic heterogeneity (12).

Muckle-Wells syndrome. In 1962, Muckle and Wells described a European family that reported transient attacks of an urticaria-like rash accompanied by chills, malaise, and limb pains. There were no identifiable triggers for the episodes that occurred intermittently and lasted several hours to days. Most of the affected patients in the original description also developed late onset sensorineural hearing loss. Additionally, some of the affected patients also developed late-onset renal failure because of systemic amyloidosis (13). Since that time there have been at least 30 reports of families and sporadic cases in Europe and North America. The classic triad of Muckle-Wells syndrome

(MWS) includes rash, deafness, and amyloidosis. However, MWS displays significant variable expression in that deafness only occurs in approximately 60% of patients, and amyloidosis is only seen in approximately 30% of affected patients. In MWS, rash is often not reported until later in childhood, hearing loss is progressive beginning in childhood, and renal disease often develops later in adulthood because of amyloid deposition. Primary morbidity and mortality are associated with the renal disease in MWS (14,15).

MWS is transmitted in a classic autosomal dominant fashion with complete or near complete penetrance. Sporadic cases have been documented as is common for autosomal dominant diseases. Two groups used genetic mapping of large families to identify a locus on chromosome 1q44 for MWS, suggesting that the gene for MWS was the same as the gene for FCAS (8,16). This was confirmed when mutations in *NLRP3* were also found in patients with MWS (17–19). At least 20 *NLRP3* mutations have been identified in patients or families with MWS (10), but as seen in FCAS, there are MWS patients for whom no *NLRP3* mutations have been found.

Chronic infantile neurologic cutaneous and articular syndrome. In 1981, Prieur and Griscelli described three patients with a rare disease characterized by a neonatal onset urticaria-like rash, chronic meningitis and other neurosensory abnormalities, significant joint deformities, and recurrent fever (20). Since that time, over 70 additional cases have been described around the world. This condition is known both as chronic infantile neurologic cutaneous and articular (CINCA) syndrome and neonatal onset multisystem inflammatory disease (NOMID), but will be referred to as CINCA in this chapter. Additional clinical features in these patients may include lymphadenopathy, hepatosplenomegaly, persistent open fontanelle, dysmorphic features, growth and developmental retardation, seizures, papilledema, hearing loss, vision loss, and hoarseness (21). One very unique feature is patellar and distal femur overgrowth resulting in significant deformity and disability (22). Leukemia has also been reported in CINCA patients (20). Rash is consistently reported in the first few months of life in patients with CINCA. Pathologic patellar and distal femur overgrowth and neurologic manifestations begin in childhood and are often progressive. Most patients have increased intracranial pressure and pleocytosis in cerebrospinal fluid. Magnetic resonance imaging (MRI) often shows ventriculomegaly, cerebral atrophy, as well as leptomeningeal and cochlear enhancement (23). Mortality is primarily associated with infection and vasculitis and systemic amyloidosis in longer-lived patients.

CINCA has been described in a few families with pedigrees consistent with autosomal dominant inheritance, but most cases are sporadic. Like MWS, there is significant variable expression in CINCA in that many patients do not display all clinical features. Several patients have been reported with no significant neurologic findings (24). The similarities between CINCA and MWS prompted two groups to search for *NLRP3* mutations in CINCA patients (24,25). At least 47 *NLRP3* mutations have been identified in CINCA patients (10), but approximately 50% of CINCA patients do not appear to possess *NLRP3* mutations (12). Several CINCA patients have been found to have somatic mosaicism, in which only some of their cells posses an *NLRP3* mutation (26).

Proposed Mechanisms

Polymorphonuclear leukocytosis is consistently observed in cryopyrinopathy patients and increases during flares. Moderate eosinophilia is also observed in some cases (25). Patients consistently have increased markers of inflammation such as elevated sedimentation rates and acute phase reactants such as C-reactive protein and serum amyloid A

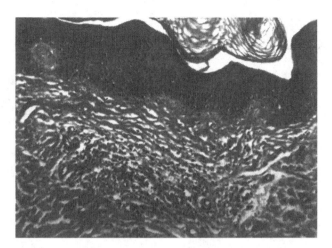

Figure 4 Skin biopsy from shoulder shows primarily neutrophils in the superficial and deep perivascular dermis (H&E: original magnification 20×).

(15,23,27). Synovial fluid samples from MWS and CINCA patients have demonstrated a primarily neutrophilic infiltrate (28,29), and interestingly, increased mast cells were noted on synovial biopsies from some CINCA patients (30).

Skin biopsies taken from cryopyrinopathy patients have shown dermal edema and perivascular and perieccrine leukocytic infiltrate consisting primarily of neutrophils (31) (Fig. 4). Increased vascularity has also been described, although vasculitis is not commonly reported. There is no increase in mast cells or histamine (32). Renal tissue from patients shows classic AA amyloidosis, a feature seen in some other inflammatory diseases (33). It is unclear why some patients develop amyloidosis, while others with equal or more evidence of inflammation do not develop amyloidosis.

Despite the association of FCAS with cold, no role for cryoglobulins has been demonstrated in FCAS. Passive transfer studies were negative, arguing against a serum factor or circulating antibody. There is no evidence for histamine release as is seen in true urticarial diseases.

Increased serum levels of IL-6 have been described in some patients. We have demonstrated elevated IL-6 levels peaking approximately four hours after an experimental cold challenge. Serum granuloctye colony-stimulating factor (GCSF) was elevated in one patient with FCAS (34). Gerbig et al. reported elevated IL-6 levels with a circadian pattern with the highest levels in the late evening in a MWS patient (35). CINCA patients have been shown to elevate levels of several serum cytokines, including IL-6 and TNF-α (23). Numerous investigators have shown that monocytes from cryopyrinopathy patients release excessive amounts of IL-1β in response to different triggers such as lipopolysaccharide and hypothermia (25,36,37).

The identification of the gene responsible for these disorders has provided several clues to the pathogenic mechanisms involved. *NLRP3* is expressed primarily in leukocytes (monocytes and granulocytes) (19,38), which is consistent with the inflammatory nature of the disease as granulocytes clearly play a significant role in these diseases. *NLRP3* codes for a protein we have termed "cryopyrin" (also known as "NALP3"), which has structural features (domains) that are similar to a number of proteins involved in innate immunity (Fig. 5). Several of these proteins have been linked to specific inflammatory diseases. The pyrin domain (PYD), located at the beginning of cryopyrin, was first identified in pyrin, a protein that when mutated causes FMF (39). This

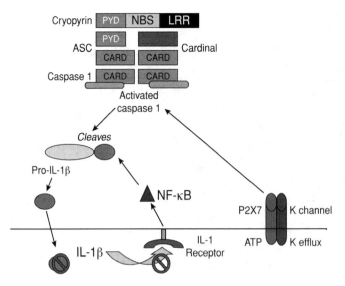

Figure 5 Cryopyrin has three conserved domains known as the pyrin domain (PYD), a nucleotide-binding site (NBS) domain, and a leucine-rich repeat (LRR). Cryopyrin forms a complex with caspase activation recruitment domain (CARD) containing adaptor proteins called ASC (Apoptosis-associated Speck-like protein with a CARD) and CARDINAL to form an intracellular protein complex with caspase 1 known as the inflammasome. Activation of the inflammasome is dependent on ATP and potassium efflux, mediated through P2×7 receptors and potassium channels, and leads to activation of caspase 1, an enzyme involved in the cleavage of pro- IL (interleukin)-1β, an inactive form of IL-1β. Cleaved IL-1β is then released from the cell where it can bind to IL-1 receptors, leading to the activation of NF-κB, a transcription factor involved in regulating the expression of many inflammatory cytokines, including pro-IL-1β. This pathway and hence disease symptoms can be effectively blocked by biologic drugs targeting IL-1β or the IL-1 receptor. *Abbreviations*: PYD, pyrin domain; NBS, nucleotide-binding site; LRR, leucine-rich repeat; CARD, caspase activation recruitment domain; ASC, apoptosis-associated speck-like protein with a CARD.

domain is structurally related to caspase activation recruitment domains (CARD) that are present in caspases. Structural features at the end of cryopyrin include a nucleotide-binding site (NBS) domain and multiple leucine rich repeats (LRR). This combination is conserved in critical proteins in organisms as distantly related as plants (plant resistance proteins) and insects (toll genes) (39). Important human genes with this structure are toll-like receptors (TLRs) and nucleotide oligomerization domain (NOD)-like proteins (NLRs), which are critical players in innate immunity (40). DNA variations in the *NOD2* gene have been implicated in a significant percentage of patients with Crohn's disease.

Significant progress has been made in unraveling the pathways involved in cryopyrin function that are consistent with inflammatory pathways seen in patients. Cryopyrin has been shown to interact with another PYD containing protein called ASC (apoptosis-associated speck-like protein with a CARD) and another adaptor protein known as CARDINAL to form an intracellular protein complex known as the inflammasome, which leads to activation of caspase 1, an enzyme involved in IL-1β release (41). The cryopyrin inflammasome is activated by a number of pathogen-associated molecular patterns (PAMPs) such as muramyl dipeptide and danger-associated molecular patterns (DAMPs) such as uric acid crystals (42,43). Adenosine triphospate (ATP) and potassium efflux, mediated through P2×7 receptors and potassium channels, also appear to play an important role in these pathways (44,45). In vitro studies suggest that cryopyrin may play a direct role in the regulation of nuclear factor kappa B (NF-κB) (38,46). NF-κB is one of the transcription factors involved in regulating many inflammatory cytokines including IL-6. Clearly, cryopyrin plays an important regulatory role in innate immune responses. However, it is still unclear how alterations in cryopyrin cause the unregulated inflammation seen in the diseases with which it has been associated.

Cryopyrin may also be involved in regulating cell death, either by apoptosis (programmed cell death) or necrosis (38,47–50). This may account for the persistent neutrophilic inflammation in all cryopyrinopathies, the hearing loss observed in MWS and CINCA, or the bony findings observed in CINCA. *NLRP3* is expressed in cartilage, which is consistent with the finding of patellar and femur overgrowth in patients and suggests a role of *NLRP3* in chondrocyte growth (24).

Differential Diagnosis and Confirmatory Tests

It is important to differentiate classic urticarial diseases such as cold urticaria and chronic urticaria as well as the other periodic fever disorders from the cryopyrinopathies. The rash may have an urticaria-like appearance, and pruritus is sometimes reported, but the additional symptoms experienced during an attack, including fever and arthralgia, are rarely seen in the true urticarial diseases. FCAS is often confused with other cold-induced urticarial diseases (discussed elsewhere), but there are several features of FCAS that are very unlike these disorders including the early age of onset, the delay of one to two hours after cold exposure, and leukocytosis. FCAS can be differentiated from classic ACU and delayed cold-induced urticaria (discussed later in this chapter) by the lack of local response to cold demonstrated by a negative ice cube test. There are some patients with atypical ACU who develop urticaria without direct contact to cold, but there is no delay of rash onset and the rash responds to antihistamines.

The main differentiating feature of FCAS from the other recurrent fever disorders is the response to cold; however, other differences include a short length of episodes (often <1 day), the early age of onset (<6 months), and lack of abdominal symptoms during attacks. Diagnostic criteria for FCAS have been proposed and validated that include one major criterion: recurrent intermittent episodes of fever and rash following generalized cold exposure and five minor criteria: (*i*) autosomal dominant pattern of inheritance (*ii*), age of onset less than six months (*iii*), duration of most attacks less than 24 hours (*iv*), presence of conjunctivitis associated with attacks, and (*v*) absence of deafness, periorbital edema, lymphadenopathy, and serositis. The presence of the major criterium and at least three of five minor criteria have been shown to be specific for FCAS (5,51).

The presence of the complete MWS triad of rash, deafness, and amyloidosis is unique among the recurrent fever disorders; however, less than a third of MWS patients have all three features. The rash is rarely pruritic and usually lasts for several hours to days, unlike most true urticarias. There are several forms of hereditary deafness, but rash is rarely an associated feature. The combination of deafness and renal disease is seen in Alport's syndrome, but in this disorder there is no amyloidosis. There are hereditary forms of amyloidosis, but AA amyloidosis is usually secondary to chronic inflammation. MWS is most often confused with other recurrent fevers such as FMF, which also has a significant frequency of amyloidosis, but is not associated with deafness or urticaria-like rash.

The primary differential diagnosis of CINCA is systemic onset juvenile idiopathic arthritis (soJIA) or Still's disease and other recurrent fever disorders, but the rash in these diseases rarely occurs in the neonatal period. Neurologic signs and patellar overgrowth are also unusual in soJIA and other recurrent fever disorders. Papilledema and optic atrophy in conjunction with other features are unique to CINCA. Inherited metabolic storage disorders may present with dysmorphic features and developmental delay, but an urticaria-like rash is rare. Classic urticarial diseases rarely present in the neonatal period.

The finding of a mutation in *NLRP3* is confirmatory of the cryopyrinopathies; however there are cases with classic clinical presentation (up to 50% of CINCA patients) that do not possess any identifiable mutations in *NLRP3*. Some of these cases display somatic mosaicism, which may be difficult to identify (50). In combination with episodic rash, demonstration of high-frequency hearing loss by audiometry or AA amyloidosis on renal biopsy would be highly suggestive of MWS. Skin biopsy may be useful, as the presence of perivascular and perieccrine neutrophilic infiltrate is usually seen in the cryopyrinopathies and less commonly in classic urticaria.

Management

In the past, many FCAS patients were misdiagnosed and inappropriately treated as cold urticaria patients, so most patients self-managed their disease by avoiding cold weather and air-conditioned rooms, dressing warmly, and sometimes moving to warmer climates. Partial responses have been observed with high dose corticosteroids in the cryopyrinopathies, but their long-term use is limited by side effects. Nonsteriodal anti-inflammatory drugs (NSAIDs) do provide some relief from arthralgias, but not other symptoms. There are also sporadic reports of clinical responses to gold, colchicine, and thalidomide (5,52).

The identification of the molecular basis of the cryopyrinopathies has directly resulted in improvement in the therapy of these disorders. The remarkable effectiveness of a recombinant IL-1 receptor antagonist called anakinra, currently approved for the treatment of rheumatoid arthritis, has completely changed the management of these patients in the last five years (53). Anakinra completely blocked symptoms and inflammatory responses when given prior to an experimental cold challenge in FCAS patients (27). It has also demonstrated long-term symptom prevention and resolution of chronic inflammation associated with amyloidosis in MWS patients (15). There are reports of resolution of amyloid-associated kidney disease as well as improvement in hearing with anakinra (54,55). Most importantly, anakinra has had spectacular success in the treatment of CINCA, resulting in the resolution of chronic inflammatory symptoms involving the skin and central nervous system (23). However, no controlled clinical trials have been performed with anakinra in the cryopyrinopathies. Recently a randomized double blind placebo-controlled trial was performed in FCAS and MWS patients with another IL-1 targeted therapy known as rilonacept with remarkable efficacy resulting in the first approved drug for the cryopyrinopathies (56). While IL-1-targeted therapies have an excellent safety profile, there is a risk of increased susceptibility to infection, so patients should be monitored closely.

Patients should be monitored for the development of amyloidosis. Urine should be monitored for the development of proteinuria, an early sign of renal amyloidosis. Dialysis is often necessary when renal function deteriorates. Transplantation is an option, but renal amyloidosis can recur in a transplanted kidney. Hearing should be monitored regularly and hearing aids should be used when appropriate. A multidisciplinary approach is necessary for managing CINCA patients, utilizing pediatric rheumatologists, opthalmologists, neurologists, audiologists, and orthopedists.

A Clinical Spectrum of One Disease

The three cryopyrin-associated diseases all share features of an atypical urticarial rash, recurrent fever, and joint manifestations. The rash is generalized, polymorphic in nature, and non-pruritic. Each disease has features that distinguish it, including cold sensitivity in

Table 1 Distinguishing Features of Cryopyrin-Associated Diseases

Feature	Familial cold autoinflammatory syndrome	Muckle-Wells syndrome	Chronic infantile neurologic cutaneous and articular syndrome
Inheritance	Autosomal dominant/ sporadic	Autosomal dominant/ sporadic	Sporadic/autosomal dominant
Age of onset	95% <6 mo	~85% <20 yr	<6 mo
Length of attacks	Usually <1 day	1–2 days	Constant inflammation
Musculoskeletal	Arthralgia, myalgia	Arthralgia, myalgia, arthritis	Arthritis, patellar/distal fibular overgrowth
Lymphadenopathy	None	Occasional	Common
Neurologic	Headache	Headache	Chronic aseptic meningitis, development delay, seizures, persistent open fontanelle
Sensory	Conjunctivitis	Conjunctivitis, deafness ~60%	Papilledema, uveitis, deafness
Amyloidosis	~2%	~30%	Occasional
Treatment	NSAIDS, IL-1 targeted therapy	NSAIDS, IL-1 targeted therapy	IL-1 targeted therapy

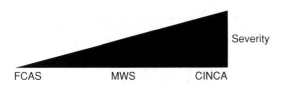

Figure 6 Continuum of cryopyrinopathy phenotypes with increasing severity.

FCAS, a significant risk of systemic amyloidosis in MWS, and epiphyseal or patellar overgrowth in CINCA (Table 1). However, there can be overlap in clinical features that blur the margins, making it difficult to differentiate between FCAS and MWS (some MWS patients report worsening with cold exposure and some families with FCAS develop amyloidosis) or MWS and CINCA (some CINCA patients have no obvious neurologic manifestations and some MWS patients have dysmorphic features consistent with CINCA). This has prompted investigators to suggest that these diseases are actually a spectrum of one disease, with FCAS being the mildest and CINCA being the most severe (12,57) (Fig. 6). We may eventually find other inflammatory diseases that fall into the spectrum of *NLPR3*-associated disorders. Further elucidation of *NLPR3* may shed light on the underlying mechanisms of other inflammatory diseases with urticaria.

Hereditary Disorders with Typical Urticaria or Angioedema

There are several case reports describing diseases with urticaria or angioedema with a significant family history consistent with inherited disease. It has been difficult to confirm inheritance pattern and identify chromosomal locations of genes responsible for these diseases because of the limited number of affected patients and family members available for study. We first discuss disorders for which there is sufficient evidence to suggest a heritable disease and then will discuss a few additional disorders that may be hereditary, but have less evidence to support this possibility.

Delayed Cold-Induced Urticaria

Clinical features and heredity. Soter et al. described a familial syndrome characterized by late onset (9–18 hours) "deep erythematous indurated swelling" also referred to as urticaria that developed at the site of a cold stimulus. The skin lesions were described as deep erythematous indurated swelling and intermittently pruritic and generally are localized to the site of the cold stimulus. They resolve leaving transient hyperpigmentation. No systemic symptoms or signs are described in the report. It is considered a benign disorder with no reports of serious clinical sequela. The age of onset was specified for only one affected family member who developed symptoms at age four. Signs and symptoms typically continue throughout life (58). Analysis of one multigenerational family suggests that the syndrome is transmitted as an autosomal dominant trait. Acquired delayed cold-induced urticaria (DCU) has also been described in sporadic cases in which a wheal response develops 18 to 24 hours following cold stimulation (59). Although the timing is slightly different, it is possible that these are new mutations in the same gene. There is apparently no discernible linkage of delayed cold urticaria to human leukocyte antigen (HLA) loci (58).

Proposed mechanisms. Skin biopsies revealed edema of the dermis with lymphocyte and monocyte/macrophage cells located around venules. No mast cell degranulation was noted, and there was no evidence of vascular necrosis. Immunofluoresence studies did not reveal deposits of immunoglobulins, complement three, or fibrin. There was no evidence of histamine release following provocation challenges with cold stimulation. Serotonin and complement components were not detected in the same studies. Passive transfer studies of the patient serum and skin tissue extract to monkey skin were negative. These studies suggest that there was no operative serum factor, such as an immunoglobulin observed with other physical urticarias (i.e., cold urticaria and solar urticaria).

Differential diagnosis and confirmatory tests. Classic ACU is characterized by an immediate response to cold stimulation (60) compared with DCU, which is associated with a delayed or biphasic response to cold. Cold urticaria with leukocytoclastic vasculitis is delayed in onset and leaves residual hyperpigmentation like DCU. However, skin lesions in this disorder persist for more than 24 to 36 hours following cold stimulation, and skin biopsy of this syndrome reveals microscopic features of leukocytoclastic vasculitis (61). In some respects, the clinical description of acquired and familial DCU is similar to the delayed swelling of deep pressure urticaria, although they are induced by different physical stimuli. The diagnostic test for DCU is a cold stimulus (ice water) applied to the forearm for about five minutes, which in the case of DCU results in a deep erythematous skin reaction typically developing 9 to 18 hours following the cold stimulation. The time of cold stimulus application needed to induce the skin reaction may vary with each individual.

Management. Avoidance of cold stimulation is the mainstay of management. Hydroxyzine appeared to have some suppressive effect but the skin lesions were not abolished. Theoretically antihistamines would not suppress symptoms in view of the fact that histamine is not released following cold exposure. The delayed inflammatory nature of this disorder may suggest a role for low dose, alternate day corticosteroids if symptoms persist in persons who cannot curtail cold exposure.

Familial Atypical Systemic Cold Urticaria

Clinical features and heredity. We have identified three multigenerational families with a history of immediate erythema, pruritic wheals, and angioedema associated with systemic cold exposure, including air and water. Some patients have described systemic symptoms such as fainting. There is no history of fever or arthralgias to suggest FCAS. Symptoms begin early in life and persist throughout life, although it appears to improve with age in some patients. A comprehensive evaluation of these patients is in progress, but pedigree analysis revealed a clear autosomal dominant inheritance pattern. The phenotype is similar to patients reported previously with systemic cold urticaria (62,63).

Proposed mechanisms. The pathophysiology appears to involve mast cell histamine release, however the underlying mechanisms are unclear at this time.

Differential diagnosis and confirmatory tests. This condition should be distinguished from typical ACU that is rarely associated with a family history. The cold stimulation time test (CSTT), the diagnostic standard for ACU, does not result in a raised wheal in these patients, although erythema occurs in some patients. This disease should also be distinguished from FCAS based on history and the nature of the rash. No confirmatory tests are currently available.

Management. Avoidance of cold is the primary management goal. Prophylactic antihistamines have been empirically effective, but have not been formally studied in this disease.

Hereditary Vibratory Urticaria

Clinical features and heredity. Patterson et al. described a familial syndrome characterized by development of urticaria and angioedema at the site of a vibratory stimulus. In general the signs and symptoms are localized to the site of the vibratory stimulus. On rare occasions, systemic symptoms may evolve as generalized or facial erythema and headaches. No hypotensive symptoms have been described, and there are no deaths ascribed to this syndrome. Signs and symptoms appear at birth and continue throughout life. Evaluation of a few families suggests that the syndrome is multigenerational and is transmitted as an autosomal dominant trait with high penetrance (64).

Proposed mechanisms. Metzger et al. confirmed that histamine is released following provocation challenges with vibratory stimulation. Other mediators such as serotonin and bradykinin were not detected in the same studies. Serum-passive transfer from affected individuals to normal individuals did not transfer vibratory-induced angioedema, suggesting that there was no operative serum factor such as an immunoglobulin, which has been observed with other physical urticarias (i.e., cold urticaria; solar urticaria). The authors concluded that this syndrome serves as a model of nonimmunologic hypersensitivity reaction that is physically induced (65).

Differential diagnosis and confirmatory tests. Dermographism should be excluded using conventional blunted instruments to stroke the skin. Diagnosis is confirmed using a vibrating tool, such as a Vortex mixer, that is applied to the forearm for about four minutes. The speed, time, and pressure of Vortex mixer application needed to induce the skin reaction may vary with each individual. Epstein et al. described a syndrome referred to as dermo-distortive urticaria. It is transmitted as an autosomal dominant trait and appears to have many of the same characteristics as hereditary vibratory angioedema.

There is a good likelihood that dermo-distortive urticaria and hereditary vibratory angioedema are the same disorder (66,67).

Management. Avoidance of vibratory stimuli would be the mainstay of management. Occupations requiring use of vibratory tools such as a jackhammer should by necessity be curtailed. There is not adequate clinical data regarding the use of suppressive antihistamines, but prophylactic use of second and third generation antihistamines would certainly be reasonable considerations.

Estrogen-Dependent Inherited Form of Angioedema (Also Referred to as: Hereditary Angioedema with Normal C1 Inhibitor Activity)

Clinical features and heredity. A unique type of HAE that affects primarily women was described initially by Binkley et al. (68) and Bork et al. (69). Clinically this type of HAE exhibits many of the same signs and symptoms that characterize HAE types I and II (discussed elsewhere in this book). Affected members exhibit angioedema without urticaria, laryngeal edema with airway compromise, and abdominal pain due to intestinal edema. This form of HAE affects primarily females who are on estrogen or contraceptives or during pregnancy, but has also been reported in men in two families (70,71). The Binkley report made the interesting observation that affected women can accurately predict pregnancy by the spontaneous appearance of angioedema. Females may experience symptoms at any age if they are on estrogen supplements or estrogen-containing contraceptives. Patients experience symptoms throughout the course of pregnancy and/or while on exogenous estrogens and remain asymptomatic during nonpregnant intervals and while off exogenous estrogens. To date there have been no reported fatalities in this variant of HAE, although affected patients require close surveillance as there is reportedly an incidence of 25% mortality from laryngeal edema in types I and II HAE.

Reported pedigrees suggest an autosomal dominant inheritance pattern with incomplete penetrance even though almost all affected members were females. Obligate male and female carriers have been identified in families. Affected individuals were identified in four generations in one family (70).

Proposed mechanisms. Measurements of C1esterase inhibitor, both antigenic and functional, and C4 levels were normal in asymptomatic patients and in one symptomatic patient who was receiving exogenous estrogens. In addition, assessment of coagulation assays for factor XII, prekallikrein, and high molecular weight kininogen were normal in three tested patients. These studies suggest that C1esterase inhibitor deficiency is not a likely cause of this disorder. Mutations were recently reported in the coagulation Factor XII gene, but the underlying mechanisms have not been fully elucidated (71,72).

Differential diagnosis and confirmatory tests. HAE types I and II can be differentiated from this third type of HAE in that this form of angioedema is usually estrogen-dependent and primarily affects females. Type I HAE can affect males and females and is associated with reduced levels of antigenic C1 esterase inhibitor. The less common type II HAE exhibits normal antigenic C1 esterase inhibitor levels but has abnormal function. Measurements of C1esterase inhibitor, both antigenic and functional, and C4 are normal in patients with this form of HAE. The diagnosis is confirmed by the identification of Factor XII mutations and by excluding types I and II HAE, observing that affected females only develop symptoms during pregnancy or while on exogenous estrogens, and noting the presence of angioedema without urticaria.

Management. Patients are advised to avoid use of estrogen supplements or estrogen-containing contraceptives and if possible to avoid pregnancy. Bork et al. noted that treatment with C1 inhibitor concentrate, steroids, and antihistamines were ineffective. Two patients received danazol and one had a remission on it, while the other was unresponsive to this androgen (69). Treatment of affected pregnant females is problematic as the use of attenuated androgens during pregnancy is contraindicated.

Exercise-Induced Urticaria and Anaphylaxis

Clinical features and heredity. Grant et al. (73) reported exercise-induced anaphylaxis involving seven male members in three generations and Longley et al. (74) described familial exercise-induced anaphylaxis involving two male siblings and a paternal nephew. Following exercise, patients typically develop pruritis, urticaria, angioedema, and cardio-respiratory symptoms occasionally culminating in hypotensive episodes. Signs and symptoms appear in early childhood and continue throughout life. All affected members of the family described by Grant et al. were male, but the most likely pattern is an autosomal dominant mode of inheritance. A linkage of HLA haplotype A-3, B-8, and DR-3 was noted in two affected siblings involving a sister and a brother in the Longley study.

Proposed mechanisms. Histamine levels during induced episodes were not elevated. Grant et al. noted that complement components (C2 and C5) were reduced in one patient at baseline, with further reduction following an exercise challenge. In the Longley et al. study, complement components remained normal during exercise challenges in two patients. The role of occult food allergy that is implicated in sporadic exercise-induced anaphylaxis has not been observed in the familial disorder.

Differential diagnosis and confirmatory tests. Exercise-induced anaphylaxis should be differentiated from cholinergic urticaria. While exercise is a common and reproducible trigger for cholinergic urticaria, the rash in exercise-induced anaphylaxis is less reproducible, but consists of large wheals, while the rash in cholinergic urticaria consists of small punctate lesions. Wheezing, angioedema, and cardiovascular collapse may develop in severe cases of exercise-induced anaphylaxis, and systemic symptoms are rare in cholinergic urticaria. A methacholine intradermal skin challenge (discussed later in the chapter) is negative. Placing an extremity in hot water (104°F), a passive warming test, will induce punctate urticaria in cholinergic urticaria, and not in exercise-induced anaphylaxis. Exercise challenge testing under controlled conditions may reproduce signs and symptoms of anaphylaxis. However a negative exercise challenge test does not rule out exercise-induced anaphylaxis. The key feature for diagnosis is confirming that symptoms occur during exercise and not with passive warming.

Management. Avoidance of vigorous exercise would be the mainstay of management. Carrying a self-administered adrenalin kit would be advisable. There is no good clinical data regarding use of suppressive antihistamines, but prophylactic use of second and third generation antihistamines would be reasonable considerations.

Familial Dermographism

Clinical features and heredity. Jedele et al. described a four-generation family with dermographism (75). Familial dermographism is similar to sporadic dermographism and is characterized by wheal-and-flare responses to scratching or minor skin trauma. Responses usually develop within several minutes after stimulation and may last several hours.

Headaches are the only systemic symptom and may occur if skin trauma affects more than 5% of the body surface area. No serious systemic signs of anaphylaxis have been observed. There is no association with other physical urticarias such as sensitivity to cold, heat, or exercise. Anecdotally affected males experience dermographism on a daily basis, as the response typically occurs after shaving with a razor blade. Signs and symptoms appear in early childhood and can affect newborns. The symptoms continue throughout life.

The dermographism described in the Jedele et al. family appears to be transmitted in an autosomal dominant manner. A total of five males and females of a four-generation family were affected with dermographism. Four of the eight children born to the affected parent exhibited dermographism, which is compatible with an autosomal dominant pattern of inheritance.

Proposed mechanisms. Mast cell degranulation in reaction to mild trauma has been observed in the sporadic type of dermographism, but the mechanism of this phenomenon is not understood. Mediator levels were not measured in this family.

Differential diagnosis and confirmatory tests. Delayed pressure urticaria is distinguished from familial dermographism by the presence of deep swelling that develops only after a delay of several hours and it requires sustained pressure to produce a reaction. The areas of swellings are diffuse and painful. Vibratory angioedema requires repetitive vibration to induce angioedema in contrast to dermographism that requires a single application of pressure. A single stroke of the skin with a blunt object will induce an immediate, linear, continuous wheal-and-flare response.

Management. Avoidance of vigorous skin trauma would be the mainstay of management. Prophylactic use of second and third generation antihistamines would be reasonable, although there is no data to support this.

Familial Localized Heat Urticaria of Delayed Type

Clinical features and heredity. Michaelsson et al. described a three-generation family with localized heat urticaria of delayed type (76). Familial localized heat urticaria of delayed type (FLHU) is characterized by delayed (2 to 14 hour) onset of wheal with erythema localized and limited to the contact site of a heat stimulus. Constitutional symptoms such as headaches have been described with FLHU, but no systemic reactions have been reported. Affected members may develop symptoms following direct contact with a warm object, such as a hot water bottle or exposure to an ambient heat source such as an open fire. Swelling and itching of the scalp may occur after use of a hair dryer. Sunlight is well tolerated, although pronounced heating of the skin from sunbathing can produce wheals on areas covered by dark clothing. Exercise does not induce urticaria in these patients. Signs and symptoms appear at early childhood and continue throughout life.

The localized heat urticaria of delayed-type family described in the Michaelsson report appears to be transmitted in an autosomal dominant manner. A total of 9 out of 14 family members (males and females) of a three-generation family were affected with FLHU.

Proposed mechanisms. Mast cell and basophil degranulation to heat stimulation has been observed in FLHU. Mediator levels were not measured by Michaellson et al. Passive transfer studies (Prausnitz-Kustner test) from an affected patient to a control were negative. These studies suggest that there was no causative serum factor, such as a transferable immunoglobulin.

Differential diagnosis and confirmatory tests. The sporadic type of localized heat urticaria has a similar description, but the wheal and erythema develops immediately following heat stimulation and has been associated with hypotensive episodes. Exercise-induced anaphylaxis and cholinergic urticaria should be considered in the differential diagnosis. An exercise-tolerance test in FLHU should not induce punctate or normal-sized urticaria and/or anaphylaxis. Methacholine skin test and passive warming test would be negative in FLHU as compared with cholinergic urticaria. Solar urticaria should also be ruled out by exposure to UV light in the absence of heat.

Diagnosis is confirmed using a heated test jar (ranging from 40–45°C) applied to different skin areas for various times, ranging from 0.5, 3, 5, 15, and 20 minutes. A wheal and erythematous response will occur two to –four hours after application and may persist up to 14 hours. Apparently each patient has a minimum threshold for temperature and time of heat stimulus application required to induce a positive skin response.

Management. Avoidance of sustained heat exposure, such as a hot tub or hot water bottle, would be the mainstay of management. As with the other disorders with limited clinical data, prophylactic use of second- and third-generation antihistamines would be reasonable. The delayed inflammatory nature of this disorder may suggest a role for low dose, alternate day corticosteroids if symptoms persist in persons who cannot curtail prolonged heat exposure.

Familial Cholinergic Urticaria

Clinical features and heredity. Onn et al. reported on four families with presumed cholinergic urticaria that have symptoms that are similar to sporadic cholinergic urticaria, namely the appearance of small, pruritic, punctate wheals following increased core body heating from exercise. None of the patients exhibited systemic symptoms of cardiovascular collapse that is occasionally observed with sporadic cholinergic urticaria. Signs and symptoms appear in mid-teens and can continue throughout life (77). A total of 9 males out of a total of 16 family members from four families, i.e., approximately 50% affected individuals, exhibited signs of this disorder. This is most consistent with autosomal dominant transmission.

Proposed mechanisms. All patients had a positive methacholine skin test that is also observed with the sporadic disorder. The exact mechanism of familial and sporadic cholinergic urticaria is not known but the presumption is that an underlying exaggerated cholinergic response develops in relation to an increase in core body temperature. The theory suggests that released acetylcholine causes mast cell degranulation and histamine mediation of urticaria.

Differential diagnosis and confirmatory tests. The diagnosis of exercise induced anaphylaxis would be a consideration if the exercise tolerance test induced large wheals and the patient exhibited a negative methacholine skin test and negative passive warming test. The diagnosis of cholinergic urticaria is confirmed if an intradermal methacholine skin test at a concentration of 0.1 mg/mL induces a wheal when compared to a negative response with a saline control. The induction of small pruritic wheals following exercise would also confirm the diagnosis.

Management. Avoidance of sustained exercise would be the mainstay of management. Prophylactic use of first, second, and third generation antihistamines would be reasonable considerations.

Other Possible Hereditary Disorders with Urticaria or Angioedema

Familial aquagenic urticaria has been described by four groups, with only two to six individuals described in each report (78–81). The symptoms began in patients in their mid-20s and are similar to sporadic aquagenic urticaria, namely the appearance of wheals following exposure to water, without systemic symptoms. One report described an association with lactose intolerance (81) and another with Bernard-Solier syndrome (80).

Pruritic urticarial papules and plaques of pregnancy (PUPPP) is a polymorphic skin eruption characterized by urticarial papular wheals and erythematous plaques that initially affect abdominal stria and then spread to other regions. It occurs during the third trimester, more commonly in the first pregnancy, and disappears a few weeks after delivery. Weiss et al., who described two small families, postulated that this is a reaction to a circulating paternal antigenic factor for which tolerance develops in subsequent pregnancies (82).

Aspirin-induced urticaria is relatively common, but is rarely reported in families. Mastalerz reported two families who had at least two affected members with documented sensitivity by oral aspirin challenge (83). They evaluated polymorphisms in the genes for leukotriene C4 (LTC_4) and glutathione S transferase ($GSTM_1$), but could not establish causality.

Chronic idiopathic urticaria (CIU) does not have a clear pattern of inheritance, but in one study there was an eightfold increased incidence in first-degree relatives of affected patients (84). The symptoms in families studied are similar to those of sporadic CIU, but there was a much higher frequency of autoantibodies to IgE and IgE high-affinity receptor in patients from these families. These observations in combination with the previously recognized association of CIU with HLA DR_4 suggest that genetic factors are involved in the pathogenesis of CIU (85,86).

SUMMARY

Relatively speaking, little work has been done in the area of hereditary urticaria or angioedema. The reports we have described, except for the cryopyrin-associated disorders, are mostly individual cases, which limit the conclusions that can be drawn. However, as more data is produced, we will undoubtedly piece together the complex puzzle of the immune responses and inflammatory processes, which lead to urticaria and angioedema. As the pathogenetic mechanisms are elucidated for more of these illnesses, we will be able to use such tools as genetic testing and modulators of inflammatory mediators to more accurately diagnose and treat these hereditary disorders.

REFERENCES

1. Strachan T, Read AP. Human Molecular Genetics. New York: John Wiley and Sons, 1996.
2. Hull KM, Shoham N, Chae JJ, et al. The expanding spectrum of systemic autoinflammatory disorders and their rheumatic manifestations. Curr Opin Rheumatol 2003; 15:61–69.
3. Brydges S, Kastner DL. The systemic autoinflammatory diseases: inborn errors of the innate immune system. Curr Top Microbiol Immunol 2006; 305:127–160.

4. Kile RL, Rusk HA. A Case of cold urticaria with an unusual family history. JAMA 1940; 114: 1067–1068.

5. Hoffman HM, Wanderer AA, Broide DH. Familial cold autoinflammatory syndrome: Phenotype and genotype of an autosomal dominant periodic fever. J Allergy Clin Immunol 2001; 108:615–620.

6. Stych B, Dobrovolny D. Familial cold autoinflammatory syndrome 9FCAS): characterization of symptomatlogy and impact on patients' lives. Curr Med Res Opin 2008; 24:1577–1582.

7. Hoffman HM, Wright FA, Broide DH, et al. Identification of a locus on chromosome 1q44 for familial cold urticaria. Am J Hum Genet 2000; 66:1693–1698.

8. Jung M, Ross B, Wienker TF, et al. A locus for familial cold urticaria maps to distal chromosome 1q: familial cold urticaria and Muckle Wells syndrome are probably allelic (abstract). Am J Hum Genet 1996; 59:A223.

9. Ting JPY, Lovering RC, Alnemri ES, et al. The NLR gene family: a standard nomenclature. Immunity 2008; 28:285–287.

10. Touitou I, Lesage S, McDermott M, et al. Infevers: an evolving mutation database for auto-inflammatory syndromes. Hum Mutat 2004; 24:194–198.

11. Jeru I, Duquesnoy P, Fernandes-Alnemri T, et al. Mutations in NALP12 cause hereditary periodic fever syndromes. Proc Natl Acad Sci U S A 2008; 105:1614–1619.

12. Aksentijevich I, Putnam CD, Remmers EF, et al. The clinical continuum of cryopyrinopathies: novel CIAS1 mutatoins and a new cryopyrin model. Arthritis Rheum 2007; 56:1273–1285.

13. Muckle TJ, Wells M. Urticaria, deafness and amyloidosis: a new heredo-familial syndrome. QJM 1962; 31:235–248.

14. Hawkins PN, Lachmann HJ, Aganna E, et al. Spectrum of clinical features in Muckle-Wells syndrome and response to anakinra. Arthritis Rheum 2004; 50:607–612.

15. Leslie KS, Lachmann HJ, Bruning E, et al. Phenotype, genotype, and sustained response to anakinra in 22 patients with autoinflammatory disease associated with CIAS-1/NALP3 mutations. Arch Dermatol 2006; 142:1591–1597.

16. Cuisset L, Drenth JP, Berthelot JM, et al. Genetic linkage of the Muckle-Wells syndrome to chromosome 1q44. Am J Hum Genet 1999; 65:1054–1059.

17. Aganna E, Martinon F, Hawkins PN, et al. Association of mutations in the NALP3/CIAS1/PYPAF1 gene with a broad phenotype including recurrent fever, cold sensitivity, sensorineural deafness, and AA amyloidosis. Arthritis Rheum 2002; 46:2445–2452.

18. Dode C, Le Du N, Cuisset L, et al. New mutations of CIAS1 that are responsible for Muckle-Wells syndrome and familial cold urticaria: a novel mutation underlies both syndromes. Am J Hum Genet 2002; 70:1498–1506.

19. Hoffman HM, Mueller JL, Broide DH, et al. Mutation of a new gene encoding a putative pyrin-like protein cause familial cold autoinflammatory syndrome and Muckle-Wells syndrome. Nat Genet 2001; 29:301–305.

20. Prieur AM, Griscelli C. Arthropathy with rash, chronic meningitis, eye lesions, and mental retardation. J Pediatr 1981; 99:79–83.

21. Prieur AM, Griscelli C, Lampert F, et al. A chronic, infantile, neurological, cutaneous and articular (CINCA) syndrome. A specific entity analysed in 30 patients. Scand J Rheumatol Suppl 1987; 66:57–68.

22. Kaufman RA, Lovell DJ. Infantile-onset multisystem inflammatory disease: radiologic findings. Radiology 1986; 160:741–746.

23. Goldbach-Mansky R, Dailey NJ, Canna SW, et al. Neonatal-onset multisystem inflammatory disease responsive to interleukin-1beta inhibition. N Engl J Med 2006; 355:581–592.

24. Feldmann J, Prieur AM, Quartier P, et al. Chronic infantile neurological cutaneous and articular syndrome is caused by mutations in CIAS1, a gene highly expressed in polymorphonuclear cells and chondrocytes. Am J Hum Genet 2002; 71:198–203.

25. Aksentijevich I, Nowak M, Mallah M, et al. De novo CIAS1 mutations, cytokine activation, and evidence for genetic heterogeneity in patients with neonatal-onset multisystem inflammatory disease (NOMID): a new member of the expanding family of pyrin-associated autoinflammatory diseases. Arthritis Rheum 2002; 46:3340–3348.

26. Saito M, Fujisawa A, Nishikomori R, et al. Somatic mosaicism of CIAS1 in a patient with chronic infantile neurologic, cutaneous, articular syndrome. Arthritis Rheum 2005; 52: 3579–3585.

27. Hoffman HM, Rosengren S, Boyle DL, et al. Prevention of cold-associated acute inflammation in familial cold autoinflammatory syndrome by interleukin-1 receptor antagonist. Lancet 2004; 364:1779–1785.

28. Hassink SG, Goldsmith DP. Neonatal onset multisystem inflammatory disease. Arthritis Rheum 1983; 26:668–673.

29. Watts RA, Nicholls A, Scott DG. The arthropathy of the Muckle-Wells syndrome. Br J Rheumatol 1994; 33:1184–1187.

30. Yarom A, Rennebohm RM, Levinson JE. Infantile multisystem inflammatory disease: a specific syndrome? J Pediatr 1985; 106:390–396.

31. Haas N, Kuster W, Zuberbier T, et al. Muckle-Wells syndrome: clinical and histological skin findings compatible with cold air urticaria in a large kindred. Br J Dermatol 2004; 151:99–104.

32. Tindall JP, Beeker SK, Rosse WF. Familial cold urticaria. A generalized reaction involving leukocytosis. Arch Intern Med 1969; 124:129–134.

33. Linke RP, Heilmann KL, Nathrath WB, et al. Identification of amyloid A protein in a sporadic Muckle-Wells syndrome. N-terminal amino acid sequence after isolation from formalin- fixed tissue. Lab Invest 1983; 48:698–704.

34. Urano Y, Shikiji T, Sasaki S, et al. An unusual reaction to cold: a sporadic case of familial polymorphous cold eruption? Br J Dermatol 1998; 139:504–507.

35. Gerbig AW, Dahinden CA, Mullis P, et al. Circadian elevation of IL-6 levels in Muckle-Wells syndrome: a disorder of the neuro-immune axis? QJM 1998; 91:489–492.

36. Agostini L, Martinon F, Burns K, et al. NALP3 forms an IL-1beta-processing inflammasome with increased activity in Muckle-Wells autoinflammatory disorder. Immunity 2004; 20:319–325.

37. Rosengren S, Mueller JL, Anderson JP, et al. Monocytes from familial cold autoinflammatory syndrome patients are activated by mild hypothermia. J Allergy Clin Immunol 2007; 119: 991–996.

38. Manji GA, Wang L, Geddes BJ, et al. PYPAF1: a PYRIN-containing Apaf1-like protein that assembles with ASC and regulates activation of NF-kB. J Biol Chem 2002; 277:11570–11575.

39. Ting JP, Kastner DL, Hoffman HM. CATERPILLERs, pyrin and hereditary immunological disorders. Nat Rev Immunol 2006; 6:183–195.

40. Creagh EM, O'Neill LA. TLRs, NLRs and RLRs: a trinity of pathogen sensors that co-operate in innate immunity. Trends Immunol 2006; 27:352–357 [epub 2006, Jun 27].

41. Martinon F, Burns K, Tschopp J. The inflammasome: a molecular platform triggering activation of inflammatory caspases and processing of proIL-beta. Mol Cell 2002; 10:417–426.

42. Martinon F, Agostini L, Meylan E, et al. Identification of bacterial muramyl dipeptide as activator of the NALP3/cryopyrin inflammasome. Curr Biol 2004; 14:1929–1934.

43. Martinon F, Petrilli V, Mayor A, et al. Gout-associated uric acid crystals activate the NALP3 inflammasome. Nature 2006; 440:237–241 [epub 2006, Jan 11].

44. Mariathasan S, Weiss DS, Newton K, et al. Cryopyrin activates the inflammasome in response to toxins and ATP. Nature 2006; 440:228–232 [epub 2006, Jan 11].

45. Petrilli V, Papin S, Dostert C, et al. Activation of the NALP3 inflammasome is triggered by low intracellular potassium concentration. Cell Death Differ2007; 14:1583–1589 [epub 2007, Jun 29].

46. O'Connor W Jr., Harton JA, Zhu X, et al. Cutting edge: CIAS1/cryopyrin/PYPAF1/NALP3/ CATERPILLER 1.1 Is an inducible inflammatory mediator with NF-kappaB suppressive properties. J Immunol 2003; 171:6329–6333.

47. Dowds TA, Masumoto J, Zhu L, et al. Cryopyrin induced IL-1 secretion in monocytic cells: enhanced activity of disease-associated mutants and requirement for ASC. J Biol Chem 2004; 279(21):21924–21928 [epub 2004, Mar 12].

48. Grenier JM, Wang L, Manji GA, et al. Functional screening of five PYPAF family members identifies PYPAF5 as a novel regulator of NF-kappaB and caspase-1. FEBS Lett 2002; 530: 73–78.

49. Willingham SB, Bergstralh DT, O'Connor W, et al. Microbial pathogen-induced necrotic cell death mediated by the inflammasome components CIAS1/cryopyrin/NLRP3 and ASC. Cell Host Microbe 2007; 2:147–159.

50. Fujisawa A, Kambe N, Saito M, et al. Disease-associated mutations in CIAS1 induce cathepsin B-dependent rapid cell death of human THP-1 monocytic cells. Blood 2007; 109:2903–2911.

51. Johnstone RF, Dolen WK, Hoffman HM. A large kindred with familial cold autoinflammatory syndrome. Ann Allergy Asthma Immunol 2003; 90:233–237.

52. Kallinich T, Hoffman HM, Roth J, et al. The clinical course of a child with CINCA/NOMID syndrome improved during and after treatment with thalidomide. Scand J Rheumatol 2005; 34: 246–249.

53. Hawkins PN, Lachmann HJ, McDermott MF. Interleukin-1-receptor antagonist in the Muckle-Wells syndrome. N Engl J Med 2003; 348:2583–2584.

54. Rynne M, Maclean C, Bybee A, et al. Hearing improvement in a patient with variant Muckle-Wells syndrome in response to interleukin 1 receptor antagonism. Ann Rheum Dis 2006; 65: 533–534.

55. Thornton BD, Hoffman HM, Bhat A, et al. Successful treatment of renal amyloidosis due to familial cold autoinflammatory syndrome using an interleukin 1 receptor antagonist. Am J Kidney Dis 2007; 49:477–481.

56. Hoffman HM, Throne ML, Amar NJ, et al. Efficacy and safety of rilonacept (IL-1 Trap) in cryopyrin-associated periodic syndromes (CAPS): results from two sequential placebo-controlled studies. Arthritis Rheum 2008; 58(8):2443–2452.

57. Neven B, Callebaut I, Prieur AM, et al. Molecular basis of the spectral expression of CIAS1 mutations associated with phagocytic cell-mediated auto-inflammatory disorders (CINCA/NOMID, MWS, FCU). Blood 2004; 103:2809–2815.

58. Soter NA, Joshi NP, Twarog FJ, et al. Delayed cold-induced urticaria: a dominantly inherited disorder. J Allergy Clin Immunol 1977; 59:294–297.

59. Back O, Larsen A. Delayed cold urticaria. Acta Derm Venereol 1978; 58:369–371.

60. Wanderer AA, Hoffman HM. The spectrum of acquired and familial cold-induced urticaria/urticaria-like syndromes. Immunol Allergy Clin North Am 2004; 24:259–286.

61. Wanderer AA, Nuss DD, Tormey AD, et al. Urticarial leukocytoclastic vasculitis with cold urticaria. Report of a case and review of the literature. Arch Dermatol 1983; 119:145–151.

62. Kaplan AP. Unusual cold-induced disorders: cold-dependent dermatographism and systemic cold urticaria. J Allergy Clin Immunol 1984; 73:453–456.

63. Sarkany I, Gaylarde PM. Negative reactions to ice in cold urticaria. Br J Dermatol 1971; 85: 46–48.

64. Patterson R, Mellies CJ, Blankenship ML, et al. Vibratory angioedema: a hereditary type of physical hypersensitivity. J Allergy Clin Immunol 1972; 50:174–182.

65. Metzger WJ, Kaplan AP, Beaven MA, et al. Hereditary vibratory angioedema: confirmation of histamine release in a type of physical hypersensitivity. J Allergy Clin Immunol 1976; 57: 605–608.

66. Epstein PA, Kidd KK. Dermo-distortive urticaria: an autosomal dominant dermatologic disorder. Am J Med Genet 1981; 9:307–315.

67. Epstein PA, Kidd KK, Sparkes RS. Genetic linkage analysis of dermo-distortive urticaria. Am J Med Genet 1981; 9:317–321.

68. Binkley KE, Davis A 3rd. Clinical, biochemical, and genetic characterization of a novel estrogen-dependent inherited form of angioedema. J Allergy Clin Immunol 2000; 106:546–550.

69. Bork K, Barnstedt SE, Koch P, et al. Hereditary angioedema with normal C1-inhibitor activity in women. Lancet 2000; 356:213–217.

70. Bork K, Gul D, Dewald G. Hereditary angio-oedema with normal C1 inhibitor in a family with affected women and men. Br J Dermatol 2006; 154:542–545.

71. Martin L, Raison-Peyron N, Nöthen MM, et al. Hereditary angioedema with normal C1 inhibitor gene in a family with affected women and men is associated with the p.Thr328Lys mutation in the F12 gene. J Allergy Clin Immunol 2007; 120:975–977 [epub 2007, Sep 7].

72. Dewald G, Bork K. Missense mutations in the coagulation factor XII (Hageman factor) gene in hereditary angioedema with normal C1 inhibitor. Biochem Biophys Res Commun 2006; 343: 1286–1289.
73. Grant JA, Farnam J, Lord RA, et al. Familial exercise-induced anaphylaxis. Ann Allergy 1985;54:35–38.
74. Longley S, Panush RS. Familial exercise-induced anaphylaxis. Ann Allergy 1987; 58:257–259.
75. Jedele KB, Michels VV. Familial dermographism. Am J Med Genet 1991; 39:201–203.
76. Michaelsson G, Ros AM. Familial localized heat urticaria of delayed type. Acta Derm Venereol 1971; 51:279–283.
77. Onn A, Levo Y, Kivity S. Familial cholinergic urticaria. J Allergy Clin Immunol 1996; 98:847–849.
78. Bonnetblanc JM, Andrieu-Pfahl F, Meraud JP, et al. Familial aquagenic urticaria. Dermatologica 1979; 158:468–470.
79. Juhlin L, Malmros-Enander I. Familial polymorphous light eruption with aquagenic urticaria: successful treatment with PUVA. Photodermatol 1986; 3:346–349.
80. Pitarch G, Torrijos A, Martinez-Menchon T, et al. Familial aquagenic urticaria and bernard-soulier syndrome. Dermatology 2006; 212:96–97.
81. Treudler R, Tebbe B, Steinhoff M, et al. Familial aquagenic urticaria associated with familial lactose intolerance. J Am Acad Dermatol 2002; 47:611–613.
82. Weiss R, Hull P. Familial occurrence of pruritic urticarial papules and plaques of pregnancy. J Am Acad Dermatol 1992; 26:715–717.
83. Mastalerz L, Setkowicz M, Sanak M, et al. Familial aggregation of aspirin-induced urticaria and leukotriene C4 synthase allelic variant. Br J Dermatol 2006; 154:256–260.
84. Asero R. Chronic idiopathic urticaria: a family study. Ann Allergy Asthma Immunol 2002; 89: 195–196.
85. Greaves M. Chronic urticaria. J Allergy Clin Immunol 2000; 105:664–672.
86. O'Donnell BF, O'Neill CM, Francis DM, et al. Human leucocyte antigen class II associations in chronic idiopathic urticaria. Br J Dermatol 1999; 140:853–858.

16

Hereditary Angioedema and Acquired C1 Inhibitor Deficiency

Allen P. Kaplan
Department of Medicine, Medical University of South Carolina, Charleston, South Carolina, U.S.A.

INTRODUCTION

The first component of complement (C1) inhibitor (INH) deficiency causes angioedema as a result of excessive bradykinin production (see chap. 5). Thus the pathways and control mechanisms for bradykinin formation and degradation are variables that one must consider in any patient with angioedema. Activated Factor XII as well as Factor XII fragment (XIIf) are inhibited by C1 INH (1,2), thus the absence of C1 INH facilitates Factor XII autoactivation, which augments the ability of Factor XIIa to convert both prekallikrein to kallikrein and Factor XI to Factor XIa. Studies estimate that over 90% of plasma inhibition of Factor XIIa and Factor XIIf is due to C1 INH (2). The remainder is due to antithrombin III and the protein C_a inhibitor. The next enzyme in the cascade is kallikrein, and it is inhibited by C1 INH and $\alpha_2$macroglobulin in approximately equal proportions (3). Minor inhibitors of kallikrein are antithrombin III and $\alpha_1$antitrypsin. Thus if there is any stimulus for activation of the plasma bradykinin-forming cascade, in the absence of functional C1 INH, there is a marked augmentation of bradykinin formation with angioedema as the result. Urticaria is not seen in patients with C1 INH deficiency, but at the inception of an episode of swelling, they may have a rash resembling erythema marginatum. When patients present with both chronic urticaria and angioedema, assays for C1 INH are generally unnecessary, and the utility of a C4 determination depends on whether an underlying vasculitis is suspected. Hereditary C1 INH deficiency, the most common and best-studied presentation of hereditary angioedema (HAE), is an autosomal dominant disorder, resulting in low plasma levels or synthesis of a dysfunctional C1 INH. A new form of HAE with normal C1 INH may be present in some families because of mutant Factor XII. Acquired C1 INH deficiency is caused by the depletion of functional C1 INH, as a result of the binding to active enzymes or the presence of antibody to C1 INH. Synthesis is insufficient to maintain a normal level. Disease associations include lymphoma, connective tissue disorder, or autoimmune processes.

C1 INHIBITOR DEFICIENCY

Causes and Inheritance

C1 INH deficiency is an important cause of angioedema, which may involve almost any portion of the body. Sometimes local trauma to an extremity can initiate an exaggerated local swelling or a more generalized episode of swelling. However, a triggering event may not be immediately evident, so that swelling appears to occur spontaneously. C1 INH deficiency can be familial (in which there is a mutant C1 INH gene) or acquired. Both the hereditary and acquired forms of C1 INH deficiency have two subgroups. For the hereditary disorder, type I HAE is typically an autosomal dominant disorder in which a mutant gene leads to markedly depressed C1 INH levels (4). Type II HAE is also inherited as an autosomal dominant disorder and has a mutation that leads to synthesis of a dysfunctional protein; the C1 INH protein level may then be normal or even elevated (5). The acquired form of C1 INH deficiency also has two forms. In the first type, there is an association with either a B-cell lymphoma or a connective tissue disease in which there is sufficient consumption of C1 INH to cause angioedema (6–8). The second form of acquired C1 INH deficiency is an autoimmune disorder, in which there is a circulating IgG antibody directed to C1 INH itself (9–11). A positive family history, the presence of a lymphoma, or an underlying connective tissue disease would each suggest C1 INH deficiency when swelling is a manifestation. The presence of visceral involvement in any patient with angioedema (in the absence of hives) is suggestive. The most severe complication is laryngeal edema, which had been a major cause of mortality in this disorder. Patients can also have abdominal attacks lasting one to three days, consisting of vomiting, severe abdominal pain, and guarding in the absence of fever, leukocytosis, or abdominal rigidity. This may nevertheless be difficult to differentiate from an acute surgical abdomen. However, the attacks are self-limited and caused by edema of the bowel wall (12). The ultrastructural lesions seen in the tissues of patients with HAE, in particular, consists of gaps in the postcapillary venule endothelial cells, edema, and almost no cellular infiltrate, consistent with the release of a vasoactive factor such as kinin (13).

Molecular Genetics

HAE is transmitted as an autosomal dominant disorder, in most instances, due to alterations of the C1 INH gene. Its prevalence is 1/50,000 (14); however, there is a high incidence of de novo mutations accounting for close to 25% of cases. Thus there may not be a family history to guide evaluation of such patients, and it is therefore reasonable to obtain a C4 and C1 INH determination in any patient presenting with recurrent angioedema in the absence of urticaria.

Figure 1, taken from a review by Tosi (14), summarizes the mutations that may be seen in patients with HAE. Gene instability due to unequal crossing over between repetitive Alu sequences causes deletions or duplications, accounting for about 20% of mutations. The remainder involves microdeletions or duplications or single nucleotide substitutions. Figure 1 summarizes the mutational spectrum seen in type I HAE in which the protein level is quantitatively low (<50%); episodes of swelling typically occur when the plasma level drops to 25% of normal or less. Point mutations and deletions or insertions are scattered along the entire C1 INH gene. Missense mutations are found along the entire coding sequence, with the exception of the 100 amino acid long N-terminal segment that is highly glycosylated and has little homology with other plasma proteinase inhibitors. The consequences of severe missense mutations have been determined by transfection of in vitro mutagenized constructs into COS cells. Amino acid substitutions seen in type I

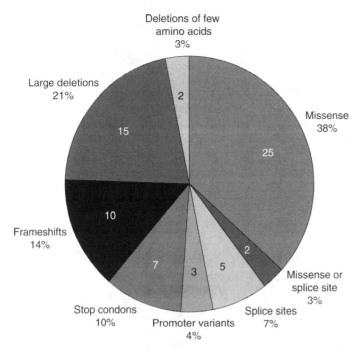

Figure 1 Distribution of 69 mutations found in 66 type I HAE patients. Forty-three kindreds are from (5) and twenty-three are irom (9). Double mutations were found in three kindreds (5). Note that only half of the changes observed (large deletions, frameshifts, and stop-codon mutations) can be considered directly as pathogenic, without the need of functional assays. *Abbreviations*: HAE, hereditary angioedema; kDa, kilodalton. *Source*: From Ref. 14.

HAE often affect intracellular transport of C1 INH (as do other mutations in type I disease) with impairment of protein secretion. Amino acid substitutions, rather than deletions, insertions, stop codons, or frameshift mutations, characterize type II disease in which there is secretion of a dysfunctional protein (i.e., plasma protein levels may appear normal, but a large fraction of the secreted protein is dysfunctional). Here the mutations cluster about the reactive site of C1 INH at Arg 444 (the protein is cleaved by the enzyme to which it will bind, exposing a reactive site that in turn covalently binds the active site serine of the enzyme, thereby inactivating it). These are sites of spontaneous deamination of methylated cytosines of a CpG dinucleotide, which account for most of the type II abnormalities. It is important to note that in types I and II HAE, there is one normal gene; thus C1 INH synthesis should theoretically be at 50% of normal. Yet in type I HAE, the total C1 INH protein is often much less (angioedema typically occurs at levels of 25% or less), and in type II disease normal and dysfunctional proteins circulate side by side. Further depletion of the normal gene product may occur because of hypercatabolism, that is, turnover as a result of the binding to plasma proteases (15) or suppression of normal C1 INH protein (transinhibition) by the mRNA or abnormal protein of the dysfunctional allele (5,16). An intermediate phenotype encompassing features of type I and II abnormalities may be seen, in which an amino acid substitution leads not only to decreased secretion of the protein but is also dysfunctional.

A very rare recessive form of the disease may be seen with mutations in the promotor region of the gene or within the first intron, in which homozygosity is required to lower the C1 INH level sufficiently to cause clinical symptoms. An estrogen-dependent form of HAE has been described in which there is no abnormality of C1 INH, and C4 levels are normal (17). Symptoms typically occur only during pregnancy or while the patient is taking exogenous estrogen (which also increases angioedema in C1 INH deficiency). The inheritance appeared to be dominant. Recently male patients have been identified in (18) some families, and a Factor XII mutation has been identified (19). There is presumed to be excessive bradykinin formation because the activated Factor XII (Factor XIIa) has a higher-specific activity than the normal protein.

Diagnosis

Patients with HAE have measurable levels of the activated C1 although this protein generally circulates as an unactivated enzyme. The serum level of C4 is diminished, even when the patient is free of symptoms, and is virtually undetectable during an attack (20). A C4 determination is therefore the simplest way to screen for the hereditary disorder. Rocket immunoelectrophoresis for C4 cleavage products, such as C4b, is a more sensitive assay more so than C4 quantitation (21). It should be noted that 5% of patients have a normal C4 level, so that assays of total and functional inhibitor still need to be done if suspicion of C1 INH deficiency exists. Levels of C2, the other substrate of C1, are usually within normal limits when the patient is asymptomatic, but the concentration is also diminished during an attack of swelling (22). When a diminished C4 level is obtained, a direct assay of the protein, C1 INH, should always be performed. A diminished or absent level of C1 INH protein would confirm the diagnosis; 80% to 85% of patients with HAE have this type of disorder (type I). However, 15% to 20% of patients will have a mutant form of C1 INH protein that renders it functionless (type II) (23). In these cases, the quantitative secretion of total C1 INH protein is typically normal and is sometimes actually increased, although the abnormal gene product may have an abnormal electrophoretic mobility. Thus an assay for functional C1 INH is necessary to confirm the diagnosis.

Pathogenesis

The pathogenesis of the swelling appears to involve primarily the plasma kinin-forming pathway rather than complement; however, it is germane to review the history of the complement data and to point out how it was first thought to be a source of a kinin and then present the more recent data that suggest otherwise. Intracutaneous injection of C1 into normal individuals was reported to cause the formation of a small wheal reaction, whereas injection into patients with HAE yields localized angioedema (i.e., an augmented response because of low C1 levels of inhibitor) (24). A kinin-like peptide was isolated from such patients and its formation appeared to be inhibited in C2 deficient plasma; C2 was therefore considered to be the source of the pathogenic peptide (25). However, direct demonstration of such a kinin-like peptide upon interaction of activated C1 with C4 and C2 or with C2 alone is lacking. Although it was originally reported that cleavage of C2b by plasmin generated kinin (26), attempts to confirm this experiment have failed (27,28). The only identifiable kinin seen in subsequent studies was bradykinin (28). On the other hand, the amino acid sequence of C2b is known, and Strang et al., (29) have synthesized peptides of various lengths and tested each for kinin-like activity. One such peptide was shown to cause edema when injected intracutaneously, reminiscent of the C2 kinin originally described. However, it has not been shown to be a cleavage product of C2b, nor has it been shown to be present during attacks of swelling in patients with HAE. Thus, at this time it seems unlikely that a kinin-like molecule is derived from C2b as a result of enzymatic cleavage, and the original data may have been artifactual (30).

On the other hand, the presence of bradykinin has been documented as described below, and it is now accepted to be the cause of the swelling. In fact when one of the proponents of the C2 kinin reexamined the kinin formation in the plasma of patients with HAE, only bradykinin was found (31). Although the plasma levels of C3 and C5 are normal in this disorder, C3 turnover is clearly enhanced (32). The lesions, however, are not pruritic, and administration of antihistamines has no effect on the clinical course of the disease. Thus, complement activation is undoubtedly occurring, perhaps even during quiescent periods to lead to a low level of C4, but the vasoactive consequences of augmented complement activation that occur during attacks of HAE do not appear to be the cause of swelling. Figure 2 is a diagrammatic representation of the plasma kinin–forming cascade, indicating the various enzymatic steps including the sites of inhibition by C1 INH. The cascade is initiated by Factor XII (Hageman factor) binding to a site of tissue injury, followed by autoactivation in which traces of activated Factor XII cleave native, i.e., unactivated Factor XII bound to the surface (33). A critical level of Factor XIIa is generated so as to convert prekallikrein to kallikrein. This autoactivation step is inhibited by C1 INH. Since native Factor XII has no measurable enzymatic activity, it is assumed that traces of Factor XIIa normally exist in human plasma (34). Concentrations as low as 10^{-13} molar are sufficient to initiate activation for the kinin system in plasma: 50% activation of the cascade can occur within 30 seconds (35).

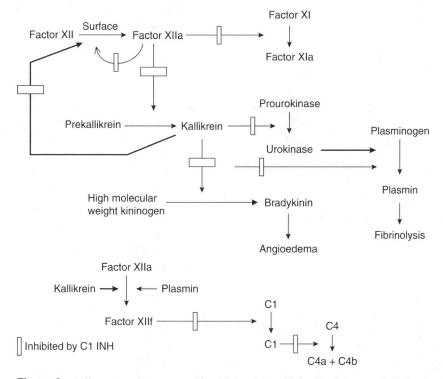

Figure 2 A diagrammatic representation of the plasma kinin–forming cascade indicating the steps inhibitable by C1 INH. All functions of Factor XIIa and kallikrein are affected. The lower figure indicates that further digestion of Factor XIIa by kallikrein and plasmin generates Factor XIIf, which is an initiator of the complement cascade. Both Factor XIIf and C1 are inhibited by C1 INH. *Abbreviations*: Factor XIIf, Factor XII fragment.

This concentration of Factor XIIa is over a million times lower than our ability to assay Factor XIIa in plasma, so that there is little hope of ever measuring it. Nevertheless, there is now evidence that the kinin cascade can be activated along the surface of endothelial cells, and that process may be a source of infinitesimal amounts of Factor XIIa under normal physiologic conditions (36,37). Factor XIIa then converts prekallikrein to kallikrein, and kallikrein (38) cleaves high molecular weight kininogen to generate bradykinin. There is also an important positive feedback in the system, in which the kallikrein generated rapidly converts unactivated Factor XII to activated Factor XII (39), and the rate of this reaction is hundreds of times faster than the rate of autoactivation (35,40). Therefore, much of the unactivated Factor XII can be cleaved and activated by kallikrein. C1 INH inhibits all functions of Factor XIIa and it is one of the two major plasma kallikrein inhibitors. Thus all functions of kallikrein are also inhibited, including the feedback activation of Factor XII, the cleavage of high molecular weight kininogen, and the activation of plasma prourokinase (41) to lead to plasmin formation. C1 INH also inhibits the fibrinolytic enzyme plasmin, although it is a relatively minor inhibitor compared with α_2 antiplasmin or α_2 macroglobulin.

Patients with HAE appear to be hyperresponsive to cutaneous injections of kallikrein as they are to C1 (42), and elevated levels of bradykinin and cleaved kininogen have been observed during attacks of swelling (43,44). There is also evidence that C1 activation observed in patients with HAE may also be dependent on Factor XII (25). Thus, a Factor XII-dependent enzyme may be initiating the classic complement cascade. Plasmin is capable of activating C1s and may represent one such enzyme (45). Ghebrehiwet et al., demonstrated that Factor XIIf can directly activate the classic complement cascade by activating C1r (46,47). This may represent a critical link between the intrinsic coagulation-kinin cascade and complement activation. The presence of kallikrein-like activity in induced blisters of patients with HAE supports this notion (48), as does the progressive generation of bradykinin upon incubation of HAE plasma in plastic (28) (noncontact-activated) tubes as well as the low prekallikrein and high-molecular-weight kininogen levels seen during the attacks (49). More recent data support these indirect observations, favoring bradykinin as the critical pathogenic peptide for HAE and for acquired C1 INH deficiency as well. One unique family has been described, in which there is a point mutation in C1 INH (Ala^{443} → Val), leading to inability to inhibit the complement cascade, but there is normal inhibition of Factor XIIa and kallikrein (50,51). No family member of this type II mutation has had angioedema. In recent studies, plasma bradykinin levels have been shown to be elevated during attacks of swelling in patients with hereditary and acquired forms of C1 INH deficiency (44,52), and local bradykinin generation has been documented at the site of the swelling (53).

The role of fibrinolysis needs also to be considered a part of the pathogenesis of the disease, since antifibrinolytic agents such as ε aminocaproic acid and tranexamic acid appear to be efficacious. As shown in Figure 1, kallikrein converts plasminogen to plasmin. Although kallikrein (Fig. 1), Factor XIa, and even Factor XIIa (not shown) have some ability to activate plasminogen directly, the plasma pathway via the prourokinase intermediate appears to be the major Factor XII–dependent fibrinolytic mechanism. Among the functions of plasmin are the activation of C1s, the ability to cleave and activate Factor XII just as kallikrein can (54), and digestion of C1 INH (55). Each of these would serve to augment bradykinin formation and further deplete the levels of C1 INH. Thus, the formation of plasmin may, in this fashion, contribute to the pathogenesis of the disease.

There are also considerable new data regarding the formation of bradykinin along the endothelial cell surface, and it is possible that this is a locus of bradykinin formation in

HAE (chap. 5, Figs. 6 and 7). The entire cascade can be activated along the surface of the cell, with gC1qR as an initiating protein capable of catalyzing Factor XII autoactivation (56). Critical for this discussion is that C1 INH can inhibit all of these reactions at the cell surface. The fact that heat shock protein 90 (HSP 90) expressed by endothelial cells can directly activate the prekallikrein-high-molecular-weight kininogen complex (57) provides a mechanism by which stress might initiate bradykinin formation. Factor XII is then converted to Factor XIIa by the kallikrein produced.

ACQUIRED C1 INHIBITOR DEFICIENCY

An acquired form of this disease has been described in patients with lymphoma who have circulating low-molecular-weight IgM and depressed C1 INH levels. This entity has an unusual complement utilization profile because C1q levels are low and C4, C2, and C3 are depleted. The low C1q level differentiates this condition from the hereditary disorder (7,8,58). The depressed C1 INH level may be caused by depletion secondary to C1 activation by circulating immune complexes or C1 interaction with a tumor cell surface antigen. For B-cell lymphoma, the most common associated malignancy, C1 fixation and C1 INH depletion, are caused by an anti-idiotypic antibody bound to immunoglubulin on the surface of the B cell (59). Other B-cell disorders associated with C1 INH depletion are acute and chronic lymphocytic leukemia, multiple myeloma, Waldenstrom's macro-globulinemia, and essential cryoglobulinemia.

Patients with connective tissue disorders such as systemic lupus erythematous or carcinoma (60,61) can present with acquired C1 INH deficiency, and, like patients with the hereditary form, will respond to androgen therapy, which enhances C1 INH synthesis. A second form of C1 INH deficiency results from the synthesis of an autoantibody directed to C1 INH itself (9,62). These patients also have low levels of C4, C1q, and C1 INH protein and function, and no family history. This form of acquired C1 INH deficiency appears to be increasingly recognized. Under normal circumstances, C1 INH is a substrate for the enzymes it inactivates: the active enzyme cleaves C1 INH, which exposes the active site in the inhibitor. The cleaved C1 INH then binds stoichiometrically to the enzyme and inactivates it. When antibody to C1 INH is present, the C1 INH is cleaved and is unable to inactivate the enzyme (11,63,64). Thus cleaved, functionless C1 INH circulates, and unopposed activation of the complement-and kinin-forming cascade takes place. Plasmin is one of the enzymes that is capable of cleaving and inactivating C1 INH, and local C1 INH degradation by plasmin may be a critical event in the loss of protease inhibition during inflammation. In a more general sense, this observation may also explain the efficacy of antiplasmin agents such as ε-aminocaproic acid or tranexamic acid in the treatment of C1 INH deficiency states.

One circumstance in which the two forms of acquired C1 INH deficiency merge is in an occasional patient with monoclonal gammopathy, indicative of an underlying lymphoproliferative disorder, in which the monoclonal imunoglobulin is in fact an antibody to C1 INH (65,66). The immune complex–mediated depletion of C1 INH and the autoantibody directed to C1 INH represent types I and II acquired C1 INH deficiency, respectively. The type II variety can be most readily determined by immunoblot with antibody to C1 INH. The presence of a C1 INH cleavage product at 95 kDa differentiates the two forms of the acquired disorder, and it is not present in the hereditary disorder.

Table 1 is a summary of the laboratory tests that may be used to identify the different forms of C1 INH deficiency. If a family history is present, one needs to differentiate the two types of HAE. Since the C4 level will be diminished in both, the

Table 1 Assays for C1 Inhibitor Deficiency

	C1 INH protein	C1 INH function	C4	C1Q	95 kDa C1 INH
Hereditary type I	↓	↓	↓	N	No
Hereditary type II	N or↑	↓	↓	N	No
Acquired type I	↓	↓	↓	↓	No
Acquired type II	↓	↓	↓	↓	Yes

distinction is usually made by comparing C1 INH protein level and C1 INH function. Both protein and function will be low in parallel in type I HAE, whereas the protein level will be normal or elevated in the type II form of this disorder with functional C1 INH diminished. Since a low C1q level characterizes types I and II acquired C1 INH deficiency and a 95 kDa cleaved C1 INH protein is seen in type II disease, the absence of these abnormalities or of any family history of swelling, in patients with low C4 and abnormally low functional C1 INH, would define a patient with a probable new mutation. As indicated above, the acquired form of C1 INH deficiency with lymphoma or connective tissue disease or cryoglobulinemeia or an occasional carcinoma is identified by low C1, and more specifically low C1q, in addition to low C4 and diminished C1 INH levels in which protein and function are diminished in parallel. Occasionally this pattern may be obtained in someone who does not have any of the aforementioned predisposing immune conditions. Such patients need to be evaluated carefully over time because there have been reports of angioedema of this sort preceding the diagnosis of the underlying disorder. The type II acquired disorder with cleaved C1 INH as assessed by immunoblot or by specific assay for antibody directed to C1 INH is the most difficult to diagnose because the tests required are not commercially available.

TREATMENT

A rational best approach for treatment of hereditary C1 INH deficiency is the replacement with purified C1 INH. This is available in Europe and Australia, and is now being evaluated in the United States. Infusions can be administered for acute attacks of swelling, but more importantly, can be administered as a biweekly or monthly infusion to prevent episodes of swelling.

   The traditional drugs of choice for treatment of HAE are agents with weak androgenic properties such as danazol or stanozolol (Winstrol). For stanozolol, the typical dosage ranges between 2 and 4 mg taken daily and for danazol somewhere between 50 and 400 mg daily (67–72). The major side effects of these are liver dysfunction, weight gain, and mild virilization (73,74). Nevertheless, these drugs have been used successfully in young women, including some passing through puberty, without adverse effect. The maintenance dosage should be minimized, and occasionally treatment every other day can be sufficient to treat the disorder. As the dosages employed have decreased, side effects, even with long-term use, are few (75). Periodic assessment of liver function is most important. The minimum dosage required, however, has to be determined and titrated for each individual patient.

   Alternative drugs used to treat HAE include antifibrinolytic drugs such as ε-aminocaproic acid or tranexamic acid (76–79). These are generally less well tolerated, and because of concern with regard to side effects, they are not recommended as first-line agents. One exception is their use to treat symptoms in children with HAE (particularly young women), where there is concern regarding androgen administration (80). Nevertheless, even in these instances, my own experience suggests safety and efficiency of low doses of androgenic agents. For acute attacks of angioedema, subcutaneous epinephrine is administered, fresh frozen plasma can be infused to replace C1 INH, or, if available, C1 INH concentrate (81,82). Initially, there was a theoretical concern that administration of plasma would provide more substrate for the production of vasoactive factors and worsen angioedema, but such an adverse effect is rarely seen. In fact replacement of C1 INH, regardless of the form in which it is given, significantly slows down the enzymatic reactions and controls the cascade. Abdominal attacks of severe cramps, guarding, and in some instances diarrhea can be rapidly controlled in this fashion, although they tend to subside spontaneously within 48 to 72 hours of observation. For severe laryngeal edema, there may be no choice but to do a tracheostomy, dependent upon the status of the patient when initially seen.

This year new agents have become available for the treatment of acute episodes including a B-2 receptor antagonist (Icatibant) (83,84) and a kallikrein inhibitor (Ecallantide) (85). These provide a physiologic approach that targets the kallikrein-kinin cascade and might eventually become available in preparations that can also be employed for prophylaxis. Treatment of acquired C1 INH deficiency requires, first, treatment of the underlying disease, if one has been identified, plus treatment with the aforementioned drugs. Their use is essentially the same as that for treatment of the hereditary disorder. Androgenic agents are typically employed. Treatment of type II acquired C1 INH deficiency with an autoantibody directed to C1 INH is indeed more difficult because the ability to replete C1 INH is significantly compromised. Plasmapheresis and use of a cytotoxic agent in addition to the use of prophylactic androgenic compounds or antifibrinolytic agents may be necessary for chronic treatment, and infusion of plasma or C1 INH concentrate is employed for acute emergency treatment. The latter is clearly preferable to prevent volume overload, and to be able to give enough C1 INH to bind the autoantibody so as to raise the C1 INH level significantly. In a practical sense, this is often not feasible. Tranexamic acid has also been successfully employed in the treatment of type II acquired C1 INH deficiency, in which activation of the bradykinin-forming cascade and fibrinolysis (the latter determined by elevated levels of plasmin-α_2 antiplasmin complexes) was observed (86). It is noteworthy that for treatment of the hereditary disorder the dosage of androgen required is based on clinical course (i.e., the frequency and severity of episodes) and not the level of C1 INH or even the increase in C4 that will result. It has been shown that the C4 level can approach normal with treatment, and C1 INH levels rise significantly beyond the critical 25% of normal levels; yet many patients are responsive to doses of androgen that are insufficient to achieve this. The reason for that is not clear, unless it is possible to achieve changes at a local level that might not be evident in the systemic circulation.

OTHER HEREDITARY AND NONHEREDITARY ANGIOEDEMA

Other hereditary forms of angioedema do not relate to C1 INH deficiency, but all of them are rare. Binkley et al., reported an estrogen-dependent but familial form of angioedema associated with pregnancy or with ingestion of estrogenic compounds (17). The disorder appears to have dominant inheritance, although initially thought to be present only in women because of the hormonal dependence. Recent studies of large families with the disorder have revealed occasional males who have symptoms (18). Peripheral angioedema is very common and gastrointestinal episodes are seen as well. Laryngeal edema, although, possible, seems less frequent compared with C1 INH deficiency. Some families have a mutant form of Factor XII, which when activated has enhanced activity

(19). Thus bradykinin may be the mediator, and therapy with newer agents that target the kallikrein-kinin system will be of interest. This has now been named HAE, type III.

There is also a familial vibratory angioedema that is a histamine-dependent (87) physically induced swelling (88) manifests when vibrating stimuli (e.g., rubbing a towel across the back after showering) are applied. Angioedema manifests frequently due to food or drug reactions and is then often associated with urticaria (in contrast to all of the aforementioned entities). Idiopathic angioedema (see chap. 22) is quite common, but little is known regarding the pathogenesis of the swelling. Cicardi et al., have classified patients with idiopathic angioedema into those that are histaminergic (i.e., respond to antihistamines), and those whose condition is refractory to antihistamines (89). A role for bradykinin release in the latter group has been reported with response to tranexamic acid, but the data have not yet been confirmed. Others propose a role for leucotreines B, C, and D secretion in patients resistant to antihistamines (Beltrani, V; personal communication) and suggest that inhibitors of leucotrene synthesis such as zeileutin (Zyflo) may be helpful. The extensive knowledge regarding the pathogenesis of hereditary and acquired C1 INH deficiency can be instructive regarding mechanisms of angioedema that are clearly distinct from allergic mechanisms, and may yet prove to be relevant for the treatment of other nonhereditary forms of swelling.

One of the most prominent causes of nonHAE is the use of ACE inhibitors, and this is now the most common cause of angioedema seen in emergency rooms. The angioedema is due to increased bradykinin levels (without urticaria) because the destruction of bradykinin by ACE is then impaired and blood levels gradually rise. It can occur at any time, but is most common within the first few months of therapy, and is particularly common in blacks (90). There may be polymorphisms of other inhibitors or changes in end organ responsiveness to bradykinin that determine who becomes symptomatic (91). These agents are not only employed for treatment of hypertension but are also indicated for congestive heart failure, diabetic neuropathy, and scleroderma renal disease. ACE is identical to kininase II and destroys bradykinin by removing the C-terminal Phe-Arg dipeptide, followed by removal of Ser-Pro, leaving the inactive pentapeptide Arg-Pro-Pro-Gly-Phe (91). With drug inhibition of ACE, the primary mechanism for bradykinin degradation is eliminated and bradykinin levels increase (52). Like C1 INH deficiency, swelling of the tongue, pharynx, and even larynx can be severe, requiring intubation for treatment of airway obstruction. In contrast to patients with C1 INH deficiency, urticaria is occasionally seen accompanying the angioedema, although the angioedema predominates. The reason for this difference is unclear and may relate to a different site of bradykinin action within the skin, or even a concomitant IgE-mediated reaction to the drug.

REFERENCES

1. Schreiber AD, Kaplan AP, Austen KF. Inhibition by C1 INH of Hageman factor fragment activation of coagulation, fibrinolysis, and kinin generation. J Clin Invest 1973; 52:1402–1409.
2. Pixley RA, Schapira M, Colman RW. The regulation of factor XII by plasma proteinase inhibitors. J Biol Chem 1985; 260:1723–1729.
3. Harpel PC, Lewin MF, Kaplan AP. Distribution of plasma kallikrein between C1 inactivator and α_2 macroglobulin-kallikrein complexes. J Biol Chem 1985; 260:4257–4263.
4. Donaldson VH, Evans RR. A biochemical abnormality in hereditary angioneurotic edema. Am J Med 1963; 35:37–44.
5. Kramer J, Katz Y, Rosen FS, et al. Synthesis of C1 inhibitor in fibroblasts from patients with Type I and Type II hereditary angioneurotic edema. J Clin Invest 1991; 87:1614–1620.

6. Cladwell JR, Ruddy S, Schur P, et al. Acquired C1 inhibitor deficiency in lymphosarcoma. Clin Immunol Immunopathol 1972; 1:39–52.

7. Hauptmann G, Lang JM, North ML, et al. Acquired C1 inhibitor deficiencies in lymphoproliferative diseases with serum immunoglobulin abnormalities. Blut 1976; 32:195–206.

8. Schreiber AD, Zweiman B, Atkins P, et al. Acquired angioedema with lymphoproliferative disorder association of C1 inhibitor deficiency with cellular abnormality. Blood 1976; 48:567–580.

9. Alsenz J, Bork K, Loos M. Autoantibody-mediated acquired deficiency of C1 inhibitor. N Engl J Med 1987; 316:1360–1366.

10. Zuraw BL, Curd JG. Demonstration of modified inactive first component of complement (C1) inhibitor in the plasmas of C1 inhibitor deficient patients. J Clin Invest 1986; 78:567–575.

11. Malbran A, Hammer CH, Frank MM, et al. Acquired angioedema: observations on the mechanism of action of autoantibodies directed against C1 esterase inhibitor. J Allergy Clin Immunol 1988; 81:1199–1204.

12. Pearson KD, Buchignani JS, Shimkin PM, et al. Hereditary angioneurotic edema of the gastrointestinal tract. Am J Roentgenol Radium Ther Nucl Med 1972; 116:256–261.

13. Sheffer AL, Craig JM, Willms-Kretschmer K. Histopathological and ultrastructural observations on tissues from patients with hereditary angioneurotic edema. J Allergy 1971; 47:292–297.

14. Tosi M. Molecular genetics of C1 inhibitor. Immunobiology 1998; 199:358–365.

15. Quastel M, Harrison R, Cicardi M, et al. Behavior in vivo of normal and dysfunctional C1 inhibitor in normal subjects and patients with hereditary angioedema. J Clin Invest 1983; 71: 1041–1046.

16. Kramer J, Rosen RS, Colter HR, et al. Transinhibition of C1 inhibitor synthesis in Type I hereditary angioneurotic edema. J Clin Invest 1993; 91:1258–1262.

17. Binkley KE, Davis III AE. Clinical, biochemical, and genetic characterization of a novel estrogen-dependent inherited form of angioedema. J Allergy Clin Immunol 2000; 106:546–550.

18. Dewald G, Bork K. Missense mutations in the coagulation factor XII (Hageman Factor) gene in heredidtary angioedema with normal C1 inhibition. Biochem Biophys Res Commun 2006; 343: 1286–1289.

19. Martin L, Raison-Peyron N, Nothem MM, et al. Hereditary angioedema with normal C1 inhibitor gene in a family with affected women and men is associated with the p.Thr328Lys mutation in the F12 gene. J Allergy Clin Immunol (Letter to Editor) 2007; 120:975–976.

20. Ruddy S, Gigli I, Sheffer AL, et al. The laboratory diagnosis of hereditary angioedema. In: Rose N, Richter M, Sehon A. et al. eds. Allergology: Proceedings of the Sixth International Congress of Allergology. Amsterdam: Excepta Medica, 1968:351–359.

21. Zuraw BL, Sugimoto S, Curd JG. The value of rocket immunoelectrophoresis for C4 activation in the evaluation of patients with angioedema or C1 inhibitor deficiency. J Allergy Clin Immunol 1986; 78:1115–1120.

22. Austen KF, Sheffer AL. Detection of hereditary angioneurotic edema by demonstration of a reduction in the second component of human complement. N Engl J Med 1965; 272:649–656.

23. Rose FS, Alper CA, Pensky J, et al. Genetic heterogeneity of the C1 esterase inhibitor in patients with hereditary angioneurotic edema. J Clin Invest 1971; 50:2143–2149.

24. Klemperer MR, Donaldson VH, Rosen FS. The vasopermeability response in man to purified C1 esterase. J Clin Invest 1968; 47:604 (abstr).

25. Donaldson VH. Mechanisms of activation of C1 esterase in hereditary angioneurotic edema plasma in vitro: the role of Hageman Factor, a clot-promoting agent. J Exp Med 1968; 127:411–429.

26. Donaldson VH, Rosen FS, Bing DH. Role of the second component of complement (C2) and plasmin in kinin release in hereditary angioneurotic edema (H.A.N.E.) Plasma Trans Assoc Am Physicians 1977; 40:174–183.

27. Curd JG, Yelvington M, Burridge N. Generation of bradykinin during incubation of hereditary angioedema plasma. Mol Immunol 1983; 19:1365.

28. Fields T, Ghebrehiwet B, Kaplan AP. Kinin formation in hereditary angioedema plasma: evidence against kinin derivation from C2 and in support of "spontaneous" formation of bradykinin. J Allergy Clin Immunol 1983; 72:54–60.

29. Strang CJ, Cholin S, Spragg J, et al. Angioedema induced by a peptide derived from complement component C1. J Exp Med 1988; 168:1685–1698.
30. Kaplan AP, Ghebrehiwet B. Does C-2 kinin exist. J Allergy Clin Immunol (Letter to Editor) 2004; 115:876.
31. Shoemaker LR, Schurman SJ, Donaldson VH, et al. Hereditary angioneurotic edema: characterization of plasma kinin and vascular permeability-enhancing activities. Clin Exp Immunol 1994; 95:22–28.
32. Carpenter CB, Ruddy S, Shehadeh IH, et al. Complement metabolism in man: hypercatabolism of the fourth (C4) and third (C3) components in patients with real allograft rejection and hereditary angioedema. J Clin Invest 1969; 48:1495–1505.
33. Silverberg M, Dunn JT, Garen L, et al. Autoactivation of human Hageman Factor: demonstration utilizing a synthetic substrate. J Biol Chem 1980; 255:7281–7286.
34. Silverberg M, Kaplan AP. Enzymatic activities of activated and Zymogen forms of Hageman Factor (Factor XII). Blood 1982; 60:64–70.
35. Tankersly DL, Finlayson JS. Kinetics of activation and autoactivation of human Factor XII. Biochem 1984; 23:273–279.
36. Schmaier AH, Kuo A, Lundberg D, et al. The expression of high molecular weight kininogen on human umbilical vein endothelial cells. J Biol Chem 1988; 263;16327–16333.
37. van Iwaarden F, DeGroot PG, Bouma BN. The binding of high molecular weight kininogen to cultured human endothelial cells. J Biol Chem 1988; 263:4698–4703.
38. Mandle RJ Jr, Kaplan AP. Hageman Factor substrates I. Human plasma prekallikrein. Mechanism of activation by Hageman Factor and participation in Hageman Factor-dependent fibrinoloysis. J Biol Chem 1977; 252:6097.
39. Cochrane CG, Revak SD, Wuepper KD. Activation of Hageman Factor in solid and fluid phase. J. Exp Med 1973; 135:1564–1583.
40. Dunn JT, Silverberg M, Kaplan AP. The cleavage and formation of activated Hageman Factor by autodigestion and by kallikrein. J Biol Chem 1982; 257:1779–1784.
41. Ichinose A, Fujikawa K, Suyama T. The activation of prourokinase by plasma kallikrein and its inactivation by thrombin. J Biol Chem 1986; 261:3486–3489.
42. Juhlin L, Michaelsson G. Vascular reactions in hereditary angioedema. Acta Derm Venereol. 1969; 49:20–25.
43. Talamo RC, Haber E, Austen KF. A radioimmunoassay for bradykinin in plasma and synovial fluid. J Lab Clin Med 1969; 74:816–827.
44. Nussberger J, Cugno M, Amstutz C, et al. Plasma bradykinin in angioedema. Lancet 1998; 351:1693–1697.
45. Ratnoff OD, Naff GB. The conversion of CN1S to CN1 esterase by plasmin and trypsin. J Exp Med 1967; 125:337–358.
46. Ghebrehiwet B, Silverberg M, Kaplan AP. Activation of the classical pathway of complement by Hageman Factor fragment (HFf). J Exp Med 1981; 153:665–676.
47. Ghebrehiwet G, Randazzo BP, Dunn JT, et al. Mechanism of activation of the classical pathway of complement by Hageman Factor fragment. J Clin Invest 1983; 71:1450–1456.
48. Curd JG, Prograis LF Jr, Cochrane CG. Detection of active kallikrein in induced blister fluids of hereditary angioedema patients. J Exp Med 1980; 152:742–747.
49. Schapira M, Silver LD, Scott CF, et al. Prekallikrein activation and high molecular weight kininogen consumption in hereditary angioedema. N Engl J Med 1983; 308:1050–1053.
50. Zahedi R, Bissler JJ, Davis III AE, et al. Unique C1 inhibitor dysfunction in a kindred without angioedema II. Identification of a Ala [443] → Val substitution and functional analysis of the recombinant mutant protein. J Clin Invest 1995; 95:1299–1305.
51. Zahedi R, Wisnieski J, Davis III AE. Role of the P2 residue of complement 1 inhibitor (Ala 443) in determination of target protease specificity: inhibition of complement and contact proteases. J Immunol 1997; 159:983–988.
52. Cugno M, Cicardi M, Coppola R, et al. Activation of Factor XII and cleavage of high molecular weight kininogen during acute attacks in hereditary and acquired C1 inhibitor deficiencies. Immunopharmacology 1996; 33:361–364.

53. Nussberger J, Cugno M, Cicardi M, et al. Local bradykinin generation in hereditary angioedema. J Allergy Clin Immunol 1999; 104:1321–1322.

54. Kaplan AP, Austen KF. A prealbumin activation of prekallikrein II. Derivation of activators of prekallikrein from activated Hageman Factor with plasmin. J Exp Med 1971; 133:696–712.

55. Wallace EM, Perkins SJ, Sim RB, et al. Degradation of C1-inhibitor by plasmin: implications for the control of inflammatory processes. Mol Med 1997; 3:385–396.

56. Joseph K, Shibayama Y, Ghebrehiwet B, et al. Factor XII-dependent contact activation on endothelial cells and binding proteins gC1qR and cytokeratin 1. J Thromb Haemost 2001; 85: 119–124.

57. Joseph K, Tholanikunnel BG, Kaplan AP. Heat shock protein 90 catalyzes activation of the prekallikrein-kininogen complex in the absence of Factor XII. Proc Natl Acad Sci 2002; 99: 896–900.

58. Caldwell JR, Ruddy S, Schur P, et al. Acquired C1 inhibitor deficiency in lymphosarcoma. Clin Immunol Immunopathol 1972; 1:39–52.

59. Geha RS, Quinti I, Austen KF, et al. Acquired C1-inhibitor deficiency associated with antiidiotypic antibody to monoclonal immunoglobulin. N Engl J Med 1985; 312:534.

60. Donaldson VH, Hess EV, McAdams PJ. Lupus-erythematosus-like disease in three unrelated women with hereditary angioneurotic edema. Ann Intern Med 1977; 86:312–313.

61. Cohen SH, Koethe SM, Kozin F, et al. Acquired angioedema associated with rectal carcinoma and its response to danazol therapy. J Allergy Clin Immunol 1978; 62:217–221.

62. Jackson J, Sim RB, Whelan A, et al. An IgG autoantibody which inactivates C1 inhibitor. Nature 1986; 323:722–724.

63. Jackson J, Sim RB, Whaley K, et al. Autoantibody facilitated cleavage of C1 inhibitor in autoimmune angioedema. J Clin Invest 1989; 83:698–707.

64. He S, Sim RB, Whaley K. Mechanism of action of anti C1 inhibitor autoantibodies: prevention of the formation of stable C1S-C1 INH complexes. Molec Med 1998; 4:119–128.

65. Cicardi M, Beretta A, Colombo M, et al. Relevance of lymphoproliferative disorders and anti C1 inhibitor autoantibodies in acquired angioedema. Clin Exp Immunol 1996; 106:475–480.

66. Chevailler A, Orland G, Ponard D, et al. C1 inhibitor binding monoclonal immunoglobulins in three patients with acquired angioneurotic edema. J Allergy Clin Immunol 1996; 97:998–1008.

67. Gelfand JA, Sherin RJ, Alling DW, et al. Treatment of hereditary angioedema with danazol; reversal of clinical and biochemical abnormalities. N Engl J Med 1976; 295:1444–1448.

68. Sheffer AL, Fearon DT, Austen KF. Clinical and biochemical effects of stanazolol therapy for hereditary angioedema. J Allergy Clin Immunol 1981; 68:181–187.

69. Warin AP, Greaves MW, Gatecliff M, et al. Treatment of hereditary angioedema by low-dose attenuated androgens: dissociation of clinical response from levels of C1 esterase inhibitor and C4. Br J Dermatol 1980; 103:405–409.

70. Sheffer AL, Fearon DT, Austen KF. Hereditary angioedema: a decade of management with stanozolol. J Allergy Clin Immunol 1987; 80:855–860.

71. Gadek JE, Hosea SW, Gellfand JA, et al. Response of variant hereditary angioedema phenotypes of danazol therapy. J Clin Invest 1979; 64:280–286.

72. Hosea SW, Santaella ML, Brown EJ, et al. Long term therapy of hereditary angioedema with Danazol. Ann Int Med 1990; 93:809–812.

73. Cicardi M, Bergamaschini L, Cugno M, et al. Long term treatment of hereditary angioedema with attenuated androgens: a survey of a 13-uear experience. J Allergy Clin Immunol 1991; 87: 768–773.

74. Cicardi M, Castelli R, Zingale LC, et al. Side effects of long-term prophylaxis with attenuated androgens in hereditary angioedema: comparison of treated and untreated patients. J Allergy Clin Immunol 1997; 99:194–196.

75. Sloane DE, Lee CW, Sheffer AL. Hereditary angioedema: safety of long-term stanozolol therapy. J Allergy Clin Immunol 2007; 120:654–658.

76. Frank MM, Sergent JS, Kane MA, et al. Epsilon-aminocarproic and therapy of hereditary angioneurotic edema: a double blind study. N Engl J Med 1972; 286:808–812.

77. Lundh B, Laurell A, Wetterqvist H, et al. A case of hereditary angioneurotic edema successfully treated with epilson-aminocarproic acid. Studies on C'1 esterase inhibitor, C'1 activation, plasminogen level and histamine metabolism. Clin Exp Immunol 1968; 3:733–745.

78. Sheffer AL, Austen KF, Rosen FS. Tranexamic acid therapy in hereditary angioneurotic edema. N Engl J Med 1972; 287:452–454.

79. Soter NA, Austen KF, Gigli I. Inhibition by epilson-aminocarproic acid of the activation of the first component of the complement system. J Immunol 1975; 114:928–932.

80. Gadek JE, Hosea SW, Glefand JA, et al. Replacement therapy in hereditary angioedema: successful treatment of acute episodes with partly purified C1 inhibitor. N Engl J Med 1980; 302:542–546.

81. Visentin DE, Yang WH, Karsh J. C1 esterase inhibitor transfusion in patients with hereditary angioedema. Ann Allergy Asthma Immunol 1998; 80:457–461.

82. Bas M, Bier H, Greve J, et al. Novel pharmacotherapy of acute hereditary angioedema with bradykinin B2-receptor antagonist Icatibant. Allergy 2006; 61:1490–1492.

83. Bork K, Frank J, Grundt B, et al. Treatment of acute edema attacks in hereditary angioedema with a bradykinin receptor–2 antagonist (Icatibant). J Allergy Clin Immunol 2007; 119:1497–1503.

84. Schneider L, Lumry W, Vegh A, et al. Critical role of kallikrein in hereditary angioedema pathogenesis: a clinical trial of ecallantide, a novel kallikrein inhibitor. J Allergy Clin Immunol 2007; 120:416–422.

85. Cugno M, Cicardi M, Agostoni A. Activation of the contact system and fibrinolysis in autoimmune acquired angioedema: a rationale for prophylactic use of tranexamic acid. J Allergy Clin Immunol 1994; 93:870–876.

86. Metzger WJ, Kaplan AP, Irons J, et al. Hereditary vibratory angioedema: confirmation of histamine release in a type of physical hypersensitivity. J Allergy Clin Immunol 1976; 57:605–608.

87. Patterson R, Mellies CJ, Blankenship ML, et al. Vibratory angioedema: a hereditary type of physical hypersensitivity. J Allergy Clin Immunol 1972; 50:174–182.

88. Cicardi M, Bergamaschini L, Zingale LC, et al. Idiopathic nonhistaminergic angioedema. Am J Med 1999; 106:650–654.

89. Kaplan AP, Greaves MW. Angioedema. J Am Acad Dermatol 2005; 53:373–388.

90. Byrd JB, Shreevatsa A, Putlur P, et al. Dipeptidyl peptidase IV deficiency increases susceptibility to angiotension-converting enzyme inhibitor-induced peritracheal edema. J Allergy Clin Immunol 2007; 120:403–408.

91. Sheikh I, Kaplan AP. The mechanism of digestion of bradykinin and lysyl bradykinin (kallidin) in human serum: the role of carboxypeptidase, angiotension converting enzyme, and determination of final degradation products. Biochem Pharmacol 1989; 38:993–1000.

17

Chronic Urticaria: Autoimmune Chronic Urticaria and Idiopathic Chronic Urticaria

Malcolm W. Greaves
St. John's Institute of Dermatology, St. Thomas' Hospital, London, U.K.

Allen P. Kaplan
Department of Medicine, Medical University of South Carolina, Charleston, South Carolina, U.S.A.

INTRODUCTION

Chronic urticaria is conventionally defined as the daily or almost-daily occurrence of wheals for six weeks or more (1). This heading encompasses a variety of different disorders that share whealing as the most prominent clinical feature (Table 1). These include the physical urticarias in which whealing occurs in response to a physical stimulus, usually applied directly to the skin. Cholinergic urticaria is usually included under the heading of a physical urticaria, although here the triggering stimulus is a rise in body temperature because of heat, exercise, or emotion. It also includes autoimmune chronic urticaria, a relatively recently described entity (2–5), which will be considered in more detail below. Chronic urticaria, which cannot be ascribed to any of the above, and for which an identifiable cause is elusive, is still a common and troublesome problem, termed "chronic idiopathic urticaria" (CIU). Of course co-existence of physical urticarias with CIU or autoimmune urticaria frequently occurs in the same individual.

Angioedema also occurs concurrently with chronic urticaria in 87% of patients with CIU and is also frequent in autoimmune urticaria (6). Urticarial vasculitis is frequently included under the heading of chronic urticaria because it is often clinically indistinguishable from CIU and is a very important differential diagnosis of the latter. However it is dealt with fully in chapter 21 and will not be considered in detail here.

How common is chronic urticaria? Accurate figures are hard to come by. In patients visiting their general practitioners, 5.1% had experienced urticaria for more than four weeks (7). An overall average lifelong prevalence of chronic urticaria of 1% to 2% is likely. Chronic urticaria is also highly disabling. Use of an internationally recognized

Table 1 Chronic Urticaria: Classification

Physical urticaria	Autoimmune urticaria
Symptomatic dermographism	Chronic idiopathic urticaria
Cold urticaria	
Cholinergic urticaria	Urticarial vasculitis
Delayed pressure urticaria	
Solar urticaria	
Heat urticaria	
Aquagenic urticaria	

quality of life instrument has recently shown that the degrees of personal, occupational, and social disability are comparable with those found in patients with triple coronary artery disease awaiting bypass surgery (8). Thus better information on etiology and pathogenesis is badly needed.

AUTOIMMUNE URTICARIA

Indirect Evidence

We know that the wheals of chronic urticaria are in part due to release of histamine and other mediators from dermal mast cells (9). The suggestion that chronic urticaria might be the result of the action of circulating histamine-releasing factors is not new and has been proposed by earlier authors. In the early 1960s, Rorsman (10) observed a paucity of circulating peripheral blood basophils in urticaria, and proposed that "antigen–antibody reactions ... bring about degranulation of basophil leucocytes."

Indirect evidence that chronic "idiopathic" urticaria might have an autoimmune basis has been with us for many years. In 1983 Lesnoff et al. reported an association between thyroid autoimmunity and CIU, and in 1989 Leznoff proposed a "syndrome" of autoimmune thyroid disease and chronic urticaria and angioedema (11,12) with thyroid autoantibodies identified in 15% of patients. Published figures for the incidence of thyroid autoantibodies in CIU range from 5% to 90%. We (13) recently reported that of 182 patients with chronic urticaria, 22 had antithyroid microsomal autoantibodies (12%), and 8 of these were autologous serum skin test positive. Kikuchi et al. reported (14) an incidence of antimicrosomal antibodies plus antithyroglobulin antibodies of 24% and the presence of those antobodies was associated with anti-IgE receptor antibodies. The incidence in the anti-IgE-receptor negative patients was 10%, while the reported incidence in the general population is 7%. Thyroid-stimulating hormone plasma levels were elevated in 14 patients, all but one of which were positive for the autologous serum skin test. Most patients with CIU and thyroid autoantibodies are euthyroid. Recently published guidelines (15) recommend that thyroid autoantibody and thyroid function testing should not be performed routinely, but only if there is clinical or family history evidence pointing toward thyroid dysfunction. That treatment of thyroid dysfunction in patients with idiopathic urticaria favorably influences the urticaria is often claimed (13), but remains unproved. It is also worth noting that determinations of the human leukocyte antigen (HLA) class 2 alleles in CIU patients revealed a significantly increased frequency of HLA DRB1*04 (corrected $p = 3.6 \times 10^{-6}$) for patients with evidence of autoimmune chronic urticaria (16), a result consistent with the view that an autoimmune basis underlies this subset of chronic urticaria patients.

Abnormal Basophil Function

In 1974, Greaves et al. (17) made the observation that basophils of patients with chronic urticaria are hyporesponsive to anti-IgE, and soon thereafter Kern and Lichtenstein (18) confirmed that blood basophil suspensions from patient with CIU had diminished basophil-releasing ability evoked by anti-IgE. This finding suggested basophil desensitization, but its significance was not appreciated. We now know that basophil desensitization together with a parallel reduction in basophil numbers in chronic urticaria is at least in part, due to the action of circulatory histamine-releasing autoantibodies (19). Recent studies have reexamined this observation, and data have emerged suggesting an abnormality in signal transduction observed in basophils of patients with chronic urticaria. Luquin et al. (20) found basophil hyporesponsiveness to anti-IgE, but paradoxically hyper-responsiveness to a serum factor. However these abnormalities were not confined to those patients with autoantibodies, thus an intrinsic abnormality in signal transduction might be present. Recently Vonakis et al. (21) reported hyporesponsiveness in a subpopulation of patients with chronic urticaria (about half) attributed to excessive activity of SHIP (Src homology 2–containing inositol phosphatase), which dephosphorylates kinases such as Syk and thereby diminishes responsiveness. The authors contend that the two basophil subpopulations (normally responsive vs. hyporesponsive) do not correspond to those patients considered to have autoimmune features versus those that are still considered to be idiopathic.

Evidence for Involvement of a Circulating Histamine-Releasing Factor

The idea that autoantibodies directed against epitopes expressed by mast cells or basophils could be an important cause of histamine release in urticaria is not a novel concept. In 1988 Gruber et al. (22) reported that patients with cold urticaria had autoantibodies of the IgG class directed against IgE as determined by enzyme immunoassay. These antibodies were also found in occasional patients with CIU and urticarial vasculitis. The serum of one cold urticaria patient was shown to release histamine from normal human basophils, but immunoabsorption studies indicated that this activity was located in the IgM fraction of the serum. None of the immunoreactive sera caused an immediate wheal and flare reaction upon intradermal injection. A role for IgG anti-IgE as an activator of mast cells and basophils was also proposed in atopic dermatitis (23). Other nonimmunoglobulin histamine–releasing factors were also proposed, notably an IgE-dependent histamine-releasing factor (24) and a cytokine-like factor (25).

Evidence that Serum Histamine-Releasing Activity in Chronic Urticaria is Due to an Autoantibody

The ability of sera from some but not all patients with CIU to cause a wheal and flare reaction upon autologous intradermal injection was first reported by Grattan et al. (1986) (26). He showed a positive response in 7 of 12 patients and noted that in these patients a positive result could only be obtained if the urticaria was currently active. Initial investigation of this activity suggested it was a histamine-releasing autoantibody with the characteristics of anti-IgE on the basis of absorption of this activity by monoclonal IgE and inhibition by lactic acid stripping of IgE from normal human basophils (27). It was supposed that in patients with positive sera, the development of urticarial wheals was because of the ability of these antibodies to cross-link dermal mast cell–bound IgE, causing mast cell activation and histamine release (Fig. 1).

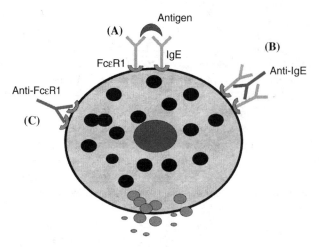

Figure 1 Activation of dermal mast cell via FcεR1. (**A**) Antigen cross-links specific IgE; (**B**) IgG anti-IgE cross-links via Fc portion of IgE; (**C**) IgG anti-FcεR1 cross-links adjacent FcεR1 directly.

Further analysis of histamine-releasing activity of sera from four patients with chronic urticaria revealed that it consisted of IgG, or less commonly IgM, with novel epitope specificities. Inhibition experiments, using the human recombinant extracellular fragment of the high-affinity IgE receptor (FcεR1) alpha subunit (α), identified IgG autoantibodies directed against FcεR1. It was proposed that these autoantibodies cross-linked adjacent α subunits of FcεR1 on dermal mast cells and basophils (2) (Fig. 1C). It was concluded that cross-linking autoantibodies against the α- chain of FcεR1, leading to mast cell activation could represent an important pathogenetic mechanism in CIU. Nimii et al. subsequently studied 165 patients with CIU, 105 of whom had a positive autologous serum skin test. Of these sera, 43 (26% of all urticaria patients studied) released histamine from high- and low-IgE donor basophils, indicating the presence of functional anti-FcεR1α autoantibodies, anti-IgE autoantibodies, or both (3). Eight patients' sera reacted only with basophils from a high-IgE donor, suggesting that these patients possessed autoantibodies reacting with IgE. Sera from 19 healthy donors were nonreactive against basophils of low- or high-IgE donors (3). In the same study, autologous serum skin test positive sera from 12 patients with CIU caused IgG-mediated histamine release from dermal mast cells of healthy donors, which could also be inhibited by human recombinant FcεR1α (3). These data, taken together with the histological finding of dermal mast cell degranulation following intradermal injection of autologous serum (28), represent persuasive evidence that anti-FcεR1α autoantibodies are relevant to the pathogenesis of CIU. Recently Sabroe et al. (2002) (29) have classified sera from 75 patients with CIU into five subsets: immunoreactive histamine-releasing anti-FcεR1 autoantibodies (26%); immunoreactive nonhistamine-releasing anti-FcεR1 autoantibodies (15%); anti-IgE autoantibodies (9%); sera containing a nonimmunoglobulin mast cell–specific histamine-releasing factor (3) (9%); and sera with no identifiable factor (41%). Positive autologous serum skin tests were strongly associated with histamine-releasing anti-FcεR1 autoantibodies and no autoantibodies were detected in healthy subjects or in patients with physical urticarias (29).

Fiebiger et al. (4) used human recombinant FcεR1α and Western blotting to demonstrate that 37% of sera of 32 patients with CIU contained immunoreactive anti-FcεR1α autoantibodies, and in most cases these antibodies showed functional histamine-releasing activity. No immunoreactivity was found in sera of healthy subjects or patients with atopic eczema. In a subsequent publication (30), the same laboratory showed that anti-FcɛR1α immunoreactivity could be detected in the serum of patients with other autoimmune diseases, including pemphigus vulgaris, bullous pemphigoid, dermatomyositis, and systemic lupus erythematosus. However unlike the anti-FcɛR1 autoantibodies found in chronic urticaria, which are mainly of the IgG1 or IgG3 subtypes, anti-FcɛR1 autoantibodies in these other autoimmune disorders were nonfunctional (nonhistamine-releasing) and predominantly of the IgG2 or IgG4 subtypes. Similar results were reported by Kaplan's group in 1996 (5). In 50 patients with CIU, these authors used a rat basophil leukemia cell line expressing FcɛR1α to demonstrate the presence of functional (β-hexosaminidase-releasing) anti-FcɛR1 autoantibodies in sera of 38 (76%). All but one of 20 healthy control subjects were negative in this assay. However when human basophils were used as indicator cells, sera from 20 of 50 patients (40%) with chronic urticaria but only one of 19 healthy controls released histamine.

Horn et al. (31) detected anti-FcɛR1α antibodies in sera from healthy donors using recombinant protein consisting of two moieties of the extracellular part of human FcɛR1α, flanking one moity of human serum albumen. Although the affinities of these autoantibodies against recombinant FcɛR1α were low, healthy donor sera containing these antibodies showed histamine-releasing activity. However these autoantibodies were cross-reactive with tetanus toxoid, and demonstration of histamine-releasing activity was dependent on pretreatment of donor basophils with interleukin (IL)-3 and stripping the cells of bound IgE. The significance of these autoantibodies, existence of which has yet to be independently confirmed, requires further examination. Attempts to eliminate patient antibody to the IgE receptor by incubation with tetanus toxoid by Kaplan's groups (unpublished observations) failed while absorption with cloned α subunit reduced or eliminated the activity.

Mode of Action of Anti-FcɛR1 Autoantibodies

Kaplan has also addressed the issue of complement involvement in autoantibody-mediated histamine release in autoimmune urticaria (32,33). Earlier work (2,3) suggested that release of histamine from mast cells and basophils by anti-FcɛR1 autoantibodies was due to direct cross-linking of adjacent α-chains of FcɛR1 on the surface of these cells, without complement involvement. That complement activation may be involved was suggested by the earlier identification of IgG1 or IgG3 as the principal immunoglobulin subtypes in autoimmune urticaria. (30). Further evidence supporting a role for complement activation derives from histamine release experiments using highly purified IgG anti-FcɛR1 and decomplemented sera that is deficient in either C2 or C5. It was found that whole sera from patients with chronic urticaria but not complement-deficient sera, released histamine from dermal mast cells. It was further found that C5a may play a key role since in vitro release of histamine from normal human basophils was dependent upon the concentration of C5a and was inhibited by an antibody to the C5a receptor. It was concluded that release of histamine from dermal mast cells (32) or basophils (33,34) by anti-FcɛR1 autoantibodies was augmented primarily by C5a activation. The involvement of C5a could also explain the otherwise puzzling lack of clinical evidence of pulmonary involvement in autoimmune urticaria, since the major subtype of pulmonary mast cell (but not dermal mast cells) are deficient in C5a receptors (35).

Chronic Urticaria as an Autoimmune Disease

At least 30% to 50% of patients with CIU have detectable functional anti-FcɛR1 or anti-IgE autoantibodies and these patients show, as already mentioned (16) an increased frequency of HLA DR alleles characteristically associated with autoimmune disease. In the subset that possesses these autoantibodies, the evidence that they are pathogenic is persuasive and can be summarized as follows: functional (histamine-releasing) anti-FcεR1 autoantibodies are not found in healthy people, allergic subjects, or in patients with other types of chronic urticaria (2,3,5); the antibodies release histamine from mast cells and basophils (2,3); they cause whealing upon intradermal injection in a healthy volunteer (36); the plasma levels of the autoantibodies correlate well with disease activity (37) and removal of the autoantibody leads to remission (38). Additional autoimmune phenomena are also seen in this subgroup, including antithyroid antibodies and a high incidence of positive antinuclear antibodies (ANAs) with speckled pattern (Kaplan AP, unpublished observation). None had systemic lupus erythematosus. Standard criteria for definition of an autoimmune disease require that, in addition to the above, reproduction of the disease in experimental animals be performed (39), and this has not yet been done using anti-FcεR1 autoantibodies; therefore strictly the evidence should be regarded as convincing, but a little short of fully proven. That autoantibodies against receptors can cause disease is by no means a novel concept, recognized examples, including myasthenia gravis (acetyl choline receptor) and insulin resistant diabetes mellitus (insulin receptor). In these and other similar examples receptor activation is blocked or downgraded. Receptor activation due to a receptor-specific autoantibody is less common and autoimmune urticaria now joins Graves' disease (autoantibody against the thyroid-stimulating hormone receptor) as an example of this less common receptor-mediated cell activation autoimmune phenomenon. These interesting issues have previously been discussed in greater detail (40). It should also be noted that virtually every autoimmune disease has some subjects with positive antibodies and no disease, which may explain the occasional positive basophil histamine release reported in subjects without urticaria (41). Nevertheless Kaplan and Joseph (42) recently reported on a typical assay in which no positives were found in 35 allergic subjects who did not have urticaria and 54 positives out of 104 chronic urticaria patients were reported (Fig. 2). The small amount of histamine seen

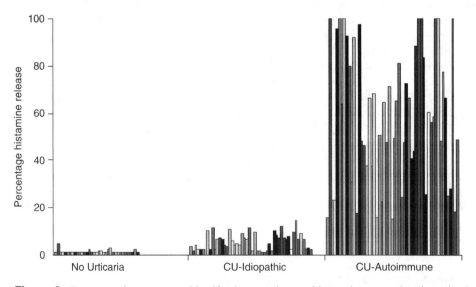

Figure 2 Representative assay to identify those patients with autoimmune chronic urticaria. Percent histamine release is shown for 35 normal controls and 104 patients with chronic urticaria. Separation into the idiopathic and autoimmune groups is evident. *Source*: Adapted from Ref. 42.

in the "idiopathic" group may represent a weak histamine-releasing factor present or more likely, represents the serum histamine level of patients, which was not subtracted. It is not present in controls.

Autoimmune Urticaria: Diagnosis

Clinical examination of the patient with CIU is generally unhelpful in distinguishing autoimmune from nonautoimmune patients (43). Although the disease is usually more severe and persistent in autoantibody positive patients, systemic symptoms are nevertheless not especially prominent in autoimmune, compared with nonautoimmune patients. Likewise, histological examination of skin biopsy material is unrewarding (44). It was observed that EG2 positive (activated) eosinophils were more profuse in older (>12 hours) wheals in autoantibody negative patients, but no diagnostically useful histological or immunocytochemical features could be discerned. Recently Ying et al. (45) reported immunopathological studies of skin biopsies from 13 patients with CIU, 6 of whom were positive for anti-FcεR1 autoantibodies. The immunopathology of skin biopsies from autoantibody positive and autoantibody negative patients did not differ significantly. Specifically the population density of CD3, CD4, CD8, and CD25 T cells, IL-4, IL-5 IFNγ mRNA + cells, eosinophils, neutrophils basophils macrophages, and tryptase positive mast cells was similar in the two groups.

The Autologous Serum Skin Test

The autologous serum skin test, which detects autoreactivity in the chronic urticaria patient's serum, has proved a useful screening test for autoimmune urticaria (46) (Fig. 3). In this test 50 µL of the patient's autologous serum is injected intradermally into the flexor surface of the forearm along with equal volumes of normal saline and histamine

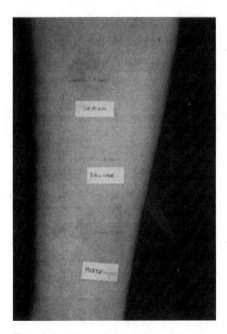

Figure 3 (*See color insert*) Autologous serum skin test.

(10 μg/mL) as negative and positive controls, respectively. Wheal and flare responses are measured at 30 minutes and their areas are calculated from measurement of two perpendicular diameters ($d1$ and $d2$) according to the formula: $\pi\ (d1 + d2)/4$. Wheal and flare measurements for serum-induced responses are corrected by subtraction of the equivalent values for the saline-induced responses in each subject. Using these measurements a positive test is defined as a red serum-induced wheal with a diameter of 1.5 mm or more than the saline-induced response at 30 minutes, and under these conditions the sensitivity and specificity of the test proved to be 65% to 81% and 71% to 78%, respectively. Despite having modest sensitivity and specificity as a screening test for histamine-releasing activity in serum and practical disadvantages, especially lack of standardization, it is a simple low-cost test that provides convincing evidence of endogenous autoreactivity in chronic urticaria. It is of value in predicting both the course and management of the disease for clinicians. However serum autoreactivity has also been detected in patients with acute urticaria because of nonsteroidal anti-inflammatory drugs (NSAIDs).

Using the basophil histamine release test as the gold standard for positivity, the test was negative in 39 of 40 healthy controls, 15 of 15 patients with symptomatic dermographism, 10 of 10 atopic patients and 8 of 9 patients with cholinergic urticaria. Although the measurements are straightforward, variations in injection technique can result in lack of reproducibility. Regular performance of the test, preferably in duplicate (right and left arms) reduces interest variation and ensures clinically useful results, which are predictive of functional anti-FcεR1 autoantibodies. However we advise that results be confirmed if possible by in vitro testing of the serum for anti-FcεR1 and anti-IgE autoantibodies. The autologous serum skin test is described in greater detail in chapter 8.

In Vitro Tests

The goal of development of a simple quantitative in vitro test for anti-FcεR1 and anti-IgE autoantibodies remains elusive. Although the use of ELISA (enzyme-linked immunosorbent assay) and immunoblotting have been reported (30,33), the correlation between functional tests (release of histamine or other mediator) and tests relying upon immunoreactivity has proved to be poor. For this reason Kikuchi and Kaplan (33) concluded, on the basis of studies in 260 patients with chronic urticaria, that immunobinding assays were not acceptable as a screening method and that functional assays are required. Assays currently in use include release of histamine from basophils of low- and high-IgE donors (2,3,33). Some published frequencies of positive results using these "gold standard" assays are listed in the Table 2.

The Basophil in Autoimmune Urticaria

That basopenia is a feature of chronic urticaria has long been recognized (10). It has also been frequently reported that basophils of CIU are unresponsive to evocation of histamine release by anti-IgE (18), especially when the urticaria is in relapse, a finding suggestive of desensitisation (50). More recently Grattan (51) was able to demonstrate an association between basopenia and histamine-releasing activity of the patient's serum in CIU. Subsequently Sabroe (19) demonstrated a close inverse correlation between levels of anti-FcεR1 autoantibodies, peripheral blood basophil numbers, and total blood histamine concentration in CIU. That counting basophils could form the basis of a useful screening test for autoimmune urticaria has been considered (52), but must await rapid and convenient methods for enumeration of peripheral blood basophils.

Table 2 Frequency of Anti-FcεR1 Autoantobodies in CIU Detected by Functional In Vitro Assays

Source	No. of CIU patients studied	Assay	Percentage positive	Reference
Tong et al.	50	RBL cells[a]	76	5
Ferrer et al.	68	BHR	48	32
Ferrer et al.	68	MCHR	46	32
Zweiman et al.	28	BHR[b]	61	47
Zweiman et al.	70	BHR	30	48
Asero et al.	121	BHR	16.5	49
Niimi et al.	165	BHR[c]	26	3
Sabroe et al.	28	BHR[c]	28	29

[a]Transfected with genes encoding for α, γ1, and γ2 chains of FcεR1.
[b]Basophils sensitized using deuterium oxide.
[c]Bsophils from both low-and high-IgE donors.
Abbreviations: CIU, chronic idiopathic urticaria; RBL, rat basophilic leukemia; BHR, basophil histamine release; MCHR, mast cell histamine release.

Prognosis and Treatment of Autoimmune Urticaria

The general principles of management of chronic urticaria from any cause apply equally to autoimmune urticaria and are dealt with in chapter 18. Although quantitative follow-up data are lacking, autoimmune chronic urticaria tends to run a more protracted course than its nonautoimmune counterpart, and is also often relatively treatment resistant. It is important to explain the nature of the disease to the patient in order to allay unjustified fears he or she may have regarding life-threatening underlying causes and to save unnecessary investigations. Use of H_1 antihistamines should always be the first line of drug treatment. In mildly or moderately affected patients fexofenadine 120–180 mg daily, or levocetirizine 5 mg, or desloratidine 5 mg daily plus a sedative H_1 antihistamine such as hydroxyzine 25 mg at night may be adequate, but it is often useful to prescribe off-label doses of such medications to control symptoms. Compliance is usually good due to the absence of adverse effects with these newer nonlipophilic, nonsedative antihistamines. Patients receiving hydroxyzine at night must be warned of the continuing effect of the drug on cognitive function throughout the following morning. However some patients with autoimmune urticaria are severely disabled by constant pruritus, wheals, and angioedema. In these patients increased employment of first generation antihistaminics (chap. 20) or recourse to immunotherapy may be necessary. Systemic corticosteroids are often disappointing and incur troublesome adverse effects if used inappropriately (chap. 20). Cyclosporin 2.5 to 5 mg/kg/day is a satisfactory alternative and has been proved to be effective in a well-controlled study (53) of patients with CIU, all of whom had a positive autologous serum skin test and serum histamine-releasing activity and therefore likely had an autoimmune basis for their disease. Contraindications to cyclosporin include a history of renal impairment, cancer, or a positive cervical smear. The drug should be used with extreme caution in patients with hypertension or hyperlipidemia. In patients in whom cyclosporin is contraindicated, poorly tolerated or ineffective, recourse can be made to intravenous immunoglobulin or plasmapheresis. The reader is referred to detailed accounts in the literature of the use of these treatments for the indication of autoimmune urticaria (36,37,54). One of the authors (Kaplan A) has, however failed to observe a response to IVIG in six out of seven patients in whom it was tried.

Does Making a Diagnosis of Autoimmune Urticaria Really Matter?

From the above account, the answer is "yes," with the caveat that in patients with mild to moderate impairment of quality of life and reasonable control of symptoms by H_1 antihistamines there may be little advantage to be gained by further investigation. However, even in these patients, elucidation of an autoimmune cause can set the patient's mind at rest and obviate fruitless quests for dietary and other causes and expenses from unnecessary tests. In severely affected patients with resultant disruption of occupational family and social activities the presence of anti-FcεR1 or anti-IgE autoantibodies should be sought, since additional therapeutic options, outlined above, are available and effective and should be considered in each case.

CHRONIC IDIOPATHIC URTICARIA

Up to 50% of patients with chronic "idiopathic" urticaria turn out to have autoimmune urticaria. This leaves a remainder of at least 50%, conventionally described as having idiopathic disease. A few of these may in fact have autoimmune urticaria, false-negative results being the consequence of timing or insufficient sensitivity of available tests, but most appear to have a nonautoimmune basis. By definition, the term "idiopathic" indicates absence of an evident cause. Nevertheless these patients are frequently widely investigated, nearly always with disappointing results.

Clinical Features

These are clinically indistinguishable from those occurring in chronic autoimmune urticaria (43). The duration of the disease is by generally accepted definition at least six weeks, during which daily, or almost daily, wheals occur, which are associated with mucocutaneous angioedema in about 90% (43), and about 50% also have concomitant delayed-pressure urticaria (chap. 7). Angioedema, though alarming to the patient, is rarely life threatening in idiopathic chronic urticaria. Individual wheals, which are associated with increased tissue levels of histamine (9), last less than 24 hours, usually about 12 hours, depending on the size. They may be annular, serpiginous, or confluent to form large plaques, and they fade without leaving any stain in the skin apart from the effects of vigorous rubbing, causing bruising. Patients rarely scratch urticaria. Smaller wheals may be surrounded by a white halo because of a steal effect consequent upon the increased blood flow within the wheals. The distribution is universal, including the palms and soles, although associated delayed-pressure urticaria may be the cause of whealing at these sites. Pruritus is invariably troublesome, especially at night (43) and is of a burning or pricking quality. Lesions of angioedema also last less than 24 hours unless they are massive, and the occurrence of itching is inconsistent. Associated systemic symptoms occur in 25% to 30% and include gastrointestinal symptoms, flushing, palpitations, headache arthralgia, and fatigue. Gastrointestinal symptoms often turn out to be because of irritable bowel syndrome and palpitations because of anxiety. If these symptoms are unusually prominent idiopathic anaphylaxis should be considered. Two thirds of patients report exacerbating factors (43) and these are listed in Table 3.

Diagnosis

The problem of diagnosis of chronic urticaria has recently been reviewed (54). A number of nonurticarial skin conditions mimic chronic urticaria with or without angioedema (pseudourticaria), and the more important of these are listed in Table 4.

Table 3 Factors Reported by Patients to Exacerbate CIU

Drugs
  NSAIDs (including aspirin), antibiotics, HRT, amphetamines, herbal remedies
Infections
  Intercurrent virus infections
Foods
  Especially sea foods, flavored and colored soft drinks, alcoholic drinks, eggs and dairy products
Stressful events
  Menses
    Premenstrual or during menses

Abbreviations: CIU, chronic idiopathic urticaria; NSAIDs, nonsteroidal anti-inflammatory drugs; HRT, hormone replacement therapy.

Table 4 Pseudourticaria: Skin Conditions Commonly Misdiagnosed as Urticaria/Angioedema

Acute contact allergic dermatitis
  Especially of the face and eyelids
Cellulitis
  Especially occurring in the setting of facial lymphoedema (Melkersson–Rosenthal syndrome)
Dermatomyositis
  Especially of the eyelids
Discoid lupus erythematosus
  Of the tumid type and on the face
Crohn's disease
  Of the lips
Hypoalbumenemia
  From any cause, especially resulting in scrotal edema
Myxoedema
Urticarial dermatitis
  An eczematous dermatitis with clinical and histological features suggestive of urticaria

Provided the presence of true urticaria is confirmed, the next step in diagnosis is to exclude a physical urticaria by appropriate skin challenge testing. A physical urticaria may occur as an isolated problem, or in association with CIU. The methodology for physical urticaria challenge testing is reviewed in chapter 7. It is important to identify patients with physical urticarias because if the latter, confirmed by challenge testing, turns out to be the patient's sole or principal problem, then further investigations are obviated. No laboratory investigations are indicated in physical urticarias, with the rare exceptions of cold-precipitating proteins in cold urticaria and action spectrum phototesting in solar urticaria. Once physical urticarias have been excluded the next step is to consider the possibility of urticarial vasculitis, described in detail in chapter 17 and recently reviewed (55). Although apparently relatively rare it is probably often missed, as inspection of the skin in this condition may reveal nothing unusual. However there are a number of useful clinical pointers (Table 5). Individual wheals invariably persist longer than the 24-hour limit of "ordinary" chronic urticaria. However this measurement may be difficult to ascertain, as most patients are poor witnesses in this respect. Wheals of urticarial vasculitis may leave residual staining of the skin because of vascular damage. Itching is inconsistent in urticarial vasculitis; indeed the lesions may be tender and painful rather than itchy. Systemic symptoms are more common than in CIU and consist of arthralgia,

Table 5 Clinical Features Helping to Distinguish Urticarial Vasculitis from Chronic Idiopathic Urticaria

Clinical feature[a]	Urticarial vasculitis	CIU
Duration of individual wheals	>24 h	<24 h
Residual skin staining	Common	Rare, except for bruising due to rubbing
Pruritus	Inconsistent	Invariable
Pain and tenderness	Common	Unusual
Systemic symptoms	Frequent	Infrequent
Response to antihistamines	Poor	Usually fairly good

[a]In at least 50% of patients with urticarial vasculitis, the clinical picture is essentially indistinguishable from CIU.
Abbreviation: CIU, chronic idiopathic urticaria.

fatigue, and weight loss. However the disease may be surprisingly asymptomatic. A lawyer patient of one of us (Greaves MW) attended out patients regularly for several years, with an invariably highly visible histologically confirmed rash of urticarial vasculitis but seemed unfazed by failure to find a cause or an effective treatment. Urticarial vasculitis should be considered in any patient whose chronic urticaria is poorly responsive to routine antihistamine treatment. The diagnosis should not be made without histological confirmation. It is important to establish the diagnosis because, if confirmed, important underlying causes will have to be excluded. These include autoimmune connective tissue diseases, especially lupus and Sjogren's syndrome, hepatitis C infection, and paraproteinemia.

Do Foods Cause Chronic Idiopathic Urticaria?

This issue has been discussed recently in some detail (56). Food allergy is a recognized cause of acute urticaria, but the role of food components in chronic urticaria is controversial. In a recent textbook on urticaria (57), Henz describes food proteins preservatives and coloring agents as major causative factors in chronic urticaria. The concept of food additives as a cause of chronic urticaria first became popularised in the European literature of the 1970s and 1980s by Juhlin and Michaelsson and later by Doeglas and by Supramanian and Warner (58–60). These studies involved challenge testing but were not adequately placebo controlled, and the reproducibility of apparently positive reactions was not investigated, although positively reacting patients were said to respond subsequently to dietary restrictions. The experience of one of us (Greaves MW) in the routine use of placebo-controlled single blind challenge testing for food additive intolerance over a period of 20 years indicates that patients who can *reproducibly* be shown to react to a food additive are extremely rare and we agree with Mathews (61) who stated in 1983 that "as a cause for chronic urticaria or angioedema food allergy can only be rarely implicated."

Thyroid Function in CIU

Hashimoto's thyroiditis and less commonly Graves' disease show a positive association with CIU (12,62). Antithyroid autoantibodies are found in 27% of patients with chronic urticaria and 19% have abnormal thyroid function (63). However there is no convincing evidence that treating the underlying thyroid dysfunction alters the course of the accompanying urticaria. Thyroid disease and chronic urticaria are frequently associated, but there is no evidence that the thyroid autoantibodies are pathogenic in the context of chronic urticaria. The significance of the association lies in the separate autoimmune mechanisms found in both disorders.

Other Claimed Causative Factors in CIU: *Helicobacter Pylori*

That numerous anecdotal reports of different "causes" of chronic urticaria continue to appear in the literature bears witness to the frustrations of clinicians dealing with the disorder. It is pointless to itemize these, but one microorganism, *Helicobacter pylori*, is worth a brief mention because of its possible significance, not as a direct cause of chronic urticaria but because of its possible relevance to autoimmunity. This topic has recently been reviewed (64). Evidence of *H. pylori* infection is found in up to 50% of the general population in most regions of the world and in at least 30% of patients with CIU. However treating the *H. pylori* has no significant effect on the course of the chronic urticaria (65). Recent evidence has demonstrated that *H. pylori* infection induces autoantibody formation because of the immunogenicity of its cell envelope polysaccharide Lewis X and Y blood group antigens. Autoantibodies are formed by molecular mimicry analogous with the role of *Campylobacter jejuni* in the Guillain–Barre syndrome. *H. pylori* also induces HLA-DR expression on gastric epithelium, enabling these cells to behave as antigen-presenting cells. The interesting possibility therefore arises that *H. pylori* might have an indirect role in the etiology of CIU as a result of the reduction of immune tolerance and the induction of autoantibody formation, including anti-FcεR1α autoantibodies.

Investigation of Patients with CIU

Patients with CIU are almost invariably over-investigated and usually present with a dossier of expensive but uninformative test results, including allergen-specific IgE determinations. Several recent publications have attempted to provide guidance on the rational investigation of these patients (66,67).

In 2005, European guidelines for the diagnosis of chronic urticaria were published (66). This group recommended use of a checklist to assist with history-taking and to ensure exclusion of physical urticarias that, when confirmed by appropriate challenge testing, usually require no further investigation, and urticarial vasculitis that requires full investigation. An erythrocyte sedimentation rate (ESR) was advised, a positive result suggested underlying systemic disease and prompting a skin biopsy to exclude urticarial vasculitis, together with a differential white blood cell count to exclude parasite infestation. In rare patients where the history yielded strong evidence of involvement of a food factor, a double blind, placebo-controlled challenge-testing procedure was advised. In the event that the above yielded negative results, the group advised further investigation for autoimmune urticaria.

In a retrospective study of 130 patients with chronic urticaria Bos (67) concluded that careful history-taking with the aid of a questionnaire elicited the cause in almost half of the patients studied. However in most of these, the diagnosis proved to be physical urticaria, although apart from dermographism, this was not routinely confirmed by physical urticaria challenge testing. Other diagnoses consisted of adverse drug reactions (3.4%), adverse food reactions (5.4%), and systemic disease (2.3%). In 55% no cause could be found. Laboratory testing was unhelpful, but the authors nevertheless recommend routine determination of the ESR and differential white blood cell count, to help exclude underlying systemic disease and parasite infestation.

Table 6 Guidelines for Investigation of Chronic Urticaria

Exclusion of physical urticaria/angioedema by history + appropriate challenge-testing
  A positive result obviates the need for further investigation, except in cold and solar urticaria (see text)
Exclusion of urticarial vasculitis by history, examination of the skin, an ESR, and skin biopsy
  Positive results should prompt full work-up for hepatitis C infection, autoimmune connective tissue diseases, paraproteinemia, and inflammatory bowel disease.
In patients with a convincing history, exclusion of reactivity to food components by placebo-controlled challenge testing
  A positive result must be tested for reproducibility
Exclusion of thyroid disease by thyroid autoantibody screen and, if positive, thyroid function tests
  A positive result strengthens the likelihood of an underlying autoimmune process
Differential white blood cell count to reveal a blood eosinophilia; a negative test enabling exclusion of parasite infestation
  Probably only worthwhile in regions where parasite infestation is endemic; stool examination for ova, parasites should not be requested in the absence of eosinophilia
Investigation for autoimmune urticaria
  Patients who are severely disabled, treatment unresponsive and in whom no causative factors have emerged

Abbreviation: ESR, erythrocyte sedimentation rate.

We are in general agreement with the above guidelines, but believe that there is a sufficiently strong association with thyroid disease to warrant additional routine laboratory screening, although we acknowledge that treatment of an underlying thyroid disorder is unlikely to influence the associated urticaria. Our recommendations are set out in Table 6.

Management of CIU

The principles of management of CIU and angioedema have recently been reviewed (63,68). They are also discussed in detail in chapters 14 and 15 and will not be considered here.

REFERENCES

1. Greaves MW. Current concepts: chronic urticaria. N Engl J Med 1995; 332:1767–1772.
2. Hide M, Francis DM, Grattan CEH, et al. Autoantibodies against the high affinity IgE receptor as a cause for histamine release in chronic urticaria. N Engl J Med 1993; 328:1599–1604.
3. Nimii N, Francis DM, Kermani F, et al. Dermal mast cell activation by autoantibodies against the high affinity IgE receptor in chronic urticaria. J Invest Dermatol 1996; 106:1001–1010.
4. Fiebiger E, Maurer D, Holub H, et al. Serum IgG autoantibodies directed against the α chain of FcεR1; a selective marker and pathogenetic factor for a distinct subset of chronic urticaria patients. J Clin Invest 1995; 96:2606–2612.
5. Tong LJ, Balakrishnan G, Kochan JP, et al. Assessment of autoimmunity in patients with chronic urticaria. J Allergy Clin Immunol 1997; 99:461–465.
6. Greaves MW, Sabroe S. Allergy and the skin. Br Med J 1998; 316:1447–1450.
7. Lamberts H, Brouwer HJ, Mohrs J. Reason for Encounter and Episode and Process-Oriented Standard Output from Transition Project; Parts 1 and 2. Amsterdam, the Netherlands: Amsterdam University Press, 1991.
8. O'Donnell BF, Lawlor F, Simpson J, et al. The impact of chronic urticaria on quality of life. Br J Dermatol 1997; 136:553–556.

9. Kaplan AP, Horakova Z, Katz SI. Assessment of tissue fluid histamine levels in patients with urticaria. J Allergy Clin Immunol 1978; 61:350–354.

10. Rorsman H. Basophilic leucopenia in different forms of urticaria. Acta Allergol 1962; 17:168–184.

11. Leznoff A, Josse RG, Denburg J, et al. Association of chronic urticaria and angioedema with thyroid autoimmunity. Arch Dermatol 1983; 119:636–640.

12. Leznoff A, Sussman GL. Syndrome of idiopathic urticaria and angioedema with thyroid autoimmunity: a study of 90 patients. J Allergy Clin Immunol 1989; 84:66–71.

13. O'Donnell BF, Francis DM, Swana GT, et al. Thyroid autoimmunity in chronic urticaria. Br J Dermatol 2005; 153:331–335.

14. Kikuchi Y, Fann T, Kaplan AP. Antithyroid antibodies in chronic urticaria and angioedema. J Allergy Clin Immunol 2003; 112:218.

15. Grattan C, Powell S, Humphreys F. Management and diagnostic guidelines for urticaria and angioedema. Br J Dermatol 2001; 144:708–714.

16. O'Donnell BF, O'Neill CM, Francis DM, et al. Human leucocyte antigen class 2 associations in chronic idiopathic urticaria. Br J Dermatol 1999; 140:853–858.

17. Greaves MW, Plummer VM, Mc Laughlan P, et al. Serum and cell bound IgE in chronic urticaria. Clin Allergy 1974; 4:265–271.

18. Kern F, Lichtenstein LM. Defective histamine release in chronic urticaria. J Clin Invest 1976; 57:1369–1377.

19. Sabroe RA, Francis DM, Barr RM, et al. Anti-FcεR1 autoantibodies and basophil histamine releasability in chronic idiopathic urticaria. J Allergy Clin Immunol 1998; 102:651–658.

20. Luquin E, Kaplan AP, Ferrer M. Increased responsiveness of basophils of patients with chronic urticaria to sera but hypo-responsiveness to other stimuli. Clin Exp Immunol 2005; 115: 815–821.

21. Vonakis BM, Vasager K, Gibbons SP Jr., et al. Basophil FcεRI Histamine release parallels expression of Src-homology 2- containing inositol phosphatases in chronic idiopathic urticaria. J Allergy Clin Immunol 2007; 119:441–448.

22. Gruber BL, Baeza ML, Marchese MJ, et al. Prevalence and functional role of anti-IgE autoantibodies in urticarial syndromes. J Invest Dermatol 1988; 90:213–217.

23. Marone G, Casolaro V, Pganelli R, et al. IgG anti-IgE from atopic dermatitis induces mediator release from basophils and mast cells. J Invest Dermatol 1989; 3:246–252.

24. MacDonald SM, Rafnar T, Langdon J, et al. Molecular identification of an IgE dependent histamine releasing factor. Science 1995; 269:688–690.

25. Claveau J, Lavoie A, Brunet C, et al. Chronic idiopathic urticaria: possible contribution of histamine releasing factor to pathogenesis. J Allergy Clin Immunol 1993; 92:132–137.

26. Grattan CEH, Wallington TB, Warin AP, et al. A serological mediator in chronic idiopathic urticaria: a clinical immunological and histological evaluation. Br J Dermatol 1986; 114: 583–590.

27. Grattan CEH, Francis DM, Hide M, et al. Detection of circulating histamine releasing autoantibodies with functional properties of anti- IgE in chronic urticaria. Clin Exp Allergy 1991; 21:695–704.

28. Grattan CEH, Boon AP, Eady RAJ, et al. The pathology of the autologous serum skin test response in chronic urticaria resembles IgE-mediated late phase reactions. Int Arch Allergy Appl Immunol 1990; 93:198–204.

29. Sabroe RA, Fiebiger E, Francis DM, et al. Classification of anti-FcεR1 and anti-IgE autoantibodies in chronic idiopathic urticaria and correlation with disease severity. J Allergy Clin Immunol 2002; 110:492–499.

30. Fiebiger E, Hammerschmid F, Stingl G, et al. Anti-FcεR1α autoantibodies in autoimmune-mediated disorders. J Clin Invest 1998; 101:243–251.

31. Horn MP, Gerster T, Ochenberger B, et al. Human anti- FcεR1alpha autoantibodies isolated from healthy donors cross react with tetanus toxoid. Eur J Immunol 1999; 29:1139–1148.

32. Ferrer M, Nakazawa K, Kaplan AP. Complement dependence of histamine release in chronic urticaria. J Allergy Clin Immunol 1999; 104:169–172.

33. Kikuchi Y, Kaplan AP. Mechanisms of autoimmune activation of basophils in chronic urticaria. J Allergy Clin Immunol 2001; 107:1056–1062.

34. Kikuchi Y, Kaplan AP. A role for C5a in augmenting IgG-dependent histamine release from basophils in chronic urticaria. J Allergy Clin Immunol 2002; 109:114–118.

35. Fureder W, Agis H, Willheim, M, et al. Differential expression of complement receptors on human basophils and mast cells. J Immunol 1995; 155:3152–3160.

36. Grattan CEH, Francis DM. Autoimmune urticaria. Adv Dermatol 1999; 12:311–340.

37. O'Donnell BF, Barr RM, Black AK, et al. Intravenous immunoglobulin in chronic autoimmune urticaria. Br J Dermatol 1998; 138:101–106.

38. Grattan CEH, Francis DM, Barr RM, et al. Plasmapheresis for severe unremitting chronic urticaria. Lancet 1992; 339:1078–1080.

39. Rose NR, Bona C. Defining criteria for autoimmune diseases (Witebsky's postulates revisited). Immunol Today 1993; 14:426–430.

40. Hide M, Greaves MW. Chronic urticaria as an autoimmune disease. In: Hertl M, ed. Autoimmune Diseases of the Skin. New York: Springer Wien, 2005:309–332.

41. Basagar K, Vonakis BM, Gober LM, et al. Evidences of in vivo basophil activation in chronic idiopathic urticaria. Clin Exp Allergy 2006; 36:770–776.

42. Kaplan AP, Joseph K. Basophil secretion in chronic urticaria. Autoantibody dependent or not? J Allergy Clin Immunol 2007; 120:729–730.

43. Sabroe RA, Seed PT, Francis DM, et al. Chronic idiopathic urticaria: comparison of clinical features of patients with and without anti-FcεR1 or anti-IgE autoantibodies. J Am Acad Dermatol 1999; 40:443–450.

44. Sabroe RA, Poon E, Orchard G, et al. Cutaneous inflammatory cell infiltrate in chronic idiopathic urticaria: comparison of patients with and without anti-FcεR1 or anti-IgE autoantibodies. J Allergy Clin Immunol 1999; 103:484–493.

45. Ying S, Kikuchi Y, Meng K, et al. Th1/Th2 cytokines and inflammatory cells in skin biopsy specimens from patients with chronic idiopathic urticaria: comparison with the allergen-induced late phase reaction. J Allergy Clin Immunol 2002; 109:694–700.

46. Sabroe RA, Grattan CEH, Francis DM, et al. The autologous serum skin test: a screening test for autoantibodies in chronic idiopathic urticaria. Br J Dermatol 1999; 140:446–452.

47. Zweiman B, Valenzano M, Atkins PC. Modulation of serum histamine releasing activity in chronic idiopathic urticaria. Immunopharmacology 1998; 39:225–234.

48. Zweiman B, Valenzano M, Atkins PC, et al. Characteristics of histamine releasing activity in the sera of patients with chronic idiopathic urticaria. J Allergy Clin Immunol 1996; 98:89–98.

49. Asero R, Tedeschi A, Lorini M, et al. Chronic urticaria: novel clinical and serological aspects. Clin Exp Allergy 2001; 31:1105–1110.

50. Lichtenstein LM, Mac Glashan DW. The concept of basophil releasability. J Allergy Clin Immunol 1986; 77:291–294.

51. Grattan CEH, Walpole D, Francis DM, et al. Flow cytometric analysis of basophil numbers in chronic urticaria: basopenia is related to serum histamine releasing activity. Clin Exp Allergy 1997; 27:1417–1424.

52. Grattan CEH, Sabroe RA, Greaves MW. Chronic urticaria. J Am Acad Dermatol 2002; 46:645–657.

53. Grattan CEH, O'Donnell BF, Francis DM, et al. Randomised double blind study of cyclosporin in chronic idiopathic urticaria. Br J Dermatol 2000; 143:365–372.

54. Amal, SM, Harbeck RJ, Dreskin SC. Effects of intravenous immunoglobulin in chronic urticaria with increased CD 203c expression. J Allergy Clin Immunol 2008; 121(suppl 1):S98.

55. O'Donnell BF, Black AK. Urticarial vasculitis. Int Angiol 1995; 14:166–174.

56. Greaves MW. Food intolerance in urticaria and angioedema and urticarial vasculitis. In: Brostoff J, Challacombe S, eds. Food Allergy and Intolerance. 2nd ed. Saunders, 2002; 623–629.

57. Henz BM, Zuberbier T. Causes of urticaria. In: Henz B, Zuberbier T, Grabbe J, et al. eds, Urticaria: Clinical Diagnostic and Therapeutic Aspects. Berlin-Heidelberg: Springer Verlag, 1998:19.

58. Michaelsson G, Juhlin L. Urticaria induced by preservatives and dye additives in food and drugs. Br J Dermatol 1973; 88:525–532.

59. Doeglas HMG. Reactions to aspirin and food additives in patients with chronic urticaria including the physical urticarias. Br J Dermatol 1975; 93:135–144.

60. Supramanian G, Warner JO. Artificial food additive intolerance in patients with angioedema and urticaria. Lancet 1986; 2:907–910.

61. Mathews KP. Urticaria and angioedema. J Allergy Clin Immunol 1983; 72:1–14.

62. Kaplan AP, Finn A. Autoimmunity and the aetiology of chronic urticaria. Can J Allergy Clin Immunol 1999; 4:286–292.

63. Kaplan AP. Chronic urticaria and angioedema. N Engl J Med 2002; 346:175–179.

64. Greaves MW. Chronic idiopathic urticaria and Helicobacter pylori : not directly causative but could there be a link? ACI Int 2001; 13:23–26.

65. Burova GP, Mallet AI, Greaves MW. Is Helicobacter pylori a cause of chronic urticaria? Br J Dermatol 1998; 139(suppl 51):42.

66. Zuberbier T, Bindslev – Jensen C, Canonica W, et al. EAACI/GA^{2}LEN/EDF guideline: definition classification and diagnosis of urticaria. Allergy 2005; 61:321–331.

67. Kozel MMA, Moein MCA, Mekkes JR, et al. Evaluation of a clinical guideline for the diagnoses of physical and chronic urticaria and angioedema. Acta Derm Venereol 2002; 82:270–274.

68. Greaves MW. Tan KT, Chronic urticaria: recent advances. Clin Rev Allergy Immunol 2007; 33:134–143.

18

Chronic Urticaria: General Principles and Management

Clive Grattan
*Dermatology Centre, Norfolk and Norwich University Hospital, and
St. John's Institute of Dermatology, St. Thomas' Hospital, London, U.K.*

DEFINITION AND NOMENCLATURE

Urticaria becomes chronic when wheals fluctuate daily or almost daily for six weeks or more. The term "chronic urticaria" includes all patterns of urticaria, whether wheals are spontaneous or induced, but is commonly restricted to spontaneous urticaria (1). This is almost synonymous with the ordinary presentation of urticaria (2).

CLINICAL SPECTRUM

Chronic urticaria has a wide spectrum of clinical presentations. It may occur daily or follow an unpredictable course with clear days. When continuous urticaria activity is punctuated by long intervals of clearance for several weeks or months, it is called episodic (syn. intermittent or recurrent). It is not uncommon to hear of multiple episodes of chronic urticaria over a long period of time in an individual patient.

Wheals occur anywhere on the body and may be very numerous. On occasions, they may be relatively localized, such as predominantly on the head and neck. This might suggest some external precipitant, such as cold exposure. Some patients describe a few large wheals several centimetres across at any one time; others describe multiple papular wheals, with or without coalescence. The morphology of wheals is not often diagnostic but may be helpful in the physical urticarias, such as the linear wheals of dermographism or the pale papules of cholinergic urticaria with a surrounding flare. Angioedema is often described by patients with chronic urticaria. The term refers to deep swellings of the skin and mucosa and is not specific to any pattern of urticaria. There is sometimes difficulty in distinguishing wheals from angioedema, for instance, the deep dermal swellings of delayed pressure urticaria or wheals affecting the face. Angioedema *without wheals*, on the other hand, tends to be episodic rather than continuous. It is worth separating from angioedema *with wheals* because some of the patients without wheals will have C1 esterase inhibitor deficiency or be on angiotensin-converting enzyme inhibitors.

Table 1 Clinical Classification of Chronic Urticaria

Ordinary urticaria
   Idiopathic
   Autoimmune
   Drug and diet related
   Infection related
Physical urticarias
   Symptomatic dermographism
   Cold urticaria
   Cholinergic urticaria
   Delayed pressure urticaria
   Others
Urticarial vasculitis
Autoinflammatory syndromes with urticaria

The etiology of individual cases can be difficult to define in the clinic, so it is useful to have a structure for subdividing patients on the strength of their history, simple investigations, and challenge tests, as shown in Table 1. The physical urticarias (chapter 11), urticarial vasculitis (chapter 21), and autoinflammatory syndromes presenting with urticaria (chapter 15) are covered outside this chapter. The remainder of this article will relate to the ordinary presentation of chronic urticaria (chronic ordinary urticaria), which includes about 70% of the patients presenting to specialist clinics with continuous urticaria for six weeks or more. Patients with this clinical pattern can be further defined by etiology (including autoimmune and idiopathic urticaria) after full evaluation (3).

ETIOPATHOGENESIS

In many patients a specific cause remains uncertain after full evaluation, and the term "idiopathic" is often used to reflect this. Current understanding of the etiopathogenesis of chronic ordinary urticaria does however allow two statements to be made with reasonable confidence: first, that allergy is probably never the cause of it and second, that autoimmunity may account for up to 50% of cases. Spontaneous remission of chronic urticaria adds to the uncertainty about the relevance of potential causes, such as drugs, diet, and infections. Very few *associations* with chronic urticaria have been validated by large, properly conducted epidemiological studies. Only thyroid autoimmunity has emerged convincingly from several studies (4–7). An association with *Helicobacter pylori* gastritis remains controversial. Aggravating factors, such as dietary pseudoallergens, drugs, viral infections, and, perhaps, stress may trigger exacerbations when they are not the primary cause. Efforts should be made to identify them by thorough history taking and investigation to lessen disease activity when possible. A structure for thinking about the causes, associations, and influences that aggravate chronic ordinary urticaria is shown in Table 2.

CAUSES OF CHRONIC ORDINARY URTICARIA

Autoimmunity

Functional and nonfunctional autoantibodies are detectable in the blood of up to 50% of patients with chronic ordinary urticaria (8–11). Debate continues about the relevance of nonfunctional autoantibodies to the high-affinity IgE receptor (FcεRI) on mast cells and

Table 2 Chronic Ordinary Urticaria: Causes, Associations, and Aggravating Factors

Causes
Idiopathic
Autoimmunity (histamine-releasing autoantibodies)
? pseudoallergens (diet and drugs)
? infections (e.g., chronic dental abscess, *Helicobacter pylori* gastritis, intestinal parasites)
Associations
Thyroid autoimmunity
Aggravating factors
Drugs (especially nonsteroidal anti-inflammatories)
Physical (overheating, local pressure, and rubbing)
Dietary pseudoallergens (especially additives, salicylates)
Alcohol
Viral infections (e.g., adeno, rhino, and enteroviruses)
? stress

basophils detected by immunoassay (12,13), but there can be no doubt about the biological activity of autoantibodies that release histamine from them in vitro. A minority of the chronic urticaria sera studied have functional anti-IgE autoantibodies (14). There is some evidence that patients whose sera do not show histamine release on the basophil assay may nevertheless have non-antibody histamine–releasing factors (15), which may be important in urticaria pathogenesis, although the nature of these remains uncertain. The lack of a widely available standardized assay has hampered evaluation of autoimmune urticaria in the clinic. The absence of clear, distinguishing clinical differences between antibody-positive and antibody-negative patients adds to the difficulty of separating autoimmune from non-autoimmune urticaria. However, those with evidence of autoimmune urticaria have more severe disease (16), longer disease duration (17), and are less responsive to H_1 antihistamines (18). HLA-DR4 is strongly associated with chronic urticaria patients, especially those with serum histamine–releasing activity on basophils (19).

Dietary Pseudoallergens

There is a long literature on food additives and salicylates aggravating chronic urticaria and, more recently, on aromatic substances in tomatoes and herbs (20), but no convincing laboratory evidence that dietary pseudoallergens cause histamine release or have a direct causative role. There is, however, evidence that dietary pseudoallergens may aggravate existing chronic urticaria, analogous to nonsteroidal anti-inflammatories (NSAIDs). Intolerance of dietary pseudoallergens appears to be important in patients with and without functional autoantibodies (21), suggesting that the expression of urticaria may be under the combined influence of several cofactors in predisposed individuals.

Infections

There is a fairly extensive literature on chronic urticaria and infection with bacteria, parasites, viruses, and fungi; but randomized controlled studies are lacking, so the strength of evidence is weak (22). The old literature on chronic sepsis as a cause of urticaria is largely based on uncontrolled series of reports of patients with dental abscesses. Infection of the bowel by candida yeasts has not been confirmed as a cause of chronic urticaria by placebo-controlled studies of eradication therapies. Hepatitis B and C infection is associated with urticarial vasculitis but not ordinary urticaria. The short-lived urticarial rashes seen at the onset of some acute viral infections, including hepatitis B and infectious mononucleosis, do not generally progress to chronic continuous urticaria. Intestinal parasitosis as a cause of urticaria is rare in developed countries but may be more prevalent in rural underdeveloped communities. A systematic review of studies of eradication therapies for chronic urticaria patients infected with *H. pylori* found that resolution of urticaria was more likely when antibiotic therapy was successful in eradication of *H. pylori* than when it was unsuccessful (23).

Associations

Thyroid autoimmunity is more likely to be seen in patients with chronic autoimmune urticaria than those without evidence of functional autoantibodies (24,25). The frequency of organ-specific autoimmune diseases (including thyroid disease, vitiligo, insulin-dependent diabetes mellitus, rheumatoid arthritis, and pernicious anemia) was found to be higher in patients with histamine-releasing autoantibodies than those without (16). The relevance of thyroid autoimmunity to the pathogenesis of urticaria remains unclear, but there may be some indirect influence as judged by the occasional response of some clinically and biochemically euthyroid patients to thyroxine. Although there have been individual reports of a wide range of malignancies in patients with urticaria, a large retrospective epidemiological survey from Sweden showed no evidence of an association with cancer (26).

AGGRAVATING INFLUENCES ON DISEASE ACTIVITY

While the cause of chronic ordinary may remain elusive to the clinician, there are a number of potentially avoidable situations that tend to make it worse, which can often be identified by careful history-taking. These include diet, some drugs, alcoholic beverages, coincidental minor viral infections, overheating, local heat and friction, and, perhaps, severe emotional stress.

Diet

Many patients with chronic ordinary urticaria attribute exacerbations to what they have eaten, but these reactions are very rarely immediate (within minutes) and commonly not reproducible. Most patients are able to eat a full diet once their urticaria has gone into remission. There is evidence from challenge studies and dietary avoidance that pseudoallergens may be important for some patients (27) but probably for those with milder forms of disease. Pseudoallergic reactions to additives, natural salicylates, and aromatic compounds seem to be dose-related. Tables listing the estimated content of salicylate in fresh foods are available (28), but it is not known how much has to be ingested to precipitate an attack, and it seems likely that this would be highly variable between and within individuals. Even when chronic urticaria patients appeared to respond to a strict low-pseudoallergen diet, only 19% of them reacted adversely to challenge capsules containing food additives and salicylic acid (27). The trace amounts of additives present in most foods would be well below the threshold amounts in challenge capsules unless eaten to excess. Although some urticaria diets have emphasized avoidance of natural amines, the contribution of dietary histamine to urticaria activity is almost certainly negligible.

Drugs

The most important drug group is the NSAIDs, including aspirin. It has been estimated that they aggravate 20% to 30% of patients with chronic ordinary urticaria during the active phase but probably not in remission (29). The effect depends on the potency and dose of the NSAID. It possibly relates to inhibition of PGE_2, which inhibited immunological mast cell degranulation in an animal model (30), or the production of cysteinyl leukotrienes, which may cause vasopermeability and erythema. Cross-reactivity between the NSAIDs is common, although the selective Cox-2 inhibitors may be safe to use instead (31). Aspirin and other NSAIDs are also an uncommon cause of acute urticaria and nonallergic anaphylaxis. The mechanism for this is unclear but does not seem to involve IgE. Aspirin may also be a cofactor with food and exercise in food and exercise-induced anaphylaxis (32). Although caution is often advised with opiates in chronic urticaria, the evidence for an adverse effect is largely indirect from in vitro studies of non-immunologically stimulated degranulation of mast cells and in vivo skin testing with codeine (33). The relevance of these findings to chronic urticaria is less certain as clinical experience suggests that opiates can be taken safely by most patients. The high frequency of reports of penicillin reactions in some retrospective surveys (34,35) may relate to the frequency of use of this antibiotic and preferential recall by urticaria patients. Clinical experience does not suggest that penicillins should be avoided in urticaria unless there is a history of previous allergy.

Physical Stimuli

Overlap between ordinary and physical urticarias is well recognized, especially between chronic ordinary and delayed pressure urticaria where concurrence of these two clinical patterns may be as high as 40% (36). Notwithstanding this, many patients with active continuous urticaria observe that overheating and local pressure of belts or clothing elastic will aggravate their condition by encouraging immediate wheals.

Alcohol

Alcoholic beverages appear to aggravate urticaria nonspecifically by encouraging vasodilatation, and this effect is probably dose-related. There have been reports of ethanol itself causing urticaria (37) presumably through direct release of histamine from mast cells and basophils, but this is probably rare. Allergic reactions to the fruit or grain and pseudoallergic intolerance of additives in the product could, in theory, contribute to exacerbations during chronic urticaria. The concentration of histamine in wine does not relate to symptoms of wine intolerance, including urticaria (38).

Viral Infections

It is common clinical experience to hear that urticaria is aggravated by minor upper respiratory or gastrointestinal viral infections, perhaps through upregulation of cytokines during the acute phase response, leading to a temporary state of enhanced mast cell releasability.

Stress

There is increasing interest in the interactions between the central and peripheral nervous systems as a potential cause of disease (39). Pathways that promote urticaria through stress might be important though any direct or indirect proof of this is lacking. It is a common belief among patients that stress is an aggravating factor in chronic urticaria, but there is no evidence for it being a cause.

DIAGNOSIS OF CHRONIC ORDINARY URTICARIA

Diagnosis is based primarily on a history of fluctuating itchy superficial wheals and deeper angioedema swellings. Duration of individual wheals is usually less than 24 hours, but very large or confluent ones may last longer. Outlining the wheals with ink or biro can be helpful to confirm this. The wheals of physical urticarias last less than an hour, with the exception of delayed pressure urticaria, which may last for 24 hours or longer. The wheals of urticarial vasculitis typically last for days because there is blood vessel damage as well as capillary leakage. Discoloration of the wheals from blood loss into the skin and burning, rather than itch, may be features. Angioedema swellings often persist for more than a day. Systemic features are usually lacking in ordinary urticaria of mild to moderate severity, although severe disease is often accompanied by nonspecific symptoms of malaise, lethargy, poor concentration, and, sometimes, indigestion (16). By contrast, systemic features can be expected in urticarial vasculitis, including arthralgia, joint swelling, fever, headache, and abdominal pain, especially in those with hypocomplementemia.

A skin biopsy is essential if urticarial vasculitis is suspected, since the diagnosis can only be confirmed histologically. Routine investigations are otherwise unnecessary to distinguish between the clinical patterns of chronic urticaria, although simple challenge tests are helpful to confirm the physical urticarias. A comprehensive questionnaire with a complete blood count and erythrocyte sedimentation rate (ESR) produced a similar diagnostic yield to a full workup, including a full blood profile, X rays of chest, sinuses, and teeth, skin biopsy, a three-week elimination diet, and appropriate drug provocation tests (40).

Classifying ordinary urticaria by etiology is more difficult and will depend on the facilities available. The best test for functional autoantibodies is currently the basophil histamine release assay, but this is only available in a few centres. Increased expression of CD63 on urticaria basophils may be a useful biomarker of autoimmune urticaria (41), although this initial work needs to be validated in other centers. Intradermal injection of the patient's own serum (the autologous serum skin test) offers a simple but time-consuming clinical test, with a sensitivity of around 70% and a specificity of 80% for basophil histamine releasing activity when compared with a saline-control injection at 30 minutes (42) (chapter 8). Thyroid autoantibodies may be a useful surrogate marker for autoimmune urticaria. Chronic infection as a cause of urticaria should only be sought with appropriate tests when clearly indicated by the history. Dietary pseudoallergens as a cause or aggravating factor in chronic urticaria can only be confirmed clinically with an appropriate diet for three weeks to look for improvement or challenge with blinded challenge capsules containing known pseudoallergens given during a period of relative disease quiescence to look for exacerbations.

MANAGEMENT

The initial management of chronic ordinary urticaria should be directed by leads from a full clinical assessment. Management plans may be different for each patient. The key features of any plan should include treatment of any identifiable cause, avoidance of aggravating factors, advice and written information on the condition, non-pharmacological approaches for relieving symptoms, and a trial of full-dose second-generation antihistamines. Second-line approaches for patients who need more help include a range of targeted

Table 3 Management Plan for Chronic Ordinary Urticaria

Removal of any identified cause
Avoidance of aggravating factors
Advice and information
Creams and lotions for symptomatic relief
First-line drugs (antihistamines)
Second-line interventions (targeted therapies)
Third-line immunosuppressive and immunomodulatory therapies

interventions determined by investigations and clinical need. Third-line management for patients with the most severe and refractory disease may include immunosuppressive and immunomodulating therapies (Table 3).

AVOIDANCE OF AGGRAVATING FACTORS

Overheating

Higher skin temperatures may encourage wheals and itching. It is best to avoid very hot baths or showers. Wearing lighter clothes and avoiding strenuous exertion may be helpful.

Pressure

Wearing comfortable, loose clothes and footwear that does not rub may be an advantage. Walking long distances or carrying heavy bags should be avoided if this brings out pressure-induced swellings over the next few hours.

Stress

Mental stress may make urticaria harder to live with. There is no evidence that worry or emotional problems cause urticaria in the first place, but it is common to hear that stressful events may aggravate it, and chronic urticaria is a major cause of stress. One study suggested that the itch of urticaria but not wheal severity may respond to hypnosis with relaxation therapy (43).

Food

Dietary pseudoallergens include food additives (colors, preservatives, antioxidants, and flavor enhancers) natural salicylates (especially in fruits, beer, and wine), and unidentified aromatic substances in tomatoes, herbs, and white wine (20). The best-known artificial food additives are the azo dyes (E102-124) and benzoate preservatives (E210-219). Processed foods should be avoided if possible in favor of fresh foods without seasoning or spices. A strict low-pseudoallergen diet for three weeks initially may be helpful for some patients with mild chronic ordinary urticaria (25) as an alternative to antihistamines in well-motivated patients or in addition to them if it lessens the dose.

Alcohol

It is common advice to avoid alcohol in urticaria, but any adverse effect is difficult to predict. It probably depends on how much is drunk, how strong the ethanol content, and the content of pseudoallergens. Being overheated or excited at the same time as drinking alcohol may aggravate urticaria further.

Drugs

Aspirin may be present in analgesics that are widely available in drug stores. The brand names of these products do not necessarily indicate their content, so it is important to check the package labeling carefully. It is also important to avoid other NSAIDs, such as ibuprofen and diclofenac, unless they are essential and can be taken without a problem. Acetaminophen is usually suitable as an alternative. Although it is commonly said that opiates, including codeine and its derivatives, should be avoided in chronic urticaria, clinical experience indicates that they can usually be taken safely.

ADVICE AND INFORMATION

A clear explanation that chronic ordinary urticaria is not allergic is often a useful starting point to address the conviction many patients hold that the cause of their problem is a food allergen. Failure to address this point often leads to dissatisfaction that allergy tests are not offered immediately. Clearly written evidence-based information and advice sheets from professional organizations can offer patients helpful initial guidance on their condition.

Creams and Lotions

Cooling lotions can be soothing when wheals erupt and are at their most pruritic, such as 1% menthol in aqueous cream, calamine lotion, and 10% crotamiton lotion. Menthol or alcohol-containing lotions may sting broken or eczematous skin. Antihistamine creams are widely used in the community but poor cutaneous absorption limits their pharmacological effectiveness. Topical steroids are of no value in routine clinical practice, although it has been shown that regular applications of a very potent steroid to localized areas of skin will reduce the wheal response to pressure, presumably through cutaneous mast cell depletion (44,45).

FIRST-LINE THERAPY WITH ANTIHISTAMINES

Antihistamines are the first-line treatment for all patients with chronic urticaria. The subject is covered fully in chapter 19. The three main groups of antihistamines that may be used singly or in combination are the "classical" sedating H_1 antihistamines, of which chlorphenamine, hydroxyzine, and diphenhydramine are typical examples, the non-sedating second generation H_1 antihistamines and their derivatives, and the H_2 antihistamines (Table 4). Antihistamines with theoretical mast cell stabilizing properties, such as ketotifen, or those with anti-serotoninergic effects, such as cyproheptadine, offer no routine advantage to classical antihistamines for chronic urticaria, and are now little used.

Treatment should be started with a non-sedating antihistamine at the licensed dose taken at the same time each day. Some patients do better with one product than another and their response may vary over the course of their disease, but there is probably little to choose between them at licensed doses. It has become common practice to try doubling or even quadrupling the dose of non-sedating antihistamines for patients who respond poorly (1) on the grounds that there may be additional antiallergic effects at these higher doses

Table 4 Antihistamines in Chronic Ordinary Urticaria

"Classical" (sedating) H_1 antihistamines
E.g., chlorphenamine, hydroxyzine, diphenhydramine, trimeprazine, promethazine
Non-sedating second-generation H_1 antihistamines
E.g., loratadine, cetirizine, rupatadine[a], mizolastine[a]
Second-generation H_1 antihistamines derivatives
E.g., desloratadine, levocetirizine, fexofenadine
H_2 antihistamines
E.g., cimetidine, ranitidine, nizatadine

[a]Only licensed for use in Europe.

(46), but the incremental benefit from doing so is usually slight. My own preference is to add an H_2 antihistamine at full dose, since H_2 receptors have been demonstrated in the skin (47) and clinical experience shows that the combination is successful in some patients who do not respond to the H_1 antihistamine alone. An H_2 antihistamine often helps the indigestion that commonly accompanies more severe urticaria and may reduce wheal severity but not itch. Adding a sedating H_1 antihistamine at night is logical if sleep is disturbed by itch and may lead to better control of the urticaria, although long-acting products, such as trimeprazine, may have a carry-over effect of sedation the following morning.

Second-Line Therapies

Around 60% of chronic urticaria patients responded well or reasonably well to antihistamines but 40% derived little or no benefit from them in a retrospective case-note analysis from a secondary referral center (48). The challenge of helping these nonresponding patients requires a thorough knowledge of the literature on alternative therapies that might be appropriate in specific circumstances and of the drugs themselves, which are often used outside their product licences and may carry an appreciable side-effect profile. The most commonly used drug therapies are listed alphabetically in Table 5, although the list is not exhaustive. It should be noted that some authorities favor high doses of a classical antihistamine (such as hydroxyzine 25 to 50 mg qid) (49) when non-sedating antihistamines do not work prior to introducing second-line therapies outlined below. Agents other than antihistamines have been addressed in detail (chapter 20) with additional recommendations, particularly with regard to steroids and ciclosporin.

SECOND-LINE DRUG (TARGETED) THERAPIES (IN ALPHABETICAL ORDER)

Dapsone

Dapsone is an old-fashioned antibacterial sulfonamide, which also has useful anti-inflammatory properties.

Evidence for using Dapsone in Urticaria

There have been surprisingly few publications on its use in severe urticaria (50,51) despite its undoubted efficacy for some patients. It can be effective for some patients with delayed pressure urticaria and as a corticosteroid-sparing drug.

Table 5 Second-Line Targeted Treatments of Chronic Ordinary Urticaria

Drug name	Drug class	Dose range	Indication
Dapsone	Sulfonamide	75–150 mg	Chronic and delayed pressure
Doxepin	Tricyclic antidepressant	10–50 mg daily	Depression
Epinephrine	Sympathomimetic	300–500 µg IM	Angioedema of the throat
Montelukast	Leukotriene receptor antagonist	10 mg daily	Aspirin-sensitive urticaria and some ordinary urticaria
Prednisolone	Corticosteroid	10–40 mg daily	Severe flares (days only) and delayed pressure urticaria
Sulfasalazine	Sulfonamide	2–4 g daily	Delayed pressure urticaria and? some steroid-dependent ordinary urticaria
Thyroxine	Thyroid replacement	50–150 µg daily	thyroid autoimmunity

Dose and Length of Treatment

The usual starting dose of dapsone is 75 mg a day. This can be increased up to 150 mg daily if there are no important side effects.

Interactions with Other Medicines

Dapsone should not usually be taken with another sulfonamide or probenecid. Concentrations in the blood increase if taken with trimethoprim. It may possibly reduce the contraceptive effect of combined oral contraceptives.

Screening Tests

A baseline CBC, liver function tests, and glucose-6-phosphate dehydrogenase should be done before starting treatment. A CBC and liver profile should be repeated a week after starting treatment, a month later, and then every three months on treatment. Dapsone should not be taken if there is a history of sulfonamide allergy.

Problems to Look out for

The commonest unwanted effect is anemia. This is more likely to be a problem at bigger doses. Bluish discoloration of the lips may be apparent at high doses of dapsone due to methemaglobinemia. Peripheral neuropathy may occur with long-term use, although this is rare. Headache and gastrointestinal side effects may occur. A few people feel unwell around three to six weeks after starting dapsone with fever, rash, and lymphadenopathy. The drug should be stopped immediately if this happens.

Doxepin

Doxepin has been used as a treatment for urticaria since the 1980s. It has very powerful properties of an antihistamine but is better known as a tricyclic antidepressant. The doses of doxepin used for depression are usually much higher than those for urticaria. There is unlikely to be any mood-lifting effect when taken in this way, although it may be helpful if depression is also a problem. Doxepin is worth trying if non-sedating antihistamines fail to help and may be most valuable when taken at night if sleep is disturbed by itching or urticaria.

Evidence for Using Doxepin in Urticaria

Doxepin was more effective than diphenhydramine at 10 mg tid (52) and as effective as mequitazine at 5 mg bid (53). It has not been compared against modern non-sedating antihistamines.

Dose and Duration of Treatment

It is best to start at 25 mg daily, and work upward to 50 or 75 mg daily as tolerated. This can either be taken as a single dose at night or divided into two or three smaller doses over the day. The highest daily dose recommended for depression is 300 mg with a maximum single dose of 100 mg, but these very high levels are probably never appropriate for urticaria. There is no time limit to taking doxepin if it helps.

Interactions with Other Medicines

One of the disadvantages of doxepin is the high number of possible interactions with other medicines (and alcohol too). These include other antidepressants, some analgesics (e.g., tramadol), antiarrythmics (e.g., amiodarone), anticonvulsants, and antihypertensives (e.g., diltiazem). A few treatments that may be used for urticaria, such as epinephrine and cimetidine, should be avoided at the same time if possible.

Problems to Look out for

Doxepin should not be taken after a recent myocardial infarction or in severe liver disease. It should be used with caution in pregnancy and in the elderly, since it may precipitate confusion, agitation, glaucoma, and urinary retention. Sedation is the commonest unwanted effect. A dry mouth and blurring of vision are more likely as the dose increases. Other side effects may include constipation, prostatism, postural hypotension, increased appetite, rashes, and, rarely, bone marrow depression.

Epinephrine (syn. Adrenaline)

Evidence for Using Epinephrine in Angioedema

Epinephrine may be essential for severe swelling of the oropharnyx, which is fortunately rare in chronic urticaria. It is said to be ineffective in hereditary angioedema.

Dose and Method of Administration

The commonest pen used by adults for self-administration is the Epipen™, delivering 300 μg of epinephrine. There is also a Junior Epipen™ for children weighing 15 to 30 kg, which delivers 150 μg. A second injection may be necessary if the swelling has not started to go down within 10 minutes.

An epinephrine "puffer" spray (Primatene Mist™) is available on a "named-patient" basis from the United States for treatment of asthma. It may also be used for angioedema of the throat as an unlicensed indication. The aerosol should be puffed four to five times *directly* onto the swelling in the throat and not inhaled (as directed for asthma attacks). The same number of puffs can be repeated after 5 to 10 minutes. An epinephrine injection can still be given if the swelling worsens despite the inhaler.

Interactions with Other Medicines

Epinephrine may cause increased blood pressure, anxiety, shaking, and pallor. These effects wear off within an hour and usually present no problems. However, they may precipitate angina or stroke by a rapid increase in blood pressure in patients at risk, especially on a background of hypertension, ischemic heart disease, and concurrent treatment with tricyclic antidepressants (e.g., amitryptilene, doxepin, trimipramine) and β-blockers (e.g., propanolol, atenolol).

Problems to Look out for

The main side effects are anxiety, tremor, tachycardia, headache, and cold extremities. These are unimportant when epinephrine is used for emergencies because the drug may be lifesaving. It should only be used when essential in patients with heart disease, high blood pressure, and stroke.

Montelukast

The development of leukotriene receptor antagonists for asthma has provided an opportunity to try these medicines for subgroups of chronic ordinary urticaria patients who respond poorly to antihistamines. Theoretically these subgroups might include patients where leukotrienes are considered to be an important mediator of whealing or there is a delayed component to the urticarial response, in which eosinophil and basophil infiltrates are prominent.

Evidence for Using Montelukast in Urticaria

Leukotriene receptor antagonists do not help all types of urticaria. The most encouraging results have been seen in patients with aspirin-sensitive urticaria (54) and autoimmune urticaria (55). In one study, montelukast seemed to benefit some chronic ordinary patients when taken with an antihistamine (56) but provided no additional benefit in another (57).

Dose and Duration of Treatment

The daily dose of montelukast is 10 mg. It is usually taken at bedtime. Benefit should be seen within one week but accrues over six. There is no time limit to treatment.

Interactions with Other Medicines

There are no currently recognized important drug interactions.

Problems to Look out for

Gastrointestinal disturbances, dry mouth, thirst, asthenia, sleep disorders, fever, arthralgia, and myalgia may occur but are unpredictable. Urticaria, angioedema, and anaphylaxis have been reported with montelukast, which may aggravate existing urticaria very occasionally.

Prednisolone

Prednisolone has predominantly glucocorticoid activity and is the corticosteroid most commonly used by mouth for long-term disease suppression.

Evidence for Using Corticosteroids in Chronic Urticaria

There are few published studies of steroids for urticaria because they were introduced many years ago and are indisputably effective. They should only be used continuously in exceptional circumstances, such as disabling delayed pressure urticaria that does not respond to other measures or urticarial vasculitis (see chapter 21). Short-term use to cover acute exacerbations of chronic ordinary urticaria may be necessary.

Dose and Length of Treatment

Taking steroids at a relatively high dose (e.g., prednisolone 30–40 mg) for one to three days can be very helpful for the most severe attacks of urticaria or bad attacks of angioedema. Some authorities believe that alternate day dosing may be more physiological than daily administration if corticosteroids need to be taken long term.

Interactions with Other Medicines

None, except aspirin and other NSAIDs, because there is an increased risk of bleeding and ulceration of the gut.

Problems to Look out for

They should be used with care in diabetics and patients with stomach ulcers, high blood pressure, and osteoporosis. A temporary increase of steroid dose should be given to cover any significant intercurrent illness, trauma, or surgical procedure. Prolonged courses of corticosteroids increase susceptibility to infections and severity of infections. Patients who have not had chickenpox should be regarded as being at risk of severe infection. Immunization with varicella-zoster hyperimmune serum is recommended for exposed nonimmune individuals within 3 days of exposure and no later than 10 days, or those who have been on chronic treatment within the previous 3 months. Numerous potential adverse effects include well-known gastrointestinal, musculoskeletal, endocrine, neuropsychiatric, and cutaneous hazards.

Sulfasalazine

Sulfasalazine is an old drug based on a long-acting sulfonamide, sulfapyridine, and a derivative of salicylic acid, 5-aminosalicylate. The sulfonamide component is regarded as a carrier molecule when sulfasalazine is used for its licensed indications, ulcerative colitis, or Crohn's disease. It is also licensed for rheumatoid arthritis.

Evidence for Sulfasalazine in Urticaria

Sulfasalazine may be effective for delayed pressure urticaria on its own (58) or help to reduce the dose of steroids needed to control it. It has also been reported for steroid-dependent chronic ordinary urticaria (59,60) in uncontrolled reports.

Dose and Length of Treatment

A usual starting dose might be 1 g bid, increasing by 500 mg daily at intervals of two weeks to a maximum regular dose of 4 g (8 tablets) daily. A complete blood count, glucose-6-phosphate dehydrogenase assay, liver, and renal profiles should be checked before starting therapy. A blood count, liver, and renal function should be checked monthly for the first three months, then three monthly.

Interactions with Other Medicines

Sulfasalazine should not be taken with methotrexate.

Problems to Look out for

Sulfasalazine should be avoided if there is a previous history of hypersensitivity to sulfonamides or aspirin. It should only be used during pregnancy and breast-feeding if there is no alternative. A wide range of adverse effects have been described including anemia, rashes including Stevens Johnson syndrome, and exfoliative dermatitis, alopecia, loss of appetite, fibrosing alveolitis, stomatitis, aseptic meningitis, peripheral neuropathy, depression, dizziness, and reduced sperm counts. The urine may be colored orange and some soft contact lenses may be stained.

Thyroxine

Evidence for Using Thyroxine in Urticaria

In an open study, seven biochemically euthyroid patients with thyroid autoimmunity responded to thyroxine treatment for four weeks initially. Five needed treatment for at least a year because the initial response disappeared when thyroxine was stopped. The other two improved over four weeks and remained clear after stopping (61). In another study, 17 of 18 patients responded to thyroxine (62). Clinical experience nevertheless suggests that a response to thyroxine is unpredictable and usually disappointing. Other treatment, including antihistamines, is often necessary.

Dose and Duration of Treatment

The dose of thyroxine used in the studies varied from as little as 50 µg to as much as 250 µg daily. A starting dose of 1.7 µg/kg body weight has been recommended (63), although smaller doses should be considered in the elderly. Thyroid function tests should be done before starting and rechecked after four to six weeks. Suppression of thyroid stimulating hormone (TSH) below normal may be acceptable in the short term, but the aim of treatment should be to maintain TSH within the normal range. If urticaria does respond, thyroxine should be stopped initially after two months to see whether more prolonged treatment is necessary, but further courses may be given.

Interactions with Other Medicines

There are few clinically important interactions. The effect of warfarin and phenindione may be enhanced. Carbamazepine, phenytoin, and rifampicin increase the metabolism of levothyroxine. An increased dose of antidiabetic drugs (including insulin) may be necessary.

Problems to Look out for

The main contraindication is thyrotoxicosis. Side effects do not occur at normal doses, but excessive thyroid replacement may result in angina, palpitations, rapid heartbeat, tremors, excitability, sweating, flushing, and weight loss.

Others

Other second-line interventions for which there is some evidence of effectiveness include narrow-band phototherapy (64) and warfarin (65).

THIRD-LINE TREATMENTS (IMMUNOTHERAPIES AND IMMUNOMODULATORY THERAPIES)

Recognition that some patients have autoimmune urticaria has justified the use of immunotherapies for the most refractory and disabling cases of chronic urticaria. Immunomodulatory therapies using intravenous immunoglobulins (IVIG) and now biologicals have shown some promise, but controlled studies are lacking. Most of the early trials looked at patients with evidence of autoantibodies in vitro using the basophil histamine release assay and the autologous serum skin test as an in vivo marker of histamine-releasing factors. The demonstration that urticaria activity could be abolished for up to a month by plasmapheresis in some patients (66) supported the concept that functional autoantibodies are important in the pathogenesis of urticaria. Trials of ciclosporin (cyclosporine A) in patients with evidence of autoimmune urticaria have strengthened the view that immunosuppressive therapies may be of value for this subgroup. Clinical experience has, however, shown that some severely affected patients without evidence of autoimmune urticaria may also respond to immunotherapies. Small open studies of mycophenolate mofetil (67) and oral tacrolimus (68) have shown similar results to ciclosporin. Interest in methotrexate as a useful long-term therapy for some patients is increasing because of its established use in dermatology for psoriasis and its generally favorable safety profile. It should be remembered that none of the above immunotherapies are licensed for urticaria.

Ciclosporin

It is a powerful inhibitor of both cell-mediated and humoral responses. Most of the immunosuppressive effects are a consequence of inhibition of interleukin-2 (IL-2) and other cytokines from activated Th1 lymphocytes. It also inhibits the release of histamine from basophils and TNF-α production by mast cells.

Evidence for Using Ciclosporin in Urticaria

There have been several studies of ciclosporin in severe chronic ordinary urticaria (69,70) showing that about two-thirds of patients clear on treatment, but the condition often relapses on stopping. Only about one-fourth of the responders were still clear or almost clear on an antihistamine six months after treatment at 4 mg/kg/day for a month (71). Relapses occurred more frequently in patients treated for 8 than 16 weeks in a large multicenter study using a higher initial starting dose of 5 mg/kg/day (72).

Dose and Length of Treatment

There is still discussion about the best dose of ciclosporin and how long it should be taken for. My preferred protocol is 4 mg/kg/day for four weeks reducing to 3 mg/kg/day for six weeks and then 2 mg/kg/day for a final six weeks, unless there is a reason to change the dose during treatment. More than one course of ciclosporin may be given, although it is probably better to look at other therapies if this proves necessary. Long-term treatment with ciclosporin for over a year should only be undertaken when there is no reasonable alternative because of concerns about increased risks of impaired renal function, skin cancers, viral warts, and lymphoma.

Interactions with Other Medicines

There is a wide range of possible interactions. These can be grouped into drugs, which increase blood levels of ciclosporin, those that reduce blood levels, and drug levels that are affected by ciclosporin. *Increased* blood levels may be seen with including anabolic steroids (danazol), allopurinol, some antibiotics (macrolides), antiarrythmics (amiodarone), antifungals (ketoconazole, itraconazole), antimalarials (chloroquine), calcium channel blockers (diltiazem, verapamil), progestagens, and grapefruit juice. *Decreased* levels of ciclosporin may be seen with anticonvulsants (phenytoin, carbamazepine) and St. John's wort. Ciclosporin may increase levels of diclofenac and prednisolone. There is an increased risk of nephrotoxicity with NSAID drugs, aminoglycosides, cotrimoxazole, quinolones, and cytotoxics and of myopathy with the statins.

Problems to Look out for

The main contraindications are impaired kidney function, uncontrolled blood pressure, active serious infections, and cancer within five years of initiating treatment (with the exception of non-melanoma skin cancer). Symptomatic adverse effects are common including slight tremor, burning sensations of the hands and feet, swelling of the gums, nausea, muscle weakness, missed periods, and increased facial hair growth. They settle on stopping treatment. Hyperlipidemia may occur in the long term and should be checked for. The effectiveness and safety of some immunizations may be reduced, and live vaccines should not be used for three months after stopping treatment.

Intravenous Immunoglobulin

IVIG is a concentrated preparation of immunoglobulins from healthy donors. It is mainly used for patients with humoral immune deficiencies. It is also licensed for idiopathic thrombocytopenic purpura, Kawasaki syndrome, and Guillan-Barré syndrome. It may reduce the formation of pathogenic autoantibodies, but the mechanism for it helping urticaria remains uncertain.

Evidence for Using IVIG in Urticaria

There have only been two studies of IVIG for urticaria (73,74). In the first, 10 patients with disabling autoimmune chronic urticaria (73) were treated with 0.4 g/kg/day for five days. Nine of the ten patients felt better after the infusion but only five cleared completely. The urticaria came back in three of them within 6 to 20 weeks but remained clear for at least three years in two. In the second, three of eight patients with severe chronic urticaria with a history of delayed pressure urticaria went into remission after IVIG (74). Two had one infusion and one had three. Two other patients improved and three failed to respond. One of the nonresponders had six infusions. Three of four with a positive ASST cleared or improved, suggesting that they had autoimmune urticaria. Studies have not been done using different groups of urticaria patients, different doses of IVIG, or comparison against placebo.

Dose and Length of Treatment

IVIG is given daily by slow infusion over three to five days in hospital to achieve a total cumulative dose of 2 g/kg. IgA deficiency must be excluded before starting treatment because there is a risk of incompatibility reactions between natural anti-IgA antibodies and IgA from the blood of the IVIG donors.

Interactions with Other Medicines

There are no known interactions with other medicines, although it would be usual to reduce or stop other treatments affecting the immune system. Antihistamines can be taken safely at the same time as IVIG.

Problems to Look out for

Blood pressure may fall rapidly during infusions. Less severe side effects include headache, nausea, sweating, chest pain, muscle and joint aches, and fever. These relate to the speed of infusion and usually improve soon after slowing or stopping it. As with all blood products, there must be slight concern about transmission of unrecognized infection from IVIG.

Methotrexate

Methotrexate is a derivative of folic acid, which interferes with dihydrofolate reductase and the production of DNA in actively dividing cells. It is also a potent inhibitor of polymorphonuclear leucocyte chemotaxis and inhibits the secretion of TNF-α, IL-6, and IL-8 by monocytes and macrophages (75).

Evidence for Using Methotrexate in Urticaria

There have only been anecdotal reports of methotrexate being used successfully for chronic urticaria (76,77). No controlled studies comparing it against placebo have been published yet. Clinical experience has shown that it may be valuable for selected urticaria patients who do not respond to antihistamines, especially those who have corticosteroid-dependent chronic urticaria.

Dose and Length of Treatment

A small test dose of methotrexate may be given before starting regular treatment. It is essential to take methotrexate weekly rather than daily, as for psoriasis. The benefit is not immediate. There is no limit to the length of time methotrexate can be taken, provided that there are no complications.

Interactions with Other Medicines

Aspirin and other NSAIDs (e.g., ibuprofen, diclofenac, meloxicam) may reduce renal elimination of methotrexate and increase the levels of methotrexate. Some antibiotics (trimethoprim, cotrimoxazole, sulfonamides and penicillins), sulfasalazine, and probenecid may increase the risk of toxicity. The antifolate effect is increased by pyrimethamine and phenytoin. Ciclosporin and acitretin should normally be avoided concurrently with methotrexate.

Problems to Look out for

Methotrexate should not normally be used if there is an underlying blood disorder, reduced kidney function, persistent liver inflammation, peptic ulceration, or ulcerative colitis. The most important adverse effects are bone marrow suppression and hepatitis. Sore throats, mouth ulcers, or unusual bruising should be regarded as an important warning of possible bone marrow suppression. Methotrexate should usually be stopped until a blood count is known. Pneumonitis may occur occasionally with prolonged treatment. Methotrexate should be stopped if breathlessness or persistent dry cough develops. Alcohol should be avoided completely if possible during treatment. Nausea may be a problem for a day or two after taking methotrexate in some people but can be reduced by dividing the dose over 36 hours and taking folic acid. Pregnancy and fathering children should be avoided on treatment and for six months after stopping.

Mycophenolate Mofetil

Mycophenolate mofetil is a potent, selective, uncompetitive, and reversible inhibitor of inosine monophosphate dehydrogenase. It inhibits the de novo synthesis of purines in T and B lymphocytes, more than in other cell types that can utilize salvage pathways.

Evidence for Using Mycophenolate in Urticaria

There has only been one small open study of nine patients with chronic urticaria and positive ASSTs to date (67). They were treated with 1000 mg mycophenolate bid for 12 weeks. There was a significant difference in the overall urticarial activity score over the study period, and all patients were able to discontinue steroids.

Dose and Length of Treatment

On the basis of the limited evidence above, patients should be given 2 g mycophenolate daily for 12 weeks and the treatment discontinued after this. Some dosing flexibility can be exercised and up to 3 g/day may be appropriate for some patients.

Interactions with Other Medicines

Mycophenolate would not normally be given with other immunosuppressives for chronic urticaria. There are no significant interactions with non-immunosuppressive drugs. Live vaccines should not be given.

Problems to Look out for

The commonest potential adverse effects are sepsis, bone marrow suppression, and abdominal symptoms. Skin cancers, agitation and confusion, dizziness, tachycardia, pleural effusion, and hepatitis may occur. A recent alert concerning some cases of progressive multifocal encephalopathy has been made by the manufacturer.

Tacrolimus

Tacrolimus binds a cytosolic protein FKBP12. The complex specifically binds to and competitively inhibits calcineurin, leading to a calcium-dependent inhibition of T-cell signal transduction pathways, preventing transcription of IL-2, IL-3, and γ-interferon and expression of the IL-2 receptor.

Evidence for Using Tacrolimus in Urticaria

There has only been one published open uncontrolled study of tacrolimus for chronic urticaria (68). Nineteen patients with H_1 antihistamine-unresponsive chronic urticaria for over a year were treated with oral tacrolimus at an initial dose of 0.05 to 0.07 mg/kg bid for four weeks followed by 0.025 to 0.035 mg/kg/day for six weeks, then 1 mg/day for two weeks before stopping. No tests for functional autoantibodies were performed. By the end of treatment 12 had made a good or moderate improvement. Of these, three were clear three months after finishing treatment and three had a mild deterioration treatable with H_1 antihistamines alone.

Dose and Length of Treatment

On the basis of the evidence above, tacrolimus should be used at a similar starting dose range and tailed off over three months.

Interactions with Other Medicines

Tacrolimus is metabolized by hepatic CYP3A4. Ketoconazole, itraconazole, erythromycin, and grapefruit juice increase tacrolimus levels. Rifampicin, phenytoin, and St. John's wort decrease tacrolimus levels. Tacrolimus is also a CYP3A4 inhibitor and may therefore increase other products known to be metabolized by CYP3A4. It may increase the nephrotoxicity or neurotoxicity of medicinal products known to have these effects.

Problems to Look out for

Commonly reported adverse effects include increased risk of viral, bacterial, and protozoal infections in line with other potent immunosuppressive agents. Anemia, leukopenia, and thrombocytopenia may occur. Metabolic problems include hyperglycemia, diabetes, and hyperkalemia. Insomnia, tremor, headache, blurred vision, and tinnitus are common. Hypertension, renal impairment, diarrhea, pruritus, and arthralgia are reported.

Future Therapies: The Biologics

The potential for biological therapies in autoimmune urticaria has yet to be realized. None are licensed for urticaria or probably will be. Expense and concern about risk are important limiting factors. The most potentially promising is omalizumab (anti-IgE), which is licensed for asthma. As well as reducing circulating IgE, omalizumab reduces the density of high-affinity IgE receptors on basophils and mast cells. It therefore has the potential to modulate chronic urticaria where functional anti-IgE or anti-FcεRI autoantibodies can be demonstrated. Two of three patients with refractory chronic urticaria cleared within one week and the third cleared after six weeks of continuous treatment (78). Twelve patients with chronic autoimmune urticaria treated with omalizumab in an open study have been reported in abstract form (79). Seven had no further urticaria, three showed marked improvement, one moderate improvement, and there was only one nonresponder. There was evidence of anti-FcεRI autoantibodies in two patients and positive basophil histamine release in one of these. In another report, three patients with angioedema without wheals were treated with omalizumab and appeared to remit (80). Safety concerns include allergic reactions, malignancies, parasitic infections, and unmasking of Churg Strauss syndrome. Side effects include headache and injection site reactions but are uncommon and, to date, have not been serious. One patient with corticosteroid-dependent chronic urticaria with evidence of functional autoantibodies did not respond to rituximab (81) and another with psoriasis and delayed pressure urticaria responded to etanercept (82).

REFERENCES

1. Zuberbier T, Bindslev-Jensen C, Canonica W, et al. EAACI/GA^{2}LEN/EDF guideline: definition, classification and diagnosis of urticaria. Allergy 2006; 61:316–320.
2. Grattan CEH, Humphreys F. Guidelines for evaluation and management of urticaria in adults and children. Br J Dermatol 2007; 157:1116–1123.
3. Grattan CEH. Towards rationalizing the nomenclature and classification of urticaria: some guidance on guidelines. Clin Exp Allergy 2007; 37:625–626.
4. Leznoff A, Josse RG, Denburg J, et al. Association of chronic urticaria and angioedema with thyroid autoimmunity. Arch Dermatol 1983; 119:636–640.
5. Lanigan SW, Short P, Moult P. The association of chronic urticaria with thyroid autoimmunity. Clin Exp Dermatol 1987; 12:335–338.
6. Leznoff A, Sussman GL. Syndrome of idiopathic chronic urticaria and angioedema with thyroid autoimmunity: a study of 90 patients. J Allergy Clin Immunol 1989; 84:66–71.
7. Turktas I, Gokcora N, Demirsoy S, et al. The association of chronic urticaria with autoimmune thyroiditis. Int J Dermatol 1997; 36:187–190.
8. Hide M, Francis DM, Grattan CEH, et al. Autoantibodies against the high affinity IgE receptor as a cause if histamine release in chronic urticaria. N Engl J Med 1993; 328:1599–1604.
9. Niimi N, Francis DM, Kermani F, et al. Dermal mast cell activation by autoantibodies against the high affinity IgE receptor in chronic urticaria. J Invest Dermatol 1996; 106:1001–1006.
10. Fiebiger E, Hammerschmid F, Stingl G, et al. Anti-FcϵRIα autoantibodies in autoimmune-mediated diseases. J Clin Invest 1998; 101:243–251.
11. Ferrer M, Nakazawa K, Kaplan AP. Complement dependence of histamine release in chronic urticaria. J Allergy Clin Immunol 1999; 104:169–172.
12. Horn MP, Pachlopnik JM, Vogel M, et al. Conditional autoimmunity mediated by human natural anti- FcϵRIα autoantibodies? FASEB J 2001; 15:2268–2274.
13. Vonakis BM, Saini SS. Syk-deficient basophils from donors with chronic idiopathic urticaria exhibit a spectrum of releasability. J Allergy Clin Immunol 2008; 121:262–264.
14. Grattan CEH, Francis DM, Hide M, et al. Detection of circulating histamine releasing autoantibodies with functional properties of anti-IgE in chronic urticaria. Clin Exp Allergy 1991; 21:695–704.
15. Sabroe RA, Fiebiger E, Francis DM, et al. Classification of anti-FcϵRI and anti-IgE autoantibodies in chronic idiopathic urticaria and correlation with disease severity. J Allergy Clin Immunol 2002; 110:492–499.
16. Sabroe RA, Seed PT, Francis DM, et al. Chronic idiopathic urticaria: comparison of the clinical features of patients with and without anti-FcϵRI or anti-IgE autoantibodies. J Am Acad Dermatol 1999; 40:443–450.
17. Toubi E, Kessel A, Avshovich N, et al. Clinical and laboratory parameters in predicting chronic urticaria duration: a prospective study of 139 patients. Allergy 2004; 59:869–873.
18. Staubach P, Onnen K, Vonend A, et al. Autologous whole blood injections to patients with chronic urticaria and a positive autologous serum skin test: a placebo-controlled trial. Dermatology 2006; 212:150–159.
19. O'Donnell BF, O'Neill CM, Francis DM, et al. Human leucocyte antigen class II associations in chronic idiopathic urticaria. Br J Dermatol 1999; 140:853–858.
20. Zuberbier T, Pfrommer C, Specht K, et al. Aromatic components of food as novel eliciting factors of pseudoallergic reactions in chronic urticaria. J Allergy Clin Immunol 2002; 109:343–348.
21. Henz BM, Zuberbier T. Most chronic urticaria is food-dependent, and not idiopathic. Exp Dermatol 1998; 7:139–142.
22. Wedi B, Raap U, Kapp A. Chronic urticaria and infections. Curr Opin Allergy Clin Immunol 2004; 4:387–396.
23. Federman DG, Kirsner RS, Moriarty JP, et al. The effect of antibiotic therapy for patients infected with *Helicobacter pylori* who have chronic urticaria. J Am Acad Dermatol 2003; 49:861–864.

24. Kikuchi Y, Fann T, Kaplan AP. Antithyroid antibodies in chronic urticaria and angioedema. J Allergy Clin Immunol 2003; 112:218.
25. O'Donnell BF, Francis DM, Swana GT, et al. Thyroid autoimmunity in chronic urticaria. Br J Dermatol 2005; 153:331–335.
26. Lindelöf B, Sigurgeirsson B, Wahlgren CF, et al. Chronic urticaria and cancer: an epidemiological study of 1155 patients. Br J Dermatol 1990; 123:453–456.
27. Zuberbier T, Chantraine-Hess S, Hartmann K, et al. Pseudoallergen-free diet in the treatment of chronic urticaria. Acta Derm Vernereol 1995; 75:484–487.
28. Swain AR, Dutton SP, Truswell AS. Salicylates in foods. J Am Diet Assoc 1985; 85:950–960.
29. Grattan C. Aspirin-sensitive urticaria. Clin Exp Dermatol 2003; 28:123–127.
30. Chan CL, Jones RL, Lau HYA. Characterisation of prostanoid receptors mediating inhibition of histamines release from anti-IgE-activated rat peritoneal mast cells. Br J Pharmacol 2000; 129:589–597.
31. Quiralte J, Sáenz de San Pedro B, Fernando Florido JJ. Safety of selective cyclooxygenase-2 inhibitor rofecoxib in patients with NSAID-induced cutaneous reactions. Ann Allergy Asthma Immunol 2002; 89:63–66.
32. Harads S, Horikawa T, Ashida M, et al. Aspirin enhances the induction of type I allergic symptoms when combined with food and exercise in patients with food-dependent exercise-induced anaphylaxis. Br J Dermatol 2001; 145:336–339.
33. Cohen RW, Rosentreich DL. Discrimination between urticaria-prone and other allergic patients by intradermal testing with codeine. J Allergy Clin Immunol 1986; 77:802–807.
34. Juhlin L. Recurrent urticaria: clinical investigation of 330 patients. Br J Dermatol 1981; 104:369–381.
35. Humphreys F, Hunter JAA. The characteristics of urticaria in 390 patients. Br J Dermatol 1998; 138:635–638.
36. Barlow RJ, Warburton F, Watson K, et al. Diagnosis and incidence of delayed pressure urticaria in patients with chronic urticaria. J Am Acad Dermatol 1993; 29:954–958.
37. Stitcherling M, Brasch J, Brüning, Christophers E. Urticarial and anaphylactoid reactions following ethanol intake. Br J Dermatol 1995; 132:464–467.
38. Kanny G, Gerbaux V, Olszewski A, et al. No correlation between wine intolerance and histamine content of wine. J Allergy Clin Immunol 2001; 107:375–378.
39. Esch T, Stefano GB, Fricchione GL, et al. An overview of stress and its impact in immunological disease. Mod Asp Immunobiol 2002; 2:187–192.
40. Kozel MA, Mekkes JR, Bossuyt PMM, et al. The effectiveness of a history-based diagnostic approach in chronic urticaria and angioedema. Arch Dermatol 1998; 134:1575–1580.
41. Frezzolini A, Provini A, Teofoli P, et al. Serum-induced basophil CD63 expression by means of a tricolour flow cytometric method for the *in vitro* diagnosis of chronic urticaria. Allergy 2006; 61:1071–1077.
42. Sabroe RA, Grattan CEH, Francis DM, et al. The autologous serum skin test: a screening test for autoantibodies in chronic idiopathic urticaria. Br J Dermatol 1999; 140:446–452.
43. Shertzer CL, Lookinbill DP. Effects of relaxation therapy and hypnotisability in chronic urticaria. Arch Dermatol 1987; 123:913–916.
44. Barlow RJ, Macdonald DM, Kobza Black A, et al. The effects of topical corticosteroids on delayed pressure urticaria. Arch Dermatol Res 1995; 287:285–288.
45. Vena GA, Cassano N, D'Argento V, et al. Clobetasol propionate 0.05% in a novel foam formulation is safe and effective in the short-term treatment of patients with delayed pressure urticaria: a randomized double-blind, placebo-controlled trial. Br J Dermatol 2006; 154:353–356.
46. Marone G, Genovese A, Granata F, et al. Pharmacological modulation of human mast cells and basophils. Clin Exp Allergy 2002; 32:1682–1689.
47. Robertson I, Greaves MW. Responses of human skin blood vessels to synthetic histamine analogues. Br J Clin Pharmacol 1978; 5:319–322.
48. Humphreys F, Hunter JAA. The characteristics of urticaria in 390 patients. Br J Dermatol 1998; 138:635–638.
49. Kaplan AP. Urticaria and angioedema. N Engl J Med 2002; 946:275–279.

50. Fox RW, Lockey RF. Treatment of severe chronic urticaria with dapsone. J Allergy Clin Immunol 1988; 81:260.

51. Boehm I, Bauer R, Bieber T. Urticaria treated with dapsone. Allergy 1999; 54:765–766.

52. Greene SL, Reed CE, Schroeter AL. Double-blind crossover study comparing doxepin with diphenhydramine for the treatment of chronic urticaria. J Am Acad Dermatol 1985; 12: 669–675.

53. Harto A, Sendagorta E, Ledo A. Doxepin in the treatment of chronic urticaria. Dermatologica 1985; 170:90–93.

54. Pacor ML, Di Lorenzo G, Corrocher R. Efficacy of leukotriene receptor antagonist in chronic urticaria. A double-blind, placebo-controlled comparison of treatment with montelukast and cetirizine in patients with chronic urticaria with intolerance to food additives and/or salicylic acid. Clin Exp Allergy 2001; 31:1607–1614.

55. Bagenstose SE, Levin L, Bernstein J. The addition of zafirlukast to cetirizine improves the treatment of chronic urticaria in patients with positive autologous serum skin test results. J Allergy Clin Immunol 2004; 113:134–140.

56. Erbagci Z. The leukotriene receptor antagonist montelukast in the treatment of chronic idiopathic urticaria: a single-blind, placebo-controlled, crossover clinical study. J Allergy Clin Immunol 2002; 110:484–488.

57. Di Lorenzo G, Pacor ML, Mansueto P, et al. Randomized placebo-controlled trial comparing desloratadine and montelukast in monotherapy and desloratadine plus montelukast in combined therapy for chronic idiopathic urticaria. J Allergy Clin Immunol 2004; 114:619–625.

58. Engler RJM, Squire E, Benson P. Chronic sulphasalazine therapy in the treatment of delayed pressure urticaria. Ann Allergy Asthma Immunol 1995; 74:155–159.

59. Jaffer AM. Sulfasalazine in the treatment of corticosteroid-dependent chronic idiopathic urticaria. J Allergy Clin Immunol 1991; 88:964–965.

60. McGirt LY, Vasagar K, Gober LM, et al. Successful treatment of recalcitrant chronic idiopathic urticaria with sulfasalazine. Arch Dermatol 2006; 142:1337–1342.

61. Rumbyrt JS, Katz JL, Schocket AL. Resolution of chronic inflammation in patients with thyroid autoimmunity. J Allergy Clin Immunol 1995; 96:901–905.

62. Gaig P, García-Ortega P, Enrique E, et al. Successful treatment of chronic idiopathic urticaria associated with thyroid autoimmunity. J Investig Allergol Clin Immunol 2000; 10:342–345.

63. Heymann WR. Chronic urticaria and angioedema associated with thyroid autoimmunity: review and therapeutic implications. J Am Acad Dermatol 1999; 40:229–232.

64. Berroeta L, Clark C, Ibbetson SH, et al. Narrow-band (TL-01) ultraviolet B phototherapy for chronic urticaria. Clin Exp Dermatol 2004; 29:91–99.

65. Parslew R, Pryce D, Ashworth J, et al. Warfarin treatment of chronic idiopathic urticaria and angioedema. Clin Exp Allergy 2000; 30:1161–1165.

66. Grattan CEH, Francis DM, Slater NGP, et al. Plasmapheresis for severe unremitting, chronic urticaria. Lancet 1992; 339:1078–1080.

67. Shahar E, Bergman R, Guttman-Yassky E, et al. Treatment of severe chronic idiopathic urticaria with oral mycophenolate mofetil in patients not responding to antihistamines and/or corticosteroids. Int J Dermatol 2006; 45:1224–1227.

68. Kessel A, Bamberger E, Toubi E. Tacrolimus in the treatment of severe chronic idiopathic urticaria: an open-label prospective study. J Am Acad Dermatol 2005; 52:145–148.

69. Barlow RJ, Kobza Black A, Greaves MW. Treatment of severe chronic urticaria with cyclosporin. Eur J Dermatol 1993; 3:273–275.

70. Toubi E, Blant A, Kessel A, et al. Low-dose cyclosporin A in the treatment of severe chronic idiopathic urticaria. Allergy 1997; 52:312–316.

71. Grattan CEH, O'Donnell BF, Francis DM, et al. Randomised double-blind study of cyclosporin in chronic 'idiopathic' urticaria. Br J Dermatol 2000; 143:365–372.

72. Vena GA, Cassano N, Colombo D, et al. and the NEO-I-30 Study Group. Cyclosporine in chronic idiopathic urticaria: a double-blind, randomized, placebo-controlled trial. J Am Acad Dermatol 2006; 55:705–709.

73. O'Donnell BF, Barr RM, Kobza Black A, et al. Intravenous immunoglobulin in autoimmune chronic urticaria. Br J Dermatol 1998; 138:101–106.
74. Dawn G, Ureclay M, Ah-Weng A, et al. Effect of high-dose intravenous immunoglobulin in delayed pressure urticaria. Br J Dermatol 2003; 149:836–840.
75. Belgi G, Friedmann PS. Traditional therapies: glucocorticoids, azathioprine, methotrexate, hydroxyurea. Clin Exp Dermatol 2002; 27:546–554.
76. Weiner MJ. Methotrexate in corticosteroid-resistant urticaria. Ann Intern Med 1989; 110:848.
77. Gach JE, Sabroe RA, Greaves MW, et al. Methotrexate-responsive chronic idiopathic urticaria: a report of two cases. Br J Dermatol 2001; 145:340–343.
78. Spector SL, Tan RA. Effect of omalizumab on patients with chronic urticaria. Ann Allergy Asthma Immunol 2007; 99:190–193.
79. Kaplan AP, Joseph K, Maykut RJ, et al. Treatment of chronic autoimmune urticaria with omalizumab. J Allergy Clin Immunol 2008; S226.
80. Sands MF, Blume JW, Schwartz SA. Successful treatment of 3 patients with recurrent idiopathic angioedema with omalizumab. J Allergy Clin Immuol 2007; 120:979–981.
81. Mallipeddi R, Grattan CEH. Lack of response of severe steroid-dependent chronic urticaria to rituximab. Clin Exp Dermatol 2007; 32:333–334.
82. Magerl M, Philipp S, Manasterski M, et al. Successful treatment of delayed pressure urticaria with anti-TNF-α. J Allergy Clin Immunol 2007; 119:752–754.

19

Urticaria: Principles of Antihistamine Treatment

F. Estelle R. Simons
Department of Pediatrics & Child Health, Department of Immunology, CIHR National Training Program in Allergy and Asthma, Faculty of Medicine, University of Manitoba, Winnipeg, Canada

Keith J. Simons
Faculty of Pharmacy and Faculty of Medicine, University of Manitoba, Winnipeg, Canada

INTRODUCTION

Histamine is an important cell-to-cell messenger in the body, with activity at four types of G protein–coupled receptors (H_1, H_2, H_3, and H_4 receptors). In this chapter, we describe the role of histamine at H_1 receptors (Table 1) and emphasize its important role in the pathogenesis of urticaria , as well as focusing on H_1 antihistamine treatment of urticaria (1–6).

All known types of histamine receptors are heptahelical transmembrane molecules that transduce extracellular signals through G proteins to intracellular second messenger systems. They have constitutive activity, defined as the ability to trigger downstream events in the absence of ligand binding (3) (Fig. 1). The active and inactive states of the receptors exist in equilibrium. Histamine, an agonist, has a preferential affinity for the active state, stabilizes the receptor in this conformation, and consequently causes a shift in the equilibrium toward the active state. H_1 antihistamines, which in the past were called histamine antagonists or histamine blockers, are now correctly described as inverse agonists. They have a preferential affinity for the inactive state of H_1 receptors, stabilize the receptors in this conformation, shift the equilibrium toward the inactive state, and downregulate constitutive H_1-receptor activity even in the absence of histamine (3).

Histamine in Human Health

Through the H_1 receptor, histamine contributes extensively to human health. It is involved in cell proliferation and differentiation, hematopoiesis, embryonic development, regeneration, and wound healing. In the central nervous system (CNS), histamine is produced in neurons with cell bodies located exclusively in the tuberomamillary nucleus of the

Table 1 Histamine H_1 Receptors in Humans

Receptor expression	Nerve cells, airway and vascular smooth muscle, endothelial cells, epithelial cells, neutrophils, eosinophils, monocytes/macrophages, DC, T cells and B cells, hepatocytes, chondrocytes
G-protein coupling	$G_{\alpha q/11}$
Activated intra- cellular signals	Ca^{2+}, protein kinase C, phospholipase C, cGMP, phospholipase D, phospholipase A_2, NFκB
Histamine function in human health	Involvement in cell proliferation and differentiation, hematopoiesis, embryonic development, regeneration, and wound healing
Histamine function in the CNS[a]	Involvement in sleep/wakefulness, food intake, thermal regulation emotions/aggressive behavior, locomotion, memory, learning
Histamine function in allergic inflammation and immune modulation	↑ antigen-presenting cell capacity, co-stimulatory activity on B cells, ↑ cellular immunity (Th1), ↑ IFN-γ, ↑ autoimmunity, ↓ humoral immunity and IgE production; ↑ release of histamine and other mediators; ↑ cell adhesion molecule expression and chemotaxis of eosinophils and neutrophils;
Histamine function, general	↑ pruritus, ↑ pain, ↑ vasodilation ↑ vascular permeability ↑ hypotension, flushing, headache, tachycardia, bronchoconstriction, stimulation of airway vagal afferent nerves and cough receptors, ↓ atrio-ventricular node conduction time
Inverse agonists (formerly called antagonists or blockers)	>40, including cetirizine, desloratadine, fexofenadine, levocetirizine, and loratadine for urticaria

[a]Also, through presynaptic H_3 receptors located on the histaminergic and nonhistaminergic neurons of the central and peripheral nervous system, histamine modulates the release of other neurotransmitters.
Abbreviations: ↑, increases; ↓, decreases; Ca^{2+}, calcium; cGMP, cyclic guanosine monophosphate; DC, dendritic cells; H^+, hydrogen; IFN-γ interferon-gamma; NFκB, nuclear factor kappa B.
Source: Adapted from Ref. 1.

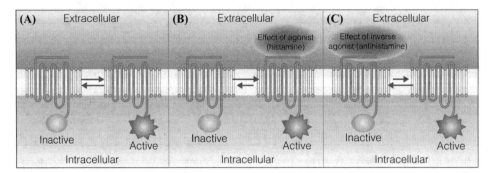

Figure 1 The histamine H_1 receptor: a simplified two-state model. (**A**) The inactive state of the histamine H_1 receptor is in equilibrium with the active state. (**B**) An agonist has a preferential affinity for the active state and stabilizes the H_1 receptor in this conformation, consequently causing a shift in the equilibrium toward the active state. (**C**) An inverse agonist such as an H_1 antihistamine has a preferential affinity for the inactive state, stabilizes the receptor in this conformation, and causes a shift in the equilibrium toward the inactive state. All H_1-antihistamines described to date function as inverse agonists. Intracellular and extracellular are defined in relation to the cell membrane. *Source*: Adapted from Ref. 3.

posterior hypothalamus, and axons that transmit histamine to the frontal and temporal cortices and other regions of the brain. In this phylogenetically old neurotransmitter system, histamine is involved in the regulation of basic body functions through the H_1 receptor, including the sleep/wake cycle, energy and endocrine homeostasis, cognition, and memory. Histamine also has natural anticonvulsant activity through the H_1 receptor. Targeted disruption of H_1 receptors in a murine model results mainly in the impairment of neurologic functions such as learning, memory and locomotion, as well as in aggressive behavior, although some immunologic abnormalities also occur (1,2).

Histamine in Human Disease

Through H_1 receptors, histamine also contributes to acute and chronic allergic inflammation. It increases antigen-presenting cell capacity, increases the release of histamine and other mediators from mast cells and basophils, upregulates cellular adhesion molecule expression and chemotaxis of eosinophils and neutrophils, upregulates Th1 priming and Th1 cell proliferation and interferon-gamma (IFN-γ) production, and downregulates humoral immunity (1,2) (Table 1).

Acting at cutaneous H_1 receptors, histamine causes itching, the predominant symptom in urticaria, via stimulation of thin, non-myelinated afferent C-fibers, which have low conduction velocity and large enervation territories (7) (Fig. 2). Acting at H_1 receptors on postcapillary venules, histamine induces the endothelium to release nitric oxide, which stimulates guanyl cyclase and increases cyclic guanosine monophosphate (cGMP) in the vascular smooth muscle, causing vasodilation and erythema and increased vascular permeability and edema, evidenced as wheals that blanch under pressure. The vasodilation is enhanced by an axon reflex resulting from the release of substance P by antidromic conduction on afferent C-fibers, evidenced as flares or erythema. This, in turn, augments histamine release (1).

Through H_1 receptors, histamine also has effects on other body organs and systems. It has a high affinity for H_1 receptors on postcapillary venules (in comparison to its affinity for H_2 receptors on postcapillary venules), and through these receptors causes flushing, hypotension, headache, and tachycardia. In addition, it causes broncho-constriction, stimulation of cough receptors, and decreased atrioventricular node conduction time (1,2).

Skin tissue fluid histamine concentrations are increased in urticarial lesions and in adjacent uninvolved skin. Although total circulating histamine concentrations are not increased in patients with chronic urticaria, clinical tolerance to histamine is reduced. If urticaria is provoked locally by challenge with a relevant stimulus, histamine concentrations in venous blood draining the urticated skin are transiently increased, peaking at 2 to 5 minutes after challenge, and declining to baseline within 30 minutes. In addition, other chemical mediators of itching and inflammation play a role in urticaria. Proteases, tachykinins, eicosanoids including leukotrienes and prostaglandins, neuro-peptides such as substance P, and other vasoactive substances lead to vascular permeability, vasodilation, whealing, and erythema. Proteases, eicosanoids, neuropeptides, and cytokines also play an important role in pruritus (2).

H_1 Antihistamines in Urticaria

The antiallergic and anti-inflammatory effects of H_1 antihistamines are classified as being either H_1-receptor *dependent* or H_1-receptor *independent* (1–6) (Fig. 3). H_1-receptor-*dependent* effects include downregulation of acute allergic inflammation,

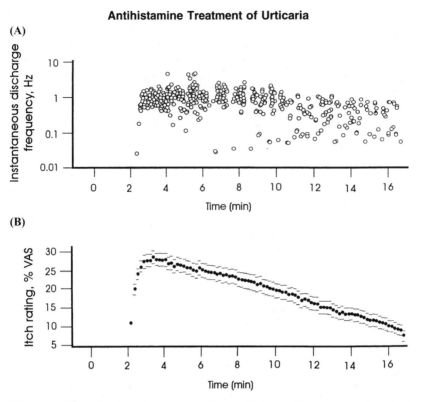

Figure 2 Histamine is an important mediator of itching. The cutaneous branch of the peroneal nerve of 21 healthy human volunteers was studied using microneurography. (**A**) Units were identified with a marking technique as "responsive" or "unresponsive" to mechanical stimulation and heat stimulation, and then tested for responsiveness to histamine 1 mA, iontophoresed for 20 seconds from a 6-mm diameter probe. (**B**) Histamine-induced itch sensations lasted several minutes. C-fibers, representing a new class of afferent nerves with extremely thin axons and excessive terminal branching, were found to mediate itch sensations. These fibers were mechanically insensitive and had low conduction velocities. Innervation territories on the lower leg were large (up to 85 mm in diameter). *Abbreviation*: VAS, visual analogue scale. *Source*: From Ref. 7.

evidenced as itching, vasodilation, vascular permeability, whealing, and erythema, as well as downregulation of chronic allergic inflammation through nuclear factor (NF)-κB, a ubiquitous transcription factor that binds to the promoter and enhancer regions of many genes involved in regulation of the production of proinflammatory cytokines and adhesion proteins. These H_1-receptor-dependent effects, which include downregulation of adhesion protein expression and of eosinophil and neutrophil migration, can be demonstrated in people taking manufacturers' recommended doses of H_1 antihistamines, and are clinically relevant in urticaria (1).

H_1-receptor-*independent* effects include antiallergic activities such as inhibition of mediator release from mast cells and basophils, through a direct effect on calcium ion channels, specifically, reduction of the inward calcium current activated by the depletion of intracellular calcium stores. In urticaria, the clinical relevance of the receptor-independent effects is uncertain, as they require high H_1 antihistamine concentrations that are unlikely to be achieved with manufacturers' recommended doses (1).

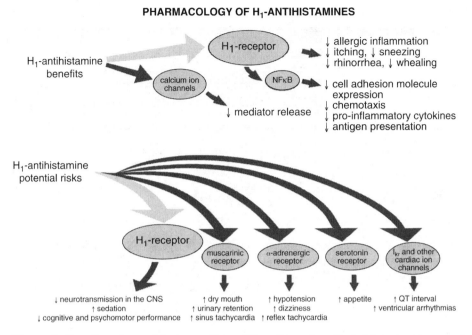

PHARMACOLOGY OF H₁-ANTIHISTAMINES

Figure 3 Benefits and potential adverse effects of H_1 antihistamines. H_1 antihistamines downregulate allergic inflammation mainly through the H_1 receptor. Most of the beneficial effects, except for relief of sneezing and rhinorrhea, are relevant to urticaria treatment. First-generation H_1 antihistamines potentially cause adverse effects not only through H_1 receptors in the central nervous system, but also through muscarinic, α-adrenergic and serotonin receptors, and cardiac ion channels. Second-generation H_1 antihistamines are relatively free from adverse effects. *Source*: Adapted from Ref. 1.

Selected H_1 antihistamines are illustrated in Figure 4. Medications in this class differ in their clinical pharmacology profiles and safety profiles, however, they have similar efficacy in urticaria treatment. In contrast to the first-generation H_1 antihist-amines, the second-generation H_1 antihistamines have high specificity for the H_1 receptor and do not bind to muscarinic, serotoninergic, α-adrenergic, or other receptors. When given in manufacturers' recommended doses, they cross the blood–brain barrier minimally or not at all, occupy $<30\%$ of CNS H_1 receptors, and are therefore less likely to cause sedation or impair cognition, memory, and psychomotor performance than are their predecessors (1,2,4,8–16).

H₁ ANTIHISTAMINES: CLINICAL PHARMACOLOGY

Clinical pharmacology (pharmacokinetic and pharmacodynamic) studies provide an objective basis for selection of an appropriate H_1 antihistamine dose and dose interval (1,2,4,8–19). They also provide the rationale for the modified dosage regimens that may be required in children, the elderly, and anyone who has impaired hepatic or renal function, or who concurrently ingests other medications or herbal products that might interfere with H_1 antihistamine elimination (17–19). H_1 antihistamine pharmacokinetics (drug concentration versus time) and pharmacodynamics (drug effect versus drug concentration) are summarized in Table 2. Pharmacodynamic studies correlate better with efficacy than pharmacokinetic studies do. The pharmacokinetics and pharmacodynamics of most first-generation H_1 antihistamines have not been optimally studied. In contrast,

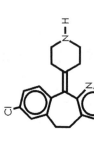

FIRST-GENERATION H₁-ANTIHISTAMINES

Diphenhydramine

Hydroxyzine

Ketotifen

SECOND-GENERATION H₁-ANTIHISTAMINES

Cetirizine

Loratadine

Fexofenadine

Levocetirizine

Desloratadine

Figure 4 Chemical formulas of representative H₁ antihistamines. Many H₁ antihistamines are structurally similar to each other. The availability of different H₁ antihistamines and different formulations of the same H₁ antihistamine varies from country to country; for example, ketotifen is available in oral formulations in some countries.

Table 2 Pharmacokinetics and Pharmacodynamics of Oral H_1 Antihistamines Differ in Healthy Young Adults

H_1 antihistamine (metabolite)	Time to maximum plasma concentration (t_{max}, hr) after a single dose[a]	Terminal elimination half-life ($t1/2\beta$, hr)	Clinically relevant drug/drug interactions[b]	Onset/ Duration of action[c] (hr)	Population in which dose adjustment may be required
First-generation					
Chlorpheniramine[d]	2.8 ± 0.8	27.9 ± 8.7	Possible	3/24	G
Diphenhydramine[d]	1.7 ± 1.0	9.2 ± 2.5	Possible	2/12	G,H
Doxepin[d]	2	13	Possible	n/a	H
Hydroxyzine[d]	2.1 ± 0.4	20.0 ± 4.1	Possible	2/24	H
Second-generation					
Cetirizine	1.0 ± 0.5	6.5–10	Unlikely	1/≥24	G,R,H
Desloratadine	1–3	27	Unlikely	2/≥24	R,H
Ebastine (carebastine)	(2.6–5.7)	(10.3–19.3)	n/a	2/≥24	R,H
Fexofenadine[b]	2.6	14.4	Unlikely	2/24	R
Levocetirizine	0.8 ± 0.5	7 ± 1.5	Unlikely	1/>24	R,H
Loratadine (descar-boethoxyloratadine)	1.2 ± 0.3 (1.5 ± 0.7)	7.8 ± 4.2 (24 ± 9.8)	Unlikely	2/24	H
Mizolastine	1.5	12.9	n/a	1/24	n/a
Rupatadine	0.75–1.0	6 (4.3–13.0)	Proven	2/24	G,R,H

Results are expressed as mean ± standard deviation, unless otherwise indicated.

[a] Time from oral intake to peak plasma concentration

[b] Clinically relevant drug-drug interactions are unlikely with most of the second-generation H_1 antihistamines; however, fexofenadine should not be administered within 15 minutes of ingestion of aluminum- and magnesium-containing antacids, which decrease its absorption.

[c] Onset/duration of action is based on wheal and flare studies.

[d] Five or six decades ago when many of the first-generation H_1 antihistamines were introduced, pharmacokinetic and pharmacodynamic studies were not required by regulatory agencies. Although they have subsequently been performed for some of these drugs, empirical dosage regimens persist; for example, the manufacturers' recommended diphenhydramine dose for urticaria is 25 to 50 mg q4-6h and the diphenhydramine dose for insomnia is 25 to 50 mg at bedtime. In addition, the use of sustained-action formulations persists despite the long terminal elimination half-life values identified for medications such as chlorpheniramine and hydroxyzine.

Abbreviations: G, geriatric; H, hepatic impairment; R, renal impairment; n/a, information not available or incomplete.

Source: Adapted from Ref. 1.

the pharmacokinetics and pharmacodynamics of the second-generation H_1 antihistamines have been systematically and thoroughly studied (1,2,8–26).

Pharmacokinetics

H_1 antihistamines are generally well absorbed after oral administration, and have variable terminal elimination half-life ($t1/2\beta$) values (1,2,8–19) (Table 2; Fig. 5). Many H_1 antihistamines, including the second-generation H_1 antihistamines ebastine, desloratadine, loratadine, mizolastine, and rupatadine, are metabolized in the hepatic cytochrome P450 (CYP450) system (1,2,10,11,14–19). Some second-generation medications are excreted largely unchanged in the urine and/or feces; for example, 60% of a cetirizine dose is eliminated unchanged in the urine; 86% of a levocetirizine dose is eliminated unchanged in the urine, and 80% of a fexofenadine dose is eliminated unchanged in the feces after biliary excretion (9,12,13). In individuals with moderate-to-severe impairment of hepatic

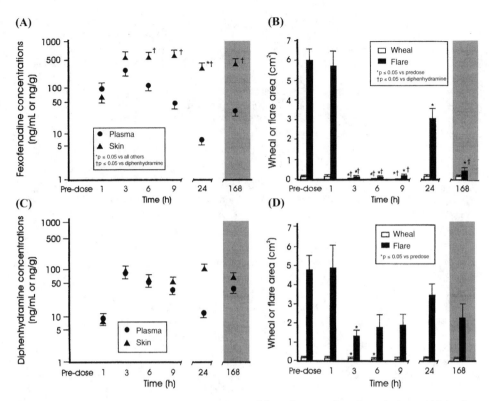

Figure 5 Correlation of skin and plasma H_1 antihistamine concentrations during multiple dose administration. In a randomized, double-blind, multiple-dose, parallel-group study, fexofenadine 120 mg/day or diphenhydramine 50 mg/day were administered for one week. At pre-dose baseline and 1, 3, 6, 9, and 24 hours after the initial H_1 antihistamine dose, skin and plasma fexofenadine concentrations were monitored and wheal and flare areas were measured after skin prick tests with histamine phosphate 1 mg/mL. Subsequently, on each of six consecutive days, participants took fexofenadine 120 mg or diphenhydramine 50 mg at 2100 hours, and all the tests were repeated at 168 hours (i.e., at steady state, which is depicted in the shaded area), exactly 12 hours after the seventh and last dose. Pre-dose plasma concentrations of both the H_1 antihistamines were zero. The values shown are mean $\pm$ standard error of the mean. Fexofenadine (**A** and **B**) achieved significantly higher concentrations in the skin, and significantly greater wheal and flare suppression than diphenhydramine (**C** and **D**). *Source*: From Ref. 23.

or renal function, and in many elderly people, H_1 antihistamines given in recommended doses potentially accumulate in plasma and tissues, necessitating a reduction in dose or dose frequency. Drug-drug interactions may occur for a variety of reasons, including interference with absorption through P-glycoprotein efflux pump activity in the gastrointestinal tract mucosa, or inhibition of metabolism in the CYP450 system (1,2,17–19).

Pharmacodynamics

The pharmacodynamics of H_1 antihistamines are medication- and dose-dependent, and are readily studied in the skin by taking advantage of the unique ability of the medications in this class to suppress the histamine- (or allergen-) induced wheal and flare (erythema) (8–17,19) (Fig. 5; Table 2). H_1 antihistamines decrease the size of the wheal directly by acting on endothelial cells to reduce postcapillary venule permeability and leakage of plasma protein, and they decrease the size of the flare indirectly by blocking the histamine-induced axon reflex. Using the standardized wheal and flare bioassay as an objective end point, dose-response curves can be identified for each H_1 antihistamine. During the first 24 hours after administration of a single dose, statistically significant, clinically relevant differences in onset, intensity, and duration of activity can be identified among these medications (8–17,19–24).

Although relatively few studies of first-generation H_1 antihistamines have been performed using the wheal and flare model; it has been documented that some of these medications such as hydroxyzine, diphenhydramine, and chlorpheniramine are significantly less effective on wheal and flare suppression than are second-generation H_1 antihistamines (1,2,23,24) (Fig. 5).

All second-generation H_1 antihistamines have been studied using the wheal and flare model (8–17, 19–24). Onset of action, as evidenced by significant suppression of the histamine-induced wheals and flares, occurs within an hour (cetirizine, levocetirizine) to two hours (desloratadine, fexofenadine, loratadine) (Table 2). Wheal and flare suppression peaks later than maximum plasma H_1 antihistamine concentrations and persists for many hours after plasma concentrations have declined below the limits of analytical detection. Where plasma and skin concentrations have been measured concurrently with wheal and flare suppression; for example, in some cetirizine or fexofenadine studies, this persistent effect is associated with high tissue–skin concentration ratios (23,24) (Fig. 5). For other H_1 antihistamines such as desloratadine and loratadine, the presence of active metabolites in skin might be important, although these metabolites have not been directly measured in tissue. Some H_1 antihistamines such as cetirizine, fexofenadine, or levocetirizine have high H_1-receptor occupancy levels in tissue throughout the dosing interval, and this correlates with their prolonged duration of action (25,26) (Fig. 6).

The duration of action of a single dose of most second-generation H_1 antihistamines in the skin is at least 24 hours; therefore, once-daily dosing is recommended (Table 2). After regular use for a week or more, these medications need to be discontinued for four to five days before allergen skin tests are performed. Loss of H_1-receptor activity and efficacy during regular daily administration of second-generation H_1 antihistamines has not been found in rigorously controlled, double-blind studies of up to 12 weeks' duration in which the suppression of skin wheals and flares has been monitored objectively, or in clinical trials of up to 6 weeks' duration during which suppression of wheals, flares, and itching has been monitored subjectively in patients with urticaria (1,2,8–17).

H_1 ANTIHISTAMINES: EFFICACY IN ACUTE AND CHRONIC URTICARIA

H_1 antihistamines are the medications of first choice medications for relieving symptoms in urticaria, in which they decrease itching and reduce the number, size, and duration of individual hives (27–30).

Acute Urticaria

In acute urticaria, defined as hives lasting less than six weeks, although H_1 antihistamines are the mainstay of symptom relief, the evidence base for their use remains small (28). In a randomized, placebo-controlled, double-blind study in 817 atopic young children, in which the effect on urticaria was a planned secondary outcome, regular treatment with cetirizine 0.25 mg/kg twice daily was significantly more efficacious than placebo in preventing and relieving episodes of acute urticaria over 18 months; however, this effect did not persist after cetirizine treatment was discontinued (31,32) (Fig. 7). In a subsequent similar 18-month randomized, controlled trial in 500 highly atopic young children, levocetirizine 0.125 mg/kg twice daily was significantly more efficacious than placebo in preventing and relieving urticaria.

(A)

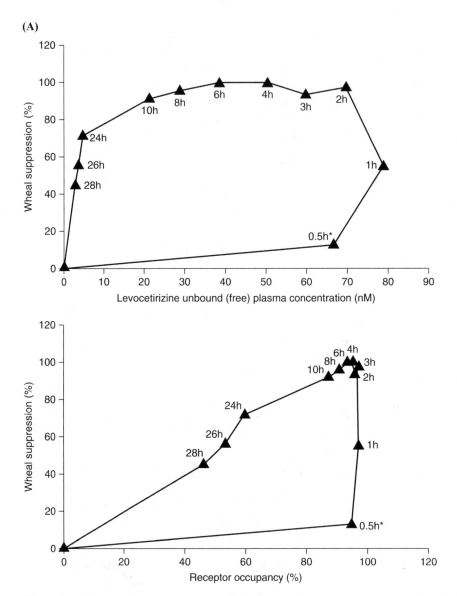

Figure 6 H_1 antihistamines and H_1-receptor occupancy. (**A**) Percent suppression of the histamine-induced wheal versus levocetirizine unbound (free) plasma concentrations. Percent suppression of the histamine-induced wheal versus percent levocetirizine H_1-receptor occupancy. (**B**) Percent suppression of the histamine-induced flare versus levocetirizine unbound (free) plasma concentrations. Percent suppression of the histamine-induced flare versus percent levocetirizine H_1-receptor occupancy. Receptor occupancy kinetics represent the time course of H_1 antihistamine pharmacodynamics better than plasma pharmacokinetics do. *Source*: From Ref. 26.

(B)

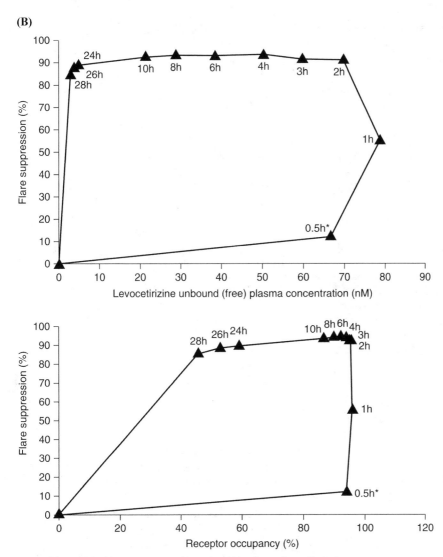

*times (h) at which skin tests were performed and blood samples collected

Figure 6 (*Continued*)

Chronic Urticaria

In chronic urticaria, defined as hives lasting at least six weeks, few first-generation H_1 antihistamines have been studied in randomized, controlled trials that meet current standards with regard to duration, and for reporting number of patients enrolled, inclusion criteria, exclusion criteria, attrition of patients, and adherence to treatment. Also, there are few randomized, placebo-controlled, double-blind studies in which a first-generation H_1 antihistamine has been compared with a second-generation H_1 antihistamine in chronic urticaria treatment. In one such study, cetirizine 10 mg once daily had a faster onset of action than hydroxyzine 25 mg three times daily in controlling itching and whealing, although the medications had similar overall efficacy (33) (Fig. 8). Cetirizine 10 mg once

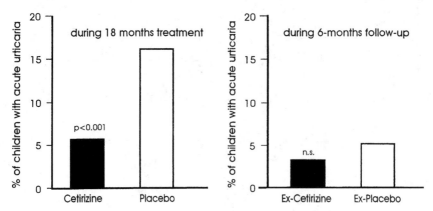

Figure 7 Cetirizine in prevention of acute urticaria. In the prospective, double-blind, parallel-group ETAC study, 817 children with atopic dermatitis who were 12 to 24 months of age at study entry were randomized to receive either cetirizine 0.25 mg/kg or placebo twice daily for 18 months. After this, they were followed for an additional 6 months, during which time the study medication code remained unbroken. In both these double-blind phases of the study, over a total of 24 months, caregivers recorded all symptoms and events, including hives, in a diary. During active treatment, acute urticaria occurred in only 5.8% of the 399 children receiving cetirizine, in contrast to 16.2% of the 396 children receiving placebo ($p < 0.001$). In this high-risk population, the protective effect of the cetirizine disappeared when treatment was stopped. *Abbreviation*: ETAC, Early Treatment of the Atopic Child study. *Source*: From Ref. 31.

daily is equivalent to hydroxyzine 30 mg once daily. Adequate double-blinding of such comparative studies is difficult to achieve, due to the sedation and/or impairment produced by the first-generation H_1 antihistamine being tested.

In contrast, the second-generation H_1 antihistamines such as cetirizine, desloratadine, ebastine, fexofenadine, levocetirizine, loratadine, mizolastine, and rupatadine have been well-studied in randomized, double-blind, placebo-controlled trials in chronic urticaria. The trials meet current standards for duration (usually 4 weeks) and for reporting number of patients enrolled, inclusion and exclusion criteria, attrition of patients, and adherence to treatment. These newer H_1 antihistamines have anti-inflammatory effects, prevent and relieve itching and whealing, and improve quality of life significantly (34–43). Some of them, for example, fexofenadine, have been studied over a wide range of doses (37) (Fig. 9).

There are few randomized, controlled trials in which the efficacy of different second-generation H_1 antihistamines has been compared in chronic urticaria. Where such studies have been conducted, it has been difficult to demonstrate statistically significant, clinically relevant differences between H_1 antihistamines. Additional comparative randomized controlled trials of second-generation H_1 antihistamines are needed (44–46). Also, additional randomized controlled trials of H_1 antihistamine efficacy are needed in young children and elderly patients with chronic urticaria.

The evidence base for the use of H_1 antihistamines in the treatment of physical urticarias including dermographism, cold-induced, solar, and delayed pressure urticaria, as well as in cholinergic urticaria, remains small. High-dose cetirizine (20 mg daily) has been reported to give some relief in cholinergic urticaria and in delayed-pressure urticaria (28).

H_1 antihistamines may be less effective in other types of urticaria; for example, in urticaria pigmentosa and cutaneous mastocytosis, in which fixed atypical urticarial lesions are manifest. They are not effective in urticarial vasculitis or in urticaria associated with cryopyrin-mediated auto-inflammatory diseases (47).

(A)

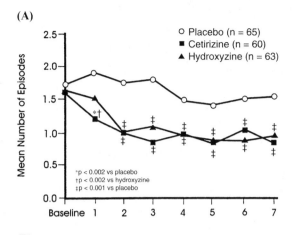

(B)

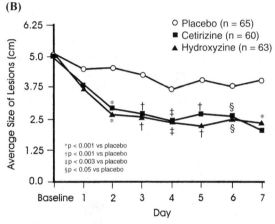

Figure 8   First- and second-generation H$_1$ antihistamines have similar efficacy in chronic urticaria. In a four-week randomized, double-blind, placebo-controlled study, 188 patients with CIU were treated with either cetirizine 10 mg once daily, hydroxyzine 25 mg three times daily, or placebo. Cetirizine had a significantly faster onset of action. Cetirizine and hydroxyzine both significantly reduced (**A**) the number of episodes of urticaria, (**B**) the size of lesions. The number of lesions and the severity of pruritus were also decreased (*not shown*). Hydroxyzine was significantly more sedating than cetirizine. *Abbreviation*: CIU, chronic idiopathic urticaria. *Source*: From Ref. 33.

Non-Allergic Angioedema

Although H$_1$ antihistamines help to relieve angioedema associated with urticaria and itching, they are not effective in relieving the non-allergic angioedemas, including hereditary angioedema types I, II, and III, and acquired angioedema associated with malignancy or with angiotensin-converting enzyme or angiotensin-receptor blocker use. Lack of response to an H$_1$ antihistamine in angioedema should therefore serve as an important diagnostic clue to the possibility of non-allergic angioedema (48) (chapter 15).

Anaphylaxis

In acute urticaria that is associated with rapid onset of upper or lower respiratory tract symptoms such as coughing, hoarseness, stridor, or wheezing; or gastrointestinal symptoms such as vomiting, diarrhea, or cramps; or cardiovascular symptoms (sudden

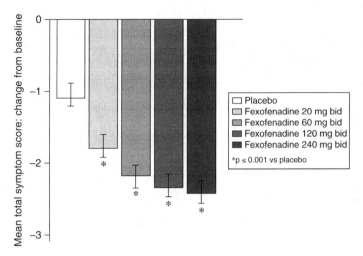

Figure 9 Fexofenadine in chronic urticaria. In a randomized, double-blind, placebo-controlled, parallel-group study, 439 patients with moderate to severe itching and hives received either fexofenadine 20 mg, 60 mg, 120 mg, or 240 mg, or placebo twice daily. The severity of itching, number of wheals, and interference with sleep/normal daily activities because of hives were assessed reflectively over the previous 12 hours. At baseline in the five different treatment groups, mean total symptom scores consisting of the sum of mean itch severity scores and mean number of wheals, ranged from 4.2 ± 1.6 to 4.6 ± 1.9 ($p = 0.3874$). All four doses of fexofenadine were superior to placebo ($p \leq 0.001$) for reducing mean total symptom score (*shown*), itch score, and wheal score from baseline over four weeks compared to placebo. *Source*: From Ref. 37.

dizziness or feeling faint), anaphylaxis is the likely diagnosis and epinephrine (adrenaline) injected intramuscularly in the mid-anterolateral aspect of the thigh is the drug of choice. In anaphylaxis, H_1 antihistamines only relieve hives and itching. They do not relieve airway obstruction, hypotension, or shock, and they do not prevent fatality (49).

Practical Aspects of H_1 Antihistamine Treatment in Chronic Urticaria

The initial treatment of choice is to use the manufacturers' recommended dose of a non-sedating second-generation H_1 antihistamine on a regular basis in order to prevent hives from appearing, rather than on an as-needed basis after hives are already present. H_1 antihistamine treatment may not relieve the wheal and flare response completely, because as noted previously, histamine acting through H_2 receptors also contributes to increased vascular permeability, as do many other vasoactive mediators. If a second-generation H_1 antihistamine is ineffective in a standard dose, a higher dose of the same non-sedating H_1 antihistamine is often recommended (27–29,50). If this fails, it may be helpful to suggest switching to another second-generation H_1 antihistamine; although clinically relevant differences between H_1 antihistamines might be difficult to document in randomized, controlled trials (44–46), individual patients might get more relief from one H_1 antihistamine than from another. Some physicians advise sequential use of two different second-generation H_1 antihistamines on the same day; however, this recommendation is made on an empirical basis, and prospective, randomized, double-blind, placebo-controlled trials are needed to support or refute it.

If various strategies involving use of second-generation non-sedating H_1 antihistamines are unsuccessful in chronic urticaria treatment, consideration should be given to use of a sedating, first-generation H_1 antihistamine. Although these older medications are often given three or four times daily (27), these regimens are based on tradition and are unnecessary for many of them. For example, hydroxyzine or chlorpheniramine have elimination half-life values of 20 and 28 hours, respectively, and suppress wheals and flares for more than 24 hours after a single dose (2) (Table 2). Moreover, the total daily doses of these old H_1 antihistamines recommended for chronic urticaria (27) are several-fold larger than the doses at which CNS adverse effects have been regularly and consistently documented (1,2,4).

Some physicians advise regular daytime use of a first-generation H_1 antihistamine, anticipating that tolerance will develop to the sedation within one week; however, on objective testing, tolerance is not necessarily confirmed. H_1 receptors in the CNS do not differ from H_1 receptors in peripheral tissues such as the skin, where, as stated previously, tolerance has never been objectively documented. Others recommend first-generation H_1 antihistamines for use only at bedtime, in anticipation that sedation will occur only at night (29). Unfortunately, the morning after the bedtime dose, an antihistamine "hangover", defined as sedation and/or impairment of cognitive and psychomotor function, may be present (2). It is important to note that none of these treatment regimens have ever been prospectively tested in randomized, placebo-controlled, double-blind trials.

Role of H_2 Antihistamines in Chronic Urticaria

In clinical pharmacology studies, concomitant administration of an H_2 antihistamine with an H_1 antihistamine may or may not lead to significantly greater suppression of the histamine-induced wheal and flare than administration of the H_1 antihistamine alone. Where increased suppression has been demonstrated, the magnitude is only about 10%. Similarly, in patients with chronic urticaria refractory to treatment with an H_1 antihistamine alone, the synergistic effect of adding an H_2 antihistamine such as cimetidine 600 mg twice daily or ranitidine 150 mg twice daily to an H_1 antihistamine has not been found in all studies, and in some patients in whom it has been demonstrated, it is too small to be clinically relevant or cost effective. Concurrent H_1 and H_2 antihistamine treatment should therefore never be suggested routinely, and if enhanced symptom relief is not apparent after a three- to four-week trial of concurrent treatment, the H_2 antihistamine should be discontinued (2,27–29).

The tricyclic antidepressant doxepin has clinically important H_1 and H_2 antihistamine properties, with greater activity than either diphenhydramine or hydroxyzine at H_1 receptors and greater activity than cimetidine at H_2 receptors. In patients with chronic urticaria, doxepin 25 mg three times daily suppresses whealing and itching significantly more than placebo does; and even in a low dose of 10 mg three times daily, doxepin is significantly more effective than diphenhydramine. Since doxepin has a t1/2β of 13 hours and is extremely sedating, a single daily dose at bedtime is often recommended. It is not approved for use in children.

Failure of Antihistamine Treatment

If antihistamines fail to relieve symptoms in chronic urticaria, a leukotriene modifier such as montelukast, or another immunomodulator such as an oral corticosteroid, cyclosporine, hydroxychloroquine, or omalizumab should be added to H_1 antihistamine treatment (chap. 20). Montelukast has been studied in large randomized, controlled trials, and cyclosporine, hydroxychloroquine, and omalizumab have been studied in small randomized, controlled trials. Recommendations for use of other immunomodulators are based on case reports, case series, and clinical experience, rather than on prospective, randomized, placebo-controlled clinical trials. With the exception of antihistamines and montelukast, pharmacologic interventions in chronic urticaria potentially cause severe adverse effects that necessitate regular monitoring of all patients treated with them (27–29).

H_1 ANTIHISTAMINES: ADVERSE EFFECTS

First-generation H_1 antihistamines, in contrast to their newer second-generation counterparts, potentially cause a variety of adverse effects, even when given in manufacturers' recommended doses (Table 3). These include antimuscarinic effects such as dry mucus membranes and urinary retention, anti-α-adrenergic effects such as dizziness and postural

Table 3 Adverse Effects of First-Generation H_1 Antihistamines Vs. Second-Generation H_1 Antihistamines

	First-generation[a,b,c]	Second-generation[b]
CNS Mechanism: Interference with neurotransmitter effect of histamine through H_1 receptor	After usual doses, may cause drowsiness, fatigue, somnolence, dizziness, impairment of cognitive function, memory, and psychomotor performance, headache, dystonia, dyskinesia, agitation, confusion, and hallucinations May cause adverse CNS effects in newborns if taken by the mother immediately before parturition May cause irritability, drowsiness, or respiratory depression in nursing infants	None with fexofenadine at doses up to 360 mg (off-label) None with desloratadine 5 mg or loratadine 10 mg, although dose-related CNS effects may occur at higher doses Cetirizine doses 10 mg or higher may cause sedation in adults No CNS adverse effects reported in newborns or nursing infants
Cardiac Mechanisms: Antimuscarinic effects α-adrenergic receptor blockade Blockade of cardiac ion currents (I_{Kr} and, less commonly, I_{Na}, I_{to}, I_{Ki}, and I_{Ks})[c]	Dose-related sinus tachycardia reflex tachycardia, prolonged atrial refractive period, and supraventricular arrhythmias Dose-related prolongation of the QTc interval and ventricular arrhythmias reported for cyproheptadine, diphenhydramine, doxepin, hydroxyzine, promethazine, and others	No major concerns in any country (such as the United States or Canada) in which regulatory approval was withdrawn for astemizole and terfenadine
Other Sites Mechanisms: Blockade of muscarinic, α-adrenergic, and serotonin receptors	After usual doses, may cause mydriasis (pupillary dilation), dry eyes, dry mouth, urinary retention and hesitancy, decreased gastrointestinal motility, constipation, erectile dysfunction, memory deficits Peripheral vasodilation, postural hypotension, dizziness Appetite stimulation and weight gain (cyproheptadine, ketotifen)	None reported

(Continued)

Table 3 Adverse Effects of First-Generation H_1 Antihistamines Vs. Second-Generation H_1 Antihistamines (*Continued*)

	First-generation[a,b,c]	Second-generation[b]
Toxicity after overdose Mechanisms:	CNS effects such as extreme drowsiness, lethargy, confusion, delirium, and coma in adults Paradoxical excitation, irritability, hyperactivity, insomnia, hallucinations, seizures, and respiratory depression/ arrest in infants and young children In both adults and children, CNS adverse effects predominate over cardiac adverse effects Death may occur within hrs after ingestion of drug in untreated patients Rhabdomyolysis has also been reported	No serious toxicity or fatality reported
Abuse of H_1 antihistamines Mechanisms: Through H_1 and other receptors in the CNS	Euphoria, hallucinations and "getting high" reported for diphenhydramine, dimenhydrinate and others	None reported
Teratogenicity after use in pregnancy[d]	FDA Category B (chlorpheniramine, diphenhydramine), or C (hydroxyzine, ketotifen)	FDA Category B (cetirizine, levocetirizine, loratadine) or C (desloratadine, fexofenadine)
Long-term safety	No studies	Studies of at least 12–18 mo duration in adults and children
Carcinogenicity/tumor promotion	None documented in humans	None documented in humans

[a]Most first-generation H_1 antihistamines have not been prospectively studied for their adverse effects. The information is based on descriptions of adverse effects in case reports and case series published during the last 60 years.

First-generation H_1 antihistamines, particularly in the phenothiazine class, have been associated with sudden infant death syndrome, although causality has never been proven.

First-generation H_1 antihistamines such as diphenhydramine or doxepin, applied topically to the skin, may cause contact dermatitis and if applied to abraded skin, they potentially cause systemic adverse effects.

[b]Rarely, both first- and second-generation H_1 antihistamines are reported to cause adverse effects for which the mechanisms are incompletely understood: fixed-drug eruption, photosensitivity, urticaria, anaphylaxis, fever, liver enzyme elevation/hepatitis, and agranulocytosis.

[c]I_{Kr}, rapid component of the delayed rectifier potassium current; I_{Na}, sodium current; I_{to}, transient outward potassium current; I_{Ki}, inward rectifying current; I_{Ks}, slow component of the delayed rectifier potassium current.

[d]FDA, Food and Drug Administration

Category A—animal studies and human studies negative; no H_1 antihistamines in this category.

Category B—animal studies negative, human data not available; or, animal studies positive, human data negative.

Category C—animal studies positive, human data not available; or, neither animal nor human data available.

Category D—animal studies positive or negative; human data positive.

H_1 antihistamines that are not approved for use in the United States (e.g., ebastine, mizolastine, rupatadine) are not categorized by the FDA.

Source: Adapted from Ref. 1.

hypotension, and antiserotonin effects such as appetite stimulation; however, the greatest concern is the adverse CNS effects that occur through the H_1 receptor (1–4,51–65).

Central Nervous System

First-Generation H_1 Antihistamines

In the CNS, first-generation H_1 antihistamines such as chlorpheniramine, diphenhydramine, hydroxyzine, ketotifen (available in some countries as an oral formulation), and promethazine penetrate the nonfenestrated endothelial lining of the CNS capillaries, the so-called blood–brain barrier. The mechanisms involved include low lipophilicity/solubility ratios, relatively low molecular weights, and lack of recognition by the P-glycoprotein efflux pump expressed on the luminal surfaces of endothelial cells in the cerebral vasculature. As demonstrated by positron emission tomography, these older H_1 antihistamines occupy >70% of the H_1 receptors in the frontal cortex, temporal cortex, hippocampus, and pons. In manufacturers' recommended doses, they all potentially cause CNS adverse effects by interfering with the normal neurotransmitter effects of endogenous histamine (52–56).

Self-reporting of adverse CNS effects caused by H_1 antihistamines or any other CNS-active medications or chemicals such as ethanol underestimates the true rate of occurrence of sedation or impairment. Lapses and errors can be documented in the absence of symptoms, regardless of the substance ingested or the objective test used to assess impairment (57). First-generation H_1 antihistamines have been implicated in loss of productivity in the workplace, on-the-job injuries, and also in motor vehicle accidents, and civil aviation accidents. Elevated postmortem blood and liver H_1 antihistamine concentrations have been found in drivers and pilots involved in fatal accidents. In some jurisdictions, drivers who have been taking a first-generation H_1 antihistamine and are found guilty of causing a traffic fatality can lose their license, and be fined or imprisoned. For obvious reasons, military pilots and commercial airline pilots are prohibited from using them before or during flights (1,2).

People who are particularly vulnerable to the adverse CNS effects of H_1 antihistamines include: the elderly, those with pre-existing CNS disease, small body mass with consequent relatively high mg/kg dose, impairment of hepatic or renal function leading to H_1 antihistamine accumulation in the CNS and other tissues, and those concomitantly using ethanol or other CNS function-impairing chemicals and drugs (1,2,64,65).

Second-Generation H_1 Antihistamines

Second-generation H_1 antihistamines such as cetirizine, desloratadine, ebastine, fexofenadine, levocetirizine, loratadine, mizolastine, and rupatadine are highly specific for H_1 receptors and penetrate the CNS poorly because of their lipophobicity, relatively high molecular weight, and for fexofenadine, recognition by the P-glycoprotein efflux pump is expressed on endothelial cells in the cerebral vasculature. As objectively documented by positron emission tomography, these newer H_1 antihistamines occupy from <1% to 30% of H_1 receptors in the CNS. Fexofenadine, in doses of up to 360 mg (2–3 times larger than the recommended daily dose), occupies less than 1% of CNS H_1 receptors. Cetirizine in an above-label dose of 20 mg occupies 26% to 30% of CNS H_1 receptors. CNS H_1 receptor occupancy by the other second-generation, nonsedating H_1 antihistamines is intermediate between that of fexofenadine and cetirizine (52–56). These objective studies of CNS H_1-receptor occupancy correlate with objective tests of psychomotor function, and with objective (EEG) and subjective evidence of drowsiness.

The second-generation H_1 antihistamines do not exacerbate the CNS effects of concomitantly ingested ethanol or other CNS-active substances, although with the exception of fexofenadine, they may potentially do so if manufacturers' recommended doses are exceeded (4,64,65). Regulatory agencies do not require screening processes or standardized protocols and objective tests for investigation of the CNS safety of new H_1 antihistamines.

Cardiac Toxicity

H_1 antihistamines are among many classes of drugs that potentially prolong the QT interval and lead to ventricular arrhythmias, including torsade de pointes. Blockade of the rapid component of delayed rectifier potassium (I_{Kr}) channels and prolongation of the monophasic action potential (QT interval) may induce the development of early after-depolarization and dispersion of repolarization, leading to torsade de pointes through reentry mechanisms. Blockade of other ion channels, for example, the I_{To} I_{Ki} and I_{Ks} channels, may also lead to prolongation of the QT interval (1–4,66).

Some people have an increased risk of developing cardiac toxicity from medications such as H_1 antihistamines; for example, females, and individuals with pre-existing organic heart disease (ischemia, cardiomyopathy), cardiac arrhythmias (congenital or acquired), or metabolic abnormalities (hypokalemia, hypocalcemia, or hypomagnesemia). Others at increased risk include those who ingest medications, herbal formulations, or foods that inhibit H_1 antihistamine elimination by the CYP450 system, or those concurrently taking another drug that by itself prolongs the QTc interval (1–4).

First-generation H_1 antihistamines such as cyproheptadine, diphenhydramine, or hydroxyzine, and the H_1/H_2 antihistamine doxepin have a dose-related effect on the QT interval and in overdose, may cause arrhythmias, including torsade de pointes. Second-generation H_1 antihistamines such as cetirizine, desloratadine, fexofenadine, levocetirizine, and loratadine have been extensively investigated for potential cardiac toxicity, which has not been detected either at therapeutic doses, or after overdose. Regulatory agencies now aim to identify the potential risk for cardiac toxicity of all medications, including H_1 antihistamines, during preclinical and early clinical development (1–4,67,68).

Safety in Special Populations (Young Children, Pregnant or Lactating Women, Elderly People)

In contrast to the absence of prospective safety studies of first-generation H_1 antihistamines in young children, the long-term safety of some of the second-generation H_1 antihistamines has been well documented in this age group; for example, randomized, placebo-controlled studies of cetirizine, levocetirizine, and loratadine lasting up to 18 months, have been published (69–71).

H_1 antihistamines such as chlorpheniramine, diphenhydramine, cetirizine, levocetirizine, and loratadine are rated by the U.S. Food and Drug Administration as Pregnancy Category B drugs and are considered to have a relatively low risk of teratogenicity (Table 3). All H_1 antihistamines are excreted in breast milk. Nursing infants receive approximately 0.1% of an orally administered maternal H_1 antihistamine dose. First-generation H_1 antihistamines potentially cause sedation and other adverse effects in these infants (1,2,72).

Elderly individuals have increased vulnerability to CNS adverse effects from drugs and chemicals that cross the blood–brain barrier. In this age group, first-generation H_1 antihistamines such as diphenhydramine, given in manufacturers' recommended doses, potentially increase the risk of sedation, cognitive dysfunction, inattention, disorganized speech, and confusion (1,2,58). In addition, polymedication is common in the elderly, and the potential for first-generation H_1 antihistamines to interact with other drugs or herbal products is therefore increased in this age group. Potential antimuscarinic effects such as mydriasis, dry eyes, dry mouth, urinary retention, urinary hesitancy, and constipation, and potential anti-α-adrenergic effects such as dizziness and hypotension from first-generation H_1 antihistamines are also a concern. These medications are contraindicated in individuals with glaucoma or prostatic hypertrophy (1,2,58).

H_1 Antihistamine: Overdose

Deaths attributed to first-generation H_1 antihistamines after accidental overdose or suicide have been reported in the medical literature for the last 60 years (51). Although CNS symptoms predominate after overdose with these medications, they also potentially cause dose-related cardiac adverse effects including sinus tachycardia, reflex tachycardia, and supraventricular arrhythmias. In large overdoses, some of them, for example, diphenhydramine 0.5 to 1.0 g, also potentially prolong the QT interval, and cause ventricular arrhythmias including torsade de pointes (1,2,67,68) (Table 3). Diphenhydramine overdoses are so frequently reported to poison control centers in the United States that evidence-based guidelines have been published to facilitate their management (67,68,73).

SUMMARY

Through the H_1 receptor, histamine plays an important physiologic role in many body functions including neurotransmission, and an important pathologic role in allergic inflammation. The mechanism of action of histamine and H_1 antihistamines at the H_1 receptor has been elucidated. H_1 antihistamines appear to have similar efficacy in chronic urticaria, although additional within-class comparative studies of efficacy are needed. There are clinically relevant differences in H_1 antihistamine clinical pharmacology profiles, and in their safety profiles. Second-generation H_1 antihistamines are preferred to first-generation H_1 antihistamines in the treatment of chronic urticaria because of their lack of sedation, impairment of cognitive and psychomotor performance, and other adverse effects. For each H_1 antihistamine, the potential benefits should be weighed against the potential risks of adverse effects.

REFERENCES

1. Simons FER. Advances in H_1-antihistamines. N Engl J Med 2004; 351:2203–2217.
2. Simons FER, Akdis CA. Histamine and antihistamines. In: Adkinson NF Jr, Busse WW, Bochner BS, et al. eds. Middleton's Allergy Principles and Practice. 7th ed. St. Louis, MO: Mosby, Inc., (an affiliate of Elsevier Science), 2008:1517–1547.
3. Leurs R, Church MK, Taglialatela M. H_1-antihistamines: inverse agonism, anti-inflammatory actions and cardiac effects. Clin Exp Allergy 2002; 32:489–498.
4. Holgate ST, Canonica GW, Simons FER, et al. Consensus group on new-generation antihistamines (CONGA): present status and recommendations. Clin Exp Allergy 2003; 33:1305–1324.
5. Akdis CA, Simons FER. Histamine receptors are hot in immunopharmacology. Eur J Pharmacol 2006; 533:69–76.
6. Jutel M, Blaser K, Akdis CA. Histamine receptors in immune regulation and allergen-specific immunotherapy. Immunol Allergy Clin North Am 2006; 26:249–259.
7. Schmelz M, Schmidt R, Bickel A, et al. Specific C-receptors for itch in human skin. J Neurosci 1997; 17:8003–8008.
8. Golightly LK, Greos LS. Second-generation antihistamines: actions and efficacy in the management of allergic disorders. Drugs 2005; 65:341–384.

9. Curran MP, Scott LJ, Perry CM. Cetirizine: a review of its use in allergic disorders. Drugs 2004; 64: 523–561.

10. Murdoch D, Goa KL, Keam SJ. Desloratadine: an update of its efficacy in the management of allergic disorders. Drugs 2003; 63:2051–2077.

11. Hurst M, Spencer CM. Ebastine. An update of its use in allergic disorders. Drugs 2000; 59: 981–1006.

12. Simpson K, Jarvis B. Fexofenadine. A review of its use in the management of seasonal allergic rhinitis and chronic idiopathic urticaria. Drugs 2000; 59:301–321.

13. Hair PI, Scott LJ. Levocetirizine: a review of its use in the management of allergic rhinitis and skin allergies. Drugs 2006; 66:973–996.

14. Haria M, Fitton A, Peters DH. Loratadine. A reappraisal of its pharmacological properties and therapeutic use in allergic disorders. Drugs 1994; 48:617–637.

15. Simons FER. Mizolastine: antihistaminic activity from preclinical data to clinical evaluation. Clin Exp Allergy 1999; 29(suppl 1):3–8.

16. Keam SJ, Plosker GL. Rupatadine: a review of its use in the management of allergic disorders. Drugs 2007; 67:457–474.

17. Simons FER, Simons KJ. Clinical pharmacology of H_1-antihistamines. In: Simons FER, ed. Histamine and H_1-Antihistamines in Allergic Disease. 2nd ed. New York: Marcel Dekker, Inc., 2002:141–178.

18. Molimard M, Diquet B, Benedetti MS. Comparison of pharmacokinetics and metabolism of desloratadine, fexofenadine, levocetirizine and mizolastine in humans. Fundam Clin Pharmacol 2004; 18:399–411.

19. Simons FER. H_1-antihistamines in children. In: Simons FER, ed. Histamine and H_1-Antihistamines in Allergic Disease. 2nd ed. New York: Marcel Dekker, Inc., 2002:437–464.

20. Denham KJ, Boutsiouki P, Clough GF, et al. Comparison of the effects of desloratadine and levocetirizine on histamine-induced wheal, flare and itch in human skin. Inflamm Res 2003; 52:424–427.

21. Purohit A, Melac M, Pauli G, et al. Twenty-four-hour activity and consistency of activity of levocetirizine and desloratadine in the skin. Br J Clin Pharmacol 2003; 56:388–394.

22. Frossard N, Strolin-Benedetti M, Purohit A, et al. Inhibition of allergen-induced wheal and flare reactions by levocetirizine and desloratadine. Br J Clin Pharmacol 2008; 65:172–179.

23. Simons FER, Silver NA, Gu X, et al. Skin concentrations of H_1-receptor antagonists. J Allergy Clin Immunol 2001; 107:526–530.

24. Simons FER, Silver NA, Gu X, et al. Clinical pharmacology of H_1-antihistamines in the skin. J Allergy Clin Immunol 2002; 110:777–783.

25. Gillard M, Benedetti MS, Chatelain P, et al. Histamine H_1 receptor occupancy and pharmacodynamics of second generation H_1 antihistamines. Inflamm Res 2005; 54:367–369.

26. Simons KJ, Strolin-Benedetti M, Simons FER, et al. Relevance of H_1-receptor occupancy to antihistamine dosing in children. J Allergy Clin Immunol 2007; 119:1551–1554.

27. Kaplan AP. Clinical practice. Chronic urticaria and angioedema. N Engl J Med 2002; 346:175–179.

28. Zuberbier T, Bindslev-Jensen C, Canonica W, et al. EAACI/GA²LEN/EDF guideline: management of urticaria. Allergy 2006; 61:321–331.

29. Powell RJ, Du Toit GL, Siddique N, et al. BSACI guidelines for the management of chronic urticaria and angio-oedema. Clin Exp Allergy 2007; 37:631–650.

30. The Medical Letter. Drugs for allergic diseases. Treatment Guidelines from The Medical Letter 2007; 60:71–80.

31. Simons FER, on behalf of the ETAC Study Group. Prevention of acute urticaria in young children with atopic dermatitis. J Allergy Clin Immunol 2001; 107:703–706.

32. Simons FER, on behalf of the Early Prevention of Asthma in Atopic Children (EPAAC) Study Group. H_1-antihistamine treatment in young atopic children: effect on urticaria. Ann Allergy Asthma Immunol 2007; 99:261–266.

33. Breneman DL. Cetirizine versus hydroxyzine and placebo in chronic idiopathic urticaria. Ann Pharmacother 1996; 30:1075–1079.

34. Monroe E, Finn A, Patel P, et al. Efficacy and safety of desloratadine 5 mg once daily in the treatment of chronic idiopathic urticaria: a double-blind, randomized, placebo-controlled trial. J Am Acad Dermatol 2003; 48:535–541.

35. Ring J, Hein R, Gauger A, et al. Once-daily desloratadine improves the signs and symptoms of chronic idiopathic urticaria: a randomized, double-blind, placebo-controlled study. Int J Dermatol 2001; 40:72–76.

36. Ortonne Jean-P, Grob Jean-J, Auquier P, et al. Efficacy and safety of desloratadine in adults with chronic idiopathic urticaria: a randomized, double-blind, placebo-controlled, multicenter trial. Am J Clin Dermatol 2007; 8:37–42.

37. Finn AF Jr, Kaplan AP, Fretwell R, et al. A double-blind, placebo-controlled trial of fexofenadine HCl in the treatment of chronic idiopathic urticaria. J Allergy Clin Immunol 1999; 104:1071–1078.

38. Nelson HS, Reynolds R, Mason J. Fexofenadine HCl is safe and effective for treatment of chronic idiopathic urticaria. Ann Allergy Asthma Immunol 2000; 84:517–522.

39. Kaplan AP, Spector SL, Meeves S, et al. Once-daily fexofenadine treatment for chronic idiopathic urticaria: a multicenter, randomized, double-blind, placebo-controlled study. Ann Allergy Asthma Immunol 2005; 94:662–669.

40. Caproni M, Volpi W, Giomi B, et al. Cellular adhesion molecules in chronic urticaria: modulation of serum levels occurs during levocetirizine treatment. Br J Dermatol 2006; 155: 1270–1274.

41. Nettis E, Colanardi MC, Barra L, et al. Levocetirizine in the treatment of chronic idiopathic urticaria: a randomized, double-blind, placebo-controlled study. Br J Dermatol 2006; 154: 533–538.

42. Kapp A, Pichler WJ. Levocetirizine is an effective treatment in patients suffering from chronic idiopathic urticaria: a randomized, double-blind, placebo-controlled, parallel, multicenter study. Int J Dermatol 2006; 45:469–474.

43. Gimenez-Arnau A, Pujol RM, Ianosi S, et al. Rupatadine in the treatment of chronic idiopathic urticaria: a double-blind, randomized, placebo-controlled multicentre study. Allergy 2007; 62: 539–546.

44. Handa S, Dogra S, Kumar B. Comparative efficacy of cetirizine and fexofenadine in the treatment of chronic idiopathic urticaria. J Dermatolog Treat 2004; 15:55–57.

45. Garg G, Thami GP. Comparative efficacy of cetirizine and levocetirizine in chronic idiopathic urticaria. J Dermatolog Treat 2007; 18:23–24.

46. Potter PC, Kapp A, Mauer M, et al. Comparison of the efficacy of levocetirizine 5 mg and desloratadine 5 mg in chronic urticaria patients. Allergy 2008 (in press).

47. Brodell LA, Beck LA. Differential diagnosis of chronic urticaria. Ann Allergy Asthma Immunol 2008; 100:181–188.

48. Frank MM. Hereditary angioedema. J Allergy Clin Immunol 2008; 121:S398–S401.

49. Sheikh A, ten Broek VM, Brown SGA, et al. H_1-antihistamines for the treatment of anaphylaxis with and without shock. Cochrane Database Syst Rev 2007; 1:CD006160.

50. Asero R. Chronic unremitting urticaria: is the use of antihistamines above the licensed dose effective? A preliminary study of cetirizine at licensed and above-licensed doses. Clin Exp Dermatol 2007; 32:34–38.

51. Wyngaarden JB, Seevers MH. The toxic effects of antihistaminic drugs. JAMA 1951; 145:277–282.

52. Okamura N, Yanai K, Higuchi M, et al. Functional neuroimaging of cognition impaired by a classical antihistamine, d-chlorpheniramine. Br J Pharmacol 2000; 129:115–123.

53. Tashiro M, Mochizuki H, Iwabuchi K, et al. Roles of histamine in regulation of arousal and cognition: functional neuroimaging of histamine H_1 receptors in human brain. Life Sci 2002; 72:409–414.

54. Tashiro M, Sakurada Y, Iwabuchi K, et al. Central effects of fexofenadine and cetirizine: measurement of psychomotor performance, subjective sleepiness, and brain histamine H_1 receptor occupancy using ^{11}C-doxepin positron emission tomography. J Clin Pharmacol 2004; 44:890–900.

55. Tashiro M, Mochizuki H, Sakurada Y, et al. Brain histamine H_1 receptor occupancy of orally administered antihistamines measured by positron emission tomography with ^{11}C-doxepin in a placebo-controlled crossover study design in healthy subjects: a comparison of olopatadine and ketotifen. Br J Clin Pharmacol 2006; 61:16–26.

56. Chen C, Hanson E, Watson JW, et al. P-glycoprotein limits the brain penetration of nonsedating but not sedating H_1 antagonists. Drug Metab Dispos 2003; 31:312–318.

57. Shamsi Z, Hindmarch I. Sedation and antihistamines: a review of inter-drug differences using proportional impairment ratios. Hum Psychopharmacol 2000; 15(suppl 1):S3–S30.

58. McEvoy LK, Smith ME, Fordyce M, et al. Characterizing impaired functional alertness from diphenhydramine in the elderly with performance and neurophysiologic measures. Sleep 2006; 29:957–966.

59. Tashiro M, Horikawa E, Mochizuki H, et al. Effects of fexofenadine and hydroxyzine on brake reaction time during car-driving with cellular phone use. Hum Psychopharmacol 2005; 20: 501–509.

60. Verster JC, de Weert AM, Bijtjes SIR, et al. Driving ability after acute and sub-chronic administration of levocetirizine and diphenhydramine: a randomized, double-blind, placebo-controlled trial. Psychopharmacology (Berl) 2003; 169:84–90.

61. Nicholson AN, Handford ADF, Turner C, et al. Studies on performance and sleepiness with the H_1 antihistamine, desloratadine. Aviat Space Environ Med 2003; 74:809–815.

62. Nicholson AN, Stone BM, Turner C, et al. Antihistamines and aircrew: usefulness of fexofenadine. Aviat Space Environ Med 2000; 71:2–6.

63. Vuurman EFPM, Rikken GH, Muntjewerff ND, et al. Effects of desloratadine, diphenhydramine, and placebo on driving performance and psychomotor performance measurements. Eur J Clin Pharmacol 2004; 60:307–313.

64. Scharf M, Berkowitz D. Effects of desloratadine and alcohol coadministration on psychomotor performance. Curr Med Res Opin 2007; 23:313–321.

65. Barbanoj MJ, Garcia-Gea C, Antonijoan R, et al. Evaluation of the cognitive, psychomotor and pharmacokinetic profiles of rupatadine, hydroxyzine and cetirizine, in combination with alcohol, in healthy volunteers. Hum Psychopharmacol 2006; 21:13–26.

66. Liu B, Jia Z, Geng X, et al. Selective inhibition of Kir currents by antihistamines. Eur J Pharmacol 2007; 558:21–26.

67. Pragst F, Herre S, Bakdash A. Poisonings with diphenhydramine: a survey of 68 clinical and 55 death cases. Forensic Sci Int 2006; 161:189–197.

68. Nine JS, Rund CR. Fatality from diphenhydramine monointoxication: a case report and review of the infant, pediatric, and adult literature. Am J Forensic Med Pathol 2006; 27:36–41.

69. Simons FER, on behalf of the ETAC Study Group. Prospective, long-term safety evaluation of the H_1-receptor antagonist cetirizine in very young children with atopic dermatitis. J Allergy Clin Immunol 1999; 104:433–440.

70. Simons FER, on behalf of the Early Prevention of Asthma in Atopic Children (EPAAC) Study Group. Safety of levocetirizine treatment in young atopic children: an 18-month study. Pediatr Allergy Immunol 2007; 18:535–542.

71. Grimfeld A, Holgate ST, Canonica GW, et al. Prophylactic management of children at risk for recurrent upper respiratory infections: the Preventia I Study. Clin Exp Allergy 2004; 34: 1665–1672.

72. Serreau R, Komiha M, Blanc F, et al. Neonatal seizures associated with maternal hydroxyzine hydrochloride in late pregnancy. Reprod Toxicol 2005; 20:573–574.

73. Scharman EJ, Erdman AR, Wax PM, et al. Diphenhydramine and dimenhydrinate poisoning: an evidence-based consensus guideline for out-of-hospital management. Clin Toxicol (Phila) 2006; 44:205–223.

20

Treatment of Chronic Urticaria: Approaches other than Antihistaminics

Allen P. Kaplan
Department of Medicine, Medical University of South Carolina, Charleston, South Carolina, U.S.A.

INTRODUCTION

The treatment of chronic urticaria, as with virtually all other types of urticaria, begins with antihistamines as described in the preceding chapter. The amount and type used depends on the severity of urticaria and can be as simple as employing one of the second-generation antihistamines such as fexofenadine (1,2), desloratidine (3), cetirizine (4,5), or levocetirizine (6) or more complex protocols employing high doses of sedating antihistamines such as hydroxyzine (50 mg four times daily) or a comparable dosage of diphenhydramine or doxepin (7). The latter agents are particularly useful for treatment of patients with severe disease in whom a double-dose of the nonsedating antihistamines provide only minimal relief. The relief of pruritis and decrease in intensity of urticaria and angioedema may be due to very large quantities of histamine released into the skin under these circumstances. Similar doses of hydroxyzine or diphenhydramine are needed to control severe dermatographism, a disorder exclusively due to histamine release into the skin, and a dose-dependent diminution of symptoms can be observed in patients who are not relieved with a double-dose of nonsedating antihistaminics. The efficacy of first-generation antihistamines used in this fashion to treat chronic urticaria or angioedema may relate to properties other than blockade of H_1 receptors, such as effects on mast cell and basophil degranulation or influx of cells [CD4(+) lymphocytes, monocytes, eosinophils, and neutrophils] characteristic of chronic urticaria and delayed pressure urticaria (8–10). Somewhat greater antihistamine effect may be observed upon addition of an H_2 receptor antagonist because approximately 15% of cutaneous venule histamine receptors are of this subtype (11). Blockade of the H_1 receptor is, however, required to observe a significant effect. H_2 receptor antagonists also are useful if corticosteroid is required to control severe chronic urticaria and angioedema, since they provide protection against the consequences of steroid-induced hyperacidity.

Sedation seen with first-generation antihistamines (12–14) may preclude their use for treatment of allergic rhinitis, but should not necessarily limit their use in chronic urticaria (7). The reason is that the side effects of corticosteroids or cyclosporine, the most effective agents identified to date, are far more serious and their employment when there is little or no response to second- or third-generation antihistamines can lead to considerable disability that can be avoided. Furthermore, the studies of sedation are also not adequate for our purposes because no such studies include patients with chronic urticaria; normal persons are typically employed. A proper study would assess sedation with q.i.d. dosage for one to two weeks (not single doses or nighttime doses or short bursts), since this is the recommended approach for maximal efficacy and production of tolerance to any sedation present (7). A meta-analysis attempting to shed further light on this issue found the second- and third-generation antihistamininics to be less sedating but also felt the data were not definitive (15) with concerns regarding deficiencies in the trials they reported (16). This chapter will deal primarily with agents other than antihistaminics and will report on studies demonstrating efficacy, and comment on the utility (or lack thereof) of modalities that require further investigation.

LEUKOTRIENE ANTAGONISTS

Although these agents were originally marketed for the treatment of asthma, new studies suggest their efficacy in allergic rhinitis as well as chronic urticaria. Both zafirlukast and montelukast have been shown to be superior to placebo in the treatment of patients with chronic urticaria (17,18), thus leukotrienes may also contribute to hives and swelling as has been suggested by recent in vitro studies (19,20). These agents have been studied when added to antihistamines to determine whether additional benefit is obtained, but the results are variable, with some studies demonstrating additional benefit (21) and others finding none (22). They are certainly worth trying because toxicity is low and may obviate the need for agents such as corticosteroids or contribute to urticaria control with a lower dosage. A leucotriene synthesis inhibitor, zileutin (Zyflor), has not been studied in chronic urticaria, but anecdotal reports suggest some efficacy in treating idiopathic angioedema that is unresponsive to antihistamines.

SYMPATHOMIMETIC AGENTS

Oral sympathomimetic agents such as terbutaline, a $\beta2$ selective adrenergic agonist, have been tried in patients with chronic urticaria and angioedema to decrease erythema and swelling. However, the effect upon urticaria is quite low and not comparable to subcutaneous epinephrine (which, for emergency use, gives prompt relief of pruritus with regression of urticaria, as well as halting progression of angioedema), and the side effects are substantial. These include difficulty in sleeping, feeling jittery, and tachycardia. In general, these agents are not recommended.

CORTICOSTEROIDS

There are many patients whose symptoms are not sufficiently controlled by any dosage of antihistamines, including the addition of H_2 receptor antagonists and leucotriene antagonists. Under such circumstances, it is reasonable to consider employment of corticosteroids. However, use in a chronic (for many months, at least) fashion must be tempered by the potential side effects. For that reason, alternate-day steroid therapy, in a starting dosage range of 20 to 25 mg every other day has been recommended (7,23). Although a tapering short course of daily corticosteroids can be employed for treatment of a severe acute exacerbation of urticaria and angioedema (e.g., 40–50 mg/day for 3 days in succession and then tapered by 5 mg/day). If this is done repeatedly it is far more dangerous and less effective than use of alternate-day steroids at a fixed dosage. Symptoms of the disease vary from day to day but the dosage of alternate-day steroids should be reassessed at two to three week intervals for optimal control of symptoms. Then the dosage can be decreased at a rate of 2.5 to 5.0 mg every 2 to 3 weeks depending on symptom control down to 10 mg every other day (q.o.d.). Other medications should be retained at a maximal dosage until the patient has been completely tapered off steroids. To decrease further from 10 mg q.o.d., the decrement can usually employ changes of 2.5 to 5.0 mg at a time, i.e., 7.5 mg q.o.d., 5.0 mg q.o.d., 2.5 mg q.o.d., etc. however some patients may become too symptomatic as very low dosages are employed. One choice is to use 1 mg prednisone tablets, to try to decrease the dosage by 1 mg every 7 to 10 days. Although use of daily steroids has not been recommended, (23) we have recently employed 10 to 12 mg each day for 3 weeks with a taper of 1 mg every 7 to 10 days as an alternative to alternate-day steroid. We are often referred patients taking 30 to 60 mg of prednisone daily for months at a time with weight gains of 30 to 100 pounds, steroid-induced diabetes, steroid myopathy, etc. Steroids should *never* be employed in this way for chronic urticaria. I have personally not prescribed a sustained daily dosage exceeding 15 mg in the last 10,000 patients.

Although the efficacy of corticosteroids as a treatment for chronic urticaria is generally accepted, there are no long-term studies that document the optimal dosage, duration, extent of side effects, or cost-effectiveness. Thus the manner in which they are employed, as recommended herein, is based on personal experience. Corticosteriods have little or no effect upon cutaneous mast cell degranulation, thus they are generally ineffective as treatment for physically-induced hives such as cold urticaria, cholinergic urticaria, or dermatographism. They would likewise not be expected to affect mast cell degranulation caused by anti-IgE receptor autoantibodies or by C5a (see chap. 17). Instead, like the allergic late-phase reaction, they would act to prevent the perivascular cellular infiltrate that characterizes chronic urticaria and delayed pressure urticaria (24–28). The persistence of symptoms over many hours or even one to two days with each outbreak of hives is dependent on this cellular infiltrate. Thus, the state of the art in treating chronic urticaria is akin to the treatment of asthma before inhaled corticosteroids were available. Unfortunately urticaria cannot be treated topically, as is true of atopic dermatitis.

The commonly encountered side effects of steroid use, as described above, are weight gain and gradual development of cushingoid features in those patients in whom tapering of the dosage is particularly slow. These can be minimized with care to diet and exercise. Symptoms abate as the dosage decreases and are reversible once steroids are eliminated. More severe side effects (e.g., hypertension, diabetes, asceptic necrosis, or thrombophlebitis) are rarely encountered if the aforementioned limits to steroid use are followed, and if none of these are present before steroid use is begun. The presence of any of these disorders in a patient with chronic urticaria is a relative contraindication to corticosteroid use, and other modalities should be employed whenever possible.

ADDITIONAL/EXPERIMENTAL AGENTS

Other anti-inflammatory drugs have been tried in patients with chronic urticaria. Success has been reported employing colchicine (29), sulfasalazine (30), hydroxychloroquine (31), dapsone (29,32), intravenous gamma globulin (33), plasmapharesis (34), and cyclosporine (35–38). There have been no long-term studies of any of these agents in large numbers of patients, thus most reports are anecdotal observations regarding particular patients with the exception of the studies of cyclosporine by Gratten et al., and Toubi et al., which are blinded and controlled (37,38).

Hydroxychloroquin has been ineffective, in general, in our experience with the exception of treatment of the hypocomplementemic urticarial vasculitis syndrome (see chap. 21) for which hydroxychloroquine may be the drug of choice (39). Dapsone has generally been the most effective for the treatment of cutaneous disorders, in which a neutrophilic infiltrate is prominent. Thus it does have efficacy in some patients with urticarial vasculitis, but its utility in those with severe chronic urticaria is questionable. Perhaps there is logic in trying it for those patients with neutrophil-predominant chronic urticaria (40), who make up an uncommon subgroup of patients who are often refractory to treatment. Intravenous gamma globulin is extremely expensive, but has been successful employed by one of us (M. Greaves) (33). Plasmapharesis has been strikingly beneficial in the series of patients in which it was tried, and provides additional evidence in favor of the pathogenicity of IgG and anti-IgE receptor antibody (34). Thus it is most likely to work if the presence of antireceptor antibody has been documented. Yet it too is an expensive, inconvenient modality that places restrictions on the patient as much as hemodialysis might, but may be employed in selected patients who are willing to try it. The latest study suggesting efficacy of sulfasalazine has no control group thus the result is not firm (41). Furthermore treatment of hives with an aspirin-like compound and a sulfa-derivative seems odd.

Thus far, the most promising has been the use of cyclosporine (25–27) in patients whose disease is refractory to a combination of antihistaminics (H_1 and H_2 antagonists), plus leucotriene inhibitors. It is recommended as an alternate to corticosteroid use. It is often essential for patients who require inordinate dosage of corticosteroid, or where there is a contraindication to the use of corticosteroids. We have each observed many striking successes using a 200 to 300 mg per day dosage range (in adults), and have rarely encountered renal toxicity or hypertension. Periodic checks of blood pressure, blood urea nitrogen (BUN), creatinine, and urinalysis are made every six weeks. A trial of three months is warranted to determine whether it is or is not efficacious in any particular patient. A stepwise general approach to the treatment of chronic urticaria is outlined in Table 1.

Table 1 Stepwise Approach to the Treatment of Chronic Urticaria

1. Maximize H_1 and H_2 receptor blockade with appropriate antihistaminics depending on severity.*
2. Consider adding a leucotriene antagonist.
3. Alternate day corticosteroids starting at 20 mg prednisone (or equivalent) every other day. Decrease by 2.5–5.0 mg every 3 wk. Daily prednisone at 10–12 mg/day with a taper of 1 mg every 7–10 days is an alternative approach.
4. If refractory to corticosteroids or the dose required to achieve reasonable control is too high, consider cyclosporine 100 mg b.i.d., maximal dose 100 mg t.i.d.

*Mildest patients—either fexofenadine 180 mg, desloratidine 5 mg or cetirizine 10 mg as a single agent.
Somewhat more severe—fexofenadine 180 mg or desloratidine 5 mg in a.m., plus cetirizine 10 mg midday, and bedtime.
Most severe—fexofenadine 180 mg or desloratidine 5 mg in a.m., plus hydroxazine 50 mg q.i.d. or diphenlydramine 50 mg q.i.d., plus ranitidine 150 mg b.i.d. or cimetidine 400 mg b.i.d.

CONTROVERSIAL MEASURES

Although there is a clear association of chronic urticaria with Hashimoto's thyroiditis, it is not clear whether thyroid hormone can be employed for treatment of chronic urticaria and angioedema. Certainly anyone who is hypothyroid should be treated; however, there are studies suggesting that raising thyroid levels in euthyroid patients possessing antithyroid antibodies will substantially improve their urticaria (42,43), while other studies are negative (44). This is an area, in which a large study is required to answer the question. However one of us (AK) has added thyroid hormone to the regimen of 10 patients with severe disease and did not observe any difference in their course and do not recommend use of thyroid hormone in this manner. It is of interest that many patients who have Hashimoto's thyroiditis requiring thyroid replacement therapy present with chronic urticaria years later. Thus replacement at an appropriate level does not seem to prevent urticaria. Hashimoto's thyroiditis also has an increased incidence in patients with autoimmune polyglandular syndrome, Type I diabetes mellitus, vitiligo, and pernicious anemia. There is no literature to suggest that thyroid hormone improves any of these other autoimmune manifestations nor does treatment of urticaria influence thyroid disease. It seems likely that these are all associated autoimmune abnormalities reflecting an underlying immune dysregulation, but that they do not cause each other; treatment of one is not likely to affect another.

The role of heliobacter pylori in the pathogenesis of chronic urticaria and angioedema is also controversial. There are studies suggesting that eradication of the organism leads to marked improvement of the urticaria (45–47), and studies in which its eradication had no significant effect upon urticaria (48,49). The rate of infection of the population at large with this organism is very high (50), thus a large proportion of patients with chronic urticaria may test positive even if gastrointestinal symptoms are not evident. One recent publication reviewed the literature and concluded that the bulk of evidence is against a causative role, but one should not rule out an indirect contribution (51). Clearly the number of persons infected by helicobacter pylori who do not have chronic urticaria is substantial, and the number of patients with chronic urticaria who are infected with heliobacter pylori is about 40% to 50%. Whether this percentage exceeds that of the general population is not clear, thus the best studies of this issue are those that treat the organism in an attempt to affect the urticaria. However, in the past, the number of patients studied has been insufficient and critical controls omitted. A large controlled, blinded study is needed which include a placebo control, preferably antibiotics that are ineffective for helicobacter pylori, as well as antibiotic treatment of *Helicobacter pylori* negative patients. The use of patient questionnaires, plus objective assessment of the frequency and severity of symptoms, is required.

Another approach to treatment of chronic urticaria is a diet omitting foods considered to be pseudoallergens (52). These are foodstuffs containing chemical agents that are thought to be responsible for sustaining chronic urticaria. There is no IgE hypersensitivity associated with this, and no molecular mechanism has been discerned. Pseudoallergens include artificial food dyes, preservatives, and sweeteners (53), aromatic compounds in wine, tomatoes, and spices (54) as well as phenols such as p-hydroxybenzoic acid, citrus and orange oil, salicylates, etc. (55). The remission rate attributed to elimination diets varies from 30% to 90%, yet double-blind, placebo-controlled food challenge with these substances contained in capsules have failed to reproduce urticaria (56,57). Studies have proposed that mixtures of pseudoallergen are needed and that the symptoms are dose-dependent. While prominent in considerations regarding chronic urticaria in Europe, pseudoallergy is not thought to be pathogenically relevant in the USA. The reasons are that proper controlled studies have not been carried out in terms of efficacy of a pseudoallergy elimination diet or reproducible symptoms on challenge with pseudoallergens. There is also a strong bias against causes of urticaria with no known molecular or immune mechanism, the fact that patients whose urticaria has remitted can eat anything without having urticaria, and a long history of putative foodstuffs as a cause of urticaria that have been proven to be erroneous. Perhaps properly controlled studies in the future will determine whether such dietary manipulation has any value.

REFERENCES

1. Finn Jr AF, Kaplan AP, Fretwell R, et al. A double-blind placebo-controlled trial of fexofenadine HCl in the treatment of chronic idiopathic urticaria. J Allergy Clin Immunol 1999; 103:1071–1078.
2. Nelson HS, Reynolds R, Mason J. Fexofenadine HCl is safe and effective for treatment of chronic idiopathic urticaria. Ann Allergy Asthma Immunol 2000; 84:517–522.
3. Ring J, Hein R, Ganger A, et al. One-daily desloratadine improves the signs and symptoms of chronic idiopathic urticaria: a randomized double-blind, placebo-controlled study. Int J Dermatol 2001; 40:1–5.
4. La Rosa M, Leonardi S, Marchese G, et al. Double-blind multicenter study on the efficacy and tolerability of ectirizine compared with oxatomide in chronic idiopathic urticaria in preschool children. Ann Allergy Asthma Immunol 2001; 87:48–53.
5. Breneman DL. Cetirizine versus hydroxizine and placebo in chronic idiopathic urticaria. Ann Pharmacol 1996; 30:1075–1079.
6. Clough GF, Boutsiouki P, Church MK. Comparison of the effects of levocetirizine and loratadine on histamine-induced wheal, flare, and itch in human skin. Int J Dermatol 2001; 70:1–5.
7. Kaplan AP. Chronic urticaria and angioedema. N Eng J Med 2002; 346:175–179.
8. Juhlin L, Pihl-Lundin I. Effects of antihistamines on cutaneous reactions and influx of eosinophils after local injection of PAF, kallikrein, and compound 48/80 and histamine in patients with chronic urticaria and health subjects. Acta Derm Venereol 1992; 72:197–200.
9. Ciprandi G, Buscaglia S, Pesce GP, et al. Cetirizine reduces inflammatory cell recruitment and ICAM-1 (or CD54) expression on conjunctival epithelium both in early and late-phase reaction after specific antigenic challenge. J Allergy Clin Immunol 1995; 95:612–621.
10. Jinquan T, Reimert CM, Deleuran B, et al. Cetirizine inhibits the in vitro and ex vivo chemotactic response of T lymphocytes and monocytes. J Allergy Clin Immunol 1995; 95:979–986.
11. Robertson I, Greaves MW. Responses of human skin blood vessels to synthetic histamine analogues. Br J Clin Pharmacol 1978; 5:319–322.
12. Weiler JM, Bloomfield JR, Woodworth GG, et al. Effects of Fexofenadine, Diphenhydramine, and alcohol on driving performance. A randomized, placebo-controlled trial in the Iowa driving simulator. Ann Int Med 2000; 132:354–363.
13. Verster JC, Volkerts ER, van Oosterwijck AW, et al. Acute and subchronic effects of levocetirizine and diphenhydramine on memory functioning, psychomotor performance, and mood. J Allergy Clin Immunol 2003; 111:623–627.
14. Bender BG, Berning S, Dudden R, et al. Sedation and performance impairment of diphenhydramine and second-generation antihistamines: a meta-analysis. J Allergy Clin Immunol 2003; 111:770–776.
15. Shapiro GG. Antihistamine meta-analysis leaves uncertainty. J Allergy Clin Immunol 2003; 111:695–696.
16. Ellis MH. Successful treatment of chronic urticaria with leukotiene antagonists. J Allergy Clin Immunol 1998; 102:876–877.
17. Spector S, Tan RA. Antileucotrienes in chronic urticaria. J Allergy Clin Immunol 1998; 101:572.

18. Erbagci Z. The leukotriene receptor antagonist montelukast in the treatment of chronic idiopathic urticaria: a single-blind placebo-controlled, crossover clinical study. J Allergy Clin Immunol 2002; 110:484–488.

19. Ferrer M, Luquin E, Sanchez-Ibarrole A, et al. Secretion of cytokines, histamine, and leukotrienes in chronic urticaria. Int Arch Allergy Appl Immunol 2002; 129:254–260.

20. Wedi B, Novacovic V, Koerner M, et al. Chronic urticaria serum induces histamine release, leukotriene production, and basophil CD63 surface expression – inhibitory effects of anti-inflammatory drugs. J Allergy Clin Immunol 2000; 105:552–560.

21. Bagenstose SE, Levin L, Bernstein JA. The addition of Zafirlukast to cetirizine improves the treatment of chronic urticaria in patients with positive autologous serum skin test results. J Allergy Clin Immunol 2004; 113:134–140.

22. Di Lorenzo G, Pacor ML, Mansueto P, et al. Randomized placebo-controlled trial comparing desloratadine and montelukast in monotherapy and desloratadine plus montelukust in combined therapy for chronic idiopathic urticaria. J Allergy Clin Immunol 2004; 114:619–625.

23. Kaplan AP. Urticaria and angioedema. In: Kaplan AP, ed. Allergy 2nd ed. Philadelphia: WB Saunders Co, 1997:573–582.

24. Natbony SF, Phillips M, Elias JM, et al. Histologic studies of chronic idiopathic urticaria. J Allergy Clin Immunol 1983; 71:177–183.

25. Elias J, Boss E, Kaplan AP. Studies of the cellular infiltrate of chronic idiopathic urticaria: prominence of T lymphocytes, monocytes, and mast cells. J Allergy Clin Immunol 1986; 78:914–918.

26. Sabroe RA, Poon E, Orchard GE, et al. Cutaneous inflammatory infiltrate in chronic idiopathic urticaria: comparison of patients with and without anti-FcεR1 or anti-IgE autoantibodies. J Allergy Clin Immunol 1991; 103:484–493.

27. Barlow RJ, Warburton F, Watson K, et al. Diagnosis and incidence of delayed pressure urticaria in patients with chronic urticaria. J Am Acad Dermatmol 1993; 29:954–958.

28. Ying S, Kikuchi Y, Meng Q, et al. T_H1/T_H2 cytokines and inflammatory cells in skin biopsy specimens from patients with chronic idiopathic urticaria: comparison with the allergen induced late-phase cutaneous reaction. J Allergy Clin Immunol 2002; 109:694–700.

29. Tharp MD. Chronic urticaria: pathophysiology and treatment approaches. J Allergy Clin Immunol 1996; 98:S325–S330.

30. Jaffa AM. Sulfasalazine in the treatment of corticosteroid-dependent chronic idiopathic urticaria. J Allergy Clin Immunol 1991; 88:964–966.

31. Reeves GEM, Boyle MJ, Bonfield J, et al. Impact of hydroxychloroquine therapy on chronic urticaria: chronic autoimmune urticaria study and evaluation. Internal Med J 2004; 34:182–186.

32. Raap U, Liekenbrocker T, Wieczorek D, et al. New therapeutic strategies for the different subtypes of urticaria. Hautarzt 2004; 55:361–366.

33. O'Donnell BF, Barr RM, Kobza Black A, et al. Intravenous immunoglobulin in autoimmune chronic urticaria. Brit J Dermatol 1998; 138:101–106.

34. Gratten CEH, Frances DM, Slater NGP, et al. Plasmapharesis for severe unremitting chronic urticaria. Lancet 1992; 339:1078–1080.

35. Barlow RJ, Black AK, Greaves MW. Treatment of severe chronic urticaria with cyclosporin A. Eur J Dermatol 1993; 3:273–275.

36. Fradin MS, Ellis CN, Goldforb MT, et al. Oral cyclosporine for severe chronic idiopathic urticaria and angioedema. J Am Acad Dermatol 1991; 25:1065–1067.

37. Gratten CEH, O'Donnell BF, Frances DM, et al. Randomized double-blind study of cyclosporin in chronic idiopathic urticaria. Brit J Dermatol 1991; 143:365–372.

38. Toubi E, Blant A, Kressel A, et al. Low-dose cyclosporin A in the treatment of severe chronic idiopathic urticaria. Allergy 1997; 52:312–316.

39. Lopez LR, Davis KC, Kohler PF, et al. The hypocomplementemic urticarial vasculitis syndrome: therapeutic response to hydroxychloroquine. J Allergy Clin Immunol 1984; 73:600–603.

40. Peters MS, Winkelmann RK. Neutrophilic urticaria. Br J Dermatol 1985; 113:25–30.

41. McGirt LY, Vasagar K, Gober LM, et al. Successful treatment of recalcitrant chronic idiopathic urticaria with sulfasalazine. Arch Dermatol 2006; 142:1337–1342.

42. Gaig P, Garcia-Ortega P, Enrique E, et al. Successful treatment of chronic idiopathic urticaria: a practice parameter. Ann Allergy Asthma Immunol 2000; 85:521–544.

43. Rumbyrt JS, Katz JL, Schocket AL. Resolution of chronic urticaria in patients with thyroid autoimmunity. J Allergy Clin Immunol 1995; 96:901–905.

44. Tedeshi A, Lorini M, Asero R. Antithyroid peroxidase IgE in patients with chronic urticaria. J Allergy Clin Immunol 2001; 108:467–468.

45. Wedi B, Wagner S, Werfel T, et al. Prevalence of helicobacter pylori-associated gastritis in chronic urticaria. Int Arch Allergy Immunol 1998; 116:288–294.

46. DiCampli C, Gasbarrini A, Nucera E, et al. Beneficial effects of helicobacter pylori eradication on chronic idiopathic urticaria. Digest Dis Sci 1998; 43:1226–1229.

47. Liutu M, Kalimo K, Uksila J, et al. Etiological aspects of chronic urticaria. Int J Dermatol 1998; 37:515–519.

48. Schnyder B, Helbing A, Pichler WJ. Chronic idiopathic urticaria: natural course and association with helicobacter pylori infection. Int Arch Allergy Immunol 1999; 119:60–63.

49. Valsecchi R, Pigatto P. Chronic urticaria and helicobacter pylori. Acta Dermato-Venereologica 1998; 78:440–442.

50. Becker H, Meyer M, Paul E. Remission ratio of chronic urticaria: "Spontaneous" healing as a result of eradication of helicobacter pylori? Hautarzt 1998; 49:907–911.

51. Greaves MW. Chronic idiopathic urticaria (C1V) and helicobacter pylori – not directly causative, but could there be a link. Allergy Clin Immunol International 2001; 13:23–26.

52. Zuberbier T, Chantraine-Hess S, Hartmann K, et al. Pseudoallergen-free diet in the treatment of chronic urticaria. A prospective study. Acta Derm Venereol 1995; 75:484–487.

53. Young E. Prevelence of intolerance to food additives. Environ Toxicol Pharmacol 1997; 4: 111–114.

54. Zuberbeir T, Pfrommer C, Specht K, et al. Aromatic components of food as novel eliciting factors of pseudoallergic reactions in chronic urticaria. J Allergy Clin Immunol 2002; 109:343–348.

55. Guerra L, Rogkakou A, Massacane P, et al. Role of contact sensitization in chronic urticaria. J of the Am Acad Dermatol 2007; 56:88–90.

56. DiLorenzo G, Pacur ML, Mansueto P, et al. Food-additive-induced urticaria: a survey of 838 patients with recurrent chronic idiopathic urticaria. Int Arch Allergy Immunol 2005; 138:235–242.

57. Supramaniam G, Warner JO. Artificial food additive intolerance in patients with angioedema and urticaria. Lancet 1986; 2:907–919.

21
Urticarial Vasculitis/Venulitis

Nicholas A. Soter
*The Ronald O. Perelman Department of Dermatology, New York University
School of Medicine; Charles C. Harris Skin and Cancer Pavilion; and Tisch
Hospital, The University Hospital of NYU, New York, New York, U.S.A.*

INTRODUCTION

Episodes of urticaria are an uncommon manifestation of cutaneous necrotizing vasculitis that involves venules. There is a spectrum of disease that ranges from cutaneous involvement to multisystem disease with extracutaneous manifestations. Although the variety of skin lesions and extracutaneous manifestations have led to a plethora of diagnostic appellations (1–20), the terms urticarial vasculitis or venulitis currently are widely used. A subset of patients with urticarial venulitis and more extensive systemic manifestations, hypocomplementemia with low C1q levels, and an anti-C1q autoantibody has been designated as the hypocomplementemic-urticarial-vasculitis syndrome (HUVS) (19). Urticarial venulitis may occur in association with a variety of medical disorders, with infections, and with the administration of therapeutic agents; however, it may be an idiopathic condition (Table 1).

CLINICAL MANIFESTATIONS

Cutaneous Features

Urticarial venulitis involves the skin and infrequently the mucous membranes.

Between 60% and 80% (19,21,22) of afflicted individuals are women. A few cases have been reported in infants and children (22–31). There is one report of urticarial venulitis that occurred in identical twins (32).

The skin lesions appear as raised, superficial, erythematous, edematous, and circumscribed wheals. Distinctive dermatologic features include wheals with foci of purpura (Fig. 1), induration, residual contusions, and transient hyperpigmentation (Table 2). When the wheals are examined by skin surface microscopy with a dermatoscope, a purpuric globular pattern on a patchy orange-brown background is noted (33). Other skin manifestations include angioedema, which is prominent in patients with HUVS (19,34), macular erythema, livedo reticularis, nodules over the olecranon process (35), bullae

Table 1 Classification

Serum sickness
Connective-tissue disorders
Hematologic and other malignant conditions
Infections
Therapeutic agents and chemicals
Physical urticarias
Schnitzler's syndrome
Idiopathic urticarial venulitis
Hypocomplementemic-urticarial-vasculitis syndrome with anti-Clq autoantibody

Table 2 Dermatologic Features

Distinctive features
   Long-lasting wheals
   Wheals with foci of purpura
   Induration
   Residual contusions and/or hyperpigmentation
Other features
   Angioedema
   Macular erythema
   Livedo reticularis
   Nodules over the olecranon process
   Bullae
   Erythema multiforme–like lesions

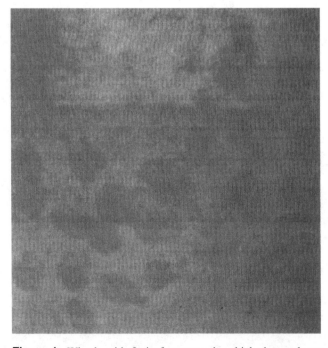

Figure 1 Wheals with foci of purpura, in which the erythema does not blanch with pressure (diascopy). Note glass slide at the top.

(5,16,17), and lesions that resemble erythema multiforme (9,16). Although the individual urticarial lesions may last fewer than 24 hours, they frequently persist for three to five days. The lesions are pruritic, burning, or painful. Occasionally there are no lesional symptoms. The episodes of urticaria are recurrent or episodic, range in duration from months to years, and vary in frequency. The lesions may be indistinguishable historically and clinically from those of chronic urticaria without vasculitis.

Extracutaneous Manifestations

General features include fever, malaise, and myalgia. Specific organ involvement may involve lymph nodes, liver, spleen, synovia, kidneys, gastrointestinal tract, respiratory tract, eyes, central nervous system, peripheral nerves, and heart (Table 3). At times, patients may experience cutaneous features without extracutaneous involvement.

Arthralgias are a major manifestation; multiple joints, especially knees, ankles, toes, elbows, wrists, and fingers, are affected. A destructive polyarthritis occasionally occurs (36). Examination of a synovial biopsy specimen in one patient showed features of necrotizing vasculitis that were similar to the vascular alterations that were observed in the skin (6). Jaccoud's arthropathy with or without valvular heart disease may occur (34,37–42).

Table 3 Extracutaneous Manifestations

General features
  Fever
  Malaise
  Myalgia
Specific organ involvement
  Lymphadenopathy
  Hepatosplenomegaly
  Synovia
    Arthralgia, arthritis, Jaccoud's arthropathy
  Kidneys
    Glomerulitis, glomerulonephritis with mesangioproliferative and membranoproliferative
      changes, crescentic membranoproliferative glomerulonephritis, nephrotic syndrome,
      end-stage renal disease
  Gastrointestinal tract
    Nausea, vomiting, pain, diarrhea
  Respiratory tract
    Laryngeal edema, dyspnea, chronic obstructive pulmonary disease, restrictive lung disease,
      interstitial lung disease, emphysema, pleural effusion, tracheal stenosis, pulmonary
      hemorrhage, pulmonary hemosiderosis
  Eyes
    Conjunctivitis, episcleritis, iridocyclitis, uveitis, vasculitis of the optic nerve and retina, optic
      atrophy, blindness
  Central nervous system
    Headache, benign intracranial hypertension (pseudotumor cerebri)
  Peripheral nerves
    Neuropathy, cranial nerve paralysis
  Heart
    Arrhythmias, valvular heart disease, pericardial effusion, congestive heart failure, myocardial
      infarct

Renal involvement usually occurs as a mild glomerulitis or glomerulonephritis (5,7,11,43,44). Nephrotic syndrome rarely may develop (45,46). In renal biopsy specimens, mesangioproliferative and membranoproliferative lesions are predominant (11,19,28,43–45,47), and crescentic membranoproliferative glomerulonephritis has been reported (48,49). Interstitial nephritis and immune complex deposition in the interstitium have been noted. In one patient with HUVS, after renal transplantation there was a flare of urticarial venulitis with the development of chronic renal failure (50). Progression to end-stage renal disease is rare (24–26,48,50,51).

Gastrointestinal tract manifestations include nausea, vomiting, pain, and diarrhea. Gastrointestinal hemorrhage is not a feature.

Involvement of the respiratory tract includes laryngeal edema, dyspnea, and chronic obstructive pulmonary manifestations (35), especially in patients with HUVS (52–54), which are more severe in individuals who smoke cigarettes. Restrictive lung disease (55), interstitial lung disease (56), emphysema (57), pleural effusion (58), tracheal stenosis, (41) pulmonary hemorrhage (25,55), and pulmonary hemosiderosis (30) are infrequent findings. Emphysema with a chest radiograph that demonstrated basilar hyperlucency was described in three patients (35,59). Necrotizing vasculitis of the pulmonary venules (60) and emphysema have been observed in lung biopsy specimens (19). In a patient with obstructive airways, histopathologic examination of an explanted lung showed patchy vasculitis and panacinar emphysema (61). In a single patient with pleural effusion, congestive heart failure, and proximal muscle weakness, a muscle biopsy specimen showed an inflammatory myositis with vasculitis (62). One patient with HUVS received a lung transplant and 15 months later was without recurrence of urticarial venulitis (19).

Conjunctivitis, episcleritis, iridocyclitis (63), uveitis, and vasculitis of the optic nerve and retina (64) occur in some individuals, especially in those with HUVS (53). Optic atrophy was reported in one patient (18), and blindness was observed in two patients (18,65).

Central nervous system involvement occurs as headaches and benign intracranial hypertension (pseudotumor cerebri) (11,18,43). Peripheral neuropathy may develop (22), and bilateral involvement of cranial nerves VIII, IX, and X was noted in one patient (66).

Cardiac manifestations include atrial fibrillation (37,67), aortic stenosis and regurgitation, mitral regurgitation, pericardial effusion (19,39), congestive heart failure (62), and myocardial infarct (34,37,41,42,67). The valvular abnormalities involve native aortic and mitral valves and homographic aortic valves (34). These cardiac manifestations may occur in association with Jaccoud's arthropathy with and without hypocomplementemia and anti-C1q autoantibody (34,37,39,42). Raynaud's phenomenon has been reported (18).

ASSOCIATED DISORDERS

Urticarial venulitis has occurred in individuals with serum sickness; with systemic lupus erythematosus (SLE) (68–76), which includes a 4-year-old girl and a 12-year-old girl (68,69); with subacute lupus erythematosus (77,78); with Sjögren's syndrome (22,69,79,80); and in single cases with systemic sclerosis (81) and relapsing polychondritis (82).

Associated hematologic malignant disorders (21), most of which are reported as single cases, include agnogenic myeloid metaplasia, diffuse large B-cell lymphoma (83), Hodgkin's lymphoma (84), B-cell non-Hodgkin's lymphoma (85,86), acute non-lymphocytic leukemia, acute myelogenous leukemia, IgG monoclonal paraproteinemia

(21,87–90), B-cell chronic lymphocytic leukemia (91), megakaryocyte leukemia (92), Castelman's disease (93), and IgA myeloma (94). Other case reports of associations include colon carcinoma (95), malignant testicular teratoma (96), nasopharyngeal carcinoma (97), renal carcinoma (98), cystic teratoma (99), polycythemia vera (100), idiopathic thrombocytopenic purpura, acquired factor VIII deficiency (101), Muckle-Wells syndrome (102), and Cogan's syndrome (103).

Urticarial venulitis has occurred in patients with hepatitis B (104,105) and C (56,106–111) virus infections; in a single patient with hepatitis A virus infection (112); in a patient with Epstein-Barr virus nuclear antigen 1 in the peripheral blood (54); in patients with infectious mononucleosis (113), *Mycoplasma pneumoniae* (114), and Lyme borreliosis (115); in the shunt nephritis syndrome with bacteremia, mixed cryoglobulinemia, and glomerulonephritis (116); and after jejunoileal bypass surgery (117). In a single patient, urticarial venulitis was associated with Hashimoto's thyroiditis and pernicious anemia (118).

Urticarial venulitis has developed after the administration of potassium iodide (119), nonsteroidal anti-inflammatory agents, trimethoprim-sulfamethoxazole (64,120), and in one instance each after the use of fluoxetine (121), paroxetine (122), procarbazine (123), procainamide (124), cimetidine (125), pemetrexed (126), the preservative butylhydroxytoluene in chewing gum (127), and nasal cocaine (128). In a single patient, urticarial venulitis and serum sickness developed after exposure to formaldehyde (129).

Urticarial venulitis has been described in rare instances of dermographism (130), cold urticaria (89,130–132), delayed-pressure urticaria (133), solar urticaria (134,135), and exercise-induced urticaria (99,136–138). The prevalence of necrotizing venulitis in individuals with physical urticaria is unknown, and the importance of this histopathologic finding for prognosis and therapy remains to be determined. Individuals with physical urticarias have provided experimental models for time-course studies of the evolution of necrotizing venulitis in human skin (130,136,137).

Schnitzler's syndrome (139–146) consists of episodes of urticarial venulitis that occur in association with a monoclonal IgM_K M component. Systemic features include fever, lymphadenopathy, hepatosplenomegaly, bone pain, and a sensorimotor neuropathy. Renal failure (145), a chronic inflammatory and demyelinating polyneuropathy (147), nodular regenerative hyperplasia of the liver (148), and the antiphospholipid syndrome with thromboses of the cerebral and coronary arteries and elevated blood levels of homocysteine (149) were reported in single patients. Three patients with an IgG_K M component (88,150,151) and three patients with type A (AA) amyloidosis have been reported (152).

Most patients with urticarial venulitis have an idiopathic disorder and those with HUVS have an anti-Clq autoantibody.

NATURAL HISTORY

The prevalence and natural history of idiopathic urticarial venulitis and its variants is unknown, although patients have been described with historical episodes of cutaneous lesions for up to 25 years (12). In one series with a follow-up period of one year, 40% of patients experienced complete resolution of skin lesions (18). In a series of patients (12), some of whom have been followed for as long as 12 years, associated diseases did not emerge. The evolution of urticarial venulitis to SLE (68,77,153) and to Sjögren's syndrome (154) has been reported. It has been suggested that some patients with idiopathic urticarial venulitis represent a subset of patients with SLE (22,80), but this hypothesis remains speculative. Evolution from urticarial venulitis with normocomplementemia or with hypocomplementemia without low C1q levels to HUVS has not been reported in retrospective and prospective observations that were made over 20 years (53). In patients with associated systemic disorders, the course of urticarial venulitis depends on the prognosis and treatment of the underlying condition. Deaths in patients with urticarial venulitis have occurred from laryngeal edema, obstructive pulmonary disease, respiratory failure, sepsis, end-stage renal disease, valvular heart disease, and myocardial infarcts (18,19,21,34).

In Schnitzler's syndrome, spontaneous remissions have not occurred, and evolution into a lymphoplasmacytic malignant condition, especially Waldenström's macroglobulinemia (155), has been reported in 15% of patients (156).

PATHOGENESIS

Studies in humans implicate immune complexes as the major pathobiologic mechanism in the production of urticarial venulitis. Various types of physical urticaria have served as models for studies on the pathogenesis of urticarial venulitis (130,136,137).

The presence of immune complexes is inferred from the occurrence of serum hypocomplementemia with activation of the classical activating pathway. Tissue immune complexes have been detected by direct immunofluorescence techniques as deposited immunoglobulins and complement proteins. Antigen has been identified in the case of hepatitis B virus. In patients with HUVS, hypocomplementemia, and a low serum C1q level, a low-molecular-weight 7s C1q-precipitin (4–6,9,23), which has been identified as an IgG (13) autoantibody that is directed against the collagen-like region of C1q (19,157–159), has been identified. Although these anti-C1q autoantibodies may contribute to the pathogenesis of urticarial venulitis by binding C1q, there is no direct evidence for their involvement (53). IgG and IgM autoantibodies against IgE, which have not been fully characterized, were detected in some patients with urticarial venulitis (160). Anti-FcεRIα autoantibodies were detected in two patients with urticarial venulitis (161,162). Circulating immune complexes that contained IgG and C3c were detected in a single patient (118).

Although present in skin biopsy specimens of patients with urticarial venulitis, the role of lymphocytes, mononuclear cells, Langerhans cells, and other infiltrating inflammatory cells in the production of urticarial venulitis remains unknown.

Evidence for the role of the mast cell is provided by an analysis of the time course of sequential histopathologic changes in the skin of an individual with circulating immune complexes and hypocomplementemia, in whom cold and acute mechanical trauma elicited urticaria as a manifestation of venulitis (130). Initial mast cell degranulation was followed by the infiltration of neutrophils and then by an influx of eosinophils and basophils, the deposition of fibrin, and venular endothelial-cell necrosis. A postulated sequence of events would be the activation of the mast cell by physical stimuli, the release of vasoactive mediators, the deposition of circulating immune complexes with activation of the complement system, the influx of neutrophils, and the development of urticarial venulitis.

Another analysis of the time course of changes in the skin is provided by a study of the cellular and molecular changes in an individual with exercise-induced urticarial vasculitis (137). At three hours, the number of mast cells decreased and eosinophils appeared around the venules with the deposition of eosinophil peroxidase at 10 hours. Tumor necrosis factor (TNF)-α levels were elevated, and E-selectin and vascular cell adhesion molecule-1 (VCAM-1) were expressed on endothelial cells. At 10 hours, an influx of neutrophils developed with the deposition of neutrophil elastase at 24 hours and the development of urticarial venulitis.

The importance of adhesion molecules in urticarial venulitis (163) was demonstrated by the detection of E-selectin on endothelial cells in skin biopsy specimens of lesions less than 48 hours old from three patients. This observation was associated with the recruitment of an infiltrate of neutrophils expressing CD11b. The endothelial cells expressed human leukocyte antigen (HLA)-DR and very-late activating antigen (VLA)-1 but not P-selectin, and the perivascular cells demonstrated VCAM-1 and HLA-DR.

In some patients with Schnitzler's syndrome (155,164,165), but not in others (166), elevated serum levels of interleukin (IL)-6 and IL-2 receptors were detected. In some patients, serum IgG autoantibodies against IL-1α (142,167,168) and against the α-chain of FcεRIα (169) have been observed.

HISTOPATHOLOGIC AND IMMUNOPATHOLOGIC FEATURES

Skin biopsy specimens stained with hematoxylin-eosin show segmental areas of fibrinoid necrosis of venules and various numbers of infiltrating neutrophils, eosinophils, and mononuclear cells; nuclear debris (leukocytoclasis); and extravasated erythrocytes (6). In one study, mast cell numbers were increased (81). In some reports, rigorous diagnostic criteria were not used, which makes the diagnosis of necrotizing venulitis questionable. Although the histopathologic features and infiltrating cell types are time dependent, one-μm sections (170–172) (Fig. 2) have allowed the recognition of a neutrophil-predominant and a less frequent lymphocyte-predominant pattern of cellular infiltration (170). Endothelial cells exhibit necrotic damage, hypertrophy, or shrinkage (170). Fibrin is deposited both in perivenular and in interstitial locations.

On direct immunofluorescence examination (18,21,173,174), immunoreactants are deposited at the dermal-epidermal junction or about the blood vessels. IgG, IgM, and C3 have been detected more frequently at the dermal-epidermal junction, although IgA, C1q, C4, factor B, properdin, and fibrin occasionally have been reported. IgM, C3, and fibrin have been detected frequently about the blood vessels, although IgG, IgA, IgE, factor B, and properdin have been occasionally noted.

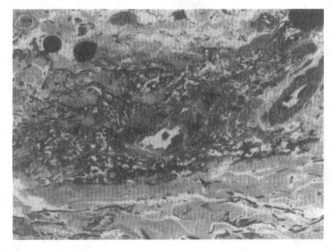

Figure 2 Venule with damaged endothelial cells and perivenular fibrin. The infiltrate contains neutrophils and mononuclear cells. (1-μm section, Giemsa, 100× in the original magnification.)

The prevalence of necrotizing venulitis in biopsy specimens obtained from patients with chronic urticaria has been reported to range from 2% to 50% (174–177), although the data are dependent on the definition of necrotizing venulitis and on reports from tertiary referral centers. Patients in some reports are assumed to have urticarial venulitis based on the presence of hypocomplementemia without histopathologic confirmation in skin biopsy specimens. The prevalence of urticarial venulitis in individuals with chronic urticaria has been suggested to be about 5% (178).

Although urticarial venulitis has been reported in 25% of patients with Schnitzler's syndrome (146), neutrophilic infiltrates without necrotizing venulitis are a more frequent observation in skin biopsy specimens (155). This finding has led to the suggestion that Schnitzler's syndrome should not be classified as urticarial venulitis (155). On direct immunofluorescence study, IgG, IgM, and C3 were detected around the superficial dermal blood vessels (140,144) and IgM along the dermal-epidermal junction (144). IgM autoantibodies of the same isotype can be present in the serum and deposited at the dermal-epidermal junction (144).

LABORATORY FINDINGS

Evaluation of patients with urticarial venulitis requires a history, physical examination, laboratory tests, and consultations (Table 4).

In patients with idiopathic urticarial venulitis and with Schnitzler's syndrome, an elevated erythrocyte sedimentation rate (ESR) is a frequent laboratory abnormality (12,19,22), and it may fluctuate with disease activity (179). Occasionally leukopenia (179) or leukocytosis (12) may occur during flares. The platelet count is normal. Although antinuclear antibodies may be present in low titre, antibodies to double-stranded DNA and Sm antigen are absent. Other laboratory abnormalities may include a positive rheumatoid factor, elevated immunoglobulin levels, cryoglobulins, and a false-positive serologic test for syphilis. Elevated serum creatinine levels and the presence of hematuria and proteinuria may indicate renal involvement. In patients with hepatitis C virus infection, cryoglobulinemia is a frequent feature. In a single patient with hepatitis C virus infection

Table 4 Patient Evaluation

Laboratory evaluation
  Erythrocyte sedimentation rate
  White-cell count with differential analysis
  Platelet count
  Urinalysis with creatinine clearance and 24-hour urine protein
  Blood chemistry profile
  Serum protein electrophoresis
  Hepatitis B antigen
  Hepatitis C antibody
  Cryoglobulins
  CH 50, C1q
  Antinuclear antibody
  Skin biopsy
Consultations with rheumatologists, nephrologists, pulmonologists, cardiologists, ophthalmologists, and neurologists when appropriate

without cryoglobulinemia, IgM anticardiolipin and anti-Ro (SS-A) antibodies were detected (112). In a single patient, there was a positive autologous serum skin test (118), and in two patients, the antibody to FcεRIα was present (162,161).

Patients have been reported with normocomplementemia, hypocomplementemia, and hypocomplementemia with low C1q levels and anti-C1q autoantibodies (6,12,18,19,21). When hypocomplementemia is present, the classical activating pathway is involved, with low levels of C1q and C4 and occasionally of C3 and C5. The complement protein factor B is rarely low (180). C1̄ inhibitor levels are normal. One patient with C2 deficiency and subacute cutaneous lupus erythematosus (71), one patient with a familial partial deficiency of C3 (181), and two patients with C3 nephritic factor activity have been reported (182,183). Patients with Schnitzler's syndrome and genetic C4 deficiency have been reported (168,184). Although individuals with hypocomplementemia have more severe disease (19,20,22,185), systemic manifestations may occur in patients without hypocomplementemia (18).

In Schnitzler's syndrome, additional laboratory tests should include a serum protein electrophoresis and bone radiographs. The patients should be followed for the emergence of a lymphoproliferative disorder.

THERAPY

Placebo-controlled, double blind trials of therapy have not been reported in patients with urticarial venulitis, in those with HUVS, or in those with Schnitzler's syndrome. Most data are reported in small case studies and anecdotal case reports. The cutaneous lesions may respond to oral H_1 antihistamines, nonsteroidal anti-inflammatory agents, colchicine, dapsone, hydroxychloroquine, and when systemic medications are administered for internal organ involvement (20,22,71,154,171,186). Oral glucocorticoids (18,21,22), hydroxychloroquine (19,21,187,188), chloroquine (118), methotrexate (62,189), colchicine (190,191), dapsone (19,28,57,154,192,193), cyclophosphamide (18,21), cyclosporine (46), mycophenolate mofetil (90,194), thalidomide (164), interferon α2a (112), interferon α2b (195), intravenous immunoglobulin (86,196), and anakinra (197) have been reported to be effective in some individuals with systemic features. The skin lesions in one patient became worse after the administration of methotrexate (198). The combination of cyclophosphamide-dexamethasone pulse therapy (199), dapsone and pentoxifylline (200), and glucocorticoids and azathioprine (51) have been reported to be effective in case reports. The combination of doxepin, interferon-α, and ribavirin (109) has been used successfully in a patient with urticarial vasculitis and hepatitis C virus infection. Plasmapheresis resulted in transient resolution in some patients (50,91,154,171). Single patients responded to intramuscular gold injections (201) and to rituximab (78). In some patients with HUVS, pharmacologic control of the cutaneous lesions was associated with increased serum complement levels and decreased levels of anti-C1q autoantibody levels (19).

In Schnitzler's syndrome, treatment with anakinra induced remission in each of eight patients (202). Therapeutic benefit has been achieved in some patients with oral glucocorticoids, hydroxychloroquine, cycloporin (151), thalidomide (202,203), and pefloxacin (204) and in a single patient with rituximab (205). One patient responded to narrow-band ultraviolet B phototherapy (166). The use of psoralen plus ultraviolet A (PUVA) photochemotherapy has allowed the reduction of the prednisone dose (155,206).

REFERENCES

1. McCombs RP, Patterson JF, McMahon HE. Syndromes associated with "allergic" vasculitis. N Engl J Med 1956; 255:251–261.
2. McDuffie FC. Serum complement levels in cutaneous diseases. Br J Dermatol 1970; 82(suppl 5): 20–23.
3. Agnello V, Winchester RJ, Kunkel HG. Precipitin reactions of the C1q component of complement with aggregated γ-globulin and immune complexes in gel diffusion. Immunology 1970; 19:909–919.
4. Agnello V, Koffler D, Eisenberg JW, et al. C1q precipitins in the sera of patients with systemic lupus erythematosus and other hypocomplementemic states: characterization of high and low molecular weight types. J Exp Med 1971; 134:228s–241s.
5. McDuffie FC, Sams WM Jr, Maldonado JE, et al. Hypocomplementemia with cutaneous vasculitis and arthritis: possible immune complex syndrome. Mayo Clin Proc 1973; 48:340–348.
6. Soter NA, Austen KF, Gigli I. Urticaria and arthralgias as manifestations of necrotizing angiitis (vasculitis). J Invest Dermatol 1974; 63:485–490.
7. Sissons JGP, Peters DK, Williams DG, et al. Skin lesions, angio-oedema, and hypocomplementaemia. Lancet 1974; ii:1350–1352.
8. Agnello V, Ruddy S, Winchester RJ, et al. Hereditary C2 deficiency in systemic lupus erythematosus and acquired complement abnormalities in an unusual SLE-related syndrome. Birth Defects Orig Artic Ser 1975; 11:312–317.
9. Oishi M, Takano M, Miyachi K, et al. A case of unusual SLE related syndrome characterized by erythema multiforme, angioneurotic edema, marked hypocomplementemia, and C1q precipitins of low molecular weight type. Int Arch Allergy Appl Immunol 1976; 50:463–472.
10. Marder RJ, Rent R, Choi EYC, et al. C1q deficiency associated with urticaria-like lesions and cutaneous vasculitis. Am J Med 1976; 61:560–565.
11. Feig PU, Soter NA, Yager HM, et al. Vasculitis with urticaria, hypocomplementemia, and multiple system involvement. JAMA 1976; 236:2065–2068.
12. Soter NA. Chronic urticaria as a manifestation of necrotizing venulitis. N Engl J Med 1977; 296:1440–1442.
13. Marder RJ, Burch FX, Schmid FR, et al. Low molecular weight C1q-precipitins in hypocomplementemic vasculitis-urticaria syndrome: partial purification and characterization as immunoglobulin. J Immunol 1978; 121:613–618.
14. Agnello V. Complement deficiency states. Medicine (Baltimore) 1978; 57:1–23.
15. Agnello V. Association of systemic lupus erythematosus and SLE-like syndromes with hereditary and acquired complement deficiency states. Arthritis Rheum 1978; 21(suppl 5): S146–S152.
16. Gammon WR, Wheeler CE Jr. Urticarial vasculitis: report of a case and review of the literature. Arch Dermatol 1979; 115:76–80.
17. Zeiss CR, Burch FX, Marder RJ, et al. A hypocomplementemic vasculitic urticarial syndrome: report of four new cases and definition of the disease. Am J Med 1980; 68:867–875.
18. Sanchez NP, Winkelmann RK, Schroeter AL, et al. The clinical and histopathologic spectrums of urticarial vasculitis: study of forty cases. J Am Acad Dermatol 1982; 7:599–605.
19. Wisnieski JJ, Baer AN, Christensen J, et al. Hypocomplementemic urticarial vasculitis syndrome: clinical and serologic findings in 18 patients. Medicine (Baltimore) 1995; 74:24–41.
20. Soter N. Urticarial venulitis. Dermatol Ther 2000; 13:400–408.
21. Mehregan DR, Hall MJ, Gibson LE. Urticarial vasculitis: a histopathologic and clinical review of 72 cases. J Am Acad Dermatol 1992; 26:441–448.
22. Davis MDP, Daoud MS, Kirby B, et al. Clinicopathologic correlation of hypocomplementemic and normocomplementemic urticarial vasculitis. J Am Acad Dermatol 1998; 38:899–905.
23. Geha RS, Akl KF. Skin lesions, angioedema, eosinophilia and hypocomplementemia. J Pediatr 1976; 89:724–727.
24. Waldo FB, Leist PA, Strife CF, et al. Atypical hypocomplementemic vasculitis syndrome in a child. J Pediatr 1985; 106:745–750.

25. Martini A, Ravelli A, Albani S, et al. Hypocomplementemic urticarial vasculitis syndrome with severe systemic manifestations. J Pediatr 1994; 124:742–744.

26. Kobayashi S, Nagase M, Hidaka S, et al. Membranous nephropathy associated with hypocomplementemic urticarial vasculitis: report of two cases and a review of the literature. Nephron 1994; 66:1–7.

27. Renard M, Wouters C, Proesmans W. Rapidly progressive glomerulonephritis in a boy with hypocomplementaemic urticarial vasculitis. Eur J Pediatr 1998; 157:243–245.

28. Cadnapaphornchai MA, Saulsbury FT, Norwood VF. Hypocomplementemic urticarial vasculitis: report of a pediatric case. Pediatr Nephrol 2000; 14:328–331.

29. Kaur S, Thami GP. Urticarial vasculitis in infancy. Indian J Dermatol Venereol Leprol 2003; 69:223–224.

30. Yuksel H, Yilmaz O, Savas R, et al. Pulmonary hemosiderosis with normocomplementemic urticarial vasculitis in a child. Monaldi Arch Chest Dis 2007; 67:63–66.

31. Koch PE, Lazova R, Rosen JP, et al. Urticarial vasculitis in an infant. Cutis 2008; 81:49–52.

32. Wisnieski JJ, Emancipator SN, Korman NJ, et al. Hypocomplementemic urticarial vasculitis syndrome in identical twins. Arthritis Rheum 1994; 37:1105–1111.

33. Vázquez-López F, Fucyo A, Sánchez-Martín J, et al. Dermoscopy for the screening of common urticaria and urticarial vasculitis. Arch Dermatol 2008; 144:568.

34. Hong L, Wackers F, Dewar M, et al. Atypical fatal hypocomplementemic urticarial vasculitis with involvement of native and homograft aortic valves in an African American man. J Allergy Clin Immunol 2000; 106:1196–1198.

35. Schwartz HR, McDuffie FC, Black LF, et al. Hypocomplementemic urticarial vasculitis: association with chronic obstructive pulmonary disease. Mayo Clin Proc 1982; 57:231–238.

36. Taillandier J, Alemanni M, Emile JF. Normocomplementemic urticarial vasculitis inaugurating destructive polyarthritis. Joint Bone Spine 2001; 68:510–512.

37. Sturgess AS, Littlejohn GO. Jaccoud's arthritis and panvasculitis in the hypocomplementemic urticarial vasculitis syndrome. J Rheumatol 1988; 15:858–861.

38. Kahn MF. Jaccoud's arthritis and urticarial hypocomplementemic vasculitis. J Rheumatol 1989; 16:252.

39. Palazzo E, Bourgeois P, Meyer O, et al. Hypocomplementemic urticarial vasculitis syndrome, Jaccoud's syndrome, valvulopathy: a new syndrome combination. J Rheumatol 1993; 20: 1236–1240.

40. Ishikawa O, Miyachi Y, Watanabe H. Hypocomplementaemic urticarial vasculitis associated with Jaccoud's syndrome. Br J Dermatol 1997; 137:804–807.

41. Chen HJ, Bloch KJ. Hypocomplementemic urticarial vasculitis, jaccoud's arthropathy, valvular heart disease, and reversible tracheal stenosis: a surfeit of syndromes. J Rheumatol 2001; 28:383–386.

42. Houser SL, Askenase PW, Palazzo E, et al. Valvular heart disease in patients with hypocomplementemic urticarial vasculitis syndrome associated with Jaccoud's arthropathy. Cardiovasc Pathol 2002; 11:210–216.

43. Ludivico CL, Myers AR, Maurer K. Hypocomplementemic urticarial vasculitis with glomerulonephritis and pseudotumor cerebri. Arthritis Rheum 1979; 22:1024–1028.

44. Moorthy AV, Pringle D. Urticaria, vasculitis, hypocomplementemia, and immune-complex glomerulonephritis. Arch Pathol Lab Med 1982; 106:68–70.

45. Saeki T, Ueno M, Shimada H, et al. Membranoproliferative glomerulonephritis associated with hypocomplementemic urticarial vasculitis after complete remission of membranous nephropathy. Nephron 2001; 88:174–177.

46. Soma J, Sato H, Ito S, et al. Nephrotic syndrome associated with hypocomplementaemic urticarial vasculitis syndrome: successful treatment with cyclosporin A. Nephrol Dial Transplant 1999; 14:1753–1757.

47. Schultz DR, Perez GO, Volanakis JE, et al. Glomerular disease in two patients with urticaria-cutaneous vasculitis, and hypocomplementemia. Am J Kidney Dis 1981; 1:157–165.

48. Messiaen T, Van Damme B, Kuypers D, et al. Crescentic glomerulonephritis complicating the course of a hypocomplementemic urticarial vasculitis. Clin Nephrol 2000; 54:409–412.

49. Enríquez R, Sirvent AE, Amorós F, et al. Crescentic membranoproliferative glomerulonephritis and hypocomplementemic urticarial vasculitis. J Nephrol 2005; 18:318–322.
50. Grimbert P, Schulte K, Buisson C, et al. Renal transplantation in a patient with hypocomplementemic urticarial vasculitis syndrome. Am J Kidney Dis 2001; 37:144–148.
51. Ramirez G, Saba SR, Espinoza L. Hypocomplementemic vasculitis and renal involvement. Nephron 1987; 45:147–150.
52. Baer MAM, McCurley T, Glick AD, et al. Evidence for immunologically mediated pulmonary injury in the hypocomplementemic urticarial vasculitis syndrome. J Am Acad Dermatol 1985; 13:509–512.
53. Wisnieski J. Urticarial vasculitis. Curr Opin Rheumatol 2000; 12:24–31.
54. Berggren MA, Heinlen L, Isaksson A, et al. EBNA 1 expression in a lung transplant recipient with hypocomplementemic urticarial vasculitis syndrome. J Med Virol 2007; 79:963–969.
55. Al Riyami BM, Al Kaabi JK, Elagib EM, et al. Subclinical pulmonary haemorrhage causing a restrictive lung defect in three siblings with a unique urticarial vasculitis syndrome. Clin Rheumatol 2003; 22:309–313.
56. Lin RY, Caren CB, Menikoff H. Hypocomplementaemic urticarial vasculitis, interstitial lung disease and hepatitis C. Br J Dermatol 1995; 132:821–823.
57. Eiser AR, Singh P, Shanies HM. Sustained dapsone-induced remission of hypocomplementemic urticarial vasculitis – a case report. Angiology 1997; 48:1019–1022.
58. Knobler H, Admon D, Leibovici V, et al. Urticarial vasculitis and recurrent pleural effusion: a systemic manifestation of urticarial vasculitis. Dermatologica 1986; 172:120–122.
59. Ghamra Z, Stoller JK. Basilar hyperlucency in a patient with emphysema due to hypocomplementemic urticarial vasculitis syndrome. Respir Care 2003; 48:697–699.
60. Falk DK. Pulmonary disease in idiopathic urticarial vasculitis. J Am Acad Dermatol 1984; 11: 346–352.
61. Hunt DP, Weil R, Nicholson AG, et al. Pulmonary capillaritis and its relationship to development of emphysema in hypocomplementaemic urticarial vasculitis syndrome. Sarcoidosis Vasc Diffuse Lung Dis 2006; 23:70–72.
62. Chew GYI, Gatenby PA. Inflammatory myositis complicating hypocomplementemic urticarial vasculitis despite on-going immunosuppression. Clin Rheumatol 2007; 26:1370–1372.
63. Corwin JM, Baum J. Iridocyclitis in two patients with hypocomplementemic cutaneous vasculitis. Am J Ophthalmol 1982; 94:111–113.
64. Batioğlu F, Taner P, Aydintuğ OT, et al. Recurrent optic disc and retinal vasculitis in a patient with drug-induced urticarial vasculitis. Cutan Ocul Toxicol 2006; 25:281–285.
65. Bielory L, Noble KG, Frohman LP. Urticarial vasculitis and visual loss. J Allergy Clin Immunol 1991; 88:819–821.
66. Koul PA, Wahid A, Shah SU, et al. Hypocomplementemic urticarial vasculitis and lower cranial nerve palsies. J Assoc Physicians India 2000; 48:536–537.
67. Jones MD, Tsou E, Lack E, et al. Pulmonary disease in systemic urticarial vasculitis: the role of bronchoalveolar lavage. Am J Med 1990; 88:431–434.
68. Soylu A, Kavukçu S, Uzuner N, et al. Systemic lupus erythematosus presenting with normocomplementemic urticarial vasculitis in a 4-year-old girl. Pediatr Int 2001; 43:420–422.
69. DeAmicis T, Mofid MZ, Cohen B, et al. Hypocomplementemic urticarial vasculitis: report of a 12-year-old girl with systemic lupus erythematosus. J Am Acad Dermatol 2002; 47(suppl 5): S273–S274.
70. O'Loughlin S, Schroeter AL, Jordon RE. Chronic urticaria-like lesions in systemic lupus erythematosus: a review of 12 cases. Arch Dermatol 1978; 114:879–883.
71. Matthews CNA, Saihan EM, Warin RP. Urticaria-like lesions associated with systemic lupus erythematosus: response to dapsone. Br J Dermatol 1978; 99:455–457.
72. Provost TT, Zone JJ, Synkowski D, et al. Unusual cutaneous manifestations of systemic lupus erythematosus. I. Urticarial-like lesions. Correlation with clinical and serological abnormalities. J Invest Dermatol 1980; 75:495–499.
73. Matarredona J, Sendagorta E, Rocamora A, et al. Systemic lupus erythematosus appearing as an urticarial vasculitis. Int J Dermatol 1986; 25:446–448.

74. Saigal K, Valencia IC, Cohen J, et al. Hypocomplementemic urticarial vasculitis with angioedema, a rare presentation of systemic lupus erythematosus: rapid response to rituximab. J Am Acad Dermatol 2003; 49:S283–S285.

75. Ruzicka T, Goerz G. Systemic lupus erythematosus and vasculitic urticaria: effect of dapsone and complement levels. Dermatologica 1981; 162:203–205.

76. Aydogan K, Karadogan SK, Adim SB, et al. Hypocomplementemic urticarial vasculitis: a rare presentation of systemic lupus erythematosus. Int J Dermatol 2006; 45:1057–1061.

77. Berti S, Moretti S, Lucin C, et al. Urticarial vasculitis and subacute lupus erythematosus. Lupus 2005; 14:489–492.

78. Holtman JH, Neustadt DH, Klein J, et al. Dapsone is an effective therapy for the skin lesions of subacute cutaneous lupus erythematosus and urticarial vasculitis in a patient with C2 deficiency. J Rheumatol 1990; 17:1222–1225.

79. Alexander EL, Provost TT. Cutaneous manifestations of primary Sjögren's syndrome: a reflection of vasculitis and association with anti-Ro (SSA) antibodies. J Invest Dermatol 1983; 80:386–391.

80. Molina R, Provost TT, Alexander EL. Two types of inflammatory vascular disease in Sjögren's syndrome: differential association with seroreactivity to rheumatoid factor and antibodies to Ro (SS-A) and with hypocomplementemia. Arthritis Rheum 1985; 28:1251–1258.

81. Kato Y, Aoki M, Kawana S. Urticarial vasculitis appearing in the progression of systemic sclerosis. J Dermatol 2006; 33:792–797.

82. Serratrice J, de Roux-Serratrice C, Ené N, et al. Urticarial vasculitis revealing relapsing polychondritits. Eur J Intern Med 2005; 16:207–208.

83. Calvo-Romero JM. Diffuse large B cell lymphoma in a patient with hypocomplementemic urticarial vasculitis. J Postgrad Med 2003; 49:252–253.

84. Strickland DK, Ware RE. Urticarial vasculitis: an autoimmune disorder following therapy for Hodgkin's disease. Med Pediatr Oncol 1995; 25:208–212.

85. Wilson D, McCluggage WG, Wright GD. Urticarial vasculitis: a paraneoplastic presentation of B-cell non-Hodgkin's lymphoma. Rheumatology 2002; 41:476–477.

86. Shah D, Rowbottom AW, Thomas CL, et al. Hypocomplementaemic urticarial vasculitis associated with non-Hodgkin lymphoma and treatment with intravenous immunoglobulin. Br J Dermatol 2007; 157:392–393.

87. Asherson RA, D'Cruz D, Stephens CJ, et al. Urticarial vasculitis in a connective tissue disease clinic: patterns, presentations, and treatment. Semin Arthritis Rheum 1991; 20:285–296.

88. Nashan D, Sunderkötter C, Bonsmann G, et al. Chronic urticaria, arthralgia, raised erythrocyte sedimentation rate and IgG paraproteinaemia: a variant of Schnitzler's syndrome?. Br J Dermatol 1995; 133:132–134.

89. Demierre M-F, Winkelman WJ. Idiopathic cold-induced urticarial vasculitis and monoclonal IgG gammopathy. Int J Dermatol 1996; 35:151–152.

90. O'Hare A, Olson JL, Connolly MK, et al. Renal insufficiency with monoclonal gammopathy and urticarial vasculitis. Am J Kidney Dis 2002; 39:203–207.

91. Alexander JL, Kalaaji AN, Shehan JM, et al. Plasmapheresis for refractory urticarial vasculitis in a patient with B-cell chronic lymphocytic leukemia. J Drugs Dermatol 2006; 5:534–537.

92. Blanco R, Martinez-Taboada V, Gonzalez-Vela C, et al. Urticarial vasculitis as clinical presentation of megakaryocytic leukaemia. J Clin Rheumatol 1996; 2:366–367.

93. Alizadeh H, Kristenssen J, El Teraifi H, et al. Urticarial vasculitis and Castelman's disease. J Eur Acad Dermatol Venereol 2007; 21:541–542.

94. Highet AS. Urticarial vasculitis and IgA myeloma. Br J Dermatol 1980; 102:355–357.

95. Lewis JE. Urticarial vasculitis occurring in association with visceral malignancy. Acta Derm Venereol 1990; 70:345–347.

96. Sprossmann A, Müller RP. Urtikaria-Vaskulitis-Syndrom Beim metastasiervenden malignen Hadenteratom. Hautarzt 1994; 45:871–874.

97. Wang CC, Chen MJ, Ho HC, et al. Urticarial vasculitis and dermatomyositis in a patient with nasopharyngeal carcinoma. Cutis 2003; 72:399–402.

98. Ducarme G, Rey D, Bryckaert PE, et al. Vasculite urticarienne paranéoplastique et carcinome rénal. Prog Urol 2003; 13:495–497.

99. Di Stefano F, Siriruttanapruk S, Di Gioacchino M. Exercise-induced urticarial vasculitis as a paraneoplastic manifestation of cystic teratoma. Rheumatology 2003; 42:1418–1419.

100. Farell AM, Sabroe RA, Bunker CB. Urticarial vasculitis associated with polycythaemia rubra vera. Clin Exp Dermatol 1996; 21:302–304.

101. Patel N, Shovel L, Moran N, et al. Acquired haemophilia in urticarial vasculitis revealed by injudicious heparin. J R Soc Med 2006; 99:151–152.

102. Grassegger A, Greil R, Feichtinger J, et al. Urtikarielle vaskulitis als Symptom des Muckle-Wells-Syndroms? Hautarzt 1991; 42:116–119.

103. Ochonisky S, Chosidow O, Kuentz M, et al. Cogan's syndrome: an unusual etiology of urticarial vasculitis. Dermatologica 1991; 183:218–220.

104. Dienstag JL, Rhodes AR, Bhan AK, et al. Urticaria associated with acute viral hepatitis type B: studies of pathogenesis. Ann Intern Med 1978; 89:34–40.

105. Popp JW Jr., Harrist TJ, Dienstag JL, et al. Cutaneous vasculitis associated with acute and chronic hepatitis. Arch Intern Med 1981; 141:623–629.

106. Hearth-Holmes M, Zahradka SL, Baethge BA, et al. Leucocytoclastic vasculitis associated with hepatitis C. Am J Med 1991; 90:765–766.

107. Kuniyuki S, Katoh H. Urticarial vasculitis with papular lesions in a patient with type C hepatitis and cryoglobulinemia. J Dermatol 1996; 23:279–283.

108. Hamid S, Cruz PD Jr., Lee WM. Urticarial vasculitis caused by hepatitis C virus infection: response to interferon alfa therapy. J Am Acad Dermatol 1998; 39:278–280.

109. Kelkar PS, Butterfield JH, Kalaaji AN. Urticarial vasculitis with asymptomatic chronic hepatitis C infection: response to doxepin, interferon-alfa, and ribavirin. J Clin Gastroenterol 2002; 35:281–282.

110. Sanli H, Özdemir E. IgM class anticardiolipin antibody and anti-Ro/SS-A positivity in urticarial vasculitis associated with hepatitis C virus infection. Int J Dermatol 2002; 41:930–932.

111. Toprak O, Cirit M, Uzunel H, et al. Hypocomplementaemic urticarial vasculitis syndrome and acute renal failure with cryoglobulin (-) hepatitis C infection. Nephrol Dial Transplant 2004; 19:2680–2682.

112. Matteson EL. Interferon alpha 2a therapy for urticarial vasculitis with angioedema apparently following hepatitis A infection. J Rheumatol 1996; 23:382–384.

113. Wands JR, Perrotto JL, Isselbacher KJ. Circulating immune complexes and complement sequence activation in infectious mononucleosis. Am J Med 1976; 60:269–272.

114. Jover F, Cuadrado JM, Ivars J, et al. Vasculitis urticariforme e infection por Mycoplasma pneumoniae. Enferm Infecc Microbiol Clin 2003; 21:218–219.

115. Olson JC, Esterly NB. Urticarial vasculitis and Lyme disease. J Am Acad Dermatol 1990; 22:1114–1116.

116. Kravitz P, Stahl NI. Urticarial vasculitis, immune complex disease, and an infected ventriculoatrial shunt. Cutis 1985; 36:135–141.

117. Stein HB, Schlappner OL, Boyko W, et al. The intestinal bypass: arthritis-dermatitis syndrome. Arthritis Rheum 1981; 24:684–690.

118. Athanasiadis GI, Pfab F, Kollmar A, et al. Urticarial vasculitis with a positive autologous serum skin test: diagnosis and successful therapy. Allergy 2006; 61:1484–1485.

119. Curd JG, Milgrom H, Stevenson DD, et al. Potassium iodide sensitivity in four patients with hypocomplementemic vasculitis. Ann Intern Med 1979; 91:853–857.

120. Feiza BA, Samy F, Asma D, et al. La vascularite urticarienne vasculitis: a propos d'une observation secondaire à une prise de sulfaméthoxazole-triméthoprime. Tunis Méd 2005; 83:714–716.

121. Roger D, Rollé F, Mausset J, et al. Urticarial vasculitis induced by fluoxetine. Dermatology 1995; 191:164.

122. Welsh JP, Cusack CA, Ko C. Urticarial vasculitis secondary to paroxetine. J Drugs Dermatol 2006; 5:1012–1014.

123. Glovsky MM, Braunwald J, Opelz G, et al. Hypersensitivity to procarbazine associated with angioedema, urticaria, and low serum complement activity. J Allergy Clin Immunol 1976; 57: 134–140.

124. Knox JP, Welykyj SE, Gradini R, et al. Procainamide-induced urticarial vasculitis. Cutis 1988; 42:469–472.

125. Mitchell GG, Magnusson AR, Weiler JM. Cimetidine-induced cutaneous vasculitis. Am J Med 1983; 75:875–876.

126. Lopes G, Vincek V, Raez LE. Pemetrexed-associated urticarial vasculitis. Lung Cancer 2006; 51:247–249.

127. Moneret-Vautrin DA, Faure G, Bene MC. Chewing-gum preservative included toxidermic vasculitis. Allergy 1986; 41:546–548.

128. Hofbauer GF, Hafner J, Trüe RM. Urticarial vasculitis following cocaine use. Br J Dermatol 1999; 141:600–601.

129. Pellizzari M, Marshman G. Formaldehyde-induced urticarial vasculitis. Australas J Dermatol 2007; 48:174–177.

130. Soter NA, Mihm MC Jr., Dvorak HF, et al. Cutaneous necrotizing venulitis: a sequential analysis of the morphological alterations occurring after mast cell degranulation in a patient with a unique syndrome. Clin Exp Immunol 1978; 32:46–58.

131. Eady RA, Keahey TM, Sibbald RG, et al. Cold urticaria with vasculitis: report of a case with light and electron microscopic, immunofluorescence and pharmacological studies. Clin Exp Dermatol 1981; 6:355–366.

132. Wanderer AA, Nuss DD, Tormey AD, et al. Urticarial leukocyclastic vasculitis with cold urticaria: report of a case and review of the literature. Arch Dermatol 1983; 119:145–151.

133. Rajka G, Mørk NJ. Clinical observations on the mechanism of delayed pressure urticaria. In: Champion RH, Greaves MW, Kobza Black A, et al. eds. The Urticarias. Edinburgh: Churchill Livingstone, 1985:191–193.

134. Armstrong RB, Horan DB, Silvers DN. Leukocytoclastic vasculitis in urticaria induced by ultraviolet irradiation. Arch Dermatol 1985; 121:1145–1148.

135. Stinco G, Di Gaetano L, Rizzi C, et al. Leukocytoclastic vasculitis in urticaria induced by sun exposure. Photodermatol Photoimmunol Photomed 2007; 23:39–41.

136. Kano Y, Orihara M, Shiohara T. Time-course analysis of exercise-induced lesions in a patient with urticarial vasculitis. Australas J Dermatol 1996; 37(suppl 1):544–545.

137. Kano Y, Orihara M, Shiohara T. Cellular and molecular dynamics in exercise-induced urticarial vasculitis lesions. Arch Dermatol 1998; 134:62–67.

138. Ramelet A-A. Exercise-induced vasculitis. J Eur Acad Dermatol Venereol 2006; 20:423–427.

139. Janier M, Bonvalet D, Blanc M-F, et al. Chronic urticaria and macroglobulinemia (Schnitzler's syndrome): report of two cases. J Am Acad Dermatol 1989; 20:206–211.

140. Borradori L, Rybojad M, Puissant A, et al. Urticarial vasculitis associated with a monoclonal IgM gammopathy: Schnitzler's syndrome. Br J Dermatol 1990; 123:113–118.

141. Berdy SS, Bloch KJ. Schnitzler's syndrome: a broader clinical spectrum. J Allergy Clin Immunol 1991; 87:849–854.

142. Lebbe C, Rybojad M, Klein F, et al. Schnitzler's syndrome associated with sensorimotor neuropathy. J Am Acad Dermatol 1994; 30:316–318.

143. Baty V, Hoen B, Hudziak H, et al. Schnitzler's syndrome: two case reports and review of the literature. Mayo Clin Proc 1995; 70:570–572.

144. Lipsker D, Spehner D, Drillien R, et al. Schnitzler syndrome: heterogeneous immunopathological findings involving IgM—skin interactions. Br J Dermatol 2000; 142:954–959.

145. Westhoff TH, Zidek W, Uharek L, et al. Impairment of renal function in Schnitzler's syndrome. J Nephrol 2006; 19:660–663.

146. de Koning HD, Bodar EJ, van der Meer JW, et al. Schnitzler syndrome: beyond the case reports: review and follow-up of 94 patients with an emphasis on prognosis and treatment. Semin Arthritis Rheum 2007; 37:137–148.

147. Blaise S, Vallat JM, Tabaraud F, et al. Syndrome de Schnitzler associé à un forme sensitive pure de polyradiculonévrite inflammatoire démyélinisante chronique. Ann Dermatol Venereol 2003; 130:348–351.

148. Lauwers A, Chouvy V, Mosnier JF, et al. A case of Schnitzler's syndrome with nodular regenerative hyperplasia of the liver. Rev Rhum Engl Ed 1999; 66:281–283.

149. Famularo G, Barracchini A, Minisola G. Severe thrombophilia with antiphospholipid syndrome and hyperhomocysteinemia in a patient with Schnitzler's syndrome. Clin Exp Rheumatol 2003; 21:366–368.

150. Sánchez G, Añó M, García-Avilés C, et al. Schnitzler syndrome: a case study. J Investig Allergol Clin Immunol 2000; 10:41–43.

151. Pascual-López M, Hernández-Núñez A, Sánchez-Pérez J, et al. Schnitzler's syndrome with monoclonal IgG kappa gammopathy: good response to cyclosporin. J Eur Acad Dermatol Venereol 2002; 16:267–270.

152. Claes K, Bammens B, Delforge M, et al. Another devastating complication of the Schnitzler syndrome: AA amyloidosis. Br J Dermatol 2008; 158:182–184.

153. Bisaccia E, Adamo V, Rozan SW. Urticarial vasculitis progressing to systemic lupus erythematosus. Arch Dermatol 1988; 124:1088–1090.

154. Aboobaker J, Greaves MW. Urticarial vasculitis. Clin Exp Dermatol 1986; 11:436–444.

155. Machet L, Vaillant L, Machet MC, et al. Schnitzler's syndrome (urticaria and macro-globulinemia): evolution to Waldenström's disease is not uncommon. Acta Derm Venereol 1996; 76:413.

156. Lipsker D, Veran Y, Grunenberger F, et al. The Schnitzler syndrome: four new cases and review of the literature. Medicine (Baltimore) 2001; 80:37–44.

157. Wisnieski JJ, Naff GB. Serum IgG antibodies to C1q in hypocomplementemic urticarial vasculitis syndrome. Arthritis Rheum 1989; 32:1119–1127.

158. Wisnieski JJ, Jones SM. Comparison of autoantibodies to the collagen-like region of C1q in hypocomplementemic urticarial vasculitis syndrome and systemic lupus erythematosus. J Immunol 1992; 148:1396–1403.

159. Wisnieski JJ, Jones SM. IgG autoantibody to the collagen-like region of C1q in hypocomplementemic urticarial vasculitis syndrome, systemic lupus erythematosus, and 6 other musculoskeletal or rheumatic diseases. J Rheumatol 1992; 19:884–888.

160. Gruber BL, Baeza ML, Marchese MJ, et al. Prevalence and functional role of anti-IgE autoantibodies in urticarial syndromes. J Invest Dermatol 1988; 90:213–217.

161. Zuberbier T, Henz BM, Fiebiger E, et al. Anti-FcεRIα serum autoantibodies in different types of urticaria. Allergy 2000; 55:951–954.

162. Sabroe RA, Fiebiger E, Francis DM, et al. Classification of anti-FcεRI and anti-IgE autoantibodies in chronic idiopathic urticaria and correlation with disease severity. J Allergy Clin Immunol 2002; 110:492–499.

163. Sais G, Vidaller A, Jucglá A, et al. Adhesion molecule expression and endothelial cell activation in cutaneous leukocytoclastic vasculitis: an immunohistologic and clinical study in 42 patients. Arch Dermatol 1997; 133:443–450.

164. Worm M, Kolde G. Schnitzler's syndrome: successful treatment of two patients using thalidomide. Br J Dermatol 2003; 148:601–602.

165. de Kleijn EM, Telgt D, Laan R. Schnitzler's syndrome presenting as fever of unknown origin (FUO): the role of cytokines in its systemic features. Neth J Med 1997; 51:140–142.

166. Gallo R, Sabroe RA, Black AK, et al. Schnitzler's syndrome: no evidence for autoimmune basis in two patients. Clin Exp Dermatol 2000; 25:281–284.

167. Saurat JH, Schifferli J, Steiger G, et al. Anti-interleukin-1α autoantibodies in humans: characterization, isotype distribution, and receptor-binding inhibition — higher frequency in Schnitzler's syndrome (urticaria and macroglobulinemia). J Allergy Clin Immunol 1991; 88: 244–256.

168. Rybojad M, Moraillon I, Cordoliani F, et al. Syndrome de Schnitzler avec déficit génétique en C4: deux observations. Ann Dermatol Venereol 1993; 120:783–785.

169. Sperr W, Natter S, Baghestanian M, et al. Autoantibody reactivity in a case of Schnitzler's syndrome: evidence of a Th1-like response and detection of IgG2 anti-Fcε RIα antibodies. Int Arch Allergy Immunol 2000; 122:279–286.

170. Soter NA, Mihm MC Jr., Gigli I, et al. Two distinct cellular patterns in cutaneous necrotizing angiitis. J Invest Dermatol 1976; 66:344–350.

171. Jones RR, Bhogal B, Dash A, et al. Urticaria and vasculitis: a continuum of histological and immunopathological changes. Br J Dermatol 1983; 108:695–703.

172. Jones RR, Eady RAJ, Schocket AL, et al. Endothelial cell pathology as a marker for urticarial vasculitis: a light microscopic study. Br J Dermatol 1984; 110:139–149.

173. Tuffanelli DL. Cutaneous immunopathology: recent observations. J Invest Dermatol 1975; 65:143–153.

174. Small P, Barrett D, Champlin E. Chronic urticaria and vasculitis. Ann Allergy 1982; 48:172–174.

175. Phanuphak P, Kohler PF, Sandford RE, et al. Vasculitis in chronic urticaria. J Allergy Clin Immunol 1980; 65:436–444.

176. Monroe EW, Schulz CI, Maize JC, et al. Vasculitis in chronic urticaria: an immunopathologic study. J Invest Dermatol 1981; 76:103–107.

177. Natbony SF, Phillips ME, Elias JM, et al. Histologic studies of chronic idiopathic urticaria. J Allergy Clin Immunol 1983; 71:177–183.

178. Champion RH. Urticaria then and now. Br J Dermatol 1988; 119:427–436.

179. Guillet G, Jeune R. Urticarial vasculitis with shock, leukopenia and thrombocytopenia, possibly due to anaphylatoxin release. Br J Dermatol 1983; 108:605–608.

180. Mathison DA, Arroyave CM, Bhat KN, et al. Hypocomplementemia in chronic idiopathic urticaria. Ann Intern Med 1977; 86:534–538.

181. McLean RH, Weinstein A, Chapitis J, et al. Familial partial deficiency of the third component of complement (C3) and the hypocomplementemic cutaneous vasculitis syndrome. Am J Med 1980; 68:549–558.

182. Borradori L, Rybojad M, Morel P, et al. Chronic urticaria and moderate leukocytoclastic vasculitis associated with C3 nephritic factor activity. Arch Dermatol 1989; 125:1589–1590.

183. Carmichael AJ, Marsden JR. Urticarial vasculitis: a presentation of C3 nephritic factor. Br J Dermatol 1993; 128:589.

184. de Castro FR, Masouyé I, Winkelmann RK, et al. Urticarial pathology in Schnitzler's (hyper-IgM) syndrome. Dermatology 1996; 193:94–99.

185. Dincy CV, Geroge R, Jacob M, et al. Clinicopathologic profile of normocomplementemic and hypocomplementemic urticarial vasculitis: a study from South India. J Eur Acad Dermatol Venereol 2008; 22:789–794.

186. Millns JL, Randle HW, Solley GO, et al. The therapeutic response of urticarial vasculitis to indomethacin. J Am Acad Dermatol 1980; 3:349–355.

187. Lopez LR, Davis KC, Kohler PF, et al. The hypocomplementemic urticarial-vasculitis syndrome: therapeutic response to hydroxychoroquine. J Allergy Clin Immunol 1984; 73:600–603.

188. Werder M, Truniger B. Hypocomplementaemic urticarial vasculitis. Nephrol Dial Transplant 1997; 12:1278–1279.

189. Stack PS. Methotrexate for urticarial vasculitis. Ann Allergy 1994; 72:36–38.

190. Wiles JC, Hansen RC, Lynch PJ. Urticarial vasculitis treated with colchicine. Arch Dermatol 1985; 121:802–805.

191. Werni R, Schwarz T, Gschnait F. Colchicine treatment of urticarial vasculitis. Dermatologica 1986; 172:36–40.

192. Nishijima C, Hatta N, Inaoki M, et al. Urticarial vasculitis in systemic lupus erythematosus: fair response to prednisolone/dapsone and persistent hypocomplementemia. Eur J Dermatol 1999; 9:54–56.

193. Fortson JS, Zone JJ, Hammond ME, et al. Hypocomplementemic urticarial vasculitis syndrome responsive to dapsone. J Am Acad Dermatol 1986; 15:1137–1142.

194. Worm M, Sterry W, Kolde G. Mycophenolate mofetil is effective for maintenance therapy of hypocomplementaemic urticarial vasculitis. Br J Dermatol 2000; 143:1324.

195. Schartz NEC, Buder S, Sperl H, et al. Report of a case of Schnitzler's syndrome treated successfully with interferon alpha 2b. Dermatology 2002; 205:54–56.
196. Staubach-Renz P, von Stebut E, Bräuninger W, et al. Hypokomplementämisches Urtkaria-Vaskulitis-Syndrom Erfolgreiche Therapie mit intravenösen Immunoglobulin. Hautarzt 2007; 58:693–697.
197. Botsios C, Sfriso P, Punzi L, et al. Non-complementaemic urticarial vasculitis: successful treatement with the IL-1 receptor antagonist, anakinra. Scand J Rheumatol 2007; 36:236–237.
198. Borcea A, Greaves MW. Methotrexate-induced exacerbation of urticarial vasculitis: an unusual adverse reaction. Br J Dermatol 2000; 143:203–204.
199. Worm M, Muche M, Schulze P, et al. Hypocomplementaemic urticarial vasculitis: successful treatment with cyclophosphamide-dexamethasone pulse therapy. Br J Dermatol 1998; 139: 704–707.
200. Nürnberg W, Grabbe J, Czarnetzki BM. Urticarial vasculitis syndrome effectively treated with dapsone and pentoxifylline. Acta Derm Venereol 1995; 75:54–56.
201. Handfield-Jones SE, Greaves MW. Urticarial vasculitis– response to gold therapy. J R Soc Med 1991; 84:169.
202. de Koning HD, Bodar EJ, Simon A, et al. Beneficial response to anakinra and thalidomide in Schnitzler's syndrome. Ann Rheum Dis 2006; 65:542–544.
203. Worm M, Kolde G. Schnitzler's syndrome: successful treatment of two patients using thalidomine. Br J Dermatol 2003; 148:601–602.
204. Asli B, Bienvenu B, Cordoliani F, et al. Chronic urticaria and monoclonal IgM gammopathy (Schnitzler syndrome): report of 11 cases treated with pefloxacin. Arch Dermatol 2007; 143:1046–1050.
205. Ramadan KM, Eswedi HA, El-Agnaf MR. Schnitzler syndrome: a case report of successful treatment using the anti-CD20 monoclonal antibody rituximab. Br J Dermatol 2007; 156:1072–1074.
206. Cianchini G, Colonna L, Bergamo F, et al. Efficacy of psoralen-UV-A therapy in 3 cases of Schnitzler syndrome. Arch Dermatol 2001; 137:1536–1537.

22

Nonhereditary Angioedema and Idiopathic Anaphylaxis

Malcolm W. Greaves
St. John's Institute of Dermatology, St. Thomas' Hospital, London, U.K.

Allen P. Kaplan
Department of Medicine, Medical University of South Carolina, Charleston, South Carolina, U.S.A.

HISTORICAL

Although John Laws Milton of St John's Hospital for Diseases of the Skin, London, used the term "giant urticaria," he provided the first definitive description of angioedema in 1876. He described in detail seven patients with typical angioedema, and none had a family history (1). Only one of these patients seems to have had accompanying "ordinary" urticaria. Six years later Quincke (2) introduced the term "angioneurotic edema" for the same condition, and this nomenclature prevailed until the latter half of the 20th century when, owing to lack of evidence of a significant neural or psychic contribution to its pathophysiology, the disease was designated "angioedema." Subsequent literature on angioedema was dominated by the original description by Osler (3) of hereditary angioedema and its subsequent molecular characterization by Donaldson (4). Consequently little attention was devoted to acquired angioedema until Caldwell (5) reported the association of nonhereditary angioedema with a lymphoproliferative disorder in 1972.

EPIDEMIOLOGY AND CLASSIFICATION

There are little or no data on the epidemiology of nonhereditary angioedema. In one review of 554 hospital outpatients with angioedema and/or urticaria (6), 11% were reported to have angioedema alone. However it is unclear how many of these, if any, had hereditary angioedema. There is no established classification of nonhereditary angioedema. The authors have found it useful and of practical value in management to classify nonhereditary angioedema into two categories: angioedema with concurrent urticaria and angioedema without urticaria (Table 1). The pathophysiology and clinical features of those types of angioedema with urticaria are discussed in detail in the relevant chapters and will

Table 1 Classification of Nonhereditary Angioedema

With urticaria[a]	Acute allergic (foods, drugs, IgE-mediated)
	Due to NSAIDs (non-IgE-mediated, idiosyncratic)
	Some physical urticarias (cold, solar, vibratory angioedema[b]) and cholinergic urticaria with angioedema
	Autoimmune urticaria (87% have concurrent angioedema (8)
	Chronic idiopathic urticaria with angioedema
	Food and exercise induced urticaria and angioedema (9)
	Episodic angioedema with eosinophilia
No urticaria	Acquired C1 esterase inhibitor (C1 INH) deficient angioedema types 1 and 2
	ACE inhibitor angioedema
	Occasional reaction to foods or drugs
	Idiopathic angioedema

[a]Members of this category are discussed in the relevant chapters.
[b]Rarely associated with urticaria.
Abbreviations: NSAIDs, nonsteroid anti-inflammatory drugs; C1 INH, C1 esterase inhibitor.

not be considered further here. The term "acquired angioedema" (types 1 and 2) is by common usage taken to mean nonhereditary angioedema due to acquired C1 INH deficiency. In this case C1 INH synthesis is normal, the lowered serum levels of C1 INH being due to increased degradation and urticaria is absent. For clarity, use of the terminology "acquired C1 inhibitor deficiency" is more meaningful.

An alternative classification for recurrent angioedema in the absence of urticaria focuses on responsiveness to antihistamines. Responders are considered "histaminergic" and the remainder "nonhistaminergic" (7). Although food and drug reactions (IgE mediated and clearly histamine dependent) can cause angioedema in the absence of urticaria, the percentage is small (probably less than 10%) compared with food and drug reactions that cause angioedema with concomitant urticaria. When no exogenous precipitant is present and hereditary angioedema, acquired C1 INH deficiency, and angiotensin-convertase (ACE)-inhibitor reactions have been ruled out, the term "idiopathic angioedema" (where the pathogenesis is unknown) is used for the remainder. This was the group studied when the "histaminergic vs. nonhistaminergic" categorization was first described (7).

PATHOPHYSIOLOGY AND CLINICAL CONSIDERATIONS

Nonhereditary angioedema, like other types of angioedema is characterized by localized increased permeability of dermal, mucosal and subcutaneous and submucosal capillaries, and post capillary venules, leading to massive localized edema. In most nonhereditary forms, the molecular basis of the increased vasopermeability has not been conclusively established. However the close resemblance pathophysiologically and clinically to the hereditary forms, in which bradykinin is recognized to be a major mediator, suggest that kinins may likewise be central to the pathomechanism of many of the nonhereditary forms. Evidence of activation of the kinin-forming enzyme kallikrein in acquired C1 esterase deficiency has been previously reported (10). Investigation of the therapeutic effect of the recently characterized selective bradykinin antagonists such as icatibant will be of interest.

The clinical features of acquired angioedema due to C1 INH deficiency closely resemble those of the hereditary forms. Mucosal involvement is common, leading to glossal, laryngeal and pharyngeal edema, with consequent respiratory obstruction, and fatalities occur. Patients may be dysarthric, so that for a case history reliance has to be obtained from relatives or caregivers. Abdominal pain due to intestinal mucosal angioedema is also common. The only significant clinical differences between the hereditary and nonhereditary forms are the age of onset of angioedema which is usually at school age in hereditary angioedema, but is much later in the nonhereditary types— usually in the fourth decade or later and of course the absence of a family history. Response to treatment, especially by C1 INH replacement is also unpredictable in the nonhereditary forms.

ACQUIRED ANGIOEDEMA TYPE 1

This type of acquired angioedema is associated with normal synthesis of functional 105-kd C1 INH. However increased catabolism of the protein, associated in most cases with lymphoproliferative disease, leads to severe depletion of C1 INH and development of angioedema (11) and increased activation of the classical complement pathway. In the laboratory, acquired angioedema type 1 and type 2, like type 1 hereditary angioedema, are associated with greatly lowered serum C1 INH and lowered C4 and C2. However in the acquired type C1q is also lowered. Thus, depletion of C1q enables distinction between acquired and hereditary angioedema, since serum C1q levels are normal in the hereditary type. Comparison of the serological values for these complement components in the hereditary and acquired forms of angioedema is discussed in detail in chapter 16.

Acquired C1 INH deficiency type 1 is associated primarily with B cell lymphoproliferative disease, which may be benign and associated with monoclonal gammopathy or malignant B cell lymphoma (12). Neoplastic lymphoma cells consume C1 INH by activating the classical complement pathway, thus explaining the laboratory findings in type 1 acquired angioedema (13).

ACQUIRED ANGIOEDEMA TYPE 2

Patients with type 2 acquired angioedema secrete normal quantities of functional 105-kd C1 INH. However they also have circulating IgG or IgM autoantibodies directed against C1 INH (14). These autoantibodies combine with C1 INH and proteinases normally bound to C1 INH cleave it leading to formation of a 96-kd fragment, with consequent impairment of its regulatory capacity. Thus, these patients have an autoimmune disease due to inactivation by autoantibodies of functional C1 INH. Occasionally, in patients with a monoclonal gammopathy, the paraprotein behaves as an autoantibody against C1 INH, leading to a similar molecular and clinical outcome.

Laboratory investigation of patients with type 2 acquired angioedema is identical with those in type 1—namely reduced serum levels of C1 INH, C4, and C1q. However type 2 acquired angioedema can be distinguished in the laboratory from type 1 by detection of the presence in serum of the 96-kd C1 INH fragment in the former but not the latter.

The clinical presentation of the two types is similar, with there being no significant differences with hereditary angioedema type 1, apart from a later age of onset and absence of family history.

ACQUIRED C1 ESTERASE DEFICIENCY
DUE TO SYSTEMIC LUPUS ERYTHEMATOSUS

Although there are several reports of severe angioedema in association with systemic lupus erythematosus (15,16), occurrence of acquired angioedema associated with C1 INH deficiency has only recently been described in lupus (17,18). In these cases activation of the classical complement pathway resulted in lowered serum C3 and C4, and this was associated with transient lowering of C1 INH (quantitative and functional). There was no evidence of lymphoproliferative disease or anti-C1 INH autoantibodies. These patients responded to immunosuppressive therapy. Similar consumption of C1 INH has been described in cryoglobulinemia (19).

ANGIOEDEMA DUE TO ANGIOTENSIN CONVERTASE INHIBITORS

In one recent series of over 7000 reports of angioedema due to drugs (20), 916 were attributed to ACE inhibitors the reaction being especially common in black patients. It has been estimated that angioedema occurs in 1 of 1000 treatment episodes. Most patients suffered from swellings of eyelids, lips, tongue, pharynx, larynx, and the angioedema was often life threatening. Abdominal pain due to intestinal angioedema is also common. Concurrent urticaria can occur but is rare. In the emergency room the diagnosis may be missed because, unlike most adverse drug reactions, episodes of angioedema due to ACE inhibitors may not occur until months or even years after commencing treatment (21). Levels of C1 INH and other complement components are normal.

The molecular mechanism is well understood (22). The components of complement activation are not involved. Bradykinin, a ubiquitous and potent vasopermeability agent acting on vascular B2 receptors, is degraded in the lungs by ACE to inactive peptide degradation products. ACE inhibitor causes reduced degradation and blood and tissue levels of bradykinin rise. Why only a tiny minority of patients receiving ACE inhibitors reacts in this way is unclear, but genetic polymorphisms in ACE or other enzymes involved in kinin degradation are suspected.

The issue of whether it is safe for patients with angioedema due to ACE inhibitors to substitute angiotensin type 11 antagonists is debated. There are several reports of patients previously suffering from angioedema in response to ACE inhibitors subsequently experiencing a reoccurrence of angioedema, following substitution of angiotensin 11 antagonists (23,24). In 2005 the *Australian Adverse Reaction Bulletin* reported 119 cases of patients developing angioedema in response to angiotensin 11 receptor antagonists (25). The mechanism is unclear, since bradykinin levels are not elevated, but increased sensitivity of the bradykinin B2 receptors has been proposed (26).

IDIOPATHIC ACQUIRED ANGIOEDEMA

Traditionally this is assumed to be a subgroup of patients with chronic urticaria and angioedema for whom the sole manifestation is angioedema. The overall incidence is about 10% of that of chronic urticaria and angioedema, i.e., 0.05%. Symptoms can vary from episodes of swelling that occur a few times a year, i.e., every few months, to those with frequent episodes a few times each week. No allergic etiology can be found (specifically no reactions to foods or drugs), their health is otherwise normal, complement studies (C4, C1 INH by protein and function) are normal, and there is no familial predisposition. However laryngeal edema and edema of the bowel is not seen, thus it differs from the angioedema associated with ACE inhibitors or the various forms of C1

INH deficiency. In this sense, it resembles closely the angioedema that is seen accompanying urticaria in those with idiopathic or autoimmune chronic urticaria. Nevertheless, differences have been noted. First, idiopathic angioedema has no sex predilection, or may be slightly more prevalent in men (Beltrani V, unpublished observations) whereas two-thirds of patients with chronic urticaria are female (27). Second, evidence of antithyroid antibodies is much less than the 25% positively associated with chronic urticaria, and antibody to the IgE receptor is rarely, if ever, seen (Kaplan AP, unpublished observation). The pathogenesis of this disorder is not known. Thus although this disorder is typically portrayed as a continuum with chronic urticaria (idiopathic or autoimmune), with or without angioedema, only a small fraction of patients may fulfill criteria of being histamine dependent with increased autoantibody synthesis.

As noted earlier, attempts to further characterize these patients have divided them into two groups depending on responsiveness to antihistamine therapy (7). The histaminergic group responds to antihistamine prophylaxis. We first employ nonsedating antihistaminics (cetrizine, desloratidine, fexofenadine, etc.) at double the usual dose. If angioedema continues, we try diphenhydramine at 25 to 50 mg q.i.d. Patients who fail to remit taking 50 mg q.i.d. are considered to be in the nonhistaminergic group. Cicardi et al. (7) found 45% of patients to be histaminergic and our data are similar. We have defined this group as being unresponsive to high doses of first generation antihistamines such as hydroxyzine or diphenhydramine employed in a prophylactic manner (28). One caveat is that effects other than blockade of histamine receptors may be contributory, so that a response is not prima facie evidence of a "histaminergic" response. But if successful, other agents are unnecessary. Anecdotal data suggests that some patients respond to addition of a leukotriene synthesis inhibitor such as Zyflo (29), and the European literature suggest efficacy of tranexamic acid in this subpopulation (7). There is evidence to implicate bradykinin release in a subpopulation of such patients (22), but the results are not definitive. Some role for the fibrinolytic pathway as another consideration. In contrast to C1 INH deficiency or ACE-induced angioedema, angioedema can be prevented with systemic corticosteroids when other approaches have failed. Such patients would not be expected to have bradykinin-induced swelling.

TREATMENT OF NONHEREDITARY ANGIOEDEMA

General measures are relevant. These include preserving the airway, administering oxygen, and establishing an intravenous line. Patients should be routinely admitted to hospital for at least 24 hours because relapses after initial improvement are common—especially in those with ACE inhibitor angioedema. Subcutaneous or even intravenous adrenaline (epinephrine) is always worth giving in any patient with severe angioedema, whatever the cause.

Patients with acquired angioedema types 1 and 2 may respond to intravenous vapor-heated C1 INH concentrate (30). However compared with hereditary angioedema, much larger dosage is usually required (11) since turnover and consumption of C1 INH is greatly enhanced in acquired angioedema types 1 and 2. If C1 INH concentrate is unavailable, tranexamic acid, an inhibitor of plasmin and plasminogen activator, is the treatment of choice for the acute attack (31). For long-term prophylaxis in type 1 acquired angioedema, the attenuated androgen stanozolol is often effective and safe (32), coupled with effective treatment of the underlying lymphoproliferative disorder. Stanozolol is ineffective in type 2 acquired angioedema (30,33), and in such cases reliance must be placed on treatment of the underlying autoimmune process (34) with approaches such as use of cytotoxic agents active on B lymphocytes and/or plasmaphoresis.

For ACE inhibitor–induced angioedema, the general measures as described above should be supplemented by subcutaneous or intravenous adrenaline. C1 INH concentrate is ineffective in ACE inhibitor–induced angioedema. It is advisable to check the C4 serum level because ACE inhibitors may evoke angioedema in patients with previously unrecognized hereditary angioedema (35,36). The risks inherent in substituting angiotensin 11 antagonists (sartans) for ACE inhibitors in patients suffering from ACE inhibitor angioedema have been alluded to above (23,24). The recent advent of bradykinin B2 receptor antagonists such as icatibant and inhibitors of the bradykinin-forming enzyme kallikrein (37), currently in phase 3 clinical trials, offer a potentially new approach to the treatment of ACE inhibitor–induced angioedema, and indeed other forms of hereditary and nonhereditary types of angioedema.

Idiopathic Anaphylaxis

Angioedema that appears to be idiopathic, yet has documented airway obstruction (no more than 1% of the patients with idiopathic angioedema) is considered to be a subgroup of patients with idiopathic anaphylaxis. We will consider this syndrome with all its ramifications.

The presence of angioedema with or without urticaria requires considerations of allergic reactions to drugs and foods as part of the differential diagnosis. Among the pathogenic hallmarks of allergy is the degranulation of cutaneous mast cells due to the bridging of IgE molecules by an allergen that is at minimum, bivalent, and also to infiltration of eosinophils as part of a late-phase reaction. Clearly the same thing can occur as a result of mast cell activation by alternative mechanisms such as occurs in the autoimmune subgroup of patients with chronic urticaria and angioedema, as well as the group that remains idiopathic because an initiating stimulus has not yet been identified. When activation of mast cells is systemic, rather than being confined to the skin, the result can be idiopathic anaphylaxis, if there is no evident exogenous precipitant, i.e., no relation to foods, drugs, or activities.

Idiopathic anaphylaxis is a diagnosis by exclusion, in which symptoms of recurrent anaphylaxis occur with no identifiable cause. Among the symptoms are flushing and urticaria and angioedema that appears similar to what one might see in a patient with food or drug allergy or in someone with chronic urticaria/angioedema whose symptoms are intermittent. The angioedema is often facial with swelling of the lips, cheeks, or periorbital area, but may also include swelling of the tongue or pharynx as well as laryngeal edema or swelling of the extremities or genitalia. It is the presence of additional, noncutaneous symptoms that prompts a diagnosis of "anaphylaxis." These may include overt wheezing (or cough or dyspnea caused by bronchospasm); gastrointestinal symptoms including any combination of nausea, vomiting, cramps, or diarrhea; with the latter two symptoms being most common; and hypotension (38–40). A classification of patients presenting with idiopathic anaphylaxis has been reported by Wong et al. (39) and is duplicated in Table 2, which divides patients into groups depending on the frequency of symptoms and the particular manifestations. It should be noted, however, that group idiopathic anaphylaxis-angioedema-infrequent (IA-A-I) and idiopathic anaphylaxis-angioedema-frequent (IA-A-F) refers to patients having angioedema, but the swelling is severe and potentially life threatening, including angioedema of the tongue and pharynx to such a degree that secretions cannot be handled. Thus there is a risk of aspiration as well as mechanical airway compromise, or edema of the glottis and/or vocal cords (laryngeal edema). Since there is no test that can be used to confirm a designation of idiopathic anaphylaxis, one might also consider such patients to be extreme versions of

Table 2 Classification of Idiopathic Anaphylaxis

Disease	Symptoms
IA-G-I	Urticaria or angioedema with bronchospasm, hypotension, syncope, or gastrointestinal symptoms with or without upper airway compromise with infrequent episodes (<6 episodes/yr).
IA-G-F	Urticaria or angioedema with bronchospasm, hypotension, syncope, or gastrointestinal symptoms with or without upper airway compromise with frequent episodes (≥6 episodes/yr).
IA-A-I	Urticaria or angioedema with upper airway compromise such as laryngeal edema, severe pharyngeal edema, or massive tongue edema without other systemic manifestations with infrequent episodes (<6 episodes/yr).
IA-A-F	Urticaria or angioedema with upper airway compromise such as laryngeal edema, severe pharyngeal edema, or massive tongue edema without other systemic manifestations with frequent episodes (≥6 episodes/yr).
IA-Q	This diagnosis is applied for a patient who is referred for management with a presumptive diagnosis of IA for which repeated attempts at documentation of objective findings are unsuccessful, response to appropriate doses of prednisone do not occur and the diagnosis of IA becomes uncertain.
IA-V	This diagnosis is applied when symptoms and physical findings of IA are variable from classic findings of IA, IA-V may subsequently be classified as IA-Q or IA excluded or IA-A or IA-G.

Abbreviations: IA-G-I, idiopathic anaphylaxis-generalized-infrequent; IA-G-F, idiopathic-anaphylaxis-generalized-frequent; IA-A-I, idiopathic anaphylaxis-angioedema-infrequent; IA-A-F, idiopathic anaphylaxis-angioedema-frequent; IA-Q, idiopathic anaphylaxis-questionable; IA-V, idiopathic anaphylaxis-variant.
Source: From Ref. 40.

idiopathic angioedema. However, as noted earlier, true airway obstruction is not seen with idiopathic angioedema even if tongue or pharyngeal edema is present, thus the authors prefer to characterize such patients as IA-A-I or IA-A-F as noted in Table 2. In all patients, C1 INH deficiency, hereditary angioedema with normal C1 INH (41), use of ACE inhibitors, or identifiable allergic precipitants, or a role for NSAIDs must be excluded before a diagnosis of idiopathic anaphylaxis can be made. Recently a subpopulation of patients with idiopathic anaphylaxis was shown to have evidence of clonal mast cell disorder with the same c-kit D816V mutation that is seen in systemic mastocytosis. Mast cells are morphologically aberrant with expression of CD20 but without cutaneous involvement (no rash) or mast cell aggregates on bone marrow biopsy (42,43). Some have a history of anaphylaxis with hymenoptera stings, particularly hypotension that is otherwise unexplained (42). Skin prick testing and/or radio-allergosorbent test (RAST) testing for food allergy is required and if positives are obtained, there must be absence of symptoms with omission of the putative allergen(s) and/or historically consistent correlation of symptoms with ingestion of the substance in question (44). It has been shown that an extensive array of food stuffs, spices, and condiments must be tested (Table 2, chapter 14). Exercise-induced anaphylaxis (with or without food hypersensitivity) (45–48) must be ruled out, i.e., there is no relationship to episodes of physical activity. To confirm the authenticity of the anaphylaxis there should be objective documentation of the anaphylactic event based on personal observation, emergency room records, pulmonary function testing, or elevated β tryptase during an episode. It is possible that some patients represent new mutations of Factor XII diagnostic of hereditary angioedema with normal C1 INH; these would be indistinguishable unless a mutation in Factor XII or specific activity of Factor XIIa is determined (49), and patients designated as IA-A-I or IA-A-F should be screened for this mutation. There is an entity designated "undifferentiated somatoform idiopathic anaphylaxis" (50) with symptoms that sound like anaphylaxis but without objective evidence of such which responds poorly (if at all) to therapy and may represent a psychiatric disorder. A combination of flushing syndrome, paradoxical motion of the vocal cords, and irritable bowel syndrome could present in this way.

Treatment of idiopathic anaphylaxis depends on the frequency and severity of the attacks. If infrequent, one may try to treat episodes as they occur, i.e., with parenteral epinephrine, a combination of H_1 and H_2 antagonists, an albuterol inhaler, and 60 to 100 mg of prednisone. However frequent symptoms require sustained treatment to prevent attacks. A useful antihistamine regimen would consist of diphenhydramine at 50 mg q.i.d, rantidine at 150 mg b.i.d., an oral sympathomimetic might be added, plus self-administered epinephrine and an albuterol inhaler for p.r.n. use. More severe episodes require the addition of corticosteroid. For the most severe cases (40), a week of prednisone at 60 mg/day is recommended, followed by q.o.d. prednisone at 40 to 60 mg/day for many months, and gradual tapering as symptoms allow. Patients with "malignant" idiopathic anaphylaxis may have to continue steroid therapy for many years, although eventually most succeed in finally eliminating it (51).

REFERENCES

1. Milton JL. On giant urticaria. Edinburgh Med J 1876; 2:513–527.
2. Quincke HI. Ueber akutes umschriebenes hautoderm. Monatshfte fur Prakt Dermat 1882; 1:129–131.
3. Osler W. Hereditary angioneurotic edema. Am J Med Sci 1888; 95:362–367.
4. Donaldson VH, Evans RR. A biochemical abnormality in hereditary angioneurotic edema: absence of serum inhibitor of C′1- esterase. Am J Med 1963; 35:37–44.
5. Caldwell JR, Ruddy S, Schur PH, et al. Acquired C1 inhibitor deficiency in lymphosarcoma. Clin Immunol Immunopathol 1972; 1:39–52.
6. Champion RH, Roberts SOB, Carpenter RG, et al. Urticaria and angioedema: a review of 554 patients. Br J Dermatol 1969; 81:588–597.
7. Cicardi M, Bergamaschini L, Zingale LC, et al. Idiopathic non-histaminergic angioedema. Am J Med 1999; 106:650–654.
8. Sabroe RA, Seed PT, Francis DM, et al. Chronic idiopathic urticaria: comparison of clinical features of patients with and without anti-FcεR1 or anti-IgE autoantibodies. J Am Acad Dermatol 1999; 40:443–450.
9. Caffarelli C, Zinelli C, Trimarco G, et al. Angioedema in a child due to eating tomatoes after exercise. Clin Exp Dermatol 2005; 31:294–295.
10. Hentges F, Humbel R, Dicato M, et al. Acquired C1 esterase-inhibitor deficiency: case report with emphasis on complement and kallkrein activation during two patterns of clinical manifestations. J Allergy Clin Immunol 1986; 78:860–867.
11. Melamed J, Alper CA, Cicardi M, et al. The metabolism of C′1 inhibitor and C′1q in patients with acquired C′1 inhibitor deficiency. J Allergy Clin Immunol 1986; 77:322–326.
12. Schrieber AD, Zweiman B, Atkins P, et al. Acquired angioedema with lymphoproliferative disorder. Association of C′1 inhibitor deficiency with cellular abnormality. Blood 1976; 48:567–580.
13. Cicardi M, Beretta A, Colombo M, et al. Relvance of lymphoproliferative disorders and of anti-C′1 inhibitor autoantibodies in acquired angioedema. Clin Exp Immunol 1996; 06:475–480.
14. Jackson J, Sim RB, Whelan A, et al. An IgG autoantibody which inactivated C′1 inhibitor. Nature 1986; 323:722–724.
15. Thong BY, Thumboo J, Howe HS, et al. Life threatening angioedema in systemic lupus erythematosus. Lupus 2001; 10:304–308.

16. Ko CH, Ng J, Kumar S, et al. Life threatening angioedema in a patient with systemic lupus. Clin Rheumatol 2006; 25:917–918.

17. Cacoub P, Fremeaux-Bacchi V, de Lacroix I, et al. A new type of acquired C′1 inhibitor deficiency associated with systemic lupus erythematosus. Arthritis Rheum 2001; 44:1836–1840.

18. Lahiri M, Lim AYN. Angioedema and systemic lupus erythematosus-a complementary association? Ann Acad Med Singapore 2007; 36:142–145.

19. Gelfand JA, Boss GR, Conley L, et al. Acquired C1 esterase inhibitor deficiency and angioedema: a review. Medicine 1979; 58:321–328.

20. Adverse Drug Reactions Advisory Committee (ADRAC). Angioedema—still a problem with ACE inhibitors. Aust Adv Drug React Bull 2005; 24(2).

21. Pavletic A. Late angioedema in patients taking angiotensin-converting-enzyme inhibitors. Lancet 2002; 360:493–494.

22. Nussberger J, Cugno M, Amstutz C, et al. Plasma bradykinin in angioedema. Lancet 1998; 351:1693–1697.

23. Howes LG, Tran D. Can angiotensin receptor antagonists be used safely in patients with previous ACE inhibitor induced angioedema? Drug Saf 2002; 25:73–76.

24. Abdi R, Dong VM, Lee CJ, et al. Angiotensin 11 receptor blocker – associated angoedema on the heels of ACE inhibitor angioedema. Pharmacotherapy 2002; 22:1173–1175.

25. Adverse Drug Reactions Advisory Committee (ADRAC). Angiotensin 11 receptor antagonists. Aust Adv React Bull 1999; 18:2.

26. Tan Y, Hutchinson FN, Jaffa AA. Mechanisms of angiotensin 11- induced expression of bradykinin B2 receptors. Am J Physiol Heart Circ Physiol 2004; 286:H926–H932.

27. Beltrani V. Non-hereditary angioedema. In: Greaves M, Kaplan AP, eds. Urticaria and Angioedema. New York : Marcel Dekker Inc., 2004:421–438.

28. Kaplan AP. Chronic urticaria and angioedema. N Engl J Med 2002; 346:175–179.

29. Beltrani VS. Angioedema: some "new" thoughts regarding idiopathic angioedema. In: Greaves MW, Kaplan AP, eds. Urticaria and Angioedema. New York: Marcel Dekker, 2004:421–439.

30. Alsenz J, Lambris JD, Bork K, et al. Acquired C′1 inhibitor (C1-INH) deficiency type 11: replacement therapy with C1-INH and analysis of patients′C1-INH and anti C1-INH autoantibodies. J Clin Invest 1989; 83:1794–1799.

31. Cugno M, Cicardi M, Agostoni A. Activation of the contact system and fibrinolysis in autoimmune angioedema: a rationale for prophylactic use of tranexamic acid. J Allergy Clin Immunol 1994; 93:870–876.

32. Sloane DE, Lee CW, Sheffer AL. Hereditary angioedema: safety of long-term stanozolol therapy. J Allergy Clin Immunol 2007; 120:654–658.

33. Alsenz J, Bork K, Loos M. Autoantibody-mediated acquired deficiency of C′1 inhibitor. N Engl J Med 1987; 316:1360–1366.

34. Donaldson VH, Bernstein DL, Wagner CJ, et al. Angioneurotic edema with acquired C′1 inhibitor deficiency and autoantibody to C′1 inhibitor: response to plasmapheresis and cytotoxic therapy. J Lab Clin Med 1992; 119:397–406.

35. Agostoni A, Cicardi M. Contraindications to the use of ACE inhibitors in patients with C′1 esterase deficiency Am J Med 1991; 90:278.

36. Kozel MMA, Mekkes JR, Bos JD. Increased frequency and severity of angioedema related to long term therapy with angiotensin convertase enzyme inhibitor in two patients. Clin Exp Dermatol 1995; 20:60–61.

37. Schneider L, Lumry W, Vegh A, et al. Critical role of kallikrein in hereditary angioedema pathogenesis: a clinical trial of ecallantide, a novel kallikrein inhibitor. J Allergy Clin Immunol 2007; 120:416–422.

38. Wiggins CA, Dykewicz MS, Patterson R. Idiopathic anaphylaxis: classification, evaluation, and treatment of 123 patients. J Allergy Clin Immunol 1988; 82:849–855.

39. Wong S, Dykewicz MS, Patterson R. Idiopathic anaphylaxis: a clonal summary of 175 patients. Arch Int Med 1990; 150:1323–1328.

40. Patterson R, Stoloff RS, Greenberger DA, et al. Algorithms for the diagnosis and management of idiopathic anaphylaxis. Ann Allergy 1993; 71:40–44.

41. Bork K, Gul D, Hurdt J, et al. Hereditary angioedema with normal C1 inhibitor: clinical symptoms and course. Am J Med 2007; 120:987–992.
42. Akin C, Scott LM, Kocabas CN, et al. Demonstration of an abberent mast cell population with clonal markers in a subset of patients with "idiopathic" anaphylaxis. Blood 2007; 110:2331–2333.
43. Sonneck K, Florian S, Mullauer L, et al. Diagnostic and subdiagnostic accumulation of mast cells – The bone marrow of patients with anaphylaxis: monoclonal mast cell activation syndrome. Int Arch Allergy Immunol 2007; 142:158–164.
44. Stricker WE, Anorve-Lopez E, Reed CE. Food skin testing in patients with idiopathic anaphylaxis. J Allergy Clin Immunol 1986; 77:516–519.
45. Sheffer AL, Soter NA, MCFadden CR Jr., et al. Exercise-induced anaphylaxis: a distinct form of physical allergy. J Allergy Clin Immunol 1983; 71:311–316.
46. Maulitz RM, Pratt DS, Schocket AL. Exercise-induced anaphylactic reaction to shellfish. J Allergy Clin Immunol 1979; 63:433–434.
47. Kidd JM III, Cohen SH, Sosman AJ. Food-dependent exercise-induced anaphylaxis. J Allergy Clin Immunol 1983; 71:407–411.
48. Novey HS, Fairshter RD, Salness K, et al. Postprandial exercise-induced anaphylaxis. J Allergy Clin Immunol 1983; 71:498–504.
49. Dewald G, Bork K. Missense mutations in the coagulation factor XII (Hageman's Factor) gene in hereditary angioedema with normal C1 inhibitor. Biochem Biophys Res Commun 2006; 343:1286–1289.
50. Choy AC, Patterson R, Patterson DR, et al. Undifferentiated somatoform idiopathic anaphylaxis: non-organic symptoms mimicking idiopathic anaphylaxis. J Allergy Clin Immunol 1995; 96:893–900.
51. Patterson R, Wong S, Dykewicz MS, et al. Malignant idiopathic anaphylaxis. J Allergy Clin Immunol 1990; 85:86–88.

23

Systemic Disorders with Urticaria and/or Angioedema

Malcolm W. Greaves
St. John's Institute of Dermatology, St. Thomas' Hospital, London, U.K.

Allen P. Kaplan
Department of Medicine, Medical University of South Carolina, Charleston, South Carolina, U.S.A.

INTRODUCTION

Urticaria and angioedema may be caused by systemic disease or, theoretically, urticaria and angioedema may themselves cause systemic disease. In practice, systemic manifestations are rather rare, and even unremitting urticaria with or without angioedema rarely causes systemic upset apart from psychological distress. Even hereditary angioedema rarely causes systemic upset apart from angioedema of the bowel, which may lead to abdominal pain due to bowel wall edema, and/or obstruction. Of the physical urticarias, only delayed pressure urticaria is regularly associated with systemic symptoms such as fatigue and arthralgia. Exceptionally, cold contact urticaria can cause headache, palpitations, bronchospasm, bowel disturbance, and even anaphylactic shock—symptoms suggestive of histamine toxicity—if cold exposure is extensive as in sea bathing. Acute urticaria and angioedema are more frequently associated with constitutional symptoms, especially if the outbreak is due to an allergic cause such as IgE-mediated hypersensitivity due to foods or drugs, especially penicillin. In this situation, systemic reactions in the cardiovascular system, lungs, and gastrointestinal tract may be the dominant clinical problem and may require urgent measures to be taken. This account will focus on systemic disease as a *cause* of, or strong association with, urticaria and angioedema.

ACUTE URTICARIA WITH ANGIOEDEMA

Acute urticaria and angioedema occur commonly in adults and children alike. The clinical picture is most familiar to the primary care or emergency room physician who may be called to the patient in the acute stage. Since the natural history of the outbreak is usually brief, the cause often evident and management straightforward, referral for a specialist's opinion may not be required. The patient often initially experiences a feeling of warmth and pruritus accompanied by facial flushing, which may become more widespread. The mouth and lips may tingle or feel numb, these symptoms heralding the development of widespread urticarial lesions with angioedema of the lips, periorbital area, and elsewhere. In more severely affected patients, systemic symptoms of acute anxiety, faintness, wheezing, bowel disturbance, and palpitations may be experienced. The most feared complications—upper respiratory obstruction and anaphylactic shock—are fortunately rare, and when they do occur the culprit is often IgE-mediated penicillin, latex, or peanut allergy. Investigation and management of acute urticaria is dealt with in detail in chapter 9 and will not be considered further here.

ACUTE URTICARIA ASSOCIATED WITH FEVER

Many infections and infestations are associated with erythematous eruptions, which superficially resemble urticaria. Only those that are genuinely urticarial will be considered here.

Systemic Infections and Infestations

Acute attacks of urticaria and angioedema can occur in response to intercurrent infection, especially in children. Sometimes unfortunately termed "acute infectious urticaria" in published reports, it is not always clear if the eruption was caused by the infection itself, by its treatment, or whether it was merely exacerbated.

Bacterial Infections

In children, acute bacterial infections may be associated with attacks of urticaria. Bivings (1) describes 22 children with acute urticaria ascribed to bacterial infections, streptococcal infection being especially common (2). A Japanese study of 50 patients with less than a week's history of urticaria and angioedema reported that 43 remitted within two weeks; 5 cleared up between two weeks and three months, and 2 were persistent for at least one year (3). In 31 the cause appeared to be infection, usually gastrointestinal or respiratory, the urticaria developing after the infection was established, although occasionally the infection was prodromal. More recently, Sakurai et al. Investigated 19 patients with acute urticaria, most of whom were children (4). They had widespread urticaria, pyrexia, neutrophil leukocytosis, raised C reactive protein, and poor response to anthistamines and systemic corticosteroids. Throat cultures were positive for bacterial pathogens in eight, negative in four, and not done in seven. These patients usually respond well to antibiotics, but poorly to antihistamines. In a large European study of 57 infants and small children (upper age limit 3 years) with acute urticaria with or without angioedema, infection was believed to be the cause in 46 (81%) (5). Thirty percent went on to suffer from chronic urticaria. In summary, infections are associated with outbreaks of acute urticaria, especially in childhood. Characteristically these patients are pyrexial with a neutrophil leukocytosis and raised C-reactive protein. They do not respond well to antihistamines but may respond to antibiotics; a few go on to chronic urticaria.

Virus Infections

Some of the pediatric cases referred to above may in fact have had virus infections. One of the possible viral culprits is the Epstein-Bar virus of infectious mononucleosis. These patients get fever, pharyngitis, lymphadenopathy, and splenomegaly. Although the exanthem is classically erythematous and maculopapular, urticarial eruptions may occur (6). Upper respiratory infections are thought to be responsible for about 40% of acute urticaria in adults (7), the viruses implicated including Coxsackie A9 and B5, ECHO 11, and Herpes virus. Hepatitis B virus infection is also associated with urticaria (8). Urticaria with hepatitis B is typically a prodrome to clinical hepatitis, frequently associated with immune complex formation (hepatitis B surface antigen complexed to IgG) with complement activation as in serum sickness.

Parasite Infestations

Parasite infestations that can cause urticaria include schistosomiasis and seabathers eruption. In patients with schistosomiasis, urticaria may develop four to eight weeks after the cercaria penetrate the skin, with fever, arthralgia, diarrhea, and a blood eosinophilia (9). This syndrome is called "urticarial fever" in some parts of the Far East, and also "swimmers Itch," and is due to the immunologically driven phase of the infestation. Seabather's eruption is due to skin contact with sea anemone and thimble jellyfish. Wheals occur at sites of penetration of skin by nematocysts; fever, abdominal pain, and arthritis may be seen (10).

Other Causes of Acute Urticaria and Angioedema with Fever in Infants and Children

Not all acute urticaria or angioedema in infancy and childhood is associated with an infectious illness. Frequently no cause can be established, but other rare but recognized syndromes should also be considered.

Acute Infantile Hemorrhagic Edema

First described by Snow in 1913 (11), this striking acute angioedema was characterized by several reports mainly in the French literature in the 1960s and 70s (12). Nowadays generally recognized as a variant of leukocytoclastic vaculitis and Henoch Schonlein purpura, it presents an alarming appearance in an infant or small child, which belies a usually benign outcome. It is characteristically preceded by an upper respiratory infection followed by cocarde (targetoid) ecchymotic urticarial and angioedematous lesions, often with a rosetted border, distributed mainly on the head, neck, and limbs and with or without accompanying fever. Histologically the lesions show a leukocytoclastic vasulitis; transitory renal involvement is followed by remission in about 10 days (13). The important differential diagnosis is meningococcal septicemia and purpura fulminans. Treatment is symptomatic.

Still's Disease

Still's disease (juvenile rheumatoid arthritis) characteristically affects children but can also occur in adults. It is a febrile arthritis of unknown etiology. The rash is transient and serpiginous (erythema marginatum) and may appear urticarial, occurring in 16% of patients (14). The rheumatoid factor is negative but the antinuclear factor may be positive. This disease in adults may present with urticaria (15).

CHRONIC URTICARIA AND SYSTEMIC DISEASE

Systemic disease is a rare but important cause of chronic urticaria in children and adults.

Autoinflammatory Syndromes (16)

When urticaria in the neonate is persistent and accompanied by fever, an autoinflammatory syndrome should be considered. Those associated with urticaria or urticaria-like rashes include familial cold autoinflammatory syndrome (FCAS), Muckle-Wells syndrome (MWS), and chronic infantile neurological cutaneous articular syndrome (CINCA). These systemic inherited disorders share the common genetic feature of a mutation in the CIAS1 gene and are together termed "cryopyrin-associated syndromes." Their pathophysiology is characterized by hyperactive neutrophils and macrophages and abnormal innate immune signaling. FACS (syn. familial cold urticaria) presents as cold urticaria at birth associated with fever and other systemic symptoms (17). MWS patients also suffer chronic urticaria from birth with sensorineural deafness and eventually renal amyloidosis (18). CINCA presents with a triad of urticaria, arthritis, and CNS disorders (19). Elevated levels of interleukin-1 (IL-1) are found in these syndromes and they may respond to the IL-1 antagonist Anakinra (20). Other inherited periodic fever syndromes that occasionally manifest urticaria include tumor necrosis factor–associated periodic syndrome (TRAPS) (21) and familial Mediterranean fever (22). These syndromes are discussed in detail in chapter 15.

Common Variable Immunodeficiency

Recently, six adult patients with combined variable immunodeficiency have been described in whom chronic urticaria with or without angioedema was the initial presentation and four had a history of recurrent infections. All had reduced IgG and IgA and four also had reduced IgM (23). Four received intravenous immunoglobulin treatment, and in all these the urticaria remitted. Combined variable immunodeficiency should be considered in patients with chronic urticaria who have a history of recurrent infections.

Schnitzler's Syndrome

The association of chronic urticaria, fever, bone pain, raised erythrocyte sedimentation rate, and macroglobulinemia was first reported by Schnitzler in 1972 (24). Since then there have been numerous reports. Pruritus is variable and angioedema is rare. Histologically, skin biopsies usually show a neutrophilic urticaria; vasculitis is rarely found. Despite some resemblances to autoimmune chronic urticaria, no autoantibodies against FcεRI have been found (25). However the great majority of patients have a monoclonal IgM gammopathy with a light chain of the κ type, but without further features of lymphoproliferative disease (26). However, presence of an IgG paraprotein has been reported (27) and was found in two (unpublished) patients of one of the authors (MWG). Bone marrow examination usually reveals normal or nonspecific results. The condition needs to be distinguished from Waldenstrom's macroglobulinemia in which urticarial lesions are rare and in which the bone marrow shows lymphoproliferative changes. The prognosis of Schnitzler's syndrome is generally good, although occasional patients have developed lymphoproliferative malignancy later in life (28).

Urticarial Vasculitis

This condition is dealt with in detail in chapter 21. Urticarial vasculitis, which presents with both chronic urticaria and angioedema, is an important differential diagnosis of chronic idiopathic urticaria, is often indistinguishable from the latter, and is significantly

Table 1   Commoner Recognized Causative Systemic Diseases in Urticarial Vasculitis

---

Autoimmune connective tissue diseases: SLE $+/-$ hypocomplementemia, Sjogren's syndrome,
   rheumatoid arthritis
Serum sickness
Infections: hepatitis C with cryoglobulinaemia, Lyme disease
Inflammatory bowel disease

---

underdiagnosed. This diagnosis should not be made in the absence of histological confirmation from a skin biopsy (29). It is due to immunoreactant deposition in the walls of the post-capillary venules leading to complement activation. Urticarial vasculitis should be looked upon as a continuous pathophysiological spectrum ranging from patients with no evident systemic disease to those with severe systemic involvement. Serum hypocomplementemia is a rather unusual finding in patients with urticarial vasculitis attending a specialist dermatology clinic, and when it occurs it is usually termed "hypocomplementaemic urticarial vasculitis syndrome." This syndrome may be associated with systemic lupus erythematosus or Sjogren's syndrome and serum sickness (30), and there is often a marked and selective reduction in C1q due to antibodies against C1q (31). Inflammatory bowel disease is another important cause (32). Other recognized causes include hepatitis C infection (often with cryoglobulins) (33) and Lyme disease (34) (Table 1). Angioedema is common, and there is associated systemic disease, including obstructive pulmonary disease, arthritis, glomerulonephritis, and also ocular inflammation. In a comprehensive review of 72 patients (32) Mehregan published figures for frequency of 40% for arthralgia, 21% for pulmonary disease, 5% to 10% for renal disease, 20% for gastrointestinal complications, and fever in 10%. However most patients presenting to the dermatology clinic with confirmed urticarial vasculitis have no detectable circulating immunoreactants, but mild systemic symptoms are common, including arthralgia and lassitude. An underlying causative disease should be sought in all patients with urticarial vasculitis (35).

Human Immunodeficiency Virus Infection

Urticaria is recognised to occur in primary human immunodeficiency virus (HIV) infection when seroconversion occurs (36). There is also one report of chronic urticaria in two HIV seropositive patients (37), although the causative relationship between HIV infection and the urticaria was not established in these cases.

ANGIOEDEMA AND SYSTEMIC DISEASE

The above-mentioned systemic diseases presenting with urticaria also manifest angioedema with few exceptions. However angioedema can present alone, without urticaria. Angioedema due to hereditary complement C1 esterase inhibitor deficiency does not manifest urticaria, although a non-urticarial prodromal erythema occasionally occurs. Urticaria is not associated with angioedema caused by angiotensin converting enzyme (ACE) inhibitors. However, apart from abdominal pain due to intestinal angioedema, neither hereditary nor ACE inhibitor–induced angioedema is associated with systemic disease. Acquired C1 esterase inhibitor deficiency is associated with lymphoproliferative disease, and rarely with an autoimmune process.

Acute Episodic Angioedema with Eosinophilia

This syndrome of recurrent attacks of angioedema, fever, and high leukocytosis with 80% to 90% eosinophilia was first described by Gleich in 1984 (38). The disease usually runs a benign course, the edema being due to release of major basic protein from degranulated eosinophils. Circulating IgG anti-endothelial antibodies are often found, but there are no systemic features. Thus the condition seems distinct from the hypereosinophilic syndrome in which there are no anti-endothelial antibodies and systemic involvement is the rule.

REFERENCES

1. Bivings L. Acute infectious urticaria. J Paediatrics 1946; 28:602–604.
2. Schuller DE, Elvey SM. Acute urticaria associated with streptococcal infection. Paediatrics 1980; 65:592–596.
3. Aoki T, Kojima M, Horiko T. Acute urticaria: history and natural course of 50 cases. J Dermatol 1994; 21:73–77.
4. Sakurai M, Oba M, Matsumoto K, et al. Acute infectious urticaria: clinical and laboratory analysis in 19 patients. J Dermatol 2000; 27:87–93.
5. Mortureux P, Leaute-Labrez C, Legrain – Liefermann V, et al. Acute urticaria in infancy and early childhood. Archs Dermatol 1998; 134:319–323.
6. Cooper KD. Urticaria and angioedema: diagnosis and evaluation. J Amer Acad Dermatol 1991; 25:146–154.
7. Zuberbier T, Ifflander J, Semmler C, et al. Acute urticaria – clinical aspects and therapeutic responsiveness Acta Dermato. Vener (Stockh) 1996; 76:295–297.
8. Vaida GA, Goldman MA, Bloch KJ. Testing for hepatitis B virus in patients with chronic urticaria and angioedema J Allergy Clin Immunol 1983; 72:193–198.
9. Gonzalez E. Schistosomiasis, cercarial dermatitis, marine dermatitis. Dermatol Clinics 1989; 7: 291–300.
10. Wong D, Meinking TL, Rosen LB, et al. Seabather's eruption. J Amer Acad Dermatol 1994; 30:
11. Snow IM. Purpura, urticaria and angioedema of the hands and feet in a nursing baby J Amer Med Ass 1913; 61:18–19.
12. Laugier F, Hunziker N, Rieffers J, et al. L'oedema aigu haemorrhagique du nourisson (purpura en cocarde avec oedeme). Dermatologica 1970; 141:113–118.
13. Nouaille J, Gautier M, Lucet P. Un cas de vascularite allergique a type d'oedema aigu haemorrhagique de la peau avec manifestations renales. Archs Fr Pediatr 1960; 17:110–113.
14. Isdale IC, Bywaters EGL. The rash of rheumatoid arthritis and Still's disease. Quarterly J Med 1956; 99:377–383.
15. Setterfield JF, Hughes GVR, Black AK. Urticaria as a presentation of adult onset Still's disease. Br J Dermatol 1998; 118:924–927.
16. Ferdman RM, Shaham B, Church JA. Neonatal urticaria as a symptom of a multisystem inflammatory disease. J Allergy Immunol 2000; 106:986–987.
17. Hoffman HM, Wanderer AA, Broide DH. Familial cold autoinflammatory syndrome: phenotype and genotype of an autosomal dominant periodic fever. J Allergy Clin Immunol 2001; 108:615–620.
18. Muckle TL, Wells M. Urticaria, deafness and amyloidosis – a new hereditofamilial syndrome. Q J Med 1962; 31:235–238.
19. Prieur AM, Griscelli C. Arthropathy with rash, chronic meningitis, eye lesions and mental retardation J Pediatr 1981; 99:79–83.
20. Hoffman HM, Rosengren S, Boyle BL, et al. Prevention of cold associated acute inflammation in familial cold autoimflammatory syndrome by interleukin – 1 – receptor antagonist. Lancet 2004; 364:1779–1785.
21. Galon J, Aksentijevich I, Mc Dermott MF, et al. TNFRS1A mutations and autoinflammatory syndromes. Curr Opin Immunol 2000; 12:479–486.

22. Ehrenfield EN, Eliakim M, Rachmilwitz M. Recurrent polyserositis (familial Mediterranean fever, periodic disease) Amer J Med 1961; 31:107–111.

23. Altschul A, Cunningham – Rundles C. Chronic urticaria and angioedema as the first presentations of common variable immunodeficiency. J Allergy Clin Immunol 2002; 110:1383–1391.

24. Schnitzler L. Lesions urticariennes chroniques permanents (erytheme petaloide?) Case cliniques n. 46B Journee Dermatologique D' Angers 1972; 28th October (Abstr. 46).

25. Gallo R, Sabroe R, Black AK, et al. Schnitzler's syndrome: no evidence for an autoimmune basis in two patients. Clin Exp Dermatol 2000; 25:281–284.

26. Almerigogna F, Giudizi MG, Capelli F, et al. Schnitzler's syndrome: what's new? J Eur Acad Dermatol 2002; 16:214–219.

27. Nashan D, Sunderkotter C, Bonsmann G, et al. Chronic urticaria, arthralgia, raised erythrocyte sedimentation rate and IgG4 paraproteinaemia: a variant of Schnitzler's syndrome? Br J Dermatol 1995; 133:132–134.

28. Lipsker D, Veran Y, Grunenberger F, et al. The Schnitzler syndrome. Four new cases and a review of the literature. Medicine 2001; 80:37–44.

29. Black AK. Urticarial vasculitis. Clin Dermatol 1999; 17:565–569.

30. Lawley TJ, Bielory L, Gascon P, et al. A study of human serum sickness. J Invest Dermatol 1985; 85:129s–132s.

31. Wisnieski JJ, Baer AN, Christensen J, et al. Hypocomplementaemic urticarial vasculitis syndrome. Medicine 1995; 74:24–41.

32. Mehregan DR, Hall MJ, Gibson LE. Urticarial vasculitis : a histopathologic and clinical review of 72 cases. J Amer Acad Dermatol 1992; 26:441–448.

33. Kuniyuki S, Katoh H. Urticarial vasculitis with papular lesions in a patient with type C hepatitis and cryoglobulinaemia. J Dermatol 1996; 23:279–283.

34. Olson JC, Esterly NB. Urticarial vasculitis and Lyme disease. J Amer Acad Dermatol 1990; 22:1114–1116.

35. O'Donnell BF, Black AK. Urticarial vasculitis. Int Angiol 1995; 14:166–174.

36. Dover, JS, Johnson RA, Cutaneous manifestations of human immunodeficiency virus infection (part 2). Arch Dermatol 1991; 127:1549–1558.

37. Friedman D, Picard – Dahan C, Grossin M, et al. Chronic urticaria revealing an HIV infection. Eur Dermatol 1995; 5:40–41.

38. Gleich GJ, Schroeter A, Marcoux JP, et al. Episodic angioedema associated with eosinophilia. New Eng J Med 1984; 310:1621–1626.

24

Systemic Mastocytosis

Barbara A. Martinez, Dean D. Metcalfe, and Todd M. Wilson
Laboratory of Allergic Diseases, National Institute of Allergy and Infectious Diseases, National Institutes of Health, Bethesda, Maryland, U.S.A.

INTRODUCTION

Mastocytosis is an uncommon disease caused by a pathologic increase of mast cells (MCs) in the connective tissue of the skin, bone marrow, gastrointestinal (GI) tract, lymph nodes, liver, and spleen. Patients experience symptoms as a result of MC degranulation and infiltration. These may include episodes of pruritus, flushing, urticaria, hypotension, nausea, vomiting, diarrhea, abdominal pain, musculoskeletal pain, and headache. Severity of disease may range from isolated skin involvement to aggressive systemic disease.

EPIDEMIOLOGY

Mastocytosis is an uncommon disorder with an unknown prevalence. There are estimated 20,000 to 30,000 patients with this disease in the United States (1). Onset of disease may occur at any age. Sixty-five percent of patients are children (2). There is a relatively equal balance between male and female patients. All ethnic groups may be affected (1).

The majority of cases of mastocytosis are sporadic in occurrence. In adult patients with systemic mastocytosis, there often exists a somatic activating mutation in the tyrosine kinase receptor Kit (3,4). Rare cases of inherited mastocytosis have been reported. Since 1891, familial urticaria pigmentosa (UP) has been described in at least 50 different families, with about half of these cases involving two or more generations (5,6). Four cases of telangiectasia macularis eruptiva perstans (TMEP) have also been reported in three generations of a single family (6).

PATHOPHYSIOLOGY

Mast Cells and Degranulation

Mastocytosis is associated with a pathologic increase in number of MCs and associated release of MC mediators. MCs originate from $CD34^+$ Kit^+ bone marrow–derived hematopoietic progenitor cells in the presence of stem cell factor (SCF) that binds and cross links its receptor Kit (4,7). As the MC progenitors mature, they move from the peripheral blood into vascularized tissues where SCF is required for survival. Mature tissue MCs are long-lived, and are found especially in association with blood vessels, glandular structures, nerves, and lymphatic tissues.

MCs are activated after contact with antigen. The antigen binds to antigen-specific IgE bound to the alpha chain of the high-affinity receptor for IgE (FcεRI). This results in aggregation of FcεRI and initiation of intracellular pathways that lead to MC degranulation, and to the generation and release of chemical mediators that induce immediate hypersensitivity reactions. MCs may also be activated by non-IgE-dependent mechanisms involving, as examples, Toll-like receptors and their ligands (i.e., lipopolysaccharide) and through receptors for anaphylatoxins (i.e., C3a and C5a) (8).

Proinflammatory mediators that contribute to symptoms in mastocytosis include histamine, tryptase, prostaglandins, and leukotrienes. Histamine exerts its effects through various histamine receptors, most notably the H_1 and H_2 receptors. H_1 receptor activation results in increased contraction of smooth muscle in the airways and GI tract, as well as increased permeability via vascular endothelial cells. H_2 receptor activation results in increased gastric acid secretion.

Role of Kit

Kit (CD117) is a tyrosine kinase transmembrane protein that acts as the receptor for SCF. It is encoded by the proto-oncogene *c-kit* on chromosome 4 (9). It is a type III tyrosine kinase receptor that contains three domains: extracellular, transmembrane, and intracellular. Dimerization of Kit, by the binding of its ligand SCF, results in the initiation of signal transduction. MCs, hematopoietic stem cells, germ cells, and melanocytes all express Kit. SCF is important for the early steps of stem cell development, but is then downregulated as hematopoietically–derived cells mature (10,11). In MCs, however, Kit remains expressed on mature cells. SCF through Kit is necessary for MC differentiation and survival. MCs will also chemotax to SCF, and SCF enhances MC degranulation (12).

Activating mutations in Kit are frequently identified in patients with systemic mastocytosis, and most often occur in the carboxy terminal tyrosine kinase domain of the intracellular segment (3,4). A point mutation, substituting aspartate for valine at the 816 codon (D816V), results in ligand-independent phosphylation and activation. This is the most common mutation observed in mastocytosis, and in one study was identified in greater than 90% of adult patients with systemic mastocytosis (13).

Genetic alterations have also been described in patients with cutaneous mastocytosis. There are reports of both activating (D816V) and inactivating Kit mutations (E839K) in children with UP (14). In addition, the substitution of phenylalanine for cysteine (F522C) in Kit was also demonstrated in a patient with skin manifestations typical of cutaneous mastocytosis. This case reported a well-differentiated MC phenotype, but lacked the diagnostic criteria for systemic mastocytosis (15). Interleukin-4 (IL-4) has been shown to increase MC apoptosis. Children with a polymorphism in the IL-4 receptor alpha chain (IL-4Rα), resulting in the substitution of glutamine for arginine (Q576R), have demonstrated less severe disease (16).

DISEASE CLASSIFICATION/DIAGNOSIS

There are seven accepted variants of mastocytosis. These include cutaneous mastocytosis (CM), indolent systemic mastocytosis (ISM), systemic mastocytosis with an associated clonal hematological non-MC-lineage disease (SM-AHNMD), aggressive systemic mastocytosis (ASM), MC leukemia (MCL), MC sarcoma (MCS), and extracutaneous mastocytoma (17,18).

Cutaneous Mastocytosis

CM is diagnosed by the presence of distinct skin lesions, but without evidence of systemic mastocytosis. This disorder is typically seen in children in the absence of systemic disease. These patients tend to have a favorable prognosis with resolution of skin lesions at or around puberty (19). Three different variants of CM have been described: maculopapular CM (MPCM), mastocytoma of the skin, and diffuse CM (DCM) (18,20).

Maculopapular Cutaneous Mastocytosis

MPCM, often referred to as UP, is the most common variant of CM, affecting approximately 85% of patients with skin limited disease (20). MPCM presents as a maculopapular rash that occurs on the trunk and later on the extremities. Lesions tend to be symmetrical but vary in size, depending upon the age of the patient. The lesions demonstrate evidence of urtication upon stroking or scratching (Darier's sign). Multiple lesions may occur; and are enduring and fawn-colored (Fig. 1). They may be seen

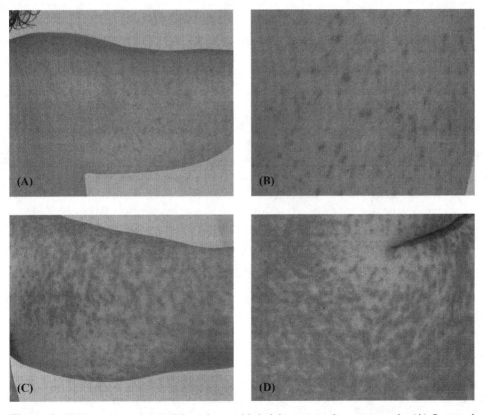

Figure 1 UP is seen on these adult patients with indolent systemic mastocytosis. (**A**) Scattered fawn-colored macules are viewed on the arm of this patient. (**B**) Close-up (**C**) Numerous macules are present on the arm of this patient to the point of confluence. (**D**) Close-up. *Abbreviation*: UP, urticaria pigmentosa

Table 1 Distinguishing Characteristics of UP Vs. Urticaria

	Maculopapular cutaneous mastocytosis/UP	Acute and chronic urticaria
Age of onset	Majority by 6 mo in children. Any age in adult population.	Any age
Time course	>6 wk	Acute <6 wk Chronic >6 wk
Individual lesion duration	Mo to yr	<48 hr (urticarial vasculitis 1–7 days)
Lesion color	Red-orange-brown, fawn-colored, hyperpigmented.	Red/white
Lesion reaction	Darier's sign[a]	Blanches with pressure
Distribution	Worse on trunk > face, scalp > palms, soles. Symmetric	Occur anywhere. May be asymmetric.
Biopsy	Multifocal MC infiltrates in dermis, >20 MCs per high power field.	Normal to slightly increase in MC number in dermis, dermal edema, dilated lymphatics, and capillaries.
Serum total tryptase	May be elevated with systemic disease.	Normal if onset not associated with systemic allergic reaction.

[a]Wheal and flare after stroking of the lesion.
Abbreviations: UP, urticaria pigmentosa; MC, mast cell.

anywhere on the skin, including mucosal membranes. Lesions tend to be less pronounced in sun-exposed areas, including the head and the neck. MPCM is rarely seen on the palms and soles. One series reports up to 25% of patients with MPCM may experience generalized symptoms from MC degranulation, including flushing, wheezing, and GI distress (20). MPCM may be mistaken for urticaria, but there are many features to differentiate MPCM from urticaria (Table 1).

Patients with MPCM will have an increase in numbers of MCs that may diffusely infiltrate the biopsied tissue or cluster in the dermal papillae and subcutaneous tissue (21). Interestingly, normal appearing dermal tissues in patients with mastocytosis will also have an increase in MCs (22). There are other subvariants of MPCM, which include papular/plaque CM and TMEP (20).

Papular/Plaque CM This form of MPCM has brown, yellow, and orange papules up to 1 cm in diameter that may coalesce to form plaques. Darier's sign is evident. These lesions present early in infancy, and half or more of the lesions resolve by puberty. It is unusual to see adults with this subvariant of MPCM (20).

Telangectasia Macularis Eruptive Perstans. TMEP is an infrequent form of MPCM. It occurs in less than 1% of mastocytosis patients and is observed mainly in adults. TMEP is characterized by generalized, reddish-brown macules with telangiectasias, and a brown background color. Lesions are small, approximately 2 to 6 mm in diameter with ill-defined borders. Darier's sign and pruritus may be present, but are less frequent compared with other variants of MPCM. TMEP patients have a lesser amount of MC infiltration observed in biopsy specimens compared with other forms of CM. MCs may be observed in increased numbers around the vessels of the superficial plexus (23).

Mastocytomas of the Skin

Another rare form of CM is mastocytoma of the skin. These lesions, also known as nodular CM, are brownish nodules usually appearing on infants less than three months of age (19,24). Nodules are typically greater than 1 cm in size, usually positioned on the extremities, and may be several in number (20). These tumors have distinct borders. Scratching such lesions may result in Darier's sign. Trauma to mastocytomas have resulted in generalized flushing, while more severe systemic symptoms are rarely reported (25). In some cases and without specific therapy, these lesions are known to spontaneously involute.

Diffuse Cutaneous Mastocytosis

DCM is another extremely rare form of CM (26). It has distinctive total body skin manifestations but usually lacks UP. This disease typically presents in children less than three years of age. The skin may be thickened with a reddish-brown *peau d'orange* appearance. Darier's sign is observed. Diffuse bullae with hemorrhage may form spontaneously or after trauma (26,27). These blisters have been described at birth after a vaginal delivery in children (28). Biopsies of the involved skin with DCM demonstrate a more diffuse and dense MC infiltration throughout the dermis and around the vasculature (22). DCM usually resolves by five years of age (20).

Evaluation of Cutaneous Disease

Cutaneous involvement in children is often not associated with systemic disease, while in adults it is typically associated with systemic mastocytosis. The current consensus recommends classifying patients temporarily as "mastocytosis in the skin" (MIS) until a complete evaluation is performed. MIS is defined by the presence of a typical exathema (major MIS criterion), and one or two of the following minor MIS criteria applied in a stepwise fashion: (*i*) mono-morphic MC infiltration that consists of large aggregates of tryptase-positive MCs (>15 cells/cluster) or scattered MCs exceeding 20 cells per high power field (40×); (*ii*) detection of the Kit mutation at codon 816 in lesional skin. If the histological exam is indeterminate, the presence of a Kit mutation at codon 816 in lesional skin will confirm the diagnosis of MIS. Adults should then be evaluated with a serum total tryptase level and bone marrow biopsy to rule out systemic disease. Children, instead, may proceed first with a serum total tryptase level. If the serum tryptase level is within normal limits and there are no other signs of systemic mastocytosis, then they are diagnosed with CM and are followed until the lesions resolve or through puberty. If the tryptase level is >20 ng/dL, a bone marrow biopsy may be required (18).

Systemic Mastocytosis

World Health Organization Criteria for Systemic Mastocytosis

For patients to be diagnosed with systemic mastocytosis there are defined criteria provided by the World Health Organization (WHO) that need to be fulfilled. The diagnosis of mastocytosis requires one major and one minor criterion, or three minor criteria to be documented (Table 2). To classify patients into more aggressive forms of systemic mastocytosis, there are additional criteria termed "B" and "C" findings. Patients with smoldering systemic mastocytosis, a subvariant of indolent mastocytosis, must possess two B findings; whereas, having one C finding is required for the diagnosis of aggressive systemic mastocytosis (Table 3) (17,29).

Table 2 WHO Criteria for Diagnosis[a] of Systemic Mastocytosis

Major	Multifocal, dense MC infiltrates with >15 MCs per aggregate detected via tryptase-immunohistochemistry or other special stains in bone marrow or extracutaneous organ biopsy.
Minor	Evidence of >25% spindle-shaped or atypical MCs in bone marrow or extracutaneous organ sections, atypical or immature MCs comprise >25% of all MCs seen on bone marrow smears.
	Genetic analysis revealing Kit point mutation at the 816 codon in the bone marrow, blood, or extracutaneous organs.
	Evidence of coexpression of Kit (CD117) with CD2 and/or CD25 surface markers on bone marrow, blood or extracutaneous organ MCs.
	Persistent elevation of serum total tryptase level >20 ng/mL (in the absence of an associated clonal myeloid disorder).

[a]Diagnosis requires one major and one minor criterion each, or three minor criteria. *Source*: From Ref. 29.

Table 3 WHO B and C Findings

B Findings	Bone marrow biopsy demonstrating >30% MC infiltration (focal, dense aggregates) with or without serum total tryptase levels >200 ng/mL.
	Evidence of myeloproliferation or dysplasia in non-MC-lineage, but with insufficient WHO criteria for the diagnosis of a hematopoietic neoplasm, and relatively normal blood counts.
	Hepatomegaly without liver impairment, and/or palpable splenomegaly without hypersplenism, and/or palpable or visceral lymphadenopathy
C Findings	Bone marrow dysfunction evident by abnormalities in the blood counts ($ANC < 1.0 \times 10^9/L$, $Hb < 10$ g/dL or platelets $< 100 \times 10^9/L$) without non-MC hematopoietic malignancy.
	Palpable hepatomegaly with liver dysfunction, ascites and/or portal hypertension.
	Palpable splenomegaly with hypersplenism.
	Skeletal abnormalities with large-sized osteolysis and/or pathologic fractures.
	Malabsorption with weight loss due to GI MC infiltration.

After meeting criteria for systemic mastocytosis, smoldering systemic mastocytosis will have two or more of the B findings, while aggressive systemic mastocytosis will have one or more C findings. *Abbreviations*: MC, mast cell; ANC, absolute neutrophil count; Hb, hemoglobin; GI, gastrointestinal tract. *Source:* From Ref. 29.

Indolent Systemic Mastocytosis

ISM is the most common form of systemic mastocytosis (27). It is a relatively stable variant and possesses a favorable prognosis. Patients fulfill all the criteria for systemic mastocytosis, but have no evidence of B or C findings. MCs may be detected in various organs throughout the body, but there is little or no evidence of end organ damage (17,29).

Smoldering systemic mastocytosis is a subvariant of ISM, in which a higher MC burden is generally found. These patients do not demonstrate organ dysfunction, but will possess two or more of the B criteria (17,29). Their long-term prognosis is unpredictable.

Systemic Mastocytosis with an Associated Clonal Hematological Non-MC-Lineage Disease

This variant of patients with systemic mastocytosis has developed an associated hematological non-MC malignancy. This disease is uncommon in children. The hematological abnormalities seen in these patients are generally myeloproliferative or myelodysplastic (30). Current recommendations stress that each disease must be treated independently (1,18).

Aggressive Systemic Mastocytosis

ASM is a rare variant of systemic mastocytosis in which MC numbers are increasing, greater infiltration of the bone marrow is observed, and there is evidence of organ dysfunction. Patients must possess one of the C criteria (17,29). Bone marrow biopsies may display varying degrees of infiltration and tryptase levels may be high. The prognosis is usually poor, and these patients will require cytoreductive therapy.

Mast Cell Leukemia

MCL is a rare, rapid, and fatal disease. The estimated average life expectancy is six to seven months (1). These patients have fulfilled the criteria for systemic mastocytosis, have evidence of biopsy proven atypical, immature MCs, possess ≥20% infiltration of their bone marrow by MCs, and have multiorgan dysfunction (29). MCs are seen in peripheral smear and may be ≥10% of circulating white cells (17). In the bone marrow of these patients, normal architecture is almost completely replaced by MCs. The peripheral blood counts reflect this in anemia and thrombocytopenia. Patients experience symptoms from MC mediator release, experience weight loss, and may suffer from severe bone pain.

CLINICAL MANIFESTATIONS

Most symptoms of mastocytosis result from the increased MC burden and release of mediators. Complaints may be similar among patients despite having different variants of disease. Patients may describe multisystem complaints, but skin (pruritus 88% and flushing 43%) and GI symptoms (80%) appear to be most common (31). Pruritus may worsen with changes in temperature or with scratching; and following ingestion of hot liquids, spicy foods, alcohol, and certain medications. Flushing is often accompanied by a warm sensation felt from an increased blood flow to cutaneous tissues secondary to vasodilatation. In mastocytosis, this vasodilatation results from release of MC mediators including histamine and arachidonic acid metabolites. There are other causes of flushing that need to be considered. Some of the more common conditions associated with flushing are perimenopausal hot flashes, pheochromocytoma, carcinoid syndrome, and infections.

Angioedema rarely occurs in mastocytosis. Angioedema is believed to occur after release of inflammatory mediators into the deeper tissues, which results in vasodilatation and increased permeability of capillaries and venules. A number of disorders are associated with angioedema with or without urticaria, and should be considered in the differential diagnosis. These include allergic reactions, autoimmune diseases, adverse reactions to certain medications, C1 inhibitor deficiency, and infections.

Anaphylaxis may be seen in patients with systemic mastocytosis, and urticaria/ angioedema, flushing, wheezing, hypotension, and/or abdominal pain may be present. Anaphylaxis has been examined in a cohort of patients with systemic mastocytosis. This study reported that 22% of adults and 6% of children had experienced at least one episode of anaphylaxis. More males appeared to be affected than females. In these patients, only 25% of the episodes of anaphylaxis were reported as IgE mediated (32).

GI complaints are common in both adult and pediatric mastocytosis patients. These include abdominal pain, nausea, vomiting, and diarrhea. Elevated blood histamine levels are associated with an increase in gastric acid secretion and peptic ulcer disease. In unusual cases, malabsorption may be present (33). Other disorders to be considered in the differential diagnosis include *Helicobacter pylori* infection, acid reflux disease, inflammatory bowel disease, vasoactive intestinal peptide-secreting tumor, and Zollinger-Ellison Syndrome.

Hepatomegaly may be seen as MCs infiltrate the liver, but severe liver dysfunction is unusual. Approximately 45% patients with ISM have been noted to have elevated liver function tests compared with normals (34). In patients with SM-AHNMD and ASM, MC infiltration may result in hepatic dysfunction, portal hypertension, ascites, and liver fibrosis (34). Splenomegaly is observed in approximately 70% of patients with systemic mastocytosis (35). In patients with ASM or SM-AHNMD, splenomegaly may be marked. MC infiltration has been observed diffusely in the red pulp, while it is more focal in the white pulp (35). Fibrosis and thrombocytopenia may result.

Osteoporosis, osteopenia, and musculoskeletal pain may occur in systemic mastocytosis. These conditions are believed to result both directly from the MC infiltration of the bone marrow and indirectly from the local and systemic release of mediators from MCs including tryptase, heparin, and IL-6. Even patients with ISM may have evidence of early osteoporosis, and should receive bone mineral density scans (36).

EVALUATION OF SYSTEMIC MASTOCYTOSIS

Systemic mastocytosis should be suspected in patients with symptoms of MC mediator release, abnormal blood counts, and hepatosplenomegaly. Most patients with systemic mastocytosis will have a serum total tryptase level of >20 ng/mL, therefore, this test is helpful in evaluating a patient for systemic mastocytosis. Elevated serum total tryptase levels are not specific to systemic mastocytosis. Other disorders, such as myeloid non-MC-lineage neoplasms and a subset of patients with hypereosinophilic syndrome, may also possess increased tryptase levels (37). Total tryptase levels also increase following a severe systemic allergic reaction.

Additional laboratory tests obtained during the evaluation include a complete blood count with differential serum chemistries and liver function tests. If the initial history, physical exam, and laboratory studies warrant a bone marrow aspiration and biopsy, then immunophenotyping and molecular analysis for the presence of the *c-kit* D816V mutation should be performed. Additional studies to aid in the patient's assessment are determined by clinical situation and include computerized tomography scans, GI evaluation via endoscopy, plain films of the bone, and bone density scans depending on clinical and laboratory findings. A generalized approach for evaluating an adult patient for mastocytosis is provided (Fig. 2).

TREATMENT

The treatment for patients with mastocytosis is determined by the specific variant of mastocytosis and patient-specific symptoms. Those with cutaneous and limited systemic disease require symptomatic therapy, while patients with aggressive systemic mastocytosis require a multidisciplinary approach and more aggressive therapy (38).

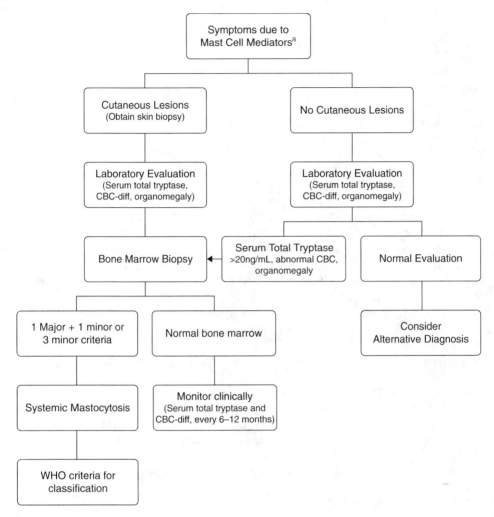

^aMediator symptoms include pruritus, flushing, anaphylaxis, diarrhea, malabsorption, etc.

Figure 2 Generalized algorithm for evaluating adult patients for mastocytosis.

Symptomatic Therapy

Controlling the symptoms that result from MC mediator release is important for the management of mastocytosis. Patient education and avoidance of potential triggers are crucial to controlling symptoms and preventing flares. Most variants of mastocytosis will require the use of the following classes of medications: antihistamines, epinephrine, glucocorticoids, and bisphosphonates.

Antihistamines are useful in the management of symptoms, but do not alter disease course. H_1 receptor blockade may help ameliorate symptoms produced by MC degranulation. The first-generation H_1 antihistamines such as diphenhydramine and hydroxyzine will reduce itching. Side effects, mainly sedation, often limit their use. Newer nonsedating second-generation antihistamines, such as cetirizine, desloratadine, fexofenadine, loratadine, and levocetirizine, may be substituted. H_2 antihistamines, including cimetidine, famotidine, and ranitidine, have also been used for symptom control. Studies have suggested their efficacy in reducing pruritis and wheal formation (39–42).

Epinephrine is critical for effective treatment of episodes of hypotension (anaphylaxis) in systemic mastocytosis. All patients with systemic mastocytosis and family members should receive instruction on the use of epinephrine autoinjectors. Medical alert bracelets stating anaphylaxis risk are routinely recommended. At the first sign of anaphylaxis, patients should receive epinephrine (self-administered or administered by someone skilled in the use of autoinjectors) and activate the emergency response system. The epinephrine injection may be repeated if needed. Emergency medicine departments should follow standard treatments for anaphylaxis. Obtaining a serum total tryptase level after patient stabilization may aid in the evaluation and diagnosis of anaphylaxis. Even in systemic mastocytosis, tryptase levels may increase above baseline. Patients with systemic mastocytosis and recurrent episodes of anaphylaxis have been reported to respond to omalizumab, but further studies are needed (43).

GI symptoms are often difficult to treat. H_2 antihistamines have been reported to be helpful in reducing gastric acid secretion and controlling gastric ulcers (33,44–46). They play a minor role in controlling malabsorption and diarrhea (45,47). Proton pump inhibitors, such as esomeprazole, lansoprazole, omeprazole, pantoprazole, and rabeprazole, may also help reduce gastric acid secretion and possibly control diarrhea (38). Oral cromolyn sodium has been reported to aid in nausea, vomiting, abdominal pain, and diarrhea, particularly in children (48–50). In ASM, glucocorticoids have been used to treat patients with ascites, portal hypertension, and problems with malabsorption (51).

There are several approaches to the treatment of cutaneous diseases. H_1 and H_2 antihistamines are used to relieve pruritus. Glucocorticoids have been used topically and intralesionally in patients with UP; however, lesions may recur upon cessation of therapy (52,53). Ultraviolet radiation in the form of oral methoxypsoralen plus ultraviolet A radiation (PUVA) has also been used as therapy for UP (54–60). Treatment may decrease the number of MCs reducing pruritus in the skin (58,59,61,62). Lesions may disappear or lessen, but often reappear after cessation of PUVA. The bullae associated with severe cutaneous disease require additional local wound care and dressing changes until healed.

Bone disease, which often results in osteopenia and osteoporosis, is treated with bisphosphonates, vitamin D, and calcium (63,64). Estrogens and androgens may be considered if appropriate. The goal is to prevent further bone loss and improve bone mineral density. Annual bone density screening should be performed in all patients with systemic mastocytosis.

Cytoreductive Therapy

Cytoreductive therapy may be mutagenic in cases of low-grade hematopoietic disorders, and is therefore reserved for more aggressive forms of systemic mastocytosis to help prevent disease progression. Their use should be limited to avoid transformation. Cytoreductive agents may be used to treat ASM, SM-AHNMD, and MCL (65).

Interferon alpha (IFN-α) has been used in systemic mastocytosis because of its known immunomodulatory effect on hematopoietic cells (66). It was first shown to be effective in mastocytosis in a case of ASM (67). While some studies have shown improvement of patient's symptoms, overall efficacy has been variable (68,69). Studies with IFN-α have shown variable reductions in MC burden and marrow infiltration, but generally no reduction in serum tryptase levels. Some patients report an improvement in their skin and GI symptoms (68,69). In cases of severe osteoporosis evident by compression fractures, IFN-α use was found to increase bone mineral density (70). Treatments are continued until symptoms are controlled or side effects occur (65). Adverse effects may be severe and include fever, fatigue, anorexia, abnormal blood counts, depression, hypothyroidism, myalgias, and bone pain (71).

2-Chlorodeoxyadenosine (cladribine or 2-CDA) is a purine nucleoside analog. After phosphorylation to 2-chlorodeoxyadenosine 5'triphosphate, this drug collects in cells (72). 2-CDA inhibits deoxyribonucleic acid (DNA) synthesis and repair in dividing lymphocytes. Further studies have shown efficacy in inhibiting monocytes and MC progenitors (73). In patients resistant to INF-α, 2-CDA may result in a reduced number of UP lesions and decreased bone marrow MC burden (74). 2-CDA may play a role in prolonging survival in MCL, as evident by cessation of MC growth in a case of MCL for over two years (75). Therapy with 2-CDA is limited by side effects, such as lowered complete blood count and infection from bone marrow suppression (76).

Imatinib mesylate is a potent ATP-competitive tyrosine kinase inhibitor with several different targets including wild-type Kit. However, the use of imatinib in systemic mastocytosis is limited because of its inability to inhibit the Kit D816V mutation (77–79). This mutation is thought to inhibit the binding of imatinib to the tyrosine kinase pocket, rendering it ineffective. Imatinib in this situation may actually inhibit wild-type Kit, and preferentially select for mutant MC clone growth and worsen disease (80). Some patients who have mutations in other areas of Kit, most notably F522C in the transmembrane portion of Kit, have demonstrated decreased bone marrow MCs with imatinib (15). Therefore, it is critical to screen patients for the *c-kit* mutation prior to initiation of therapy with imatinib and ex vivo inhibition studies using patient-specific cells may be performed to determine efficacy (38).

Clinical trials with tyrosine kinase inhibitors that target the Kit D816V mutation are in progress. Dasatinib was recently evaluated in 30 patients with systemic mastocytosis. Two complete remissions were induced, although both lacked the D816V Kit mutation and exhibited low tryptase levels. Significant systemic side effects, including pleural effusions, were reported (81). Midostaurine (PKC412) has produced slightly more promising results. Although no complete remissions were observed, 11 of 15 patients (73%) with ASM demonstrated a response (5 major and 6 partial) in a recent interim report. Nausea and vomiting were the most frequent nonhematologic toxicities (82). In vitro combinational therapeutic approaches are also under investigation and may prove more effective than single agent therapy (80).

SUMMARY

Mastocytosis is an unusual disorder with a variety of clinical manifestations. The diagnosis and management of mastocytosis pose a challenge to physicians. A careful history, physical examination, supporting laboratory analysis, and a bone marrow biopsy with aspirate are often necessary to confirm the diagnosis, and determine disease severity and variant. Often, therapy is directed at symptomatic control, but in certain patients cytoreductive therapy is required. As our understanding of the genetics and molecular pathogenesis of MC disease increases, new, and perhaps, targeted therapies will be developed.

ACKNOWLEDGMENTS

This work was supported by the Intramural Research Program of the National Institute of Allergy and Infectious Diseases at the National Institutes of Health.

REFERENCES

1. Robyn J, Metcalfe DD. Systemic mastocytosis. Adv Immunol 2006; 89:169–243.
2. Hartmann K, Metcalfe DD. Pediatric mastocytosis. Hematol Oncol Clin North Am 2000; 14(3): 625–640.
3. Longley BJ, Tyrrell L, Lu SZ, et al. Somatic c-KIT activating mutation in urticaria pigmentosa and aggressive mastocytosis: establishment of clonality in a human mast cell neoplasm. Nat Genet 1996; 12(3):312–314.
4. Nagata H, Worobec AS, Oh CK, et al. Identification of a point mutation in the catalytic domain of the protooncogene c-kit in peripheral blood mononuclear cells of patients who have mastocytosis with an associated hematologic disorder. Proc Natl Acad Sci U S A 1995; 92(23): 10560–10564.
5. Anstey A, Lowe DG, Kirby JD, et al. Familial mastocytosis: a clinical, immunophenotypic, light and electron microscopic study. Br J Dermatol 1991; 125(6):583–587.
6. Chang A, Tung RC, Schlesinger T, et al. Familial cutaneous mastocytosis. Pediatr Dermatol 2001; 18(4):271–276.
7. Rottem M, Okada T, Goff JP, et al. Mast cells cultured from the peripheral blood of normal donors and patients with mastocytosis originate from a CD34+/Fc epsilon RI-cell population. Blood 1994; 84(8):2489–2496.
8. Mekori YA. Lymphoid tissues and the immune system in mastocytosis. Hematol Oncol Clin North Am 2000; 14(3):569–577.
9. Yarden Y, Kuang WJ, Yang-Feng T, et al. Human proto-oncogene c-kit: a new cell surface receptor tyrosine kinase for an unidentified ligand. Embo J 1987; 6(11):3341–3351.
10. Ogawa M, Matsuzaki Y, Nishikawa S, et al. Expression and function of c-kit in hemopoietic progenitor cells. J Exp Med 1991; 174(1):63–71.
11. Okada S, Nakauchi H, Nagayoshi K, et al. Enrichment and characterization of murine hematopoietic stem cells that express c-kit molecule. Blood 1991; 78(7):1706–1712.
12. Akin C, Metcalfe DD. The biology of Kit in disease and the application of pharmacogenetics. J Allergy Clin Immunol 2004; 114(1):13–19; quiz 20.
13. Garcia-Montero AC, Jara-Acevedo M, Teodosio C, et al. KIT mutation in mast cells and other bone marrow hematopoietic cell lineages in systemic mast cell disorders: a prospective study of the Spanish Network on Mastocytosis (REMA) in a series of 113 patients. Blood 2006; 108(7): 2366–2372.
14. Longley BJ Jr, Metcalfe DD, Tharp M, et al. Activating and dominant inactivating c-KIT catalytic domain mutations in distinct clinical forms of human mastocytosis. Proc Natl Acad Sci U S A 1999; 96(4):1609–1614.
15. Akin C, Fumo G, Yavuz AS, et al. A novel form of mastocytosis associated with a transmembrane c-kit mutation and response to imatinib. Blood 2004; 103(8):3222–3225.
16. Daley T, Metcalfe DD, Akin C. Association of the Q576R polymorphism in the interleukin-4 receptor alpha chain with indolent mastocytosis limited to the skin. Blood 2001; 98(3): 880–882.
17. Valent P, Horny HP, Escribano L, et al. Diagnostic criteria and classification of mastocytosis: a consensus proposal. Leuk Res 2001; 25(7):603–625.
18. Valent P, Akin C, Escribano L, et al. Standards and standardization in mastocytosis: consensus statements on diagnostics, treatment recommendations and response criteria. Eur J Clin Invest 2007; 37(6):435–453.
19. Caplan RM. The natural course of urticaria pigmentosa. Analysis and follow-up of 112 cases. Arch Dermatol 1963; 87:146–157.
20. Wolff K, Komar M, Petzelbauer P. Clinical and histopathological aspects of cutaneous mastocytosis. Leuk Res 2001; 25(7):519–528.
21. Garriga MM, Friedman MM, Metcalfe DD. A survey of the number and distribution of mast cells in the skin of patients with mast cell disorders. J Allergy Clin Immunol 1988; 82(3 Pt 1): 425–432.

22. Carter MC, Metcalfe DD. Biology of mast cells and the mastocytosis syndromes. In: Wolff K, Goldsmith LA, Katz SI, Gilchrest BA, Paller AS, Leffell DJ, eds. Fitzpatrick's Dermatology in General Medicine. 7th ed. New York: McGraw, 2003:1434–1443.

23. Soter NA. Mastocytosis and the skin. Hematol Oncol Clin North Am 2000; 14(3):537–555, vi.

24. Chargin L, Sachs PM. Urticaria pigmentosa appearing as a solitary nodular lesion. AMA Arch Derm Syphilol 1954; 63(3):345–355.

25. Birt AR, Nickerson M. Generalized flushing of the skin with urticaria pigmentosa. Arch Dermatol 1959; 80:311–317.

26. Golitz LE, Weston WL, Lane AT. Bullous mastocytosis: diffuse cutaneous mastocytosis with extensive blisters mimicking scalded skin syndrome or erythema multiforme. Pediatr Dermatol 1984; 1(4):288–294.

27. Valent P, Akin C, Sperr WR, et al. Mastocytosis: pathology, genetics, and current options for therapy. Leuk Lymphoma 2005; 46(1):35–48.

28. Orkin M, Good RA, Clawson CC, et al. Bullous mastocytosis. Arch Dermatol 1970; 101(5): 547–564.

29. Valent P, Horny HP, Li CY, et al. Mastocytosis. World Health Organization Classification of Tumours: Pathology and Genetics of Tumours of the Haematopoietic and Lymphoid Tissues. Lyon: IARC Press, 2001:292–302.

30. Horny HP, Sotlar K, Sperr WR, et al. Systemic mastocytosis with associated clonal haematological non-mast cell lineage diseases: a histopathological challenge. J Clin Pathol 2004; 57(6):604–608.

31. Cherner JA, Jensen RT, Dubois A, et al. Gastrointestinal dysfunction in systemic mastocytosis. A prospective study. Gastroenterology 1988; 95(3):657–667.

32. Gonzalez de Olano D, de la Hoz Caballer B, Nunez Lopez R, et al. Prevalence of allergy and anaphylactic symptoms in 210 adult and pediatric patients with mastocytosis in Spain: a study of the Spanish network on mastocytosis (REMA). Clin Exp Allergy 2007; 37(10):1547–1555.

33. Jensen RT. Gastrointestinal abnormalities and involvement in systemic mastocytosis. Hematol Oncol Clin North Am 2000; 14(3):579–623.

34. Mican JM, Di Bisceglie AM, Fong TL, et al. Hepatic involvement in mastocytosis: clinicopathologic correlations in 41 cases. Hepatology 1995; 22(4 Pt 1):1163–1170.

35. Horny HP, Ruck MT, Kaiserling E. Spleen findings in generalized mastocytosis. A clinicopathologic study. Cancer 1992; 70(2):459–468.

36. Kushnir-Sukhov NM, Brittain E, Reynolds JC, et al. Elevated tryptase levels are associated with greater bone density in a cohort of patients with mastocytosis. Int Arch Allergy Immunol 2006; 139(3):265–270.

37. Maric I, Robyn J, Metcalfe DD, et al. KIT D816V-associated systemic mastocytosis with eosinophilia and FIP1L1/PDGFRA-associated chronic eosinophilic leukemia are distinct entities. J Allergy Clin Immunol 2007; 120(3):680–687.

38. Wilson TM, Metcalfe DD, Robyn J. Treatment of systemic mastocytosis. Immunol Allergy Clin North Am 2006; 26(3):549–573.

39. Fenske NA, Lober CW, Pautler SE. Congenital bullous urticaria pigmentosa. Treatment with concomitant use of H1- and H2-receptor antagonists. Arch Dermatol 1985; 121(1):115–118.

40. Frieri M, Alling DW, Metcalfe DD. Comparison of the therapeutic efficacy of cromolyn sodium with that of combined chlorpheniramine and cimetidine in systemic mastocytosis. Results of a double-blind clinical trial. Am J Med 1985; 78(1):9–14.

41. Gasior-Chrzan B, Falk ES. Systemic mastocytosis treated with histamine H1 and H2 receptor antagonists. Dermatology 1992; 184(2):149–152.

42. Kurosawa M, Amano H, Kanbe N, et al. Heterogeneity of mast cells in mastocytosis and inhibitory effect of ketotifen and ranitidine on indolent systemic mastocytosis. J Allergy Clin Immunol 1997; 100(6 Pt 2):S25–S32.

43. Carter MC, Robyn JA, Bressler PB, et al. Omalizumab for the treatment of unprovoked anaphylaxis in patients with systemic mastocytosis. J Allergy Clin Immunol 2007; 119(6):1550–1551.

44. Berg MJ, Bernhard H, Schentag JJ. Cimetidine in systemic mastocytosis. Drug Intell Clin Pharm 1981; 15(3):180–183.

45. Hirschowitz BI, Groarke JF. Effect of cimetidine on gastric hypersecretion and diarrhea in systemic mastocytosis. Ann Intern Med 1979; 90(5):769–771.

46. Johnson GJ, Silvis SE, Roitman B, et al. Long-term treatment of systemic mastocytosis with histamine H2 receptor antagonists. Am J Gastroenterol 1980; 74(6):485–489.

47. Bredfeldt JE, O'Laughlin JC, Durham JB, et al. Malabsorption and gastric hyperacidity in systemic mastocytosis. Results of cimetidine therapy. Am J Gastroenterol 1980; 74(2):133–137.

48. Alexander RR. Disodium cromoglycate in the treatment of systemic mastocytosis involving only bone. Acta Haematol 1985; 74(2):108–110.

49. Horan RF, Sheffer AL, Austen KF. Cromolyn sodium in the management of systemic mastocytosis. J Allergy Clin Immunol 1990; 85(5):852–855.

50. Soter NA, Austen KF, Wasserman SI. Oral disodium cromoglycate in the treatment of systemic mastocytosis. N Engl J Med 1979; 301(9):465–469.

51. Reisberg IR, Oyakawa S. Mastocytosis with malabsorption, myelofibrosis, and massive ascites. Am J Gastroenterol 1987; 82(1):54–60.

52. Barton J, Lavker RM, Schechter NM, et al. Treatment of urticaria pigmentosa with corticosteroids. Arch Dermatol 1985; 121(12):1516–1523.

53. Guzzo C, Lavker R, Roberts LJ, 2nd, et al. Urticaria pigmentosa. Systemic evaluation and successful treatment with topical steroids. Arch Dermatol 1991; 127(2):191–196.

54. Mackey S, Pride HB, Tyler WB. Diffuse cutaneous mastocytosis. Treatment with oral psoralen plus UV-A. Arch Dermatol 1996; 132(12):1429–1430.

55. Godt O, Proksch E, Streit V, et al. Short- and long-term effectiveness of oral and bath PUVA therapy in urticaria pigmentosa and systemic mastocytosis. Dermatology 1997; 195(1):35–39.

56. Christophers E, Honigsmann H, Wolff K, et al. PUVA-treatment of urticaria pigmentosa. Br J Dermatol 1978; 98(6):701–702.

57. Czarnetzki BM, Rosenbach T, Kolde G, et al. Phototherapy of urticaria pigmentosa: clinical response and changes of cutaneous reactivity, histamine and chemotactic leukotrienes. Arch Dermatol Res 1985; 277(2):105–113.

58. Kolde G, Frosch PJ, Czarnetzki BM. Response of cutaneous mast cells to PUVA in patients with urticaria pigmentosa: histomorphometric, ultrastructural, and biochemical investigations. J Invest Dermatol 1984; 83(3):175–178.

59. Smith ML, Orton PW, Chu H, et al. Photochemotherapy of dominant, diffuse, cutaneous mastocytosis. Pediatr Dermatol 1990; 7(4):251–255.

60. Stege H, Schopf E, Ruzicka T, et al. High-dose UVA1 for urticaria pigmentosa. Lancet 1996; 347(8993):64.

61. Vella Briffa D, Eady RA, James MP, et al. Photochemotherapy (PUVA) in the treatment of urticaria pigmentosa. Br J Dermatol 1983; 109(1):67–75.

62. Kettelhut BV, Metcalfe DD. Pediatric mastocytosis. J Invest Dermatol 1991; 96(3):15S–18S.

63. Cundy T, Beneton MN, Darby AJ, et al. Osteopenia in systemic mastocytosis: natural history and responses to treatment with inhibitors of bone resorption. Bone 1987; 8(3):149–155.

64. Marshall A, Kavanagh RT, Crisp AJ. The effect of pamidronate on lumbar spine bone density and pain in osteoporosis secondary to systemic mastocytosis. Br J Rheumatol 1997; 36(3): 393–396.

65. Valent P, Akin C, Sperr WR, et al. Aggressive systemic mastocytosis and related mast cell disorders: current treatment options and proposed response criteria. Leuk Res 2003; 27(7):635–641.

66. Clemens MJ. Interferons and apoptosis. J Interferon Cytokine Res 2003; 23(6):277–292.

67. Kluin-Nelemans HC, Jansen JH, Breukelman H, et al. Response to interferon alfa-2b in a patient with systemic mastocytosis. N Engl J Med 1992; 326(9):619–623.

68. Czarnetzki BM, Algermissen B, Jeep S, et al. Interferon treatment of patients with chronic urticaria and mastocytosis. J Am Acad Dermatol 1994; 30(3):500–501.

69. Kolde G, Sunderkotter C, Luger TA. Treatment of urticaria pigmentosa using interferon alpha. Br J Dermatol 1995; 133(1):91–94.

70. Weide R, Ehlenz K, Lorenz W, et al. Successful treatment of osteoporosis in systemic mastocytosis with interferon alpha-2b. Ann Hematol 1996; 72(1):41–43.

71. Hauswirth AW, Simonitsch-Klupp I, Uffmann M, et al. Response to therapy with interferon alpha-2b and prednisolone in aggressive systemic mastocytosis: report of five cases and review of the literature. Leuk Res 2004; 28(3):249–257.
72. Goodman GR, Beutler E, Saven A. Cladribine in the treatment of hairy-cell leukaemia. Best Pract Res Clin Haematol 2003; 16(1):101–116.
73. Carrera CJ, Terai C, Lotz M, et al. Potent toxicity of 2-chlorodeoxyadenosine toward human monocytes in vitro and in vivo. A novel approach to immunosuppressive therapy. J Clin Invest 1990; 86(5):1480–1488.
74. Tefferi A, Li CY, Butterfield JH, et al. Treatment of systemic mast-cell disease with cladribine. N Engl J Med 2001; 344(4):307–309.
75. Penack O, Sotlar K, Noack F, et al. Cladribine therapy in a patient with an aleukemic subvariant of mast cell leukemia. Ann Hematol 2005; 84(10):692–693.
76. Kluin-Nelemans HC, Oldhoff JM, Van Doormaal JJ, et al. Cladribine therapy for systemic mastocytosis. Blood 2003; 102(13):4270–4276.
77. Heinrich MC, Griffith DJ, Druker BJ, et al. Inhibition of c-kit receptor tyrosine kinase activity by STI 571, a selective tyrosine kinase inhibitor. Blood 2000; 96(3):925–932.
78. Ma Y, Zeng S, Metcalfe DD, et al. The c-KIT mutation causing human mastocytosis is resistant to STI571 and other KIT kinase inhibitors; kinases with enzymatic site mutations show different inhibitor sensitivity profiles than wild-type kinases and those with regulatory-type mutations. Blood 2002; 99(5):1741–1744.
79. Pardanani A, Elliott M, Reeder T, et al. Imatinib for systemic mast-cell disease. Lancet 2003; 362(9383):535–536.
80. Jensen BM, Akin C, Gilfillan AM. Pharmacological targeting of the KIT growth factor receptor: a therapeutic consideration for mast cell disorders. Br J Pharmacol 2008; 154:1572–1582.
81. Verstovsek S, Kantarjian H, Cortes J, et al. Dasatinib (Sprycel (TM)) therapy for patients with systemic mastocytosis. Blood 2006; 108:1036a.
82. Gotlib J, George TI, Corless C, et al. The KIT tyrosine kinase inhibitor midostaurine (PKC412) exhibits a high response rate in aggressive systemic mastocytosis (ASM): interim results of a Phase II trial. Blood 2007; 110:1035a.

25

Hypereosinophilic Syndromes

Florence Roufosse
Department of Internal Medicine, Erasme Hospital, Université Libre de Bruxelles, Brussels and Institute for Medical Immunology, Université Libre de Bruxelles, Gosselies, Belgium

Michel Goldman
Institute for Medical Immunology, Université Libre de Bruxelles, Gosselies, Belgium

Elie Cogan
Department of Internal Medicine, Erasme Hospital, Université Libre de Bruxelles, Brussels, Belgium

INTRODUCTION

Hypereosinophilic syndromes (HESs) are a heterogeneous group of rare disorders characterized by persistent hypereosinophilia associated with eosinophil-mediated tissue and organ damage. The skin is frequently targeted by eosinophils, and among possible clinical manifestations, urticaria and angioedema may be observed, generally associated with systemic complications of chronic hypereosinophilia. In some cases, angioedema is the predominant symptom, occurring episodically with associated weight gain, and regressing spontaneously. This clinical entity is known as episodic angioedema with hypereosinophilia, or Gleich's disease, and is typically associated with an increased serum IgM level. Prognosis of hypereosinophilic syndromes is highly variable, ranging from good for patients with Gleich's disease, to very poor or even fatal in patients with corticosteroid-resistant disease and progressive endomyocardial fibrosis. Furthermore, long-term prognosis is overshadowed by the development of haematological malignancies, such as acute myelogenous leukemia and peripheral T-cell lymphoma, in some patients. It is therefore essential to recognize this group of diseases in patients presenting with cutaneous symptoms, in order to identify, prevent, and/or treat systemic complications in a timely manner.

In this chapter, we will review the definition, classification, and clinical manifestations of HESs, discuss current knowledge on underlying pathogenic mechanisms, and formulate recommendations regarding treatment.

DEFINITION OF HYPEREOSINOPHILIC SYNDROMES

Hypereosinophilia is commonly observed in clinical practice, and can generally be ascribed to an underlying disorder, namely an allergic drug reaction, parasitic infection, or malignancy. Table 1 summarizes underlying etiologies of hypereosinophilia. The eosinophil is a predominantly tissue-dwelling leucocyte, which is able to produce and release a number of cytotoxic and pro-inflammatory substances upon activation (1,2). When eosinophil levels are significantly increased ($>1.5 \times 10^9$/L) for a prolonged period of time, infiltration of tissues and organs, such as the heart, lungs, gastrointestinal tract, skin, and central/peripheral nervous systems, may lead to marked damage and

Table 1 Causes of Hypereosinophilia

Diseases associated with hypereosinophilia	Eosinophil-mediated diseases
Parasitosis	Eosinophilic pneumonia (acute, chronic)
Mostly helminths	Eosinophilic esophagitis
Others (isospora belli, dientamoeba fragilis)	Eosinophilic gastrointestinal disorders
Allergic disease	Eosinophilic fasciitis (Shulman's syndrome)
Atopy	Eosinophilic cellulitis (Well's syndrome)
Drug allergy	Kimura's disease
Malignancy	Angiolymphoid hyperplasia with eosinophilia
Hematological disorders	Eosinophilic cystitis
Myeloproliferative (CML, CMML-Eo, SMCD-Eo)	Episodic angioedema with eosinophilia (Gleich's syndrome)
Non-myeloproliferative (HD, CTCL, PTCL, ATLL, T-cell lymphoblastic lymphoma, pre-B-cell acute lymphoblastic leukemia)	Hypereosinophilic syndrome
Solid tumors (lung, colon, cervix)	
Systemic immune-mediated inflammatory disorders	
Vasculitidis (Churg-Strauss, juvenile temporal arteritis)	
Connective tissue disorders (rheumatoid arthritis, dermatomyositis)	
Nonparasitic infections	
HIV, HTLV	
Scabies	
ABPA	
Coccidioidomycosis	
Immunodeficiency states	
Omenn's syndrome; HyperIgE or Job's syndrome	
Toxic	
Eosinophilia-myalgia syndrome; Toxic oil syndrome	
Miscellaneous	
Adrenal insufficiency	
Cholesterol embolization	
Irritation/Irradiation of serosal surfaces	
Chronic GVHD	
Psoriasis, bullous pemphigoid	

Abbreviations: CML, chronic myelogenous leukemia; CMML-EO, chromic myelomonocytic leukemia with eosinophilia; SMCD-DO, systemic mast cell disease with eosinophilia; HD, Hodgkin's disease; CTCL, cutaneous T-cell lymphoma; PTCL, peripheral T cell lymphoma; ATLL, adult T cell leukemia/lymphoma; ABPA, allergic bronchopulmonary aspergillosis; GVHD, graft versus host disease.

dysfunction. Prompt identification and treatment of the underlying cause is therefore essential for prevention of potentially life-threatening complications. However, in some cases, thorough evaluation fails to reveal a cause, and therapeutic control of eosinophil levels to avoid further damage becomes a goal in itself. It is in this setting that the term "hypereosinophilic syndrome" was coined in 1968 by Hardy and Anderson, regrouping patients with chronically increased peripheral blood eosinophil levels, and organ damage associated with and presumably due to eosinophilic infiltration (3).

A working definition of "idiopathic" HES was proposed by Chusid in 1975 (4): sustained peripheral blood eosinophilia of unknown origin, exceeding 1.5×10^9/L for more than six consecutive months, and direct involvement of eosinophils in the development of organ dysfunction and/or damage. Initial publications reporting characteristics of affected patients showed great clinical heterogeneity in terms of disease complications, prognosis, and response to therapy (4–6). Since then, several important advances in understanding mechanisms underlying hypereosinophilia in well-defined patient subgroups have been made, revealing pathogenic heterogeneity as well.

Besides the multisystem involvement observed in HES, a series of organ-specific eosinophil-mediated diseases, such as chronic eosinophilic pneumonia, eosinophilic gastro-enteritis, and eosinophilic fasciitis, have classically been singled out from this group of patients, despite the fact that peripheral blood eosinophil levels are increased in the HES range in many cases, and that they respond to similar treatment strategies. Mechanisms of tissue damage are thought to be the same as in HES (i.e., liberation of toxic granule proteins and pro-inflammatory substances by eosinophils), and it is likely that overlapping mechanisms of eosinophilia exist. Moreover, some patients with isolated organ involvement eventually develop other complications of hypereosinophilia, leading to a revised diagnosis of HES.

The definition of HES is evolving, to integrate diseases wherein eosinophils play a central role in pathogenesis, while taking pathogenic heterogeneity in consideration. It is now considered more appropriate to refer to a group of HESs (7), defined on the basis of persistent hypereosinophilia and/or eosinophil-mediated tissue and organ damage and dysfunction, unrelated to secondary causes of hypereosinophilia such as parasitosis, allergy, non-eosinophilic hematological malignancies, solid tumors, etc. This new wider definition encompasses HES variants with well-characterized pathogenic mechanisms, idiopathic HES, familial HES, organ-specific eosinophil-mediated disease, as well as so-called associated disorders with additional complex pathogenic mechanisms, but wherein eosinophils are thought to contribute to disease complications (e.g., Churg Strauss syndrome). Although the lower limit of 1.5×10^9 eosinophils/L has been retained in the modern definition of HESs, the six-month duration criterion is no longer applied because exclusion of secondary causes of hypereosinophilia takes less time than it used to, and there is no reason to withhold treatment in a patient with sustained and potentially deleterious hypereosinophilia, once underlying diseases have been excluded. This approach to defining HESs offers the advantage of providing physicians with the full array of second-line differential diagnoses of chronic hypereosinophilia, once classical underlying causes have been excluded. It also provides a basis for developing a diagnostic and therapeutic management algorithm of chronic eosinophil-mediated disease. The following paragraphs focus on HES subgroups that fulfill Chusid's criteria (excluding 6-month duration).

CLINICAL FEATURES OF PATIENTS
WITH HYPEREOSINOPHILIC SYNDROMES

Although initially reported patient series indicated that HES predominantly affects males (male:female ratio 9:1) (8), current estimations of the male to female ratio are closer to 1 (Ogbogu et al., manuscript in preparation). Age of diagnosis of HES is classically, but not restricted to, between 20 and 50 years. Clinical presentations of HES are notoriously variable and unpredictable (Table 2), and are related to liberation of various substances by activated eosinophils, including highly cationic granule proteins [major basic protein (MBP), eosinophil cationic protein (ECP), eosinophil-derived neurotoxin (EDN), and eosinophil peroxydase (EPO)], lipid mediators (responsible for smooth muscle contraction, and increased vascular permeability), free oxygen radicals, cytokines, and chemokines (1,2).

Table 2 Clinical and Laboratory Features of HES

Clinical features and complications	Immuno-hematological features
Constitutional symptoms	Hematological
Weakness, fatigue, anorexia, fever, night sweats, weight loss	Splenomegaly (40%), enlarged lymph nodes
Cardiac (>50%)	Increased WBC counts
Acute myocardial necrosis	Anemia, thrombocytopenia
Mural thrombosis (peripheral embolism)	Circulating myeloid precursors
Endomyocardial fibrosis (restrictive cardiomyopathy, valvular remodeling)	Increased serum vitamin B_{12} level
Muco-cutaneous (>50%)	Bone marrow hypereosinophilia, left shift of myeloid precursors
Eczema, papulo-nodular pruritic lesions	Immunological
Urticaria, angioedema	Increased serum IgE
Erythroderma	Polyclonal hypergammaglobulinemia
Mucosal ulcers (mouth, nose, pharynx, genital)	Low-grade inflammation (ESR, CRP)
Neurological (>50%)	
Diffuse encephalopathy	
Intracranial sinus thrombosis (hypercoagulant state)	
Embolic stroke, transient ischemia (cardiac thrombus)	
Sensory/motor polyneuropathy, mononeuritis	
Pulmonary (>40%)	
Chronic dry cough	
Obstructive syndrome with paroxystic dyspnea	
Interstitial infiltrates	
Restrictive syndrome with pulmonary fibrosis	
ARDS	
Digestive and hepatic	
Eosinophilic gastro-enteritis	
Ascitis	
Chronic active hepatitis	
Hepatomegaly	
Eosinophilic cholangitis	
Ocular	
Choroidal abnomalities	
Rheumatologic	
Arthralgia, myalgia	
Eosinophilic (teno)synovitis	
Vascular	
Microvascular thrombosis, digital necrosis	
Hypercoagulant state	
Urinary	
Eosinophilic cystitis	

Cutaneous involvement is observed in more than 50% of patients (9), and may present as eczema (involving hands, flectural areas, or dispersed plaques), erythroderma, more or less generalized thickening of the skin (lichenification), dermographism, recurrent urticaria, including immediate-pressure urticaria (10), and angioedema. These manifestations may be accompanied by pruritis and/or a burning or tingling sensation. Angioedema generally involves the distal extremities, face and neck; it may be frequent or occasional and fluctuate in intensity over time (11). Mechanisms that contribute to swelling include direct effects of eosinophil granule proteins on vasopermeability, and indirect effects of these proteins on mast cells and basophils, leading to histamine release (9).

Major target organs include lungs, gastrointestinal tract, heart, and nervous system (8) (Table 2). Eosinophilic infiltration of other tissues and organs, including liver, spleen, articulations, muscles, eyes, and kidneys occurs with variable frequency. Microvascular occlusion due to eosinophil-related damage to endothelium combined with activation of coagulation is a preoccupying complication that warrants urgent therapeutic intervention. Patients who present with Raynaud's phenomenon may develop digital necrosis if left untreated. Chronic hypereosinophilia also appears to favor venous thrombosis, and studies have shown that coagulation pathways may be targeted at different levels (12), although their respective contribution to hypercoagulability remains elusive.

Organ dysfunction induced by eosinophils may be more or less reversible, depending on the type of damage incurred. Production of eicosanoids and cytokines by eosinophils in the lungs induce asthma-like symptoms, all of which resolve if eosinophils are cleared by treatment. In contrast, endomyocardial fibrosis induced by eosinophils is largely irreversible (13), and progressively compromises heart function despite long-term therapeutic control of eosinophil levels. Similarly, prolonged presence of eosinophils in the intestinal wall may cause tissue remodelling and damage to the enteric nervous system (14), both affecting motility well after eosinophils have been cleared.

Published series underscore the great clinical heterogeneity and highly variable prognosis of HES, ranging from paucisymptomatic disease requiring no treatment and associated with prolonged survival, to rapidly fatal disease course due to development of congestive heart failure or occurrence of acute leukaemia (4,5,8). Ideally, treatment should be adapted to the level of risk for each patient, meaning that overtreatment of patients who are unlikely to develop severe complications should be avoided, whereas aggressive treatment should be initiated rapidly for patients with a risk of life-threatening or disabling disease, before the occurrence of irreversible complications. Unfortunately, to date, there are no validated biomarkers for predicting the severity and/or nature of complications of hypereosinophilia in a given patient. There is no correlation between eosinophil levels and disease severity when the HES patient population is considered as a whole. However, in a given patient, disease flares are likely to occur when eosinophil levels increase beyond a threshold, for example during tapering of therapy; and in most cases, they will be accompanied by similar clinical manifestations. Also, recent characterization of distinct pathogenic mechanisms underlying HES has led to the definition of patient subgroups, within which disease complications are more homogenous and thus more predictable, although not entirely.

PATHOGENIC MECHANISMS OF HYPEREOSINOPHILIA AND HYPEREOSINOPHILIC SYNDROME VARIANTS

Eosinophils belong to the myeloid lineage and differentiate from myeloid progenitors (GEMM-CFU) in the marrow. Among the three cytokines that act as eosinophil growth factors and apoptosis inhibitors, i.e., granulocyte-macrophage colony-stimulating factor

(GM-CSF), IL-3, and IL-5, only the latter displays specificity for eosinophils (1). The major source of this eosinophil-specific cytokine is represented by so-called type 2 helper T cells (15). Recent studies have shown that two distinct underlying mechanisms may lead to chronic unexplained hypereosinophilia in HES patient subgroups: occurrence of a sporadic hematopoïetic stem cell mutation, leading to primitive clonal expansion of cells belonging to the myeloid lineage with preferential eosinophilic differentiation (as such, hypereosinophilia belongs to the group of chronic myeloproliferative disorders), or overproduction of eosinophilopoietic cytokine(s) by an activated population of T cells (in the "lymphocytic variant" of HES, or L-HES).

Primitive or Clonal Eosinophilia

Chusid and others singled out a subgroup of patients with clinical and biological features reminiscent of chronic myeloproliferative disorders (i.e., increased serum vitamin B_{12}, hepatomegaly, splenomegaly, anemia, and thrombocytopenia), as presenting a more aggressive disease variant, with a higher incidence of disease-related morbidity and mortality (essentially development of endomyocardial fibrosis or blastic transformation) (4,8). However, until recently, evidence that a true myeloproliferative disorder existed in such patients was scarce; only a few authors were able to demonstrate the existence of chromosomal abnormalities adjacent to eosinophil granules or skewed methylation patterns of X-linked genes in purified granulocytes, suggesting the eosinophils were indeed monoclonal (16,17).

Although abnormal karyotypes are extremely rare in patients with HES, impeding detection of eosinophil clonality using conventional methods, recent studies have shown that a cryptic cytogenetic rearrangement is mechanistically responsible for clonal hypereosinophilia in a subgroup of patients. Indeed, an interstitial deletion on chromosome 4q12 results in fusion of two genes that are normally 800 kb apart, FIP1L1 and PDGFRA (18). The fusion gene encodes a FIP1LI-PDGFRA (F/P) protein, displaying constitutive tyrosine kinase activity, which is involved in clonal expansion of eosinophils that appear mature. Furthermore, the F/P fusion is implicated in malignant transformation of mutated cells, as indicated by its ability to render a murine hematopoietic cell line independent of growth factors in vitro following transfection, and by its presence in a cell line derived from a patient with acute eosinophilic leukemia (19). Although eosinophils are by far the predominant leukocyte in blood and tissues from patients with the F/P fusion, this clonal abnormality has been demonstrated in a number of other cell lineages (20), including mast cells, which display morphological changes and which may be the source of increased serum tryptase levels frequently observed in these patients (21). Importantly, the F/P fusion is exquisitely sensitive to the tyrosine kinase inhibitor commonly used to treat patients with chronic myelogenous leukemia (CML), imatinib mesylate (18).

Clinically, patients with the F/P rearrangement are predominantly males and are likely to develop fibrotic complications of hypereosinophilia, such as endomyocardial fibrosis and restrictive lung disease (21,22); increased reticulin staining may be observed on bone marrow biopsies. Other clinical complications that appear to be common in this HES subgroup include dermatitis and mucosal ulcers, splenomegaly, and peripheral neuropathy. Routine blood testing may show any of the following: markedly increased vitamin B_{12} levels, anemia, thrombocytopenia, and circulating myeloid precursors, although none of these are considered diagnostic hallmarks of this variant. Overall, natural disease course and prognosis in F/P$^+$ HES patients is poor, with a high prevalence of disease-related morbidity or death due to development of cardiac complications and possible progression toward acute leukemia (21).

The proportion of patients initially fulfilling diagnostic criteria for HES in whom the F/P mutation is detected varies among reports, ranging between 17% (23) and 56% (18). This variability reflects biased reporting by authors according to their medical subspecialties, because of which they are more or less likely to recruit patients with features of myeloproliferative disease. In a recent retrospective multicenter study, including patients recruited across a wide spectrum of specialists, the percentage appears to be closer to 10% (Ogbogu et al, manuscript in preparation).

Besides FIP1L1, other fusion partners for PDGFRA have been reported in a small number of patients with chronic hypereosinophilia. In one study, two patients with chromosomal translocations involving 4q were investigated further for fusion genes involving PDGFRA, leading to the discovery of two new partners, STRN and ETV6 (24). In another study, the authors developed a reverse transcription polymerase chain reaction (RT-PCR) test to detect over-expression of the PDGFRA kinase domain as a possible indicator of the presence of a fusion gene (25). Among nine F/P$^-$ hypereosinophilic patients in whom this domain was over-expressed, one was studied further, leading to the identification of KIF5B on chromosome 10p11 as a new fusion partner for PDGFRA. Such cases account for only a minority of observed imatinib-responses in F/P$^-$ patients. It is therefore likely that other cytogenetic rearrangements will be identified in HES patients with features of myeloproliferative disease in the years to come.

In the meantime, the term "myeloproliferative HES" (M-HES) has been proposed for patients with a presumptive, but not formally demonstrated, underlying primitive myeloproliferative disorder, on the basis of presence of at least four of the following criteria (7): presence of dysplastic eosinophils, increased serum B12, increased serum tryptase, anemia/thrombocytopenia, hepato/spleno-megaly, increased bone marrow cellularity with an increased proportion of immature cells, myelofibrosis, and dysplastic mast cells in bone marrow. Patients with no detectable PDGFRA rearrangements who respond to a trial with imatinib could be included in this definition.

According to the most recent WHO classification, patients with clonal rearrangements involving PDGFRA should be classified as chronic eosinophilic leukemia (CEL) (26); however, other terms still in use include "F/P-associated HES or disease," "F/P$^+$ HES," or "M-HES." Whether this well-defined patient subgroup should remain under the umbrella diagnosis of HES or not remains a controversial issue.

T Cell–Mediated Hypereosinophilia

In L-HES, over-production of eosinophil growth factors by T cells leads to increased cycling, differentiation, and maturation of eosinophil precursors, as well as prolonged survival of eosinophils in the periphery, resulting in non-clonal hypereosinophilia (27,28). Interleukin-5 (IL-5)-producing T-cell subsets have been described in blood of approximately 35 patients with HES, and a rough estimate would be that 15% to 20% of HES patients present this variant. The allegedly pathogenic T cells display an aberrant surface phenotype in all reported cases, and while CD3$^-$CD4$^+$ cells represent the most frequently encountered subset in this setting (29), CD3$^+$CD4$^-$CD8$^-$ (28), CD4$^+$CD7- (30) and other populations have also been reported. In addition to IL-5, the CD3$^-$CD4$^+$ cells produce other Th2 cytokines such as IL-4 and IL-13 (29), as well as GM-CSF. Effects of the Th2 cytokines IL-4 and IL-13 on other cells account for associated biological features of L-HES. Indeed, B-cell stimulation leads to increased IgE synthesis and polyclonal hypergammaglobulinemia; and effects on other cells lead to high-level production of the chemokine TARC (thymus and activation-regulated chemokine), which is frequently increased in serum from such patients (31). Clonality of phenotypically aberrant T cells has been demonstrated in many cases, by analysis of T-cell receptor (TCR) gene rearrangement patterns. Karyotypes are generally normal, although rare cases with 16q breakage (32), partial 6q or 10p deletions (33), and trisomy 7 have been reported. Although this is an initially benign lymphoproliferative disorder, several authors have reported indolent progression toward full-blown T-cell lymphoma (28,29).

Clinically, L-HES affects females at least as much as males, and cutaneous manifestations, including pruritus, eczema, erythroderma, angioedema, and urticaria generally dominate the clinical picture, whereas endomyocardial fibrosis is a rare complication despite high eosinophil levels. Lymphocytosis may be present (due to increased absolute numbers of aberrant T cells), serum IgE levels are often increased, and polyclonal IgG and/or IgM hypergammaglobulinemia may be observed. Although patients with L-HES rarely experience life-threatening end-organ damage and have better short-term prognosis than F/P$^+$ patients, some may develop peripheral T-cell lymphoma many years after diagnosis.

Idiopathic Hypereosinophilic Syndrome

Despite these important advances, up to 75% of patients with HES remain unclassified, and present truly *idiopathic* hypereosinophilia. Among these, some present features of myeloproliferative disease similar to those encountered in F/P$^+$ individuals, whereas others appear to have more of an "immuno-allergic" disorder, suggesting possible involvement of T cells. Possible clinical complications are those listed in Table 2. Prognosis is extremely variable, but has gradually improved for a number of reasons including earlier detection of complications, better surgical management of cardiac and valvular disease, and use of a wider spectrum of therapeutic molecules for controlling hypereosinophilia. Future investigations focusing on eosinophils and T cells in these idiopathic cases will very likely lead to identification of novel molecular mechanisms ultimately leading to hypereosinophilia.

DIAGNOSTIC EVALUATION OF HYPEREOSINOPHILIC SYNDROMES

Initial work-up of chronic hypereosinophilia requires rigorous step-wise progression through a diagnostic algorithm (Fig. 1). All diseases known to be associated with hypereosinophilia, and that are pertinent in a given clinical situation, must be excluded before considering diagnosis of HES (Table 1). Secondly, complications of chronic hypereosinophilia per se must be assessed. And thirdly, an attempt should be made to determine whether hypereosinophilia arises in the context of a primitive myeloid versus lymphoid disorder, i.e., to classify patients with regard to disease variant, as therapeutic strategies differ (Fig. 1).

Detection of eosinophil-induced end-organ damage should obviously be guided by clinical assessment and physical examination, with special emphasis on the systems known to be targeted by eosinophils: cutaneous, cardiovascular, nervous (peripheral and central), respiratory, and digestive systems. Minimal investigations when diagnosis of HES is established include measurement of liver enzymes, urea, and creatinin in blood, an electrocardiogram, an echocardiogram, plethysomographic pulmonary function test, a chest X ray, and abdominal ultrasound. Other imaging studies and/or biopsies should be performed on the basis of clinical findings.

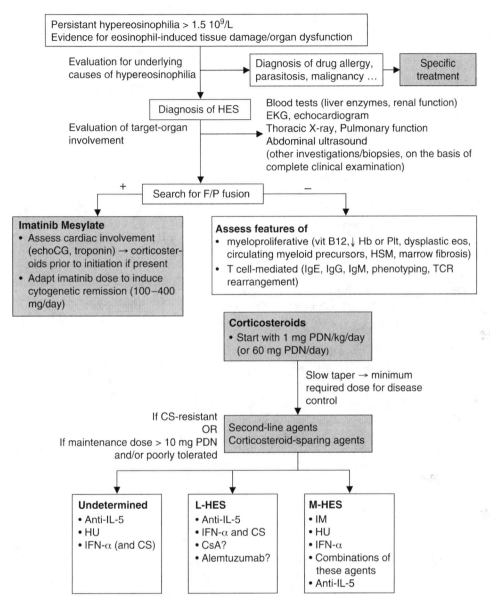

Abbreviations : CS corticosteroid, PDN prednisone, HU hydroxycarbamide, IFN-α interferon alpha, CsA cyclosporin A

Figure 1 Management strategy for patients with chronic hypereosinophilia.

Pathogenic classification of HES patients remains difficult in a routine setting, and often requires shipment of blood and/or marrow samples to qualified laboratories for optimal evaluation. Clinically, predominant cutaneous manifestations in absence of heart involvement, associated with serum hyperIgE and/or polyclonal hypergammaglobuline-mia should arouse suspicion of L-HES. Likewise, splenomegaly, heart involvement, mucosal ulcerations, increased vitamin B_{12} levels, anemia and/or thrombocytopenia, and presence of myeloid precursors in peripheral blood may be indicative of F/P-associated

HES. However, these features are neither sensitive nor specific for a disease variant, and further testing is warranted for classification and treatment of patients. Optimal care demands that the three following tests be performed on peripheral blood and/or bone marrow for all patients: 1/search for the F/P fusion gene using RT-PCR (preferably nested for increased sensitivity) and/or FISH (fluorescent in situ hybridization) for the CHIC2 locus (absence of this locus is considered a surrogate marker for F/P), 2/lymphocyte phenotyping, and 3/analysis of TCR gene rearrangement patterns using Southern Blot and/or PCR amplification of variable regions. Detection of the F/P fusion clearly identifies patients with a distinct disease variant that responds dramatically to treatment with the tyrosine kinase inhibitor imatinib. On the other hand, detection of a phenotypically aberrant monoclonal T-cell subset (principally $CD3^-CD4^+$, $CD3^+CD4^-CD8^-$, and $CD4^+CD7^-$) is sufficient for considering that hypereosinophilia is driven by a primitive T-cell disorder, which should be monitored carefully for the possible development of malignant lymphoma.

Despite adherence to the preceding guidelines, a number of patients will remain unclassified. Additional investigations in a research setting that may help identify patients with a clonal eosinophilic disorder include measurement of serum tryptase, cytogenetic analysis focusing on imatinib-targeted tyrosine kinases, and quantification of PDGFRA kinase domain expression by RT-PCR. As for identification of T-cell–mediated disease, additional surface markers may be studied on CD4 and CD8 T cells by flow cytometry (including CD2, CD5, CD7, CD25, CD27, and CD45RO, all of which may have modified expression levels on pathogenic T-cell subsets), and production of eosinophilopoietic factors and/or type 2 cytokines (IL-3, GM-CSF, IL-4, IL-5, IL-13) by T cells can be analyzed using flow cytometry or various assays that measure cytokine levels in supernatants of cultured cells. Although abnormal T cells from patients with L-HES produce enormous amounts of IL-5 in vitro when stimulated, measurement of serum or plasma IL-5 has no value for identification of this variant; patients with L-HES may have normal (undetectable) or increased serum IL-5 levels (29), just like any other patient with HES. In contrast, preliminary studies indicate that elevated serum TARC levels represent a sensitive and potentially specific diagnostic biomarker for this variant (31), although this remains to be validated on a larger and more comprehensive patient population.

TREATMENT OF HYPEREOSINOPHILIC SYNDROMES

HES are chronic long-standing diseases that develop in young to middle-aged patients, meaning that therapeutic options should take long-term toxicity into consideration. Corticosteroids and hydroxycarbamide have been the cornerstones of management since definition of the syndrome in 1975, and interferon alpha (IFN-α) was introduced in the early 1990s on the basis of several encouraging studies. The proportion of patients that respond to each of these agents is currently unknown, as longitudinal prospective studies on such a rare group of diseases have been difficult to conduct in single centers. These compounds have numerous well-known side effects that are often dose-limiting. Thus, there is a strong need for new therapeutic alternatives, which specifically target molecular mechanisms underlying hypereosinophilia, while causing as little unintentional damage as possible. With the recent description of the F/P fusion in a subgroup of patients, and the development of anti-IL-5 monoclonal antibodies, therapeutic perspectives have changed radically in the past few years.

Treatment of Chronic Hypereosinophilia Associated with Constitutive PDGFRA Tyrosine Kinase Activity

Patients in whom the F/P chromosomal rearrangement is detected should be treated with the tyrosine kinase inhibitor imatinib (Gleevec[®]) as first-line therapy. A number of clinical studies showing the striking rapidity and potency of its effects in this selected patient population have been published (18,22,34,35), and to date, no case of primary resistance to the molecule has been reported. Response to therapy in terms of eosinophil levels occurs within days in most cases, and many clinical manifestations can be reversed (including dermatitis, mucosal ulcers, restrictive lung disease, GI involvement, central nervous system manifestations, certain cardiac manifestations, anemia, thrombocytopenia, and splenomegaly). Effects of imatinib on clinical manifestations related to heart involvement are variable, and although disappearance of mural thrombi has been observed, some authors have reported that endomyocardial fibrosis and related loss of function are not reversible (22,35). Reversal of bone marrow pathology and molecular remission (35,36) (i.e., disappearance of the F/P fusion gene), a major endpoint when dealing with disease mediated by constitutively activated tyrosine kinases, can be achieved in most patients.

The dose required to induce and maintain remission is generally lower (100–400 mg/day) than for patients with CML (400 mg), meaning that dose-related adverse events including hematological toxicity, edema, muscle pain, and fatigue, are uncommon, and overall tolerance is excellent. However, there is some concern regarding side effects of imatinib on heart function. Firstly, 2 F/P[+] HES patients developed severe congestive heart failure within days after initiation of therapy, and this was presumably due to massive liberation of cytotoxic molecules following imatinib-induced eosinophil death (37,38). Rapid administration of corticosteroids was effective in reversing this preoccupying complication. To prevent its occurrence, serum troponin level should be measured prior to initiation of therapy, and an echocardiogram should be performed if this hasn't been done in the previous months. If either test is suggestive of cardiac involvement, administration of corticosteroids immediately prior to imatinib is recommended. Furthermore, serial serum troponin measurements should be done during the first days of treatment, during which eosinophil levels decrease rapidly, even in patients with no prior evidence of cardiac involvement, to detect development of acute cardiomyopathy. Secondly, a study investigating cardiomyocytes from CML patients who developed left ventricular dysfunction within months after introduction of imatinib (400–800 mg/day) has shown presence of membrane whorls and pleomorphic mitochondria with effaced cristae (39). The mechanisms underlying imatinib-induced myocyte toxicity were investigated in mice, in which mitochondria were also identified as the chief target of this compound. The conclusion of this study, i.e., that energy rundown due to mitochondrial dysfunction was responsible for imatinib-induced cardiotoxicity, is a subject of controversy.

Despite its ability to induce complete molecular remission in the majority of patients with F/P[+] disease, imatinib appears not to be curative, in that interruption of therapy is followed by recurrence of the molecular defect within months (36,40). Although re-introduction of imatinib has consistently re-induced molecular remission in such cases, one study has shown that the dose of imatinib required to maintain remission may be higher than the dose that initially achieved this endpoint (40). Altogether, these observations suggest that a contingent of F/P[+] stem cells persists during treatment with imatinib, and that emergence of imatinib-resistant sub-clones may be favored by temporary withholding of treatment. In addition, relapse of hypereosinophilia during treatment with imatinib has been reported in two F/P$^+$ patients, and was associated with appearance of a T674I point mutation in the ATP-binding site of the PDGFRA moiety (18,41), similar to the T315I mutation observed in patients with CML that become refractory to treatment. To prevent development of acquired resistance to treatment, it has been recommended that the dose of imatinib used for patients with F/P$^+$ HES should be adjusted to ensure molecular remission (7,40). The current tendency to taper imatinib to doses as low as 100 mg/week may not be optimal in this respect.

Several alternative tyrosine kinase inhibitors have been tested in vitro and in vivo (on a murine model of F/P-associated disease) for effects on F/P$^+$ cells. One molecule, nilotinib (AMN107), is able to inhibit kinase activity of wild-type F/P. Two other compounds, PKC412, which is structurally unrelated to imatinib, and sorafenib, which has been approved for treatment of advanced renal cell carcinoma, are able to inhibit kinase activity of both wild-type F/P and its imatinib-resistant T674I mutant form (42,43). Allogeneic stem cell transplantation (SCT) is another alternative for imatinib-resistant cases.

Treatment of Hypereosinophilic Syndrome in Absence of Constitutive PDGFRA Tyrosine Kinase Activity

To date, no general consensus has been reached on the ideal treatment algorithm for HES patients without the F/P fusion. In general, corticosteroids are administered as first-line therapy, starting with a daily dose of 1 mg/kg or 60 mg prednisone (7). If a response is observed, prednisone is carefully tapered to the lowest possible dose that maintains eosinophil counts and/or clinical manifestations under control, defining the level of corticosteroid-dependency. Depending on the dose of corticosteroids required and on patient tolerance, physicians frequently attempt to further reduce the dose by introducing a corticosteroid-sparing agent. If no response to corticosteroids is observed (i.e., corticosteroid-resistance), second-line therapy is warranted.

Compounds that are used for corticosteroid-sparing and for second-line purposes include hydroxycarbamide, IFN-α, and imatinib. Recent studies indicate that monoclonal anti-IL-5 antibodies represent an interesting therapeutic alternative. Other compounds such as cyclosporin, vincristine, and anti-CD52 antibody (alemtuzumab, or Campath®) have been used successfully in individual cases. Reports on administration of cytotoxic molecules such as cyclophosphamide, methotrexate, busulfan, and chlorambucil are scarce and arouse little, if any, enthusiasm for further assessment of their effectiveness in the setting of clinical trials. The following paragraphs review briefly the characteristics of molecules with observed efficacy as well as those that appear promising, to help guide clinicians in the choice of which agent to use for a given patient.

Hydroxycarbamide has been used extensively for treating HES, generally at doses between 1 and 2 g/d (7,8). The effect of hydroxycarbamide on eosinophilia is central, meaning that reduction of eosinophil levels are not to be expected before two weeks after initiation of therapy. Adverse events are frequently observed at doses needed to control disease, including hematological toxicity and gastrointestinal intolerance. Combining hydroxycarbamide with corticosteroids (44) or IFN-α (45) allows for lower dosing of each compound, thereby increasing tolerance while maintaining a response. Published reports on successful treatment of HES with hydroxycarbamide lack detailed clinical and diagnostic information that would allow speculations on which disease variants could benefit from therapy. Theoretically, this compound would appear more useful for treating patients with myeloproliferative features; however, it effectively lowered eosinophil levels in one patient with a CD3$^-$CD4$^+$ clone (46). Overall, hydroxycarbamide is a readily accessible molecule, which appears efficacious in a satisfactory proportion of patients with HES, but its use at doses required to induce remission may be precluded by poor tolerance.

Interferon-α has also been used successfully for management of HES (47). Although highly variable dosing regimens have been used, it appears that average doses of 1 to 2 million units/day are often sufficient to control eosinophil levels (7). Given its delayed action, together with dose-related side effects at the initiation of therapy, it may take months before a stable effective dose is reached. Common side effects include flu-like symptoms that tend to improve over time, depression, fatigue, thyroid dysfunction, induction of auto-antibodies, and increased liver transaminases. Many IFN-α responders reported in the literature present a number of features suggestive of myeloproliferative disease, but these reports pre-date description of the F/P fusion. It is noteworthy that some of these patients had karyotype abnormalities that disappeared during treatment. IFN-α displayed a corticosteroid-sparing effect in two of our patients with $CD3^-CD4^+$ clones, one of which eventually achieved complete disease remission with disappearance of circulating $CD3^-CD4^+$ cells (unpublished data). Although IFN-α has been shown to inhibit IL-5 production (48) and proliferation of $CD3^-CD4^+$ cells in vitro, it also inhibits their death by apoptosis (49), and may therefore provide these cells with a selective advantage. Overall, IFN-α represents a good alternative for patients with F/P^- HES, irrespective of disease presentation, but it is not easily accessed in all countries, and side effects are common. Importantly, IFN-α should not be used as monotherapy for L-HES, but rather should be combined with corticosteroids, which display pro-apoptotic effects on aberrant T cells.

Imatinib has been administered to patients with F/P^- HES, with a success rate that has been estimated to be 21% complete responses and 12% partial responses (50). These observations support the existence of other as of yet unidentified cytogenetic rearrangements associated with imatinib-sensitive tyrosine kinase activation in some patients with HES. However, apart from patients with other rearrangements involving PDGFRA, they tend to require higher doses of imatinib than F/P^+ patients, and the response may be transient. Although potential biomarkers that would help identify F/P^- patients with imatinib-sensitive disease remain to be formally identified in the setting of a well-designed clinical study, a short course of imatinib, 100 to 400 mg daily, could be proposed to patients with clinical and biological findings typically encountered in myeloproliferative disease (see those listed above for M-HES) and those resistant to therapy with corticosteroids (7). Given the rapidity of action of this agent, if a hematological response is not observed within two to four weeks, treatment should be interrupted. Imatinib should not be administered to patients with L-HES.

There is strong scientific rationale for treating HES with monoclonal anti-IL-5 or anti-IL-5R antibodies, given the specificity of this cytokine for the eosinophil lineage, and the assumption that tissue damage in HES is directly related to presence of activated eosinophils. Anti-IL-5 targets eosinophils by binding to IL-5 and preventing its ligation to the IL-5Rα-chain expressed on the eosinophil membrane. Several open-label studies evaluating effects of intravenous anti-IL-5 in HES patients showed a rapid decline of blood eosinophil counts shortly after administration (51–53), associated with improvement of a range of clinical manifestations (including rash, angioedema, mucosal ulcers, myalgia, arthralgia, dysphagia, vomiting, nasal congestion, and polyposis), correlating with significant reductions of eosinophil numbers in the skin and esophagus of patients with eosinophilic dermatitis (53) and severe eosinophilic esophagitis (51), respectively. Efficacy of the anti-IL-5 antibody, mepolizumab, as a corticosteroid-sparing agent in F/P^- HES patients has recently been confirmed in the setting of a randomized double blind, placebo-controlled clinical trial (54). In this study, the daily prednisone dose required to stabilize disease and eosinophil levels could durably be tapered down to a predefined threshold value in a significantly higher proportion of patients under 750 mg intravenous mepolizumab compared with those in the placebo arm. Mepolizumab was shown to be well tolerated and safe in this short-term study. Long-term safety is currently being evaluated in an open-label extension of this clinical trial, together with the optimal dosing interval between mepolizumab infusions.

An interesting therapeutic target in patients with L-HES is the CD52 antigen, which is expressed both on T cells and eosinophils. In a recent report, alemtuzumab, a monoclonal anti-CD52 antibody, was shown to be effective treatment for a patient with a $CD3^-CD4^+$ T-cell subset, inducing rapid normalization of eosinophil levels and clinical remission (55). Alemtuzumab can be administered subcutaneously, generally at very low doses for a few days to ensure tolerance, then doses are increased to 10 to 30 mg, at variable frequencies (on alternate days, once a week) until a response is observed; the dosing interval can then be extended to once every three weeks. Potential side effects include profound hematological toxicity with immunosuppression, leading to an increased risk of opportunistic infections, namely severe cytomegalovirus infection. The possible therapeutic benefit of this molecule in patients with HES should be weighed against the risks of dose-related immunosuppression. In this regard, a recent study conducted on patients with Sezary syndrome showed that low-dose alemtuzumab was as effective as the standard dosing regimen (10 vs. 15 mg on alternate days), with decreased toxicity (56). In addition, once the absolute Sezary cell count decreased below a given threshold, treatment was withheld; subsequent doses of alemtuzumab were tailored for each patient on the basis of regular immunological monitoring of aberrant cell counts. This is of particular interest for patients with L-HES, given the presence of phenotypically aberrant cells in blood, which could guide patient-tailored treatment in a similar fashion.

Cyclosporin interferes with calcium-mediated intracellular signaling pathways and inhibits nuclear translocation of the transcription factor NF-AT, which is essential for a number of T-cell functions including cytokine synthesis. Cyclosporin is classically used for treating autoimmune disorders, by targeting T cells. A few authors have reported successful use of cyclosporin as a corticosteroid-sparing agent in a limited number of HES patients. Given the pathogenic role of T cells in L-HES, and dependence of $CD3^-CD4^+$ T cells on IL-2 for proliferation and cytokine production (57), cyclosporin or other agents interfering with IL-2/IL-2R interactions, may theoretically be useful for this HES variant. This remains entirely to be assessed.

Vincristine is a cytotoxic agent that is rarely used for management of HES. It may prove useful for rapidly lowering eosinophilia in patients with extremely high eosinophil counts ($>100 \times 10^9$/L), and has been proposed in some pediatric cases that are refractory to classical therapeutic regimens (7). The recommended dose for adults is 1 to 2 mg intravenously.

Finally, HES patients who are refractory to classical therapy and who present progressive life-threatening end-organ damage may be candidates for allogeneic SCT (7). Obviously, this strategy requires careful thought given the inherent morbidity and mortality related to the procedure. Potential indications for SCT may include patients with F/P-associated disease who are intolerant to or no longer respond to imatinib, and patients initially presenting L-HES who develop peripheral T-cell lymphoma, as eradication of malignant T cells is not easily achieved using classical chemotherapeutic regimens.

Concluding Remarks

Overall, management of patients with HES has improved significantly, especially since the introduction of imatinib for patients with F/P^+ disease, as these are the patients that fare worst. As for L-HES, there is now increased awareness that despite the clinically benign presentation with relative sparing of end-organs, patients should be closely monitored for development of T-cell malignancy. However, T-cell–specific molecular targets for therapy remain to be identified, meaning that in the meantime therapy relies largely on corticosteroids, with eventual addition of corticosteroid-sparing agents such as IFN-α. Careful administration of alemtuzumab aiming to decrease lymphocytosis could be beneficial in such patients, although this has not yet been assessed. For the large majority of patients fulfilling current HES diagnostic criteria, pathogenesis remains unknown. Well-conducted prospective trails are needed to assess the efficacy of the available agents with previously shown efficacy such as hydroxycarbamide and IFN-α. Importantly, collection of comprehensive clinical and biological data of enrolled patients is essential for identification of biomarkers with predictive value for response to a given agent. The recently conducted mepolizumab clinical trial has proven that it is possible to achieve sufficient patient recruitment to draw statistically sound conclusions, despite the fact that HES is an orphan disease. In addition to these "text-book classics," novel therapeutic agents have become available in clinical settings sharing pathogenic characteristics with HES and its variants, such as allergic disease, myeloproliferative disorders, and cutaneous T-cell lymphoma. Their relevance for treating HES should now be examined carefully by experts, and those that appear most promising should be evaluated in the setting of clinical trials.

REFERENCES

1. Rothenberg ME, Hogan SP. The eosinophil. Annu Rev Immunol 2006; 24:147–174.
2. Jacobsen EA, Taranova AG, Lee NA, et al. Eosinophils: singularly destructive effector cells or purveyors of immunoregulation? J Allergy Clin Immunol 2007; 119(6):1313–1320.
3. Hardy WR, Anderson RE. The hypereosinophilic syndromes. Ann Intern Med 1968; 68(6): 1220–1229.
4. Chusid MJ, Dale DC, West BC, et al. The hypereosinophilic syndrome: analysis of fourteen cases with review of the literature. Medicine (Baltimore) 1975; 54(1):1–27.
5. Fauci AS, Harley JB, Roberts WC, et al. NIH conference. The idiopathic hypereosinophilic syndrome. Clinical, pathophysiologic, and therapeutic considerations. Ann Intern Med 1982; 97(1): 78–92.
6. Spry CJ, Davies J, Tai PC, et al. Clinical features of fifteen patients with the hypereosinophilic syndrome. Q J Med 1983; 52(205):1–22.
7. Klion AD, Bochner BS, Gleich GJ, et al. Approaches to the treatment of hypereosinophilic syndromes: a workshop summary report. J Allergy Clin Immunol 2006; 117(6):1292–1302.
8. Weller PF, Bubley GJ. The idiopathic hypereosinophilic syndrome. Blood 1994; 83(10): 2759–2779.
9. Leiferman KM, Gleich GJ, Peters MS. Dermatologic manifestations of the hypereosinophilic syndromes. Immunol Allergy Clin North Am 2007; 27(3):415–441.
10. Parillo J, Lawley T, Frank M, et al. Immunologic reactivity in the hypereosinophilic syndrome. J Allergy Clin Immunol 1979; 64(2):113–121.
11. Gleich GJ, Schroeter AL, Marcoux JP, et al. Episodic angioedema associated with eosinophilia. N Engl J Med 1984; 310(25):1621–1626.
12. Wang JG, Mahmud SA, Thompson JA, et al. The principal eosinophil peroxidase product, HOSCN, is a uniquely potent phagocyte oxidant inducer of endothelial cell tissue factor activity: a potential mechanism for thrombosis in eosinophilic inflammatory states. Blood 2006; 107(2):558–565.
13. Ogbogu PU, Rosing DR, Horne MK III. Cardiovascular manifestations of hypereosinophilic syndromes. Immunol Allergy Clin North Am 2007; 27(3):457–475.
14. Schappi MG, Smith VV, Milla PJ, et al. Eosinophilic myenteric ganglionitis is associated with functional intestinal obstruction. Gut 2003; 52(5):752–755.

15. Mosmann TR, Coffman RL. TH1 and TH2 cells: different patterns of lymphokine secretion lead to different functional properties. Annu Rev Immunol 1989; 7:145–173.

16. Chang HW, Leong KH, Koh DR, et al. Clonality of isolated eosinophils in the hyper-eosinophilic syndrome. Blood 1999; 93(5):1651–1657.

17. Luppi M, Marasca R, Morselli M, et al. Clonal nature of hypereosinophilic syndrome. Blood 1994; 84(1):349–350.

18. Cools J, DeAngelo DJ, Gotlib J, et al. A tyrosine kinase created by fusion of the PDGFRA and FIP1L1 genes as a therapeutic target of imatinib in idiopathic hypereosinophilic syndrome. N Engl J Med 2003; 348(13):1201–1214.

19. Griffin JH, Leung J, Bruner RJ, et al. Discovery of a fusion kinase in EOL-1 cells and idiopathic hypereosinophilic syndrome. Proc Natl Acad Sci U S A 2003; 100(13):7830–7835.

20. Robyn J, Lemery S, McCoy JP, et al. Multilineage involvement of the fusion gene in patients with FIP1L1/PDGFRA-positive hypereosinophilic syndrome. Br J Haematol 2006; 132(3): 286–292.

21. Klion AD, Noel P, Akin C, et al. Elevated serum tryptase levels identify a subset of patients with a myeloproliferative variant of idiopathic hypereosinophilic syndrome associated with tissue fibrosis, poor prognosis, and imatinib responsiveness. Blood 2003; 101(12):4660–4666.

22. Vandenberghe P, Wlodarska I, Michaux L, et al. Clinical and molecular features of FIP1L1-PDFGRA (+) chronic eosinophilic leukemias. Leukemia 2004; 18(4):734–742.

23. Roche-Lestienne C, Lepers S, Soenen-Cornu V, et al. Molecular characterization of the idiopathic hypereosinophilic syndrome (HES) in 35 French patients with normal conventional cytogenetics. Leukemia 2005; 19(5):792–798.

24. Curtis CE, Grand FH, Musto P, et al. Two novel imatinib-responsive PDGFRA fusion genes in chronic eosinophilic leukaemia. Br J Haematol 2007; 138(1):77–81.

25. Score J, Curtis C, Waghorn K, et al. Identification of a novel imatinib responsive KIF5B-PDGFRA fusion gene following screening for PDGFRA overexpression in patients with hypereosinophilia. Leukemia 2006; 20(5):827–832.

26. Fletcher S, Bain B. Diagnosis and treatment of hypereosinophilic syndromes. Curr Opin Hematol 2007; 14(1):37–42.

27. Roufosse F, Cogan E, Goldman M. Lymphocytic variant hypereosinophilic syndromes. Immunol Allergy Clin North Am 2007; 27(3):389–413.

28. Simon HU, Plotz SG, Dummer R, et al. Abnormal clones of T cells producing interleukin-5 in idiopathic eosinophilia. N Engl J Med 1999; 341(15):1112–1120.

29. Roufosse F, Schandene L, Sibille C, et al. Clonal Th2 lymphocytes in patients with the idiopathic hypereosinophilic syndrome. Br J Haematol 2000; 109(3):540–548.

30. Vaklavas C, Tefferi A, Butterfield J, et al. 'Idiopathic' eosinophilia with an Occult T-cell clone: prevalence and clinical course. Leuk Res 2007; 31(5):691–694.

31. de Lavareille A, Roufosse F, Schmid-Grendelmeier P, et al. High serum thymus and activation-regulated chemokine levels in the lymphocytic variant of the hypereosinophilic syndrome. J Allergy Clin Immunol 2002; 110(3):476–479.

32. Kitano K, Ichikawa N, Shimodaira S, et al. Eosinophilia associated with clonal T-cell proliferation. Leuk Lymphoma 1997; 27(3-4):335–342.

33. Ravoet M, Sibille C, Roufosse F, et al. 6q- is an early and persistent chromosomal aberration in CD3-CD4+ T-cell clones associated with the lymphocytic variant of hypereosinophilic syndrome. Haematologica 2005; 90(6):753–765.

34. Gleich GJ, Leiferman KM, Pardanani A, et al. Treatment of hypereosinophilic syndrome with imatinib mesilate. Lancet 2002; 359(9317):1577–1578.

35. Klion AD, Robyn J, Akin C, et al. Molecular remission and reversal of myelofibrosis in response to imatinib mesylate treatment in patients with the myeloproliferative variant of hypereosinophilic syndrome. Blood 2004; 103(2):473–478.

36. Jovanovic JV, Score J, Waghorn K, et al. Low-dose imatinib mesylate leads to rapid induction of major molecular responses and achievement of complete molecular remission in FIP1L1-PDGFRA-positive chronic eosinophilic leukemia. Blood 2007; 109(11):4635–4640.

37. Pardanani A, Reeder T, Porrata LF, et al. Imatinib therapy for hypereosinophilic syndrome and other eosinophilic disorders. Blood 2003; 101(9):3391–3397.
38. Pitini V, Arrigo C, Azzarello D, et al. Serum concentration of cardiac Troponin T in patients with hypereosinophilic syndrome treated with imatinib is predictive of adverse outcomes. Blood 2003; 102(9):3456–3457.
39. Kerkela R, Grazette L, Yacobi R, et al. Cardiotoxicity of the cancer therapeutic agent imatinib mesylate. Nat Med 2006; 12(8):908–916.
40. Klion AD, Robyn J, Maric I, et al. Relapse following discontinuation of imatinib mesylate therapy for FIP1L1/PDGFRA-positive chronic eosinophilic leukemia: implications for optimal dosing. Blood 2007; 110(10):3552–3556.
41. von Bubnoff N, Sandherr M, Schlimok G, et al. Myeloid blast crisis evolving during imatinib treatment of an FIP1L1-PDGFR alpha-positive chronic myeloproliferative disease with prominent eosinophilia. Leukemia 2005; 19(2):286–287.
42. Cools J, Stover EH, Boulton CL, et al. PKC412 overcomes resistance to imatinib in a murine model of FIP1L1-PDGFRalpha-induced myeloproliferative disease. Cancer Cell 2003; 3(5): 459–469.
43. Lierman E, Folens C, Stover EH, et al. Sorafenib is a potent inhibitor of FIP1L1-PDGFRalpha and the imatinib-resistant FIP1L1-PDGFRalpha T674I mutant. Blood 2006; 108(4):1374–1376.
44. Dahabreh IJ, Giannouli S, Zoi C, et al. Management of hypereosinophilic syndrome: a prospective study in the era of molecular genetics. Medicine (Baltimore) 2007; 86(6):344–354.
45. Butterfield JH. Interferon treatment for hypereosinophilic syndromes and systemic mastocytosis. Acta Haematol 2005; 114(1):26–40.
46. Sugimoto K, Tamayose K, Sasaki M, et al. More than 13 years of hypereosinophila associated with clonal CD3-CD4+ lymphocytosis of TH2/TH0 type. Int J Hematol 2002; 75(3):281–284.
47. Butterfield JH, Gleich GJ. Interferon-alpha treatment of six patients with the idiopathic hypereosinophilic syndrome. Ann Intern Med 1994; 121(9):648–653.
48. Schandene L, Del Prete GF, Cogan E, et al. Recombinant interferon-alpha selectively inhibits the production of interleukin-5 by human CD4+ T cells. J Clin Invest 1996; 97(2):309–315.
49. Schandene L, Roufosse F, de Lavareille A, et al. Interferon alpha prevents spontaneous apoptosis of clonal Th2 cells associated with chronic hypereosinophilia. Blood 2000; 96(13): 4285–4292.
50. Bain BJ, Fletcher SH. Chronic eosinophilic leukemias and the myeloproliferative variant of the hypereosinophilic syndrome. Immunol Allergy Clin North Am 2007; 27(3):377–388.
51. Garrett JK, Jameson SC, Thomson B, et al. Anti-interleukin-5 (mepolizumab) therapy for hypereosinophilic syndromes. J Allergy Clin Immunol 2004; 113(1):115–119.
52. Klion AD, Law MA, Noel P, et al. Safety and efficacy of the monoclonal anti-interleukin-5 antibody SCH55700 in the treatment of patients with hypereosinophilic syndrome. Blood 2004; 103(8):2939–2941.
53. Plotz SG, Simon HU, Darsow U, et al. Use of an anti-interleukin-5 antibody in the hypereosinophilic syndrome with eosinophilic dermatitis. N Engl J Med 2003; 349(24):2334–2339.
54. Rothenberg ME, Klion AD, Roufosse FE, et al. Treatment of patients with the hypereosinophilic syndrome with mepolizumab. N Engl J Med 2008; 358(12):1215–1228.
55. Pitini V, Teti D, Arrigo C, et al. Alemtuzumab therapy for refractory idiopathic hypereosinophilic syndrome with abnormal T cells: a case report. Br J Haematol 2004; 127(5):477.
56. Bernengo MG, Quaglino P, Comessatti A, et al. Low-dose intermittent alemtuzumab in the treatment of Sezary syndrome: clinical and immunologic findings in 14 patients. Haematologica 2007; 92(6):784–794.
57. Roufosse F, Schandene L, Sibille C, et al. T-cell receptor-independent activation of clonal Th2 cells associated with chronic hypereosinophilia. Blood 1999; 94(3):994–1002.

Index